Rosai and Ackerman's

Surgical Pathology Review

Commissioning Editor: Michael Houston
Development Editor: Louise Cook
Editorial Assistant: Elizabeth Brown
Project Manager: Kathryn Mason
Senior Designer: Sarah Russell
Marketing Managers (UK/USA): John Canelon and Kathy Neely

Rosai and Ackerman's

Surgical Pathology Review

Edited by

Ivan Damjanov MD, PhD

Professor of Pathology

The University of Kansas School of Medicine

Kansas City, KS, USA

Marin Nola MD, PhD

Assistant Professor of Pathology

University of Zagreb School of Medicine

Zagreb, Croatia

Consulting Editor

Juan Rosai MD

Professor, Department of Pathology

Weill Medical College of Cornell University

New York, NY, USA

MOSBY

ELSEVIER

MOSBY
ELSEVIER

An affiliate of Elsevier Inc.

First published 2007

ISBN-13: 9780323044998
ISBN-10: 0-323-04499-9

British Library Cataloguing in Publication Data

A catalogue record for this book is available from the British Library

Library of Congress Cataloging in Publication Data

A catalog record for this book is available from the Library of Congress

Notice

Medical knowledge is constantly changing. Standard safety precautions must be followed, but as new research and clinical experience broaden our knowledge, changes in treatment and drug therapy may become necessary or appropriate. Readers are advised to check the most current product information provided by the manufacturer of each drug to be administered to verify the recommended dose, the method and duration of administration, and contraindications. It is the responsibility of the practitioner, relying on experience and knowledge of the patient, to determine dosages and the best treatment for each individual patient. Neither the Publisher nor the author assume any liability for any injury and/or damage to persons or property arising from this publication.

Printed in China

Last digit is the print number: 9 8 7 6 5 4 3 2 1

Contents

Preface

Many of the leading textbooks of medicine have grown in size to the point where it is almost impossible to read them from cover to cover. For those texts that serve only as reference or for consultation, the size is of no significance; in many cases, the fatter books fare even better than the slimmer volumes. However, for books that are supposed to be read systematically, the size may be a daunting deterrent discouraging many students from undertaking the long, time-consuming (or 'chronophagic', as a friend of ours used to say), and often lonesome journey from page one to the index.

Rosai and Ackerman's Surgical Pathology is one of those hybrid books that were conceived to serve as both an instructional text and a reference manual for solving problems in daily practice. The present *Review* is aimed primarily at those who have decided to read the entire textbook and attempt to learn surgical pathology systematically. In spirit and in format it is a companion to *Rosai and Ackerman's Surgical Pathology* and we have dedicated it to residents and all those who are trying to learn surgical pathology systematically from the main textbook. We hope that pathologists in training will welcome it enthusiastically and find it useful for mastering the theory of surgical pathology.

Our primary goal was to produce a study guide which would help students of surgical pathology focus on the most important topics in each chapter of the two volumes of the Rosai and Ackerman's textbook. Each question in our *Review* is accompanied by a short answer to provide the reader with an instantaneous feedback. For a more detailed explanation and discussion of the problem identified in the question, we hope that the reader will go back to the main textbook. The page numbers to which you should direct your attention in the textbook are given at the end of each answer.

To stimulate active learning and a more efficient reading of the textbook, the material in this review is presented in the form of true/false (T/F) statements. For most of us, there is no need to explain the T/F statements in great detail. Suffice it to say that T/F statements are a form of objective test questions, which fall somewhere between the open-ended ('uncued') questions on one hand side and multiple choice questions (MCQ) on the other. In contrast to open-ended questions, these T/F statements prompt the students to focus on the expected answer. Thus answering T/F statements requires less time than thinking about open-ended questions for which no answers are offered. Most importantly, the T/F statements are a very efficient way of finding out whether you do or do not know the correct answer, whether you understand the basic premises and concepts or whether you need to study more. In the opinion of many educational experts, T/F statements are excellent for stimulating active learning, and are a very effective way of providing instantaneous feedback and guidance to the learner. In contrast to the MCQs, no 'test-taking skills' are actually required, and one does not waste time sorting the right answer from the incorrect ones included by the 'tricky professor' to confuse the unwary student. Finally, by using T/F statements, we were able to cover much more material from the textbook, and we could do it much more systematically than if we had used the MCQ format. Please note that the *Review* contains over 4000 questions altogether, amounting to at least two questions per page of the textbook.

We hope that this short paragraph about the advantages of T/F statements is convincing. However, for those who remain skeptical and prefer MCQs, we would like to point out that each T/F statement can be easily transformed into the 'stem' of an MCQ. Many a teacher knows this fact, and thus we hope that our *Review* will be used not only by students but also by the examiners to test their students. Here is an example of how a T/F statement can be transformed into an MCQ:

True false statement (from chapter 8):

Embryonal carcinoma is the most common type of mediastinal germ cell tumor.

Multiple choice question, prepared ad hoc from the same T/F statement:

Which one of the following is the most common mediastinal germ cell tumor?

A. Embryonal carcinoma
B. Dysgerminoma
C. Mature cystic teratoma
D. Choriocarcinoma
E. Yolk sac carcinoma

The T/F statement in this case is *false*, and in the MCQ question the correct answer is *C. Mature cystic teratoma.*

At the end of the book the reader will find a final examination comprising 125 board-style MCQs. Some questions, like some of those in the preceding chapters, pertain to figures. Some questions are tough and some are easy, like the questions on the actual Anatomic Pathology Boards Examination. A student who has studied most of the T/F statements in the 31 chapters of this *Review* should have no problems passing the final exam with a score of 65%–70%. A score over 85% deserves commendation and should be considered to be outstanding.

On behalf of our contributors we would like to thank our residents who have helped us write, proofread and test some of these questions. We also thank the entire team at Elsevier and especially Michael Houston, the commissioning editor, who helped us, in more ways than one, to complete this project.

Ivan Damjanov MD, PhD
Marin Nola MD, PhD
2007

List of contributors

Ivan Damjanov MD, PhD
Professor
Department of Pathology
The University of Kansas School of Medicine
Kansas City, KS, USA

Chapters 9, 13, 17, 26, 27, 31 and 32

Michael den Bakker MD
Assistant Professor
Department of Pathology
Erasmus University School of Medicine
Rotterdam, The Netherlands

Chapters 7 and 8

Katherine DeSchryver MD
Adjunct Faculty
Washington University
St Louis, MO, USA

Chapter 11

Fang Fan MD, PhD
Assistant Professor
Director of Cytology
The University of Kansas School of Medicine
Kansas City, KS, USA

Chapter 17

Zoran Gatalica MD, DSc
Professor and Director of Anatomic Pathology
Department of Pathology
Creighton University Medical Center
Omaha, NE, USA

Chapters 24 and 25

Don Hayes MD
Pathologist
Afdeling Pathologie/RPCL
Meander Medisch Centrum
Amersfoort, The Netherlands

Chapter 4

Peter A. McCue MD
Professor
Department of Pathology
Thomas Jefferson University Hospital
Philadelphia, PA, USA

Chapters 5, 6, 10 and 12

Brian E. Moore MD
Staff Pathologist
Memorial Medical Center;
Assistant Clinical Professor
Southern Illinois University School of Medicine
Springfield, IL, USA

Chapters 28, 29 and 30

Mario Mosunjac MD
Assistant Professor
Department of Pathology
Emory University;
Autopsy Director and Surgical Pathologist
Grady Memorial Hospital
Atlanta, GA, USA

Chapters 19 and 20

Marina Mosunjac MD
Assistant Professor
Department of Pathology
Emory University;
Director of Surgical Pathology
Grady Memorial Hospital
Atlanta, GA, USA

Chapters 19 and 20

Marin Nola MD, PhD
Assistant Professor
University of Zagreb School of Medicine
Zagreb, Croatia

Chapters 21, 22, 23 and 32

Emina Torlakovic MD, PhD
Associate Professor
Department of Pathology
Royal University Hospital
Saskatoon, SK, Canada

Chapters 14, 15, 16 and 18

Goran Torlakovic MD, PhD
Associate Professor
Department of Pathology
Royal University Hospital
Saskatoon, SK, Canada

Chapters 14, 15, 16 and 18

I-Tien Yeh MD
Professor
Department of Pathology
University of Texas Health Science Center at San Antonio
San Antonio, TX, USA

Chapters 1, 2 and 3

Dedication

To our residents, fellows and all other students of pathology, irrespective of their age.

Introduction: Surgical pathology and the surgical pathology report

1

Q1

The clinical functions of surgical pathologists should be limited to diagnosing the disease correctly and informing the clinician whether a lesion is benign or malignant.

Q2

The pathology requisition form should be filled out by a nurse.

Q3

The housing of specialized areas of pathology within clinical specialties should be encouraged, as the exponential growth of knowledge precludes any pathologist from the detailed knowledge needed.

Q4

The ideal surgical pathology report should be prompt, accurate, and brief.

Q5

The most important factor in the completeness of the surgical pathology report is the number of surgical specimens seen in the department each year.

Slide review and consultation

Q1

Slides sent for second review to a second hospital in which the patient is undergoing therapy should be retained by the second hospital.

Q2

It is good medical practice to document intradepartmental consultations.

Q3

The best biopsy is always a cleanly excised, uncrushed wedge that includes both normal and lesional tissue.

Q4

The larger the lesion, the more samples that should be taken during the biopsy procedure.

Q5

The surface of the biopsy should be scraped by the pathologist prior to fixation to improve diagnostic yield.

Q6

Frozen sections are performed for several indications, including establishing the presence and nature of a lesion, determining the adequacy of margins, and to determine whether diagnostic material was obtained.

Q7

Mohs' surgery refers to removing skin tumors at a 45° angle and orienting the tumor en face, then evaluating margins by frozen sections, with the surgeon serving as his own pathologist.

Diagnostic cytology

Q1

Surgical biopsy confirmation of cytologic results is generally recommended prior to definitive therapy.

Q2

The Papanicolaou grading system is highly specific and should be used for cytologic reporting.

QUESTIONS

Digital pathology, telepathology and information systems

Q1

Virtual microscopy refers to digitalization of microscopic slides that almost duplicates the examination of slides on a physical microscope.

Q2

Basic design criteria for automated information systems in surgical pathology include mandatory pathologist participation.

Q3

Each laboratory needs to build its own information system to customize its reporting needs.

Q4

The quality of work in surgical pathology should be routinely monitored; this is known by terms such as quality assurance, quality control, and total quality assessment.

Legal aspects of surgical pathology

Q1

The most common reasons for surgical pathologists to be sued include misdiagnoses.

Q2

The basic elements of malpractice are: 1) duty, 2) breach, 3) proximal cause, and 4) damage.

Q3

A pathologist can be held liable for a diagnostic error made by an expert consultant.

A1. False

The surgical pathologist needs to understand the clinician's needs and respond to them accordingly. It is not enough to tell the clinician whether a lesion is benign or malignant. The surgical pathologist must be able to tell about the adequacy of the biopsy, the grade of malignancy, the extent of the disease, and provide all other pertinent information needed under certain circumstances. **(p. 3)**

A2. False

The requisition form should be filled out by a physician familiar with the patient who is able to give a pertinent history, such as a past history of malignancy. **(p. 3)**

A3. False

Although subspecialty pathology is increasingly practiced today, the subspecialization should occur within pathology departments rather than clinical departments, as pathologic processes are not confined to organ systems. In addition, the practice of 'self-referral' represents a conflict of interest. **(p. 4)**

A4. True

The surgical pathology report should be brief but complete, and concentrate on details that relate to therapy and prognosis. The necessity for promptness and accuracy should be inherently obvious. **(p. 5)**

A5. False

Completeness of reports is dependent on the use of a standard form rather than on any other parameter. **(p. 6)**

Slide review and consultation

A1. True

Recuts should be sent for second review so that they can be retained by the treating hospital to allow comparison with subsequent material and interdepartmental conferences. If only one slide contains the diagnostic material, the slides should be photographed prior to return (and prior to send out). **(p. 7)**

A2. True

Although traditional practice has been to show slides informally within a department without documenting such action, the reality of today's legal and medical climates make the practice of documentation imperative. **(p. 7–8)**

A3. False

Although these characteristics are often taught to clinicians, sometimes the edge of the tumor may not be diagnostic and much effort is wasted trying to over-interpret a tiny area of lesion at the edge of the biopsy specimen. **(p. 8)**

A4. True

Larger lesions may be more variable, and diagnostic areas may only be present focally. **(p. 9)**

A5. False

Immediate fixation is almost always preferable. Scraping the surface of a small biopsy may introduce artifacts that impair later microscopic interpretation. **(p. 9)**

A6. True

Frozen sections should only be requested/performed if the results will influence the surgical procedure. Most of the time a specific diagnosis is neither needed nor expected. **(p. 10)**

A7. True

This method has inherent difficulties in interpretation and is usually performed by surgeons without any formal pathology training. **(p. 11)**

Diagnostic cytology

A1. True

Although diagnostic cytology is highly reliable when performed by well-trained pathologists, in many instances a confirmatory conventional biopsy is still recommended prior to a major surgical procedure or irradiation therapy. **(p. 12)**

A2. False

The Papanicolaou grading system is nonspecific and should be replaced by a specific diagnosis, such as those used in surgical pathology, whenever possible. **(p. 12)**

Digital pathology, telepathology and information systems

A1. True

Virtual microscopy allows the user to change magnifications, fields, even the focus, usually by having the slide scanned into a digital format, or by remote operation. **(p. 13–14)**

A2. False

Pathologist participation should not be compulsory, so that pathologists may work independently of the computer if they so choose. However, the more knowledgeable the pathologist, the more likely it is that the information system will be helpful to him or her. Other basic design criteria include the elimination of redundant entry, real-time integration of data, online permanent and safe storage of primary data, rapid response time, and flexible, modifiable design. **(p. 15)**

A3. False

It is not necessary to reinvent the wheel in every laboratory, and standard systems are available with modifiable components. **(p. 15)**

A4. True

This monitoring helps detect inadequacies, updates procedures, and improves the final report. **(p. 19)**

Legal aspects of surgical pathology

A1. True

Misdiagnoses include misinterpretations of the slides, sampling failures, and failure of the pathologic diagnosis to convey the nature or extent of the lesion. An analysis of claims showed that high-risk areas include breast fine-needle aspiration and biopsy, malignant melanoma, lymphoma, prostatic biopsy, frozen section diagnosis, urinary bladder, and branchial cleft cyst. Slightly over half the claims were for false positive diagnoses, such as overdiagnosis of ductal carcinoma in situ, or interpretation of proliferative breast disease as carcinoma. **(p. 19–20)**

A2. True

Duty is the obligation of the physician to treat the patient, so a plaintiff must first be recognized as a patient of the pathologist. Breach refers to negligence to treat within the standard of care. The definition of standard of care is within a community at a particular time. The alleged error or omission should result directly in physical, emotional or financial damage to the patient. **(p. 19)**

A3. True

Vicarious liability refers to liability of the submitting pathologist for errors made by their consultant pathologist. **(p. 20)**

Gross techniques in surgical pathology

2

Surgical pathology gross room

Q1

Autopsy pathology is gross pathology, whereas surgical pathology is histopathology.

Q2

A table, chair, cutting board, sink and shelf are the only necessary elements of a grossing station.

Handling of specimens

Q1

All specimens, including small needle biopsies, should be submitted fresh for examination.

Q2

A pathologist's assistant may photograph specimens, X-ray specimens, and cut and stain frozen sections, as well as make diagnoses on 'gross only' specimens.

Q3

Buffered formalin fixative is still the most inexpensive, best fixative for most special techniques.

Q4

Preservation of nucleic acids is improved by fixation in Bouin's, Zenker's or B-5.

Q5

The volume of formalin fixative that is needed is at least 10× the amount of tissue to be fixed.

Q6

The speed of tissue penetration by formalin is approximately 1 mm/h, and this is equivalent to the speed of fixation.

Q7

An unlabeled specimen should not be processed until the physician obtaining the tissue or his assistant has identified and labeled the specimen.

Q8

The external appearance of the specimen is the most important, so before sectioning, a photograph should be taken.

Q9

Specimens that contain cysts or hollow organs may have the original fluid removed, then be injected with formalin for optimal fixation.

Q10

Floaters should be suspected whenever a tissue fragment stains differently, is in a different plane, or shows an unexpected pathologic process.

Q11

HLA antigen matching and DNA testing can be carried out on suspected floaters to see if the material matches the remainder of the tissue.

Specimen photography and radiography

Q1

Specimen identification should always be in the photograph to prevent specimen mix-ups.

Q2

The gross photograph is the best permanent record of the gross features of the specimen.

Q3

Specimen radiography should be only performed by trained radiologists.

Sampling for histologic examination

Q1

Carnoy's solution can clear the fat while fixing the nodes in lymph node dissection specimens.

Q2

Tissue should be no thicker than 3 mm for submission in cassettes.

Q3

The orientation of organs with folded mucosa, such as bowel, can be better maintained by submitting sections parallel to the folds.

Q4

Once a specimen is fixed, one cannot paint the surgical margins.

Q5

A manual of gross procedures should be in the surgical pathology office, so that it stays clean of tissue and blood contaminants.

Surgical pathology gross room

A1. False

The gross examination is critical to the proper sampling and interpretation of surgical specimens, and microscopic examination is often required for proper interpretation of autopsy material. Gross pathology and histopathology are thus integral parts of both autopsy and surgical pathology. **(p. 25)**

A2. False

The elements listed above are essential, but a gross station must be properly ventilated as well. Many other features are ideal, including access to formalin, dictation equipment, computer terminal, instruments etc. **(p. 26)**

Handling of specimens

A1. False

Large specimens should be received fresh and examined as soon as possible, but small biopsy specimens can be submitted in fixative. **(p. 26)**

A2. False

A pathologist's assistant may help perform the gross examination, but the pathologist is always responsible for making the diagnosis. **(p. 27)**

A3. True

It is compatible with most special techniques, including immunohistochemistry and molecular diagnostics. **(p. 27)**

A4. False

Preservation of nucleic acids is very poor with Bouin's, Zenker's and B-5. Ordinary buffered formalin better preserves nucleic acids, particularly at 4°C. Other fixatives containing alcohol may be superior for DNA preservation. **(p. 28)**

A5. True

Inadequate fixation of specimens may occur with lesser ratios of formalin. **(p. 28)**

A6. False

Formalin does penetrate tissue at approximately 1mm/h, but additional time is needed for the fixation process. **(p. 28)**

A7. True

Although we wish to expedite the diagnostic process and keep our physician clients/friends, an unlabeled specimen should not be processed until properly identified. **(p. 29)**

A8. False

Although at times the external appearance is crucial, in most instances a properly taken cross-section better demonstrates the pathologic process. **(p. 29)**

A9. True

Fixation of the external and internal portions should be performed simultaneously. This can be accomplished by opening the cyst or hollow organ in its fresh state, or by replacing the original fluid with formalin and then sectioning after fixation. By fixing before sectioning, the original configuration is maintained for orientation, teaching, and photography. **(p. 29–30)**

A10. True

Being alert for differences will minimize the chance of making incorrect diagnoses because of floaters. **(p. 31)**

A11. True

However, these tests will not be useful in the case of contamination of the patient's own tissue to another block or area (knife metastases). Occasionally, entire specimens may be mislabeled and HLA or DNA testing of patients may be necessary to verify the identity of tissues. **(p. 31)**

ANSWERS

Specimen photography and radiography

A1. False

The use of identifiers is prohibited by patient information protection laws in photographs that will later be used for teaching purposes, publication etc. Identifiers may be distracting when viewing the photograph. Perhaps one photograph can be taken with identifiers, but others should be taken without them. Adequate record-keeping and labeling should prevent specimen mix-ups. **(p. 32)**

A2. True

The gross description, even when well done, is a poor substitute for a gross photograph of the specimen. The photographs may be marked to record dimensions and to show where sections were taken. **(p. 32)**

A3. False

Radiologic–pathologic correlation is often necessary in bone lesions, breast biopsies, calcified soft tissue lesions etc. A self-contained shielded X-ray machine designed for use by pathologists is available. **(p. 32)**

Sampling for histologic examination

A1. True

There are numerous clearing techniques available, including Carnoy's, which clears the fat by the action of chloroform. Nodes can also be dissected fresh. **(p. 33)**

A2. True

Tissue pieces should be no more than 10–15 mm on the sides and no more than 3 mm in thickness to ensure adequate paraffin infiltration. Fatty tissue should be thinner. **(p. 33)**

A3. False

Orientation is better maintained by sections perpendicular to the folds. **(p. 33)**

A4. False

The margins can be painted on either fresh or fixed specimens, and in both cases care must be taken to avoid ink getting on to surfaces that are not true surgical margins. **(p. 34)**

A5. False

Although it is true that the manual would stay clean in the office, it is not very useful to the dissecting pathologist unless it is available at the bench to refer to during gross examinations. **(p. 34)**

Special techniques in surgical pathology

3

Special stains

Q1

PAS (periodic acid–Schiff) staining demonstrates neutral mucosubstances.

Q2

Gram staining separates bacteria into two groups: those that retain the purple color of the crystal violet–iodine complex, and those that are decolorized by alcohol and stain with safranin or fuchsin.

Q3

Congo Red staining is chemically specific for amyloid.

Q4

Silver-based reticulin stains are used to demonstrate reticular cells.

Q5

Trichrome stains primarily evaluate extracellular material.

Q6

Fat stains can be performed on paraffin-embedded material.

Q7

To demonstrate mucosubstances of neutral and acidic types, it is best to use a combination of PAS and Alcian blue stains.

Q8

Giemsa staining can only be performed on smears, not on paraffin-embedded material.

Q9

Luxol fast blue stains elastic fibers.

Enzyme histochemistry

Q1

Enzyme histochemistry is technically complex, needs fresh material, and many of the reactions are nonspecific and therefore it no longer has any place in a modern laboratory.

Q2

Immunohistochemical techniques can demonstrate enzymes.

Other special procedures

Q1

Neuroblastoma can form neurites within 24 hours after being placed in appropriate culture media, thus aiding in the diagnosis of tumor type.

Q2

Measurements can be made from photographs, projected images or eyepiece graticules.

Q3

X-ray microanalysis cannot be used on paraffin-embedded material.

Q4

Limitations of electron microscopy include sampling issues and lack of specific ultrastructural features.

Q5

Electron microscopy is useful in differentiating among carcinoma, melanoma and sarcoma.

Immunohistochemistry

Q1

The biotin–avidin immunohistochemical technique depends on the lack of affinity of avidin for biotin.

Q2

Antigen retrieval techniques have improved the sensitivity of immunohistochemistry.

Q3

False negative immunohistochemical results may be caused by prolonged fixation in formalin.

Q4

False positive results may be due to expired antibody.

Q5

Transcription factors, such as TTF-1, are located in the cytoplasm of cells.

Q6

ALK is useful for the evaluation of alkaline phosphatase.

Q7

α-Fetoprotein is present in the fetal liver and visceral endoderm of the yolk sac.

Q8

α-Methylacyl-CoA racemase is expressed exclusively in prostate tumors.

Q9

B72.3 reacts to adenocarcinomas but not benign adult tissues.

Q10

Both E- and N-cadherins are frequently deficient in carcinomas.

Q11

Calretinin is a calcium-binding protein that is useful in distinguishing mesothelioma from adenocarcinoma.

Q12

Carcinoembryonic antigen (CEA) is present in mucinous adenocarcinomas, as well as medullary carcinomas of the thyroid.

Q13

CD15 and CD31 are good markers for endothelial differentiation.

Q14

Type IV collagen is the major component of basement membranes, along with laminin.

Q15

Desmin is an intermediate filament found in striated muscles only.

Q16

Chromogranin can be used as a 'pan-endocrine' marker.

Q17

Epidermal growth factor receptor (EGFR) is an important prognostic indicator for breast tumor progression.

Q18

Factor VIII-related antigen is found in endothelial cells, megakaryocytes, platelets and mast cells.

Q19

Benign fibrous histiocytomas of skin strongly mark with factor XIIIa.

Q20

FLI-1 is present in most small round blue cell tumors.

Q21

Glial fibrillary acidic protein (GFAP) is present in neoplastic astrocytes but not in normal and reactive astrocytes.

Q22

Gross cystic disease protein-15 (GCDFP-15) is an excellent marker of pancreatic cysts.

Q23

HMB-45 marks only tumors of melanocytic differentiation.

Q24

Only the β chain of human chorionic gonadotropin (hCG) is hormone specific.

Q25

Ia-like antigens are only found on cells with immune function.

Q26

Intermediate filament proteins can be co-expressed in fetal and neoplastic tissues.

Q27

Cytokeratin 7+/20+ tumors include those from the pancreas, bile duct, urothelium, and some gastric carcinomas.

Q28

Cytokeratin 5/6 is usually negative in squamous carcinomas.

Q29

Mart-1 is related to melanosomes, therefore is useful for detecting tumors of melanocytic origin.

Q30

MOC-31 is positive in most primary and metastatic adenocarcinomas found in the lung, but only rarely in mesotheliomas, and is therefore useful in the differential diagnosis between the two entities.

Q31

Of the myogenic proteins found in tumors of skeletal muscle, myogenin is the most useful in paraffin-embedded tissues.

Q32

Neurofilament is more specific than neuron-specific enolase for cells of neural origin.

Q33

p53 is expressed in basal/stem cells and can be used in the identification of myoepithelial cells of breast and salivary gland origin.

Q34

Prostatic acid phosphatase is more specific for prostate tissue than prostate-specific antigen is for prostate tissues.

Q35

S100 can be found in both the cytoplasm and nucleus, but if tissue shows only cytoplasmic localization of the S100 protein it should be considered negative for S100.

Q36

Synaptophysin is expressed in normal, reactive and neoplastic cells of neuroectodermal and neuroendocrine origin.

Q37

Thyroglobulin is nuclear protein produced by thyroid follicular cells.

Q38

In tumors of unknown origin, thyroid transcription factor-1 (TTF-1) is often used to implicate lung as the primary site, after thyroid origin is ruled out.

Q39

Vimentin is found in cells of mesenchymal origin, but may also be found in epithelial and neural cells.

Q40

WT-1 is found in Wilms' tumor, as well as rhabdomyosarcoma, mesothelioma and ovarian serous carcinoma.

Flow cytometry

Q1

Flow cytometry can evaluate cellular features such as size, granularity, viability, cell cycle time, DNA content, and surface marker phenotypes.

Q2

Flow cytometry is performed on single cell suspensions and thus cannot be performed on solid tumors.

Other methods for analysis of cell proliferation

Q1

Mitotic count, as defined by the number of mitoses per 10 high-power fields, is a very reproducible method for defining cell proliferation.

Q2

Immunohistochemical staining for nuclear antigens related to cell growth and proliferation include MIB-1 and PCNA.

Q3

Nucleolar organizer region (NOR) is a region around which nucleoli organize during metaphase and thus is useful for evaluation of cell proliferation.

Cytogenetics

Q1

Cytogenetics can be used to help classify tumors and determine their causation.

Q2

Comparative genomic hybridization can be performed only on freshly frozen tissues.

Q3

Specific chromosomal translocations are useful for specific diagnosis of malignant fibrous histiocytoma but are not found in inflammatory myofibroblastic tumors.

Molecular pathology

Q1

Molecular techniques have been developed for formalin-fixed paraffin-embedded materials, making the frozen tissue bank obsolete.

Q2

Filter hybridization (Southern blot) can detect gene rearrangements, amplifications, deletions and point mutations.

Q3

In situ hybridization (ISH) is used for the detection of specific DNA sequences in tissue sections, but cannot be used for RNA detection.

Q4

Cytogenetic analysis must be performed on cells in division, requiring tissue culture of cells.

Q5

Reverse transcriptase polymerase chain reaction (RT-PCR) is a form of the polymerase chain reaction that can be used to amplify RNA fragments.

DNA microarrays

Q1

A gene expression profile produced from a DNA microarray can include tens of thousands of genes.

Q2

Laser microdissection allows the analysis of a pure cell population, which may consist only of a single cell.

Q3

An example of an important tumor suppressor gene is the *ras* gene.

Q4

DNA replication and repair genes include the mismatch repair genes in hereditary non-polyposis colon cancer and *BRCA1/2* in breast cancer.

Special stains

A1. True
In addition, PAS will stain glycogen, basement membranes, and most fungi and parasites. **(p. 38)**

A2. True
There are several modifications of the Gram stain that are used in sections, including the Brown and Brenn stain. Those bacteria that retain the purple color are known as Gram-positive, and those that are decolorized are known as Gram-negative. **(p. 38)**

A3. False
Although we use the Congo Red stain for amyloid, it does not in fact have chemical specificity and is dependent on the molecular arrangement of the amyloid molecule (β-pleated sheets). **(p. 38)**

A4. False
Reticulin stains demonstrates reticular fibers and basement membrane material, but not reticular (or dendritic) cells. **(p. 39)**

A5. True
Although the three dyes that are used in the trichrome stain demonstrate nuclei, cytoplasm and extracellular collagen, only the extracellular collagen is somewhat specific. **(p. 39)**

A6. False
Clearing solutions, including xylene that is used in processing formalin-fixed material, will solubilize fat, so that fat stains, such as Oil red O, can only be performed on frozen sections or smears. **(p. 40)**

A7. True
The term mucin comprises a large group of compounds composed of a protein core and a carbohydrate moiety. Mucicarmine and Alcian blue stains will demonstrate acidic mucins, whereas PAS will stain neutral mucins (see Question 1). **(p. 40)**

A8. False
Giemsa can demonstrate hematopoietic cells, such as mast cells, on paraffin-embedded material and can also be used to stain microorganisms. **(p. 40)**

A9. False
Luxol fast blue is a myelin stain. Elastic fibers are best stained by Weigert or Verheoeff–van Gieson (VVG) stains. **(p. 41)**

Enzyme histochemistry

A1. False
Although the first part of the statement is true, there are a few histochemical methods that are still useful today, including skeletal muscle-related enzymes for myopathy studies, acetylcholinesterase for Hirschsprung's disease, and chloroacetate esterase for myeloid/mast cells. **(p. 41)**

A2. True
Enzymes are proteins and therefore immunogenic. Immunohistochemical techniques have largely supplanted many of the histochemical tests used in the past because immunohistochemistry can identify enzymes even when these proteins are not enzymatically active. **(p. 41)**

Other special procedures

A1. True
This observation of in vitro differentiation was justification for maintaining a tissue culture laboratory in some surgical pathology laboratories. However, the application of tissue culture is limited to a few rare tumors, and molecular pathology/immunohistochemical techniques have proved more useful. **(p. 42)**

A2. True
Current applications of image analysis include the determination of DNA ploidy, proliferative index, nuclear grading, dysplasia grading and hormone receptor analysis. **(p. 43)**

A3. False

Although it is preferable to use glutaraldehyde-fixed material, paraffin-embedded tissue can be used. In surgical pathology specimens this technique is most often used to analyze crystalline material. **(p. 43)**

A4. True

The few cells that are examined ultrastructurally may not be representative of the whole specimen. Only a few subcellular structures are specific to cell or tissue types. **(p. 43)**

A5. True

Epithelial cells can be identified by their intercellular connections, melanosomes can be detected in melanomas, and sarcomas may have some specific cytoplasmic filaments etc. **(p. 44)**

Immunohistochemistry

A1. False

The high affinity of avidin to biotin is the basis of the biotin–avidin immunohistochemical technique. Antibody is coupled to biotin, and peroxidase is coupled to avidin. The resulting complex is stable and visible on light microscopy. **(p. 45)**

A2. True

Epitopes are unmasked through a variety of methods, including heat/pressure, proteolytic enzymes, and treatment with microwaves. **(p. 46)**

A3. True

It is preferable to perform stains on original paraffin-embedded material that has been fixed for a limited time than on tissue left in formalin for extended periods. **(p. 46)**

A4. False

Generally, expired antibody results in loss of reactivity rather than increased reactivity. False positive results may be due to cross-reactivity of the antibody, nonspecific binding, endogenous peroxidase, or entrapment of normal tissue by tumor cells. **(p. 46)**

A5. False

Transcription factors are nuclear proteins needed for the transcription of genes, some of which are tissue specific. The advantages of nuclear transcription factors include greater specificity and lack of diffusion. **(p. 47)**

A6. False

ALK is the anaplastic lymphoma kinase protein and is detectable in anaplastic large cell lymphoma, as well as soft tissue neoplasms such as inflammatory myofibroblastic tumor. Alkaline phosphatases are widely distributed enzymes, useful in the characterization of germ cell tumors, as well as others. **(p. 48)**

A7. True

Alphafetoprotein is an oncofetal protein present in endodermal sinus and other germ cell tumors, as well as hepatocytic neoplasms, acinar pancreatic tumors, and carcinomas with germ cell-like features. **(p. 48)**

A8. False

Although it is overexpressed in prostatic adenocarcinomas, racemase is also found in other types of carcinoma. **(p. 48)**

A9. False

There is limited reactivity in adult tissues, but the antibody cannot be reliably used to distinguish benign from malignant. **(p. 49)**

A10. True

The cadherins are cell adhesion molecules located in desmosomes, including the epithelial (E) and neural (N) types. E-cadherin is lost in lobular carcinoma of the breast. **(p. 49)**

A11. True

Calretinen is almost always positive in mesotheliomas, and usually negative in lung adenocarcinomas. **(p. 49–50)**

A12. True

CEA is an oncofetal protein expressed in carcinomas and present only in minor quantities in normal adult tissues. **(p. 50)**

A13. False

CD31 identifies endothelial cells, but CD 15 (LeuM1) is a marker of myelomonocytic cells and adenocarcinomas. **(p. 50)**

A14. True

Type IV collagen is a non-fibril forming collagen that can be useful in the distinction between in situ and invasive carcinomas. Type VII collagen is also associated with basement membranes of epithelial cells. **(p. 51)**

A15. False

Desmin can also be found in smooth muscle cells and myofibroblasts. **(p. 51)**

A16. True

Chromogranin stains nearly all types of neuroendocrine tumor. **(p. 51)**

A17. False

Another tyrosine kinase receptor, HER-2, is important for breast cancer prognosis, but EGFR is more useful as an indicator for therapeutic response to EGFR inhibitors. **(p. 52)**

A18. True

Factor VIII-related antigen is often used as a marker of endothelial cells, to identify vascular invasion or as a marker for vascular tumors. **(p. 52)**

A19. True

Dermal dendrocytes are scattered throughout the dermis, at the dermoepidermal junction, and in dermal blood vessels. **(p. 52)**

A20. False

FLI-1 is overexpressed in Ewing sarcoma/PNET and lymphoblastic lymphomas, but usually not in other small round blue cell tumors. **(p. 53)**

A21. False

GFAP is an intermediate filament protein present in normal, reactive and neoplastic astrocytes, as well as oligodendrocytes, peripheral nerve sheath tumors and benign mixed tumors of the salivary gland. **(p. 53)**

A22. False

GCDFP-15 is a marker of apocrine differentiation and can be found in skin and breast apocrine glands, as well as glandular tumors, some of which do not show apocrine morphology. **(p. 53)**

A23. False

Although initially thought to be specific for melanocytic differentiation, HMB-45 is also found in other tumors, including others derived from the neural crest, renal angiomyolipomas and some carcinomas. **(p. 54)**

A24. True

The α chain of hCG is common to follicle-stimulating hormone (FSH), luteinizing hormone (LH) and thyroid-stimulating hormone (TSH). Many hCG antibodies detect total hCG, so to detect specific trophoblastic differentiation the marker should be specific to β-hCG. **(p. 54)**

A25. False

Ia-like antigens correspond to HLA-DR antigens and can be found on histiocytes, B lymphocytes and activated T lymphocytes. However, these antigens have also been detected in non-immune related cells, such as epithelial and endothelial cells. **(p. 54)**

A26. True

Intermediate filament proteins include cytokeratin, vimentin, desmin, glial fibrillary acidic protein and neurofilaments, characterized by their intermediate size between actin (thin) and tubulin (thick). **(p. 55)**

A27. True

The combination of CK7 and CK20 has been used to define the primary site of metastatic tumors. CK7 is typically present in lung carcinomas, and may also be present in tumors of the breast, endometrium, ovary, thyroid and salivary gland. CK20 is typically seen in tumors of colorectal origin, Merkel cell carcinomas and some gastric carcinomas. Tumors on the adrenal cortex, liver, kidney and adrenal gland are usually negative for both CK7 and CK20. **(p. 55)**

A28. False

Cytokeratin 5/6 is usually positive in squamous carcinoma, mesothelioma, salivary gland tumors and thymoma. CK 5/6 is usually negative in lung adenocarcinoma and is therefore useful in differentiating between mesothelioma and lung adenocarcinoma. **(p. 56)**

A29. False

Mart-1 is not related to melanosomes, although it is useful for detecting tumors of melanocytic origin. Like HMB-45, it stains tumors of neural crest origin, but in addition stains steroid-producing neoplasms, such as adrenal cortical tumors. **(p. 57)**

A30. True

The MOC-31 antibody stains almost all lung adenocarcinomas and 80% of non-pulmonary adenocarcinomas, but only about 5% of mesotheliomas. **(p. 57)**

A31. True

Myogenin is a nuclear protein that is expressed in all types of rhabdomyosarcoma. MyoD1 performs well in frozen tissues but not in paraffin-embedded tissues. Although myoglobin does work in paraffin-embedded tissues, it shows low sensitivity. Myosin can be found in both smooth muscle and skeletal muscle. **(p. 58)**

A32. True

Although neuron-specific enolase is found in neurons and neuroendocrine cells, it is also found in many other types of normal and neoplastic cell. Neurofilament expression has been found primarily in tumors of neuronal and neuroendocrine origin. **(p. 58)**

A33. False

P63, a homolog of p53, is expressed in basal/stem cells and can be used in the identification of myoepithelial cells of breast and salivary gland origin. *p53* is a nuclear tumor suppressor gene and mutations of it are the most common genetic alteration in human tumors. *p53* gene mutations produce a stable nuclear protein that can be detected immunohistochemically. **(p. 59)**

A34. False

Prostatic acid phosphatase can be found in bladder carcinomas and carcinoids, as well as prostate tissue. Prostate-specific antigen is more specific for normal, hyperplastic and neoplastic prostatic tissue. **(p. 60)**

A35. True

The more specific expression of S100 is nuclear, and isolated cytoplasmic staining should *not* be considered a positive result. **(p. 60)**

A36. True

Synaptophysin is commonly used to define tumors of neuroendocrine and neuroectodermal origin. **(p. 61)**

A37. False

Thyroglobulin is produced by thyroid follicular cells, but is found in the cytoplasm and in thyroid gland lumina. Thyroglobulin is specific for thyroid origin. **(p. 61)**

A38. True

TTF-1 is a nuclear transcription factor found in both pulmonary and thyroid tissue. It is often used to distinguish primary lung tumors from metastatic tumors; however, some neuroendocrine tumors of non-pulmonary origin can also be positive. **(p. 61)**

A39. True

Although tumors of mesenchymal origin have the most diffuse distribution of vimentin, it can also be found in other cells, in conjunction with other intermediate filaments. Vimentin is found in so many tissues that it is sometimes used as a control to prove that tissue is immunoreactive. **(p. 62)**

A40. True

WT-1 is a nuclear transcription factor expressed in kidney, and is useful in the differential diagnosis in small round blue cell tumors. **(p. 62)**

Flow cytometry

A1. True

All the above features can be measured by flow cytometry, as well as enzyme content. More than one cellular feature may be measured at the same time. **(p. 63)**

A2. False

Although flow cytometry must be performed on single cell suspensions, techniques are available to make cell suspensions from paraffin-embedded tissues. **(p. 64)**

Other methods for analysis of cell proliferation

A1. False

Mitotic count is highly variable, subject to differences in the fields chosen, type of microscope used, thickness of section, fixation, and identification of mitotic figures. Many attempts have been made to standardize the mitotic count, but there is no universally accepted standard. **(p. 65)**

A2. True

Ki-67 is a nuclear antigen that is expressed by cells in all phases of the cell cycle except G0. The formalin-resistant epitopes of Ki-67 are MIB-1 and MIB-3. PCNA is also used, but can sometimes be found in G0 tumor cells and so is not as specific as Ki-67. **(p. 65)**

A3. True

NORs contain ribosomal genes and acidic proteins with a high affinity for silver. These regions are related to the proliferative activity of the cells, but the technique is not frequently used today. **(p. 66)**

Cytogenetics

A1. True

Other contributions of cytogenetics to tumor pathology include: defining tumor subsets, suggesting connections between tumor types, highlighting specific changes in tumor subtypes, and defining the primary site. **(p. 66)**

A2. False

Comparative genomic hybridization can be performed and can be applied to fresh-frozen tissue, cell lines, and also DNA extracted from formalin-fixed tissue. **(p. 66)**

A3. False

Specific chromosomal translocations are found in several tumors, such as synovial sarcoma or Ewing sarcoma, but not in malignant fibrous histiocytomas. On the other hand, inflammatory myofibroblastic tumors have typical translocations t(2;19) (p23;p13.1) involving the ALK-TPM4 genes, and t(1;2) (q22-23;p23) involving TPM3-ALK genes. **(p. 67)**

Molecular pathology

A1. False

Although techniques are available for molecular analysis of formalin-fixed paraffin-embedded tissues, frozen material is still superior for DNA and RNA extraction. **(p. 67)**

A2. True

However, filter hybridization is time-consuming, may require radioactive compounds, and is subject to artifacts. **(p. 67–68)**

A3. False

ISH can be used for both DNA and RNA detection. It is most commonly used for viral infections, but is also useful in tumor analysis. **(p. 69)**

A4. False

Interphase cytogenetics can be performed on cells in non-dividing cells. This technique can be performed on both frozen and paraffin-embedded tissues. Specific DNA probes are available for a variety of genes that may have diagnostic and prognostic utility, such as HER-2 in breast cancer analysis. **(p. 69)**

A5. True

RT-PCR can amplify small amounts of extracted RNA, which is converted to cDNA for analysis. **(p. 70)**

DNA microarrays

A1. True

However, practically speaking, targeted gene profiles contain a defined subset of genes, which may be much smaller in scope. **(p. 71)**

A2. True

The concept of microdissection utilizing needles or razor blades has been around since the 1960s, but by using laser technology single cells may be lifted from tissue sections for analysis. **(p. 71)**

A3. False

The *ras* gene is a tumor proto-oncogene, not a tumor suppressor gene. The most important tumor suppressor genes include *p53* and the retinoblastoma (*Rb*) genes. Loss of function of tumor suppressor genes may result in tumor growth. **(p. 71)**

A4. True

Oncogenes and tumor suppressor genes can be categorized as those involved with mitogenic signal transduction pathways, cell cycle regulation, DNA replication and repair, and apoptosis. **(p. 72)**

4 Skin

Normal anatomy

Q1

The epidermis contains four layers: basal, prickle (malpighian), granular and cornified (horny).

Q2

The eosinophilic aspect of cells of the prickle (malpighian) layer is due to the accumulation of intracytoplasmic glycogen.

Q3

The cornified layer of the epidermis contains keratohyaline granules.

Q4

The cornified layer is thinner and looser on acral sites.

Q5

The major proteins of basal keratinocytes are keratins 5 and 14.

Q6

Parakeratosis is a form of abnormal keratinization in which cells in the cornified layer retain their nuclei.

Q7

In the skin, Langerhans' cells are exclusively found in the dermis.

Q8

Merkel cells stain positively for S100 and CD1a but not for keratin.

Q9

The eccrine sweat gland is one of the components of the pilar unit.

Q10

Proliferation within the hair follicle is a cyclic process involving an anagen, a catagen and a telogen phase.

Q11

Trichilemmal keratinization is characterized by abrupt keratinization without a granular layer.

Q12

Eccrine sweat glands are responsible for thermoregulation and have both a secretory and an excretory portion.

Q13

Apocrine glands are most frequent on the fingers and toes.

Q14

The thickness of the dermis is fairly constant, and varies little between anatomic sites.

Q15

Within the dermis, two distinct layers can be appreciated: the adventitial and the reticular dermis.

Q16

Glomus cells are modified smooth muscle cells present in specialized arteriovenous anastomoses (Sucquet–Hoyer canals).

Q17

Pacinian corpuscles have a tactile function in the skin and are located mainly on the palms and soles.

Q18

Aging and sunlight cause collagen and elastic tissue to undergo structural and tinctorial changes.

Q19

Dermal dendritic cells tend to decrease in number in inflammatory and neoplastic conditions.

Viral, bacterial and mycobacterial diseases

Q1

The lesion shown is a verruca plana.

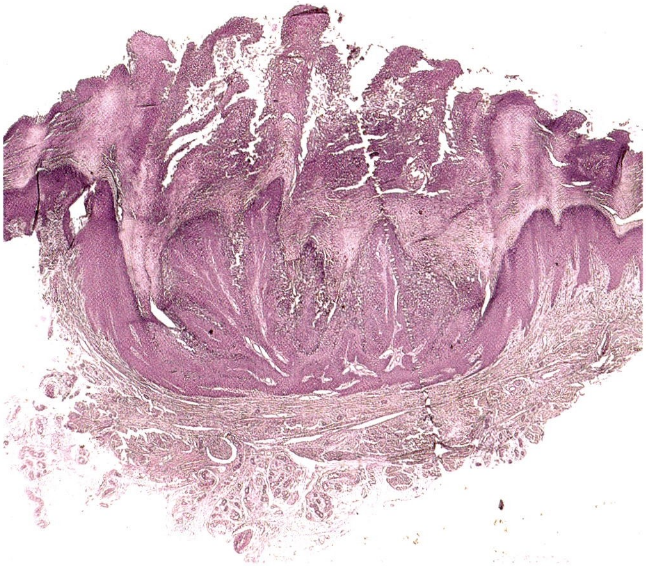

Fig. 4.1

Q2

Warts are caused by infection by human papilloma viruses (members of the papova group of viruses)

Q3

Benign or malignant skin tumors may be superimposed on HPV lesions.

Q4

Molluscum contagiosum is usually large, solitary, and clinically suspicious for deeply invasive squamous cell carcinoma.

Q5

Lesions of herpes zoster are often unilateral and in the distribution of a single dermatome.

Q6

Deep folliculitis always has an infectious etiology.

Q7

Eosinophilic folliculitis is a distinct condition seen in HIV infection.

Q8

Hidradenitis suppurativa is a destructive, inflammatory process affecting eccrine sweat glands.

Q9

The histologic changes shown are consistent with cutaneous tuberculosis.

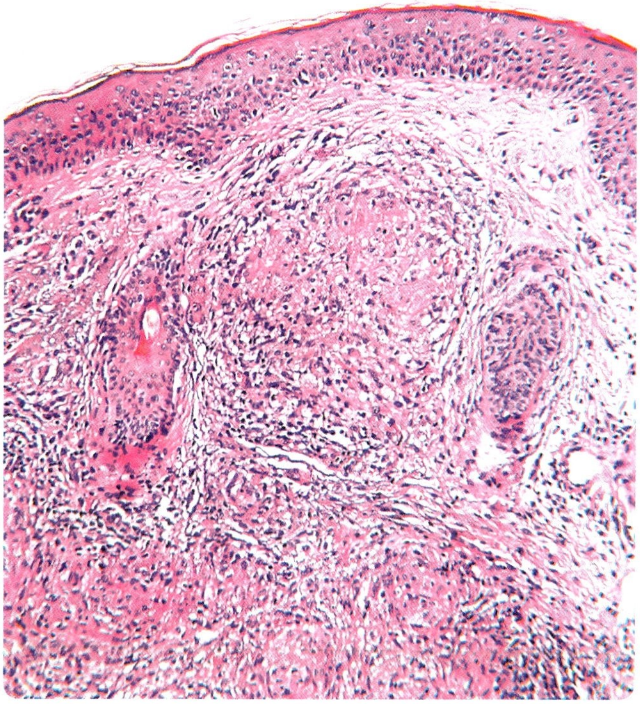

Fig. 4.2

Q10

Acid-fast bacilli are usually easily found in stained sections of lupus vulgaris.

Q11

Erythema induratum (Bazin type) usually occurs on the face.

Q12

Cutaneous infection by atypical mycobacteria may produce a variety of clinical lesions, including ulceration, abscesses and granulomas.

Q13

In tuberculoid and borderline leprosy, acid-fast bacilli are numerous in skin sections.

QUESTIONS

Q14

This type of dermal infiltrate may be seen in some subtypes of leprosy.

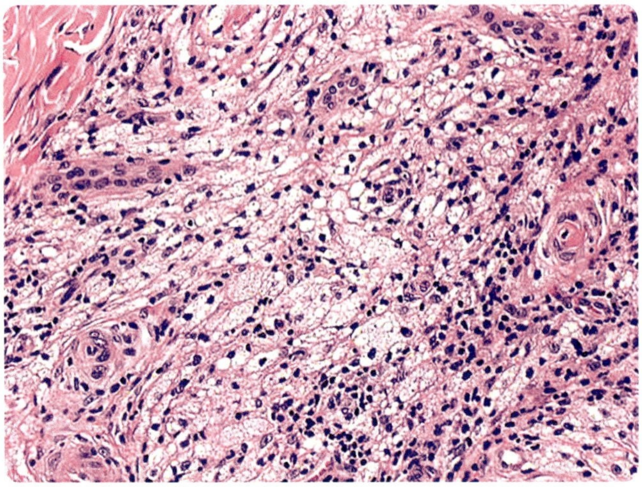

Fig. 4.3

Spirochetal and fungal diseases

Q1

Secondary syphilis is clinically very distinctive and is rarely confused with other inflammatory dermatoses.

Q2

A dermal inflammatory infiltrate containing prominent plasma cells may be a useful hint in diagnosing secondary syphilis.

Q3

Spirochetes are almost never found in tissue sections stained with a Steiner silver stain in secondary syphilis.

Q4

Lyme disease is a multisystem disease caused by the spirochete *Borrelia burgdorferi.*

Q5

Cutaneous Lyme disease characteristically shows a superficial and deep perivascular inflammatory infiltrate including plasma cells.

Q6

Severe epidermal changes with necrosis and ulceration are usual in dermatophyte infections.

Q7

Cutaneous blastomycosis (North American blastomycosis) is usually an isolated cutaneous disease.

Q8

Chromoblastomycosis, although sometimes clinically misdiagnosed as carcinoma, is an indolent cutaneous disease.

Other granulomatous diseases

Q1

A dermal infiltrate of non-caseating granulomas with little associated inflammation is typical of sarcoidosis.

Q2

Asteroid bodies, when seen, are extremely helpful, as they are specific for sarcoidosis.

Psoriasis and exfoliative dermatitis

Q1

This is the typical histologic appearance of psoriasis.

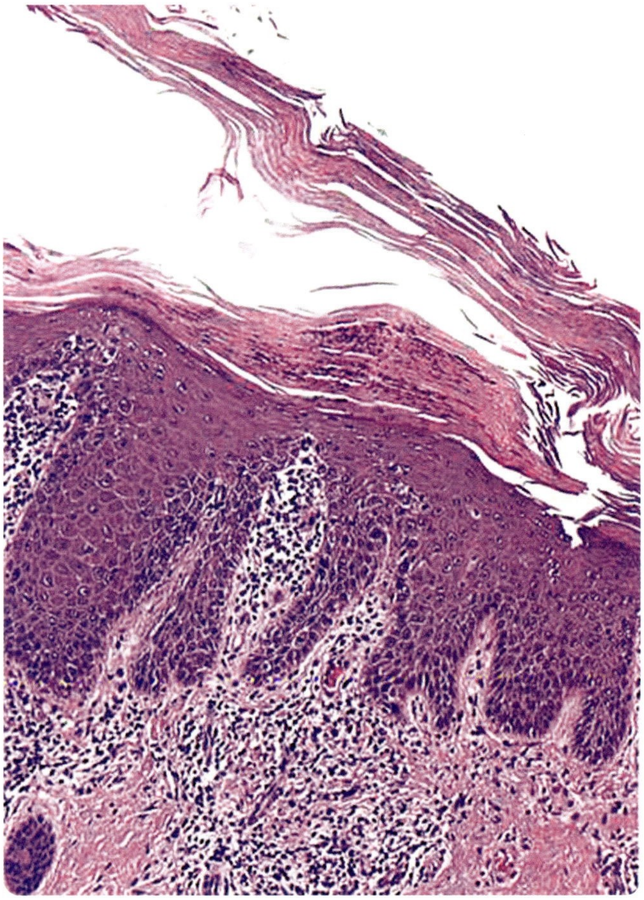

Fig. 4.4

Q2

Munro microabscesses are small groups of haloed mononuclear cells in the lower epidermis.

Q3

The histology of psoriasis is very typical and rarely causes diagnostic difficulties.

Q4

Psoriatic patients treated with long-term photochemotherapy (PUVA) do not have an increased risk of cutaneous squamous cell carcinoma or melanoma.

Q5

Erythroderma may be caused by a wide variety of malignant and inflammatory conditions.

Lichen planus and graft-versus-host disease

Q1

The lesions of lichen planus typically affect the flexor surfaces of the arms and legs.

Q2

The inflammatory infiltrate in lichen planus is largely confined to the reticular dermis, with extension around skin adnexae.

Q3

A follicular form of lichen planus is recognized (lichen planopilaris).

Q4

A similar morphologic pattern to that seen in lichen planus (the lichenoid reaction pattern) may be seen in regressing malignant melanoma.

Q5

A brisk inflammatory infiltrate is typically present in acute graft-versus-host disease and is an important clue to the diagnosis.

Vasculitis and related conditions

Q1

Vasculitis in the skin is always an expression of multiorgan vascular injury.

Q2

Most cases of vasculitis in the skin are due to the direct invasion of vascular endothelium by infectious agents.

Q3

The inflammatory infiltrate in vasculitis may be neutrophilic, lymphocytic or granulomatous.

Q4

This is an example of pigmented purpuric dermatosis.

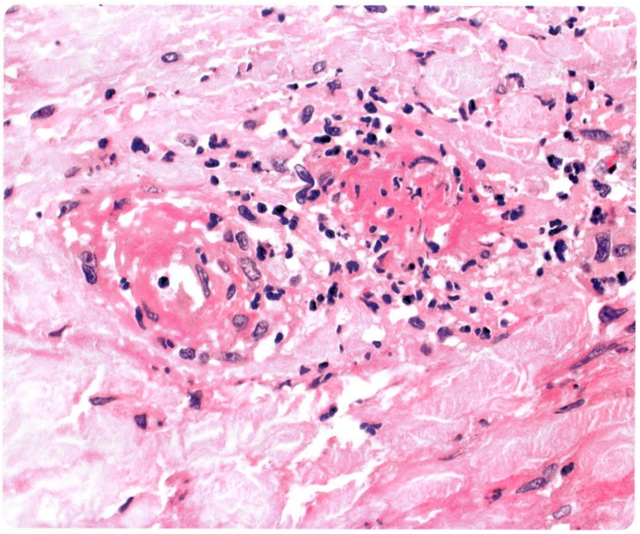

Fig. 4.5

Q5

Essential mixed cryoglobulinemia may be associated with leukocytoclastic vasculitis in the skin.

Q6

Sweet's syndrome (acute febrile neutrophilic dermatosis) shows the histologic pattern of acute leukocytoclastic vasculitis.

Q7

The inflammatory infiltrate in granuloma faciale usually extends into hair follicles and the overlying epidermis.

Q8

In granuloma faciale the dermis contains lymphocytes, histiocytes and large numbers of eosinophils.

Q9

Late lesions of erythema elevatum diutinum may show little vasculitis, but prominent storiform or concentric dermal fibrosis.

QUESTIONS

Panniculitis

Q1

Erythema nodosum is commonly associated with one of the following conditions: streptococcal infection, tuberculosis and sarcoidosis.

Q2

The inflammatory infiltrate in erythema nodosum typically extends diffusely throughout lobules of subcutaneous fat.

Q3

Chronic pancreatitis and α1-antitrypsin deficiency may present as a septal panniculitis.

Granuloma annulare and necrobiosis lipoidica

Q1

This is an example of necrobiosis lipoidica.

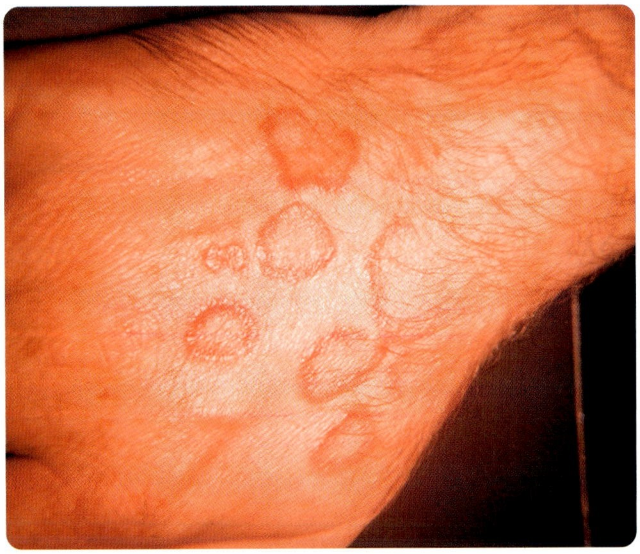

Fig. 4.6

Q2

The key histologic abnormality in granuloma annulare is so-called necrobiotic collagen with palisading granuloma formation.

Q3

Occasionally, children may present with deep-seated nodules showing a similar histology to that of granuloma annulare.

Q4

Necrobiosis lipoidica is always associated with diabetes mellitus.

Mastocytosis

Q1

Urticaria pigmentosa is the commonest clinical form of cutaneous mastocytosis.

Q2

The histologic appearance of urticaria pigmentosa on biopsy is sometimes very subtle and can be missed.

Lupus erythematosus and dermatomyositis

Q1

Skin involvement by lupus erythematosus may represent either part of a systemic disease or a condition limited to the skin.

Q2

Epidermal atrophy, hyperkeratosis and liquefactive degeneration of the basal layer are important clues to chronic discoid lupus erythematosus.

Q3

Linear deposition of immunoglobulin and complement along the dermoepidermal junction (the lupus band) is highly specific for cutaneous lupus erythematosus.

Q4

Dermatomyositis is an inflammatory disorder characterized clinically by proximal muscle weakness and cutaneous lesions.

Q5

There is no association between dermatomyositis and underlying malignancy.

Scleroderma, drug eruptions and pyoderma gangrenosum

Q1

Scleroderma may present clinically as localized or systemic disease.

Q2

Allergic reactions to drugs may present a clinical picture similar to that of another well-defined dermatosis.

Q3

Chemotherapeutic agents may result in acute necrotizing changes in sweat glands (neutrophilic eccrine hidradenitis).

Q4

In drug-induced coma the first cutaneous structure to undergo necrosis is the epidermis.

Q5

Pyoderma gangrenosum is only very rarely associated with a systemic disease.

Vesiculobullous diseases

Q1

Dermatitis herpetiformis is a symmetric pruritic disease, frequently associated with gluten-sensitive enteropathy.

Q2

The most consistent histologic findings in bullous pemphigoid are a multilocular blister with necrosis of dermal papillae.

Q3

In epidermolysis bullosa the site of cleavage may be very variable (in the lower epidermis, dermis or dermoepidermal junction) depending on the clinical type.

Q4

Dermatitis herpetiformis characteristically shows linear basement membrane staining with IgA.

Q5

In bullous impetigo and pemphigus foliaceus the level of the split is high in the epidermis.

Q6

This epidermal staining pattern for IgG on direct immunofluorescence is consistent with herpes gestationis.

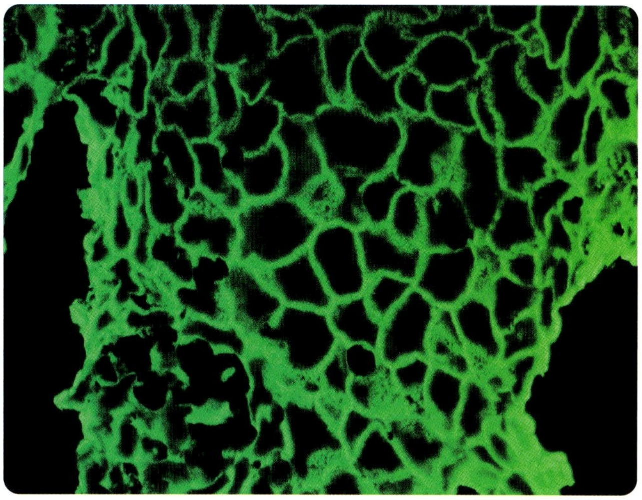

Fig. 4.7

Q7

Bullous pemphigoid, bullous SLE and epidermolysis bullosa acquisita often show an identical staining pattern on direct immunofluorescence.

Q8

Some cases of pemphigus are associated with malignancies of internal organs.

Q9

In Hailey–Hailey disease the mechanism of cell separation is spongiosis.

Q10

Clinically, Grover's disease (transient acantholytic dermatosis) presents with pruritic, excoriated papules and vesicles on the trunk.

Q11

The histologic finding of acantholysis and dyskeratosis is always of clinical significance.

Miscellaneous conditions

Q1

Lichen sclerosus et atrophicus most often occurs on the anogenital region, upper trunk, neck and flexor surfaces of the wrist.

Q2

In elastosis perforans, abnormally coarse elastic fibers are eliminated through a hyperplastic epidermis.

Q3

Pseudoxanthoma elasticum is in most cases an acquired condition of the skin, related to exaggerated aging of connective tissue.

Q4

Pretibial myxedema is most often associated with hypothyroidism.

Q5

The dermal mucinoses show separation of collagen by basophilic material that stains with Mayer's mucicarmine and Hale's colloidal iron.

Q6

The reaction pattern of follicular mucinosis is always a benign condition.

Q7

Cutaneous myxomas are part of Cowden's syndrome.

Q8

Acanthosis nigricans may be associated with internal malignancies.

Q9

The pigmentation visible clinically in acanthosis nigricans is due to increased melanin production by epidermal melanocytes.

Q10

This is an example of severe psoriasis.

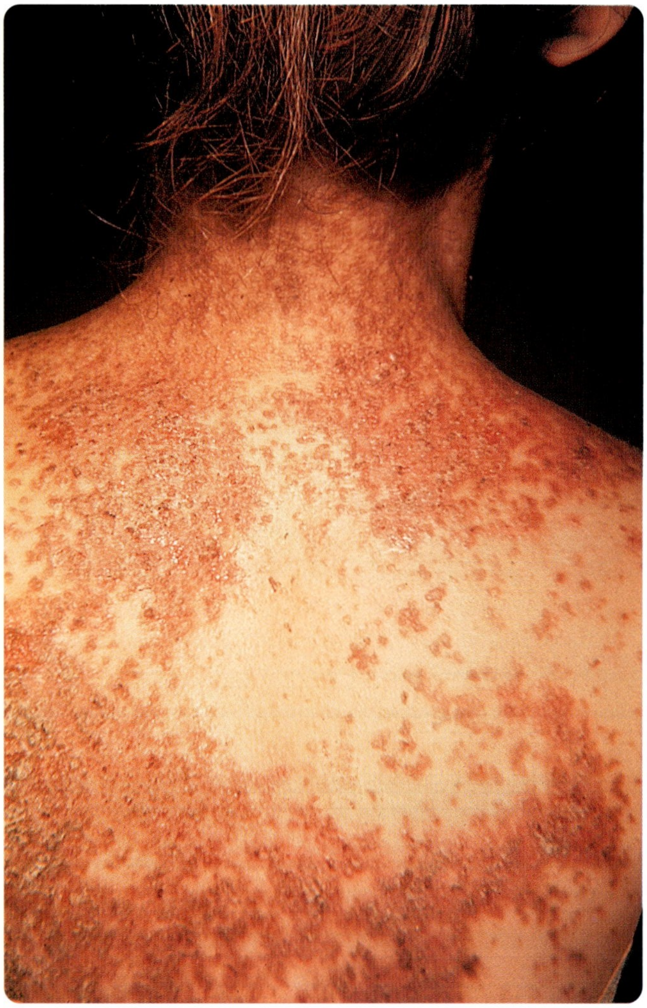

Fig. 4.8

Q11

In the setting of HIV infection, seborrheic dermatitis may be more severe and clinically more widespread.

Epidermal tumors

Q1

Internal malignant disease may be associated with the sudden appearance or increase in size of seborrheic keratoses.

Q2

p53 accumulation is not seen in actinic keratoses.

Q3

A cutaneous horn may overlie benign or malignant epidermal proliferations.

Q4

The changes shown represent psoriasis.

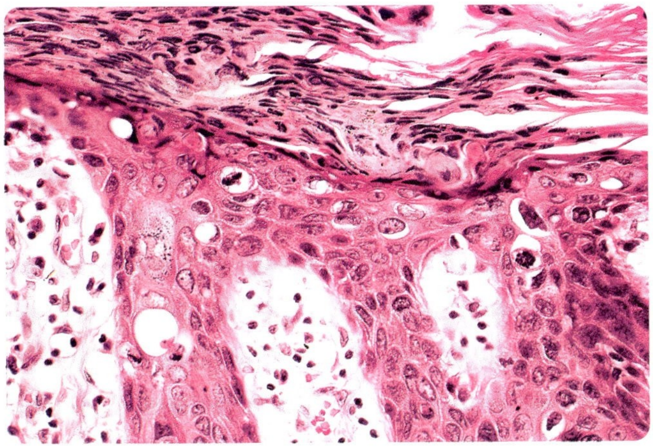

Fig. 4.9

Q5

Some cases of Bowen's disease may microscopically mimic Paget's disease.

Q6

Squamous cell carcinoma may complicate xeroderma pigmentosum.

Q7

Squamous cell carcinoma may be composed of spindle cells on histology.

Q8

Verrucous carcinoma is a highly aggressive subtype of squamous cell carcinoma.

Q9

Acantholytic (adenoid) squamous cell carcinoma is the cutaneous equivalent of mucoepidermoid carcinoma in the salivary gland.

Q10

Vertical tumor thickness and level of dermal invasion are important prognostic indicators in squamous cell carcinoma.

Q11

Multiple squamous cell carcinomas occur in the setting of Gorlin's syndrome.

Q12

Immunohistochemically, basal cell carcinomas are usually positive for EMA but show only weak, focal staining for bcl-2.

Q13

Superficial basal cell carcinoma exhibits a high recurrence rate.

Q14

Basal cell carcinoma never metastasizes.

Adnexal tumors

Q1

Eccrine poromas may be purely intradermal.

Q2

Eccrine syringomas are usually solitary and are most often found on acral sites.

Q3

Chondroid syringomas have an appearance comparable to that of mixed tumors of salivary origin.

Q4

Eccrine cylindromas may be multiple and associated with a specific genetic mutation.

Q5

The tumor shown is an intradermal poroma.

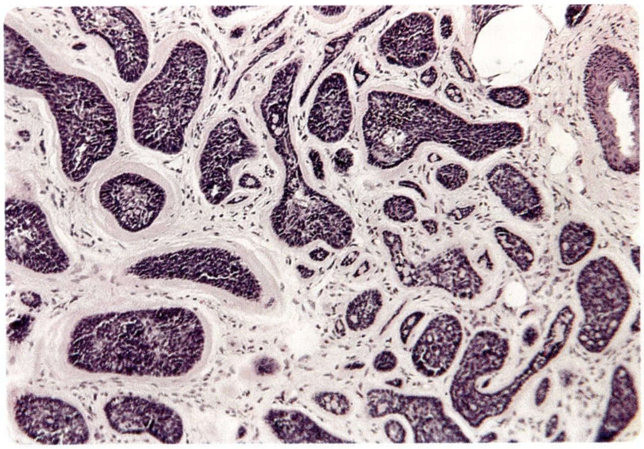

Fig. 4.10

Q6

Eccrine spiradenoma may be confused clinically with a vascular tumor.

Q7

Papillary syringoadenoma (syringocystadenoma papilliferum) may arise in a nevus sebaceus.

Q8

Malignant sweat gland tumors are microscopically very distinctive and are unlikely to be confused with another tumor type.

Q9

Porocarcinoma (malignant eccrine poroma) may show marked epidermotropism.

Q10

Microcystic adnexal carcinoma (sclerosing sweat duct carcinoma) is a highly malignant tumor that commonly shows regional and distant metastases.

Q11

Electron microscopic examination has shown that the cells in extramammary Paget's disease are altered keratinocytes.

Q12

The lesion shown is a nevus sebaceus.

A

B

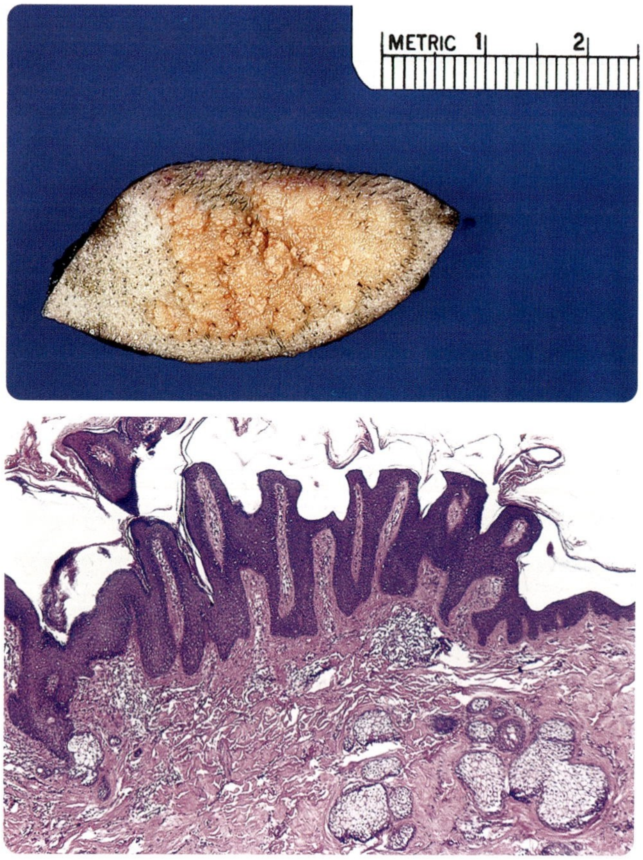

Fig. 4.11

Q13

Sebaceous adenomas are associated with tuberous sclerosis.

Q14

Sebaceous carcinoma of the eyelid is a relatively indolent malignancy.

Q15

Sebaceous adenomas and carcinomas both show expression of EMA and androgen receptor.

Q16

Sebaceous tumors may be a component of Muir–Torre syndrome.

Q17

The tumor shown is an inverted follicular keratosis.

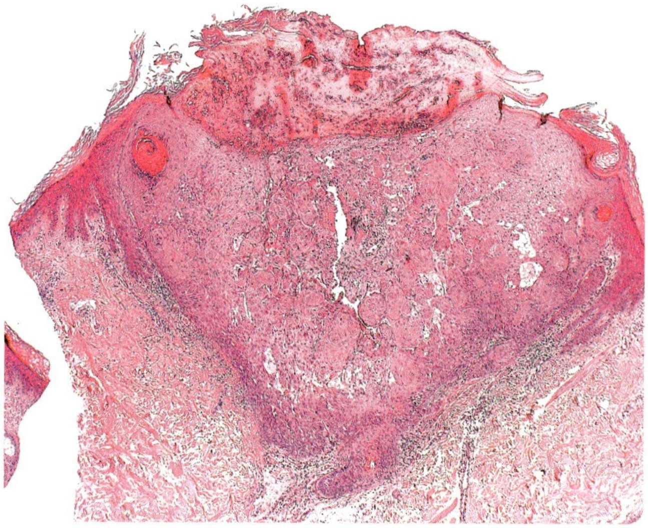

Fig. 4.12

Q18

Trichoepitheliomas may be multiple, and can occur in a familial setting.

Q19

Merkel cells are usually not present in benign hair follicle tumors.

Q20

Assessment of architecture in a keratoacanthoma is just as important as the cytonuclear features in the differential with traditional squamous cell carcinoma.

Q21

Keratoacanthoma is always solitary and on sun-exposed parts.

Q22

Pilar (trichilemmal) cysts show an intact granular cell layer in their wall.

Q23

Cutaneous cysts may develop from the ductal portion of a sebaceous gland.

Q24

Pilar tumors have a predilection for the scalp.

Q25

Pilomatrixoma is a benign hair follicle tumor that differentiates toward the outer root sheath of the follicle.

Q26

Ghost or shadow cells are specific for pilomatrixoma and are not found in any other primary cutaneous tumor.

Melanocytes, their benign tumors and tumor-like conditions

Q1

Racial differences in skin pigmentation are due to differences in the number of melanocytes in the basal epidermis.

Q2

The average Caucasian adult has between three and five nevi.

Q3

Most nevi of the palms and soles are of junctional type.

Q4

Nevi on some anatomic sites may be larger and microscopically atypical.

Q5

The histologic hallmark of a common blue nevus is the dendritic dermal melanocyte.

Q6

Blue nevi are confined to the dermis.

Q7

Epithelioid blue nevus may be part of the Carney complex.

Q8

By definition, Spitz nevi are compound melanocytic proliferations, with a prominent epidermal component.

Q9

Kamino bodies are a useful histologic finding in diagnosing Spitz nevus.

Q10

Some Spitz nevi may show predominantly intraepidermal growth.

Q11

Immunohistochemical stains are very valuable in distinguishing Spitz nevus from malignant melanoma.

Q12

Some cutaneous tumors fulfilling the morphologic criteria for Spitz nevus behave in a malignant fashion.

Q13

In general, congenital nevi are smaller than acquired nevi.

Q14

Giant congenital nevi may give rise to malignant melanoma.

Q15

This is the typical clinical appearance of a Spitz nevus.

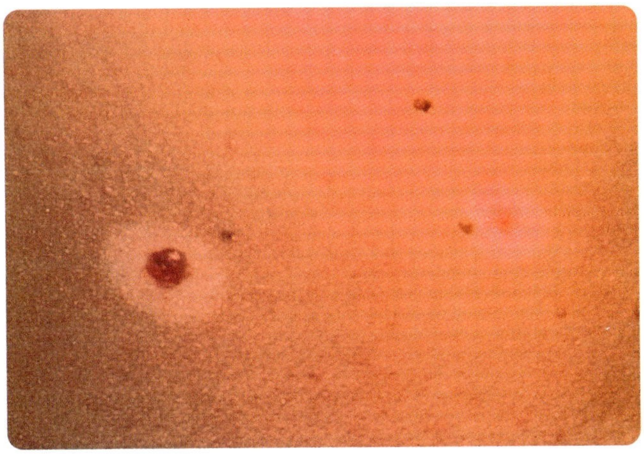

Fig. 4.13

Q16

When a benign nevus recurs after inadequate excision, the histology in the re-excision may be very different from that in the original lesion.

Q17

Nevi that have been exposed to ultraviolet light or excessive sunlight may appear histologically different from other nevi.

Q18

The patient shown also has a father and brother with morphologically similar nevi; he is at risk of developing malignant melanoma.

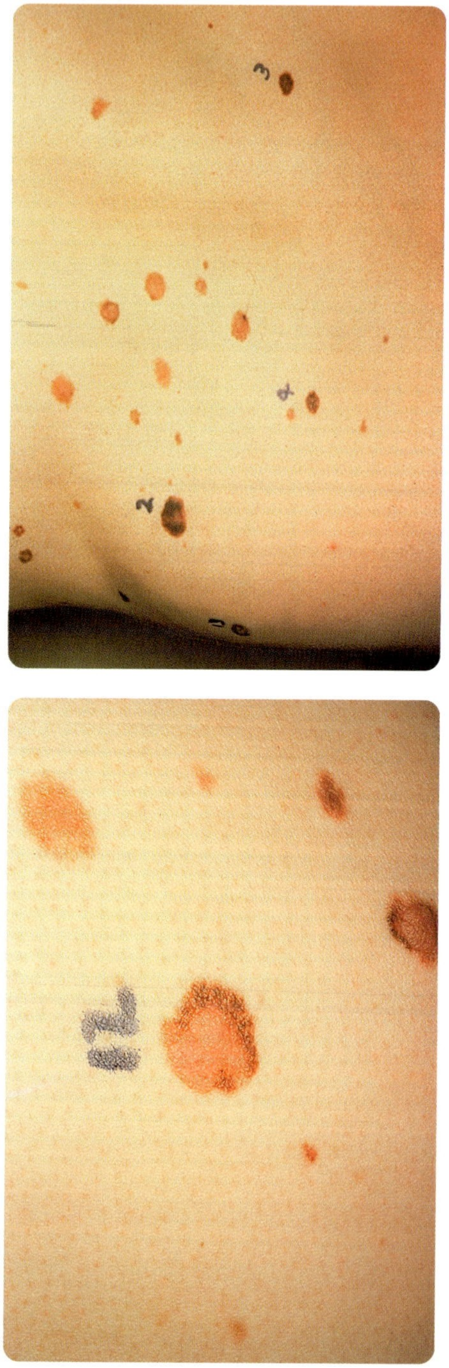

A

B

Fig. 4.14

Q19

The majority of clinically atypical nevi show the features of dysplastic nevi on biopsy.

Q20

Dysplastic nevi differ from banal nevi only by their cytonuclear features.

Malignant melanoma

Q1

The presence of a large number of nevi is a risk factor for the development of melanoma.

Q2

This is an example of a compound nevus.

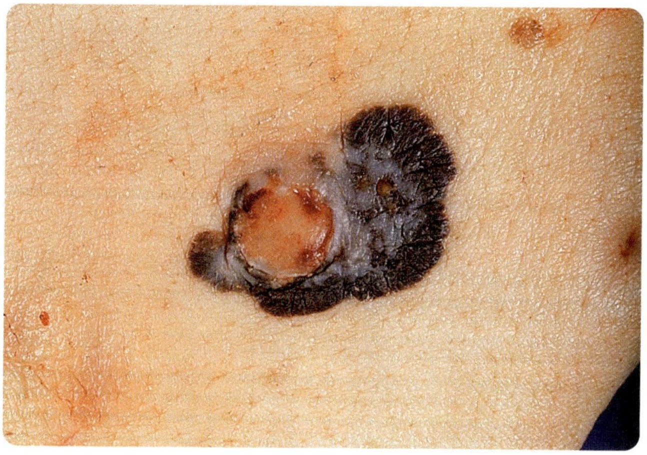

Fig. 4.15

Q3

Desmoplastic melanoma may be misdiagnosed as a benign lesion.

Q4

Atypical mitoses in a melanocytic proliferation are a good clue to malignancy.

Q5

Immunohistochemical markers are very useful in distinguishing nevi from melanomas.

Q6

HMB-45, a pan-melanoma marker, is positive in all melanoma subtypes.

Q7

Microphthalmia transcription factor (MiTF) is a useful marker for tumors of melanocytic origin.

Q8

Immunohistochemical positivity for keratin effectively excludes melanoma.

Q9

Consistent gene mutations have been identified in a subset of melanomas.

Q10

Patients with metastatic melanoma in whom a primary tumor is never found represent cases of carcinoma or sarcoma that were incorrectly diagnosed.

Q11

These structures were found on EM in a cytologically malignant tumor that was negative for S100, HMB-45 and Melan-A. The diagnosis is melanoma.

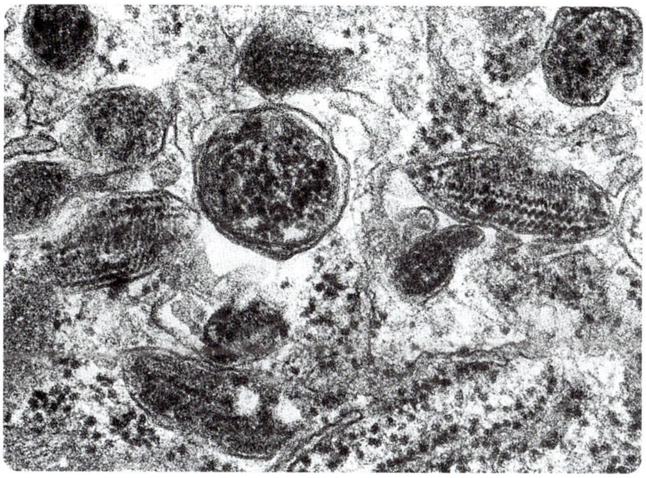

Fig. 4.16

Q12

Cutaneous metastases from melanoma elsewhere are confined to the deep dermis.

Q13

The presence of S100-positive cell clusters in a sentinel node biopsy for melanoma means metastatic disease is present.

Q14

Tumor stage is the most important prognostic parameter for melanoma.

Q15

After tumor stage, the most powerful predictors of survival in melanoma are tumor diameter and histologic subtype.

Q16

Clinical factors affecting prognosis in melanoma include tumor site, patient age and gender.

Q17

The presence of an inflammatory infiltrate in primary cutaneous melanoma has no influence on prognosis.

Q18

The detection of microscopic satellites in primary cutaneous melanoma has an adverse effect on prognosis.

Other tumors and tumor-like conditions

Q1

This EM photograph shows melanosomes from a malignant melanoma.

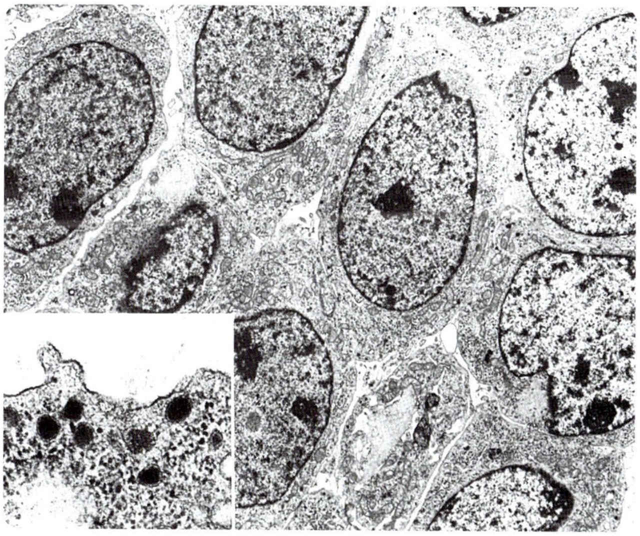

Fig. 4.17

Q2

Merkel cell carcinoma is a locally aggressive tumor, similar in its behavior to basal cell carcinoma.

Q3

This pattern of cytokeratin 20 staining is typical of a Merkel cell carcinoma.

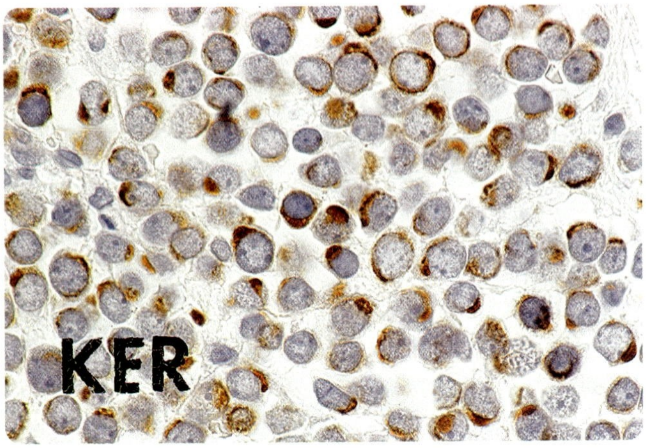

Fig. 4.18

Q4

Keloid occurs more often in African-American patients than in caucasians.

Q5

Fibrous papule of the face is a cutaneous marker for tuberous sclerosis.

Q6

Dermatofibromas (fibrous histiocytomas) are usually positive for factor XIIIa and negative for CD34.

Q7

This is a variant of fibrous histiocytoma (dermatofibroma).

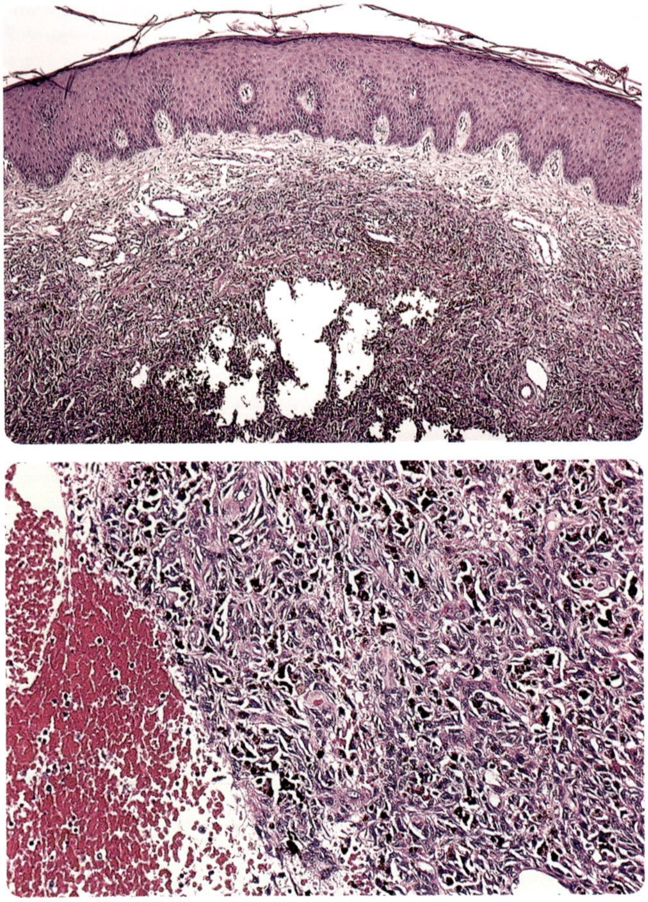

A

B

Fig. 4.19

Q8

An epithelioid variant of fibrous histiocytoma (dermatofibroma) is described.

Q9

Atypical fibroxanthoma is another variant of dermatofibroma with scattered large atypical cells.

Q10

In addition to cytologic atypia, atypical fibroxanthoma often shows deep, destructive growth and necrosis.

Q11

Atypical fibroxanthoma is a clinically and histologically distinctive lesion which is unlikely to be confused with another tumor.

Q12

The growth pattern in the subcutis of this predominantly intradermal spindle cell proliferation is consistent with dermatofibrosarcoma protuberans (DFSP).

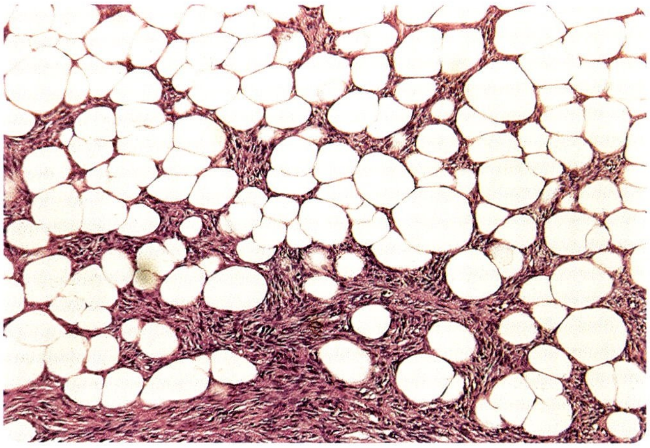

Fig. 4.20

Q13

Dermatofibrosarcoma protuberans is a highly aggressive sarcoma that metastasizes widely.

Q14

Cytogenetic studies may help in diagnosing dermatofibrosarcoma protuberans.

Q15

This is a form of cutaneous xanthoma.

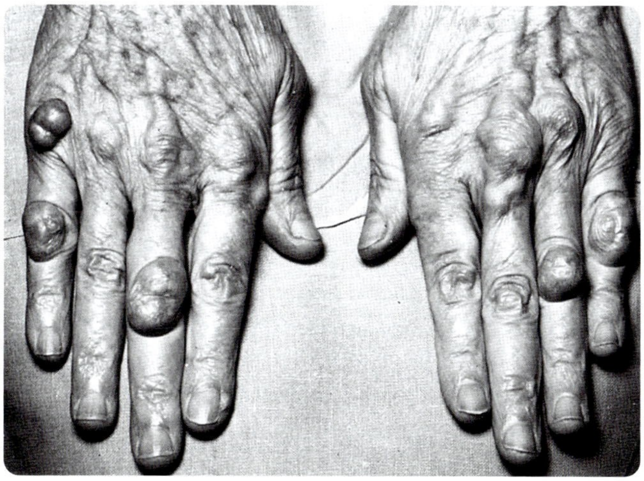

Fig. 4.21

Q16

Juvenile xanthogranuloma represents a proliferation of S100-positive histiocytic cells.

Q17

Juvenile xanthogranuloma may occur at any body site.

Q18

Leiomyosarcomas arising in the dermis metastasize in up to 25% of cases.

Q19

S100 is consistently positive in neurothekeoma.

Q20

Perineurioma shows immunoreactivity for EMA.

Q21

This vascular lesion is often associated with an underlying syndrome.

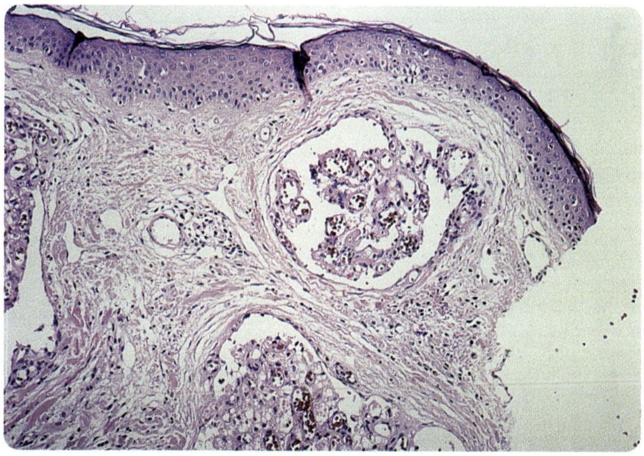

Fig. 4.22

Q22

Cutaneous vascular tumors with an epithelioid morphology are always benign.

Q23

Masson's tumor (intravascular papillary endothelial hyperplasia) is most likely a reactive process.

Q24

HHV-6 is found in almost 100% of cases of Kaposi's sarcoma.

Q25

Intracytoplasmic hyaline bodies are diagnostic for Kaposi's sarcoma.

Q26

Bacillary angiomatosis is a vascular proliferation closely related to Kaposi's sarcoma and caused by the same virus.

Q27

The lesions of primary cutaneous angiosarcoma and classic Kaposi's sarcoma have a similar anatomic distribution.

Q28

Cutaneous angiosarcoma may be difficult to distinguish microscopically from a benign process.

Q29

Cutaneous lymphoid hyperplasia may be difficult to distinguish from low-grade B-cell lymphoma.

Q30

This histology is consistent with early mycosis fungoides.

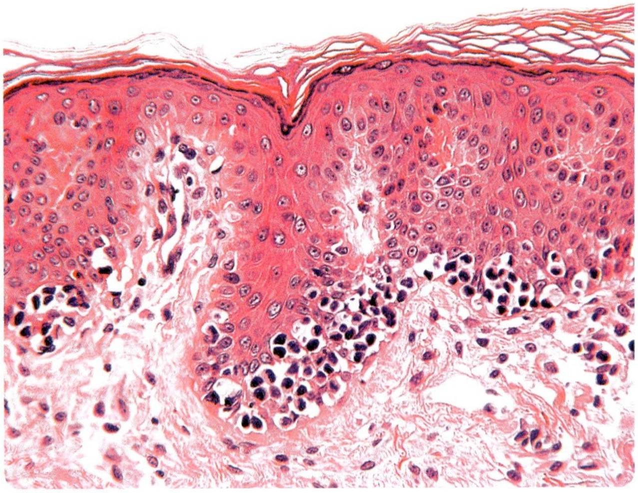

Fig. 4.23

Q31

Sparing of the skin adnexae is a helpful sign in mycosis fungoides.

Q32

Small convoluted T cells with a cerebriform (cerebroid) appearance are diagnostic of mycosis fungoides.

Q33

The atypical cells in mycosis fungoides are always T lymphocytes.

Q34

Mycosis fungoides may show loss of T-cell differentiation antigens.

Q35

Pagetoid reticulosis is a type of cutaneous T-cell lymphoma with an excellent prognosis.

Q36

This patient had similar lesions on the trunk and legs. Histology showed many CD30-positive atypical cells. The diagnosis is anaplastic large cell lymphoma.

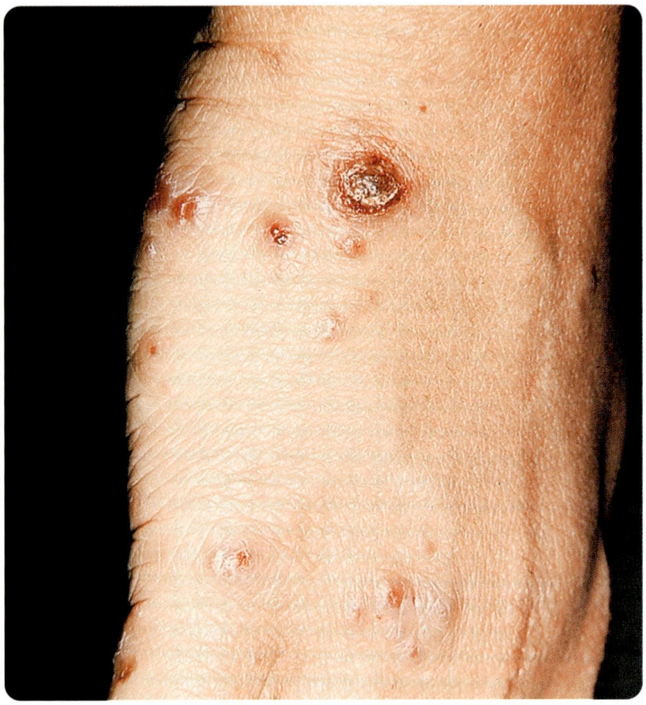

Fig. 4.24

Q37

Large cells in the dermis showing CD30-positivity are diagnostic for either anaplastic large cell lymphoma or lymphomatoid papulosis.

Q38

Intravascular lymphoma is not a true lymphoma but a neoplasm of endothelial cells.

Q39

Leukemia may sometimes present in the skin without evidence of disease on examination of the peripheral blood.

Q40

On biopsy, cutaneous endometriosis may mimic malignancy.

Q41

The most common sites for skin metastases are the chest and abdomen.

Normal anatomy

A1. True
The relative prominence of these various layers depends not only on the anatomic location but also the type of disease process affecting the skin. **(p. 94)**

A2. False
The eosinophilic appearance correlates with the accumulation of filaments, which are the precursors of keratin. **(p. 94)**

A3. False
The *granular* layer contains basophilic granules known as keratohyaline granules. Keratohyaline granules contain the precursor of fillagrin, which is important for the aggregation of keratin filaments. Abnormalities in fillagrin can lead to defects in desquamation and are found in some forms of ichthyosis. **(p. 94)**

A4. False
The cornified layer is thickest on acral sites. **(p. 94)**

A5. True
Defects in these keratin types are found in some types of epidermolysis bullosa. Terminally differentiated keratinocytes in the epidermis express keratins 1 and 10. **(p. 94)**

A6. True
This can be associated with reduced transit time through the epidermis in hyperproliferative disorders (e.g. psoriasis) or overlying areas of previous spongiosis. **(p. 94)**

A7. False
The important immunologic function of Langerhans' cells explains the presence of significant numbers in the epidermis as well as the dermis. Langerhans' cells are characterized ultrastructurally by the presence of Birbeck granules – these are very distinctive rod-shaped structures, sometimes with a bulbous end (likened to a tennis racket). **(p. 94)**

A8. False
Langerhans' cells stain with S100 and CD1a; these markers are negative in Merkel cells. Keratin positivity is an important characteristic of Merkel cells, particularly CK20. **(p. 95)**

A9. False
In certain anatomic regions the apocrine sweat gland forms part of the pilar unit. The eccrine sweat gland has no direct association with hair follicles and opens by way of its own duct on to the epidermis. **(p. 95)**

A10. True
The cyclical nature of folliculogenesis is important for understanding hair growth and alopecia: active hair growth occurs during anagen, involution during catagen, and telogen represents the resting phase. **(p. 95)**

A11. True
This type of keratinization is seen in the isthmus region of hair follicles and is recapitulated in some cysts (trichilemmal cysts) and tumors (pilar tumors). Keratinization in the infundibular region of follicles resembles that in the epidermis and includes keratohyaline granules. **(p. 95)**

A12. True
The intraepidermal portion of the eccrine sweat duct is known as the acrosyringium. **(p. 95)**

A13. False
Apocrine glands are typically found in the axillae, groins and perineum; smaller numbers are found on the face. **(p. 95)**

A14. False
The thickness of the dermis varies considerably from area to area and is particularly thick on the back. The dermis is a connective tissue structure composed of collagen and elastic fibres bathed in ground substance. **(p. 95)**

A15. True
The adventitial dermis is a delicate network of collagen which includes the papillary dermis (just under the epidermis) and the periadnexal dermis; the reticular dermis contains thick bundles of type I collagen admixed with thick elastic fibers. **(p. 95)**

A16. True
These structures are particularly present on acral skin; proliferation of glomus cells can give rise to tumors (e.g. glomus tumors or glomangiomas). **(p. 96)**

A17. False
Pacinian corpuscles are sensitive to pressure and are located on weightbearing parts: Wagner–Meissner corpuscles have a tactile function and are found on the palms and soles. **(p. 96)**

A18. True
Elastic tissue in particular can be seen to undergo basophilic degeneration and accumulation in large amorphic masses (solar/actinic elastosis). **(p. 96)**

A19. False
These cells are believed to act as antigen-presenting cells and are in fact increased in inflammatory and reactive conditions. They express coagulation factor XIIIa. **(p. 96)**

Viral, bacterial and mycobacterial diseases

A1. False
This is a verruca vulgaris, which shows the characteristic epidermal hyperplasia; verruca plana is not exophytic. **(p. 96)**

A2. True
Many different HPV types have been isolated from verrucae, but HPV-2 is commonly associated with verruca vulgaris and HPV-10 with verruca plana. **(p. 96)**

A3. True
These include seborrheic keratoses, Bowen's disease and invasive squamous cell carcinoma. **(p. 97)**

A4. False
These lesions are usually small and multiple, often with distinctive central umbilication. Cells in molluscum contagiosum show large, eosinophilic viral inclusions (similar to poxviruses) that displace the nucleus and enlarge the cell. **(p. 97)**

A5. True
This is the classic presentation, but more severe infection may cause herpetic keratitis and corneal ulceration. Herpes zoster is caused by the same virus that causes chickenpox (varicella). **(p. 97)**

A6. False
Some forms of deep folliculitis are indeed caused by infection (e.g. bacterial or fungal), but initially sterile lesions of acne conglobata or cases of perforating folliculitis must also be considered. **(p. 97)**

A7. True
It is also important to exclude an infectious etiology in cases showing this reaction pattern. **(p. 98)**

A8. False
This condition affects *apocrine* glands, not eccrine glands, which explains its frequent occurrence in the axillae, groins and perineum. This condition tends toward chronicity and often leads to scarring, fistulae and sinuses. **(p. 98)**

A9. True
Cutaneous tuberculosis has varied clinical and morphologic forms, depending on the mode of entry and whether it is a primary or secondary infection. Although a relatively uncommon disease, it should always be borne in mind in cases of granulomatous inflammation. **(p. 99)**

A10. False
Cultures or PCR may be necessary to demonstrate the bacilli. Microscopically, cutaneous tuberculosis may show either necrotic or non-necrotic granulomatous inflammation. Lupus vulgaris often involves the face. **(p. 99)**

A11. False
This is regarded by many as a type of tuberculid (TB-associated skin lesion) presenting as tender subcutaneous nodules on the calves of women. **(p. 99)**

A12. True
The range of histologic changes seen is broad, and well-formed granulomas are often absent. *Mycobacterium marinum* and *M. ulcerans* are well known pathogens. **(p. 99)**

A13. False
Organisms are often plentiful in lepromatous leprosy, but in these other forms PCR techniques may be required for demonstration of the bacilli. **(p. 99)**

A14. True
Lepromatous leprosy (shown here) is characterized histologically by a diffuse dermal infiltrate of parasitized macrophages. Cutaneous leprosy should be suspected when a granulomatous and lymphocytic dermal infiltrate is seen to surround nerves and infiltrate the arrectores pilorum muscle. **(p. 99)**

Spirochetal and fungal diseases

A1. False
Secondary syphilis is a great mimic and may clinically resemble lichen planus, psoriasis, drug eruption or many other named conditions. The microscopic appearances in secondary syphilis may be entirely nonspecific, especially so in macular lesions, and a degree of clinical suspicion is required if a diagnosis is to be reached. **(p. 100)**

A2. True
Some cases, however, contain very few plasma cells. **(p. 100)**

A3. False
Some studies report a high rate of positivity with the Steiner stain (of the order of 70%). PCR-based techniques are also available. **(p. 100)**

A4. True
Besides the skin, the heart, joints and nervous system may be affected. Lyme disease may become manifest in the skin as erythema chronicum migrans, acrodermatitis chronica atrophicans or cutaneous lymphoid hyperplasia. **(p. 100)**

A5. True
Spirochetes can sometimes be demonstrated with the Warthin–Starry silver stain in cutaneous Lyme disease. A PCR-based test is also available. **(p. 100)**

A6. False

Mild epidermal changes are common, and some clinically atypical forms of dermatophyte infection may be easily overlooked on biopsy. A PAS or Gomori's methenamine silver stain will highlight the organisms; a sharp eye may also discern them on H&E staining. **(p. 101)**

A7. False

Usually the skin lesion is secondary to pulmonary involvement – which may be subclinical. Typically there is pseudoepitheliomatous epidermal hyperplasia with mixed suppurative and granulomatous inflammation. **(p. 102)**

A8. True

It is very rare for hematogenous dissemination to occur. In tissue sections spores of chromoblastomycosis are brown and show septation with cross-wall formation instead of budding. **(p. 102)**

Other granulomatous diseases

A1. True

Microscopically, sarcoidosis is a diagnosis of exclusion and may be mimicked by a variety of diseases. **(p. 102)**

A2. False

These are relatively uncommon and are not specific for sarcoidosis. **(p. 102)**

Psoriasis and exfoliative dermatitis

A1. True

Psoriasis is a common dermatosis, affecting between 0.5% and 1.5% of the population. A histologic hallmark of psoriasis is parakeratosis, reflecting markedly shortened epidermal cell turnover time. Lesions of psoriasis typically show regular elongation of the rete ridges, suprapapillary thinning and prominent capillaries in the papillary dermis. **(p. 103)**

A2. False

Munro microabscesses are subcorneal and intracorneal collections of neutrophils. The description given refers to Pautrier's microabscesses, seen in mycosis fungoides. **(p. 104)**

A3. False

Cases biopsied are usually clinically atypical and a similar histologic reaction pattern (the psoriasiform pattern) can be produced by irritation of the epidermis in a variety of conditions (e.g. lichen simplex chronicus, seborrheic dermatitis). **(p. 104)**

A4. False

Patients are at an increased risk for these cancers, depending on the total dose of radiation received. **(p. 104)**

A5. True

These include Sézary's syndrome, psoriasis, drug reaction, pityriasis rubra pilaris and contact dermatitis. Exfoliative dermatitis often shows nonspecific histology; for this reason some clinicians have questioned the value of biopsy in this condition. **(p. 104)**

Lichen planus and graft-versus-host disease

A1. True

The oral cavity may also be affected and lesions are typically pruritic. The histology of lichen planus shows irregular epidermal hyperplasia, hyperkeratosis and a prominent granular cell layer. **(p. 104)**

A2. False

The papillary dermis contains a band-like infiltrate that erodes the basal epidermis; degenerating basal keratinocytes (Civatte and colloid bodies) are seen. Deep dermal or periadnexal extension are not features – they should suggest lupus erythematosus. **(p. 104)**

A3. True

Other variants include hypertrophic, atrophic, bullous and pemphigoid (lichen planus pemphigoides). **(p. 105)**

A4. True

It may also be seen in other regressing tumors – important to remember. **(p. 105)**

A5. False

The earliest changes in acute graft-versus-host disease are vacuolation of the basal epidermis and individual cell necrosis. These may be very subtle and inflammation is often very mild. Chronic graft-versus-host disease may clinically and histologically resemble scleroderma. **(p. 105)**

Vasculitis and related conditions

A1. False

Many cases are restricted to the skin, and may be generalized or limited to a single focus. The extension of vasculitis into the deep dermis and subcutaneous fat should raise the possibility of the presence of systemic disease. **(p. 105)**

A2. False

Immune-mediated injury and the action of immune complexes have an important pathogenic role in many cases of cutaneous vasculitis. Direct immunofluorescence often shows deposits of immunoglobulin, complement and fibrin in and around vessel walls. **(p. 105)**

A3. True

The type of infiltrate is often helpful in determining the likely cause of the vascular changes, but it is important to remember that fibrinoid necrosis is not always present. **(p. 105)**

A4. False

Pigmented purpuric dermatosis is an example of lymphocytic, non-necrotizing vasculitis. These vessels clearly show fibrinoid necrosis and granulocytic nuclear debris. **(p. 106)**

A5. True

In some cases this may look identical to allergic (leukocytoclastic) vasculitis of the skin, but extension into the deep reticular dermis and subcutis may suggest systemic disease. **(p. 106)**

A6. False

This condition shows a massive outpouring of neutrophils in the dermis, unaccompanied by bona fide necrotizing vasculitis. Sweet's syndrome may occur as a paraneoplastic manifestation in patients with hematologic malignancies (e.g. AML). **(p. 106)**

A7. False

The adventitial dermis is typically spared in granuloma faciale, unlike erythema elevatum diutinum. **(p. 107)**

A8. True

Prominent eosinophils are a helpful clue to the diagnosis; fewer eosinophils occur in erythema elevatum diutinum. A mild vasculitis may be seen in some cases, but this is usually not prominent. **(p. 107)**

A9. True

This can give the impression of a primary mesenchymal proliferation. Nuclear dust or subtle clues to vasculitis may still remain and should be carefully sought. **(p. 107)**

Panniculitis

A1. True

There are many other associations and in some cases the cause is unknown. **(p. 107)**

A2. False

This is the classic example of septal panniculitis – inflammation extends along the fibrous septa of the panniculum and not diffusely through the fatty lobules. **(p. 107)**

A3. False

These are examples of lobular panniculitis, where diffuse involvement of subcutaneous fatty lobules is characteristic. Foci of fat necrosis with 'ghosts' of fat cells are a clue to pancreatitis-associated panniculitis. **(p. 109)**

Granuloma annulare and necrobiosis lipoidica

A1. False

Multiple annular lesions on the back of the hand are typical of granuloma annulare. Granuloma annulare may also occur in generalized form (often in middle-aged women). Necrobiosis lipoidica typically presents as atrophic, yellowish plaques on the legs. **(p. 108–109)**

A2. True

Areas of altered dermal collagen are positive with mucin stains. In some cases the alterations are more diffuse and subtle in the dermis (incomplete or interstitial types of granuloma annulare). **(p. 108)**

A3. True

These lesions share some features of the nodules of rheumatoid arthritis and rheumatic fever. **(p. 108)**

A4. False

This is an important clinical association, but some patients have (and continue to have) normal glucose tolerance. **(p. 109)**

Mastocytosis

A1. True

Other forms include solitary mastocytoma, diffuse and erythrodermic cutaneous mastocytosis and telangiectasia macularis eruptiva perstans (TMEP). **(p. 109)**

A2. True

Special histochemical stains for mast cells may be necessary: these include toluidine blue, Giemsa or Leder stains (chloroacetate esterase). Mast cells may also be identified by immunostaining with CD117 (c-kit). **(p. 109)**

Lupus erythematosus and dermatomyositis

A1. True

Systemic lupus erythematosus is an immune-mediated multiorgan disease with protean symptomatology and antibodies against DNA, whereas chronic discoid lupus is milder, is confined to the skin, and occurs more frequently in women. **(p. 110)**

A2. True

The degree to which any one of these changes is present in a biopsy depends on the stage and type of lesion sampled. **(p. 110)**

A3. False

This is a useful test in diagnosing lupus, but is not always positive. Importantly, it can also be seen in sun-exposed normal skin and some blistering and non-blistering diseases. Direct immunofluorescence is usually negative in cases of polymorphous light eruption (which can be very helpful). **(p. 111)**

A4. True

Microscopically, the skin changes in dermatomyositis may closely resemble those of SLE. In dermatomyositis the lupus band test is usually negative. **(p. 111)**

A5. False

Although it is true that most patients with dermatomyositis do not have a malignancy, some studies have shown an association – elderly patients in particular who present with this condition should be investigated for an underlying tumor. **(p. 111)**

Scleroderma, drug eruptions and pyoderma gangrenosum

A1. True

In the systemic form of scleroderma the lungs and esophagus are often affected. Histology shows increased dermal collagen, which appears normal. Early lesions often show inflammation and some evidence of vascular damage. Direct IF is usually negative. **(p. 111)**

A2. True

Drug reactions may mimic urticaria, erythema multiforme, folliculitis, purpura, hyperpigmentation and many other conditions. Numerous eosinophils in the dermal infiltrate are often a clue to a drug etiology. **(p. 112)**

A3. True

This may eventually result in syringosquamous metaplasia – this change can also follow necrosis and ulceration of the overlying epidermis independent of medication use. **(p. 112)**

A4. False

The first cutaneous structure to undergo necrosis is the secretory portion of the eccrine sweat coil; the epidermis is the very last structure to necrose. **(p. 112)**

A5. False

About half of all cases have some disease association, e.g. inflammatory bowel disease or a hematologic malignancy. **(p. 112)**

Vesiculobullous diseases

A1. True

Microscopically, dermatitis herpetiformis typically shows papillary microabscesses and a multilocular subepidermal bulla. **(p. 113)**

A2. False

The blister is typically unilocular and dermal papillae are preserved (so-called festooning of dermal papillae). **(p. 113)**

A3. True

The levels of cleavage described above refer to the epidermolytic, dermolytic and junctional forms, respectively. Some forms of epidermolysis bullosa may be complicated by squamous cell carcinoma (notably the Hallopeau–Siemens recessive dystrophic form). **(p. 114)**

A4. False

Dermatitis herpetiformis shows *granular* deposits of IgA, mainly at the tips of the dermal papillae. The pattern described in the question is seen in linear IgA disease. **(p. 115)**

A5. True

These are examples of subcorneal blistering diseases, where the level of the split is in the granular or cornified layer. Subcorneal pustular dermatosis is another example. **(p. 113)**

A6. False

This is a case of pemphigus vulgaris showing intraepidermal, intercellular staining with IgG. On direct immunofluorescence, herpes gestationis shows linear C3 along the epidermal basement membrane zone. **(p. 115)**

A7. True

These are all examples of subepidermal blistering diseases. Although the nature of the inflammatory infiltrate will help differentiate these conditions, clinical correlation is essential. **(p. 114)**

A8. True

Paraneoplastic pemphigus is the name given to this association. Histologically, cases show some overlap between the changes of erythema multiforme and pemphigus vulgaris. **(p. 115)**

A9. False

In this condition, acantholysis is the mechanism of cell separation; there is less dyskeratosis than in Darier's disease. **(p. 115)**

A10. True

This condition may histologically mimic Darier's disease, pemphigus vulgaris or Hailey–Hailey disease. The combination of acantholysis and spongiosis is a clue to the diagnosis of Grover's disease. **(p. 115)**

A11. False

These changes may be seen incidentally in biopsies taken for other reasons, e.g. next to a melanocytic nevus, dermatofibroma or basal cell carcinoma. **(p. 115)**

Miscellaneous conditions

A1. True

Epidermal atrophy, hyperkeratosis and hydropic degeneration of the basal epidermal layer are the hallmarks of lichen sclerosus. In older lesions the upper dermis shows a pale-staining hypocellular band of connective tissue, increased capillaries and purpura. **(p. 116)**

A2. True

This condition typically occurs in adolescent boys, often on the neck. **(p. 116)**

A3. False

This is a heritable disease in which ocular and vascular abnormalities may occur in addition to skin lesions. Clinically, there are yellowish streaks or plaques in skin creases (e.g. axillae or neck). There is dystrophic calcification of dermal elastic fibers. **(p. 116)**

A4. False

Pretibial myxedema is most often associated with thyrotoxicosis; generalized myxedema is associated with hypothyroidism. **(p. 117)**

A5. True

The dermal mucinoses represent a very disparate group of diseases including myxoid cyst, focal mucinosis, myxedema (pretibial and generalized), papular mucinosis and many more. Adequate clinical information is essential to reach the correct diagnosis. **(p. 117)**

A6. False

Although often associated with localized alopecia (alopecia mucinosa), this reaction pattern may also be seen in cutaneous lymphoma (e.g. mycosis fungoides). The exact relation between follicular mucinosis and cutaneous T-cell lymphoma is a topic of debate. **(p. 117)**

A7. False

They form part of Carney's syndrome (cardiac myxomas, spotty pigmentation and endocrine overactivity). Trichilemmomas may be associated with Cowden's syndrome. **(p. 117)**

A8. True

There is an association with carcinomas of the gastrointestinal tract. It may also be associated with diabetes, obesity, and other forms of tissue resistance to insulin. Acanthosis nigricans manifests clinically as brown, velvety plaques in flexural areas. **(p. 117)**

A9. False

This is an example of increased cutaneous pigmentation due to conformational changes of the epidermis – in this case, hyperkeratosis and papillomatosis. Melanocyte numbers and melanin content remain unchanged. **(p. 117)**

A10. False

This is Darier's disease, a genodermatosis that presents with keratotic, reddish-brown papules over the seborrheic areas of the body. Histologically, there is suprabasal clefting associated with dyskeratotic cells in the form of *corps ronds* and *corps grains*. **(p. 117)**

A11. True

This is a common complication of HIV infection. Severe psoriasis and drug reactions may also occur in this clinical setting. **(p. 118)**

Epidermal tumors

A1. True

This is known as the Leser–Trelat sign. Seborrheic keratoses are very common tumors and, when heavily pigmented, may be confused clinically with malignant melanoma. **(p. 131)**

A2. False

Approximately three-quarters of actinic keratoses show p53 accumulation, which often correlates with the degree of atypia. **(p. 132)**

A3. True

Most cases are caused by an actinic keratosis, but others may surmount a verruca, seborrheic keratosis or squamous cell carcinoma. **(p. 132)**

A4. False

This is Bowen's disease. There is psoriasiform epidermal hyperplasia and parakeratosis, but the full-thickness atypia of the epidermis represents a form of squamous cell carcinoma in situ. These lesions are often clinically scaly and psoriasiform in character. **(p. 133)**

A5. True

This is called pagetoid Bowen's disease and is sometimes seen at the edge of the lesion. **(p. 133)**

A6. True

This is due to diminished capacity for DNA repair in these patients. Other associated conditions include arsenic exposure, epidermodysplasia verruciformis, organ transplantation and HIV infection. **(p. 133)**

A7. True

These tumors may be difficult to distinguish from atypical fibroxanthoma or melanoma. Keratin positivity is the rule in these carcinomas but they may also stain for vimentin. **(p. 134)**

A8. False

This is an extremely well differentiated tumour, often located on the sole of the foot, which invades locally but rarely gives rise to metastases. It may be positive for HPV. **(p. 135)**

A9. False

In this type of squamous cell carcinoma the pseudoglandular spaces are the result of acantholysis (hence the name 'acantholytic squamous cell carcinoma'). There are no true glandular spaces, nor is there mucin production. **(p. 135)**

A10. True

(p. 136)

A11. False

Gorlin's syndrome (basal cell nevus syndrome) is characterized by multiple basal cell carcinomas, palmar pits, keratinous cysts of the jaws and other anomalies of the skeletal, nervous and endocrine systems. **(p. 136)**

A12. False

Strong, diffuse staining for bcl-2 is typical in many basal cell carcinomas, which are usually negative for EMA. BerEP4 is also usually positive in basal cell carcinoma but negative in squamous cell carcinoma. Basal cell carcinomas also overexpress p53. **(p. 138)**

A13. True

This is one common subtype of basal cell carcinoma; others include nodular, granular and clear cell variants, as well as basosquamous (metatypical) carcinoma and fibroepithelioma (of Pinkus). **(p. 138)**

A14. False

Although exceptionally rare, it can occur in large, neglected, deeply invasive tumors. Metastases are more likely in the basosquamous subtype and those tumors showing perineural spread. **(p. 139)**

Adnexal tumors

A1. True

These tumors, which share features with the acrosyringium, may be either intraepidermal, purely intradermal or (most commonly) mixed. They are typically EMA positive and contain glycogen. **(p. 140)**

A2. False

These tumors are often multiple and are typically found on the neck and face of women. They have a distinctive microscopic appearance, with small ducts and comma-like structures in a sclerotic background. **(p. 141)**

A3. True

These tumors are also called mixed tumors of the skin and show varying proportions of epithelial and myoepithelial cells. Tumors lacking an epithelial element are known as myoepitheliomas. **(p. 141)**

A4. True

Cylindromas may give rise to large, multicentric tumors of the scalp known as 'turban tumors.' There is an association between the development of multiple tumors and a mutation in the *CLYD* gene on chromosome 16. **(p. 142)**

A5. False

This is the classic appearance of an eccrine cylindroma. Note the compact nests of tumor cells surrounded by thick basement membrane. **(p. 142)**

A6. True

These tumors are very vascular, sometimes painful, and can look worryingly cellular on biopsy. A heavy infiltration of lymphocytes may simulate the appearance of a thymoma. Sometimes features of cylindroma and spiradenoma exist in the same lesion. **(p. 142)**

A7. True

Up to one-third of cases may show juxtaposed nevus sebaceus. A glandular papillary proliferation connected to the skin surface is characteristic, as are numerous plasma cells. **(p. 143)**

A8. False

Eccrine adenocarcinomas in particular may be difficult (or even impossible) to differentiate from metastatic carcinoma, especially from the breast. Positivity for estrogen receptor in these sweat gland malignancies can further confuse the issue, and clear cell eccrine adenocarcinomas may mimic metastatic renal cell carcinoma. **(p. 144)**

A9. True

Epidermotropism is a common feature of this tumor and the resulting picture may closely simulate extramammary Paget's disease. **(p. 144)**

A10. False

This tumor is of low-grade malignancy, having a strong tendency for local recurrence but metastases are extremely rare. However, its anatomic location (often at the angle of the mouth or eye) can cause disfigurement and severe problems in achieving local control. **(p. 145)**

A11. False

These cells show glandular differentiation, differentiating towards glandular structures native to the anatomic location (e.g. apocrine or colorectal glands). **(p. 146)**

A12. True

These lesions occur on the scalp and face and are present from infancy. A variety of benign and malignant tumors may arise in them, including various adnexal tumors (including trichoblastoma), basal cell carcinoma and, rarely, squamous cell carcinoma. **(p. 147)**

A13. **False**
The so-called adenoma sebaceum of tuberous sclerosis is, in fact, a fibrovascular proliferation known as an angiofibroma. **(p. 148)**

A14. **False**
Sebaceous carcinomas of the eyelid and orbit are usually more aggressive than those occurring elsewhere in the skin. The pattern of sebaceous differentiation in these tumors is much less orderly than in sebaceous hyperplasia or adenoma, and carcinomas typically show invasive growth, atypia and mitoses. **(p. 148)**

A15. **True**
The latter can be very useful in poorly differentiated tumors where sebaceous differentiation is difficult to appreciate. **(p. 148)**

A16. **True**
This syndrome is associated with multiple internal malignancies and in many patients is an expression of DNA microsatellite instability. Sebaceous tumors often have a cystic appearance in this syndrome – an important clue. **(p. 148)**

A17. **True**
These are benign follicular lesions, most often occurring on the face of the elderly. The presence of numerous keratotic (squamous) 'eddies' is characteristic. **(p. 149)**

A18. **True**
These benign tumors often show follicular differentiation in the form of papillary mesenchymal bodies, recapitulating the papillary mesenchyme of hair follicles. A desmoplastic variant may be difficult to separate from morphea-like basal cell carcinoma. **(p. 149)**

A19. **False**
Merkel cells are usually demonstrable in trichoblastomas, trichofolliculomas and trichoepitheliomas. Their presence may be helpful in differentiating from basal cell carcinoma. **(p. 150)**

A20. **True**
The symmetric cup-shaped invagination is an important feature of keratoacanthoma, one that is difficult to assess in small biopsies or currettings. The exact relation between keratoacanthoma and squamous cell carcinoma is controversial, but many authorities agree that they do show clinical and pathological differences that justify a distinction. **(p. 151)**

A21. **False**
Although most cases conform to the description given, eruptive multiple lesions are described in some rare syndromes; the distribution in these cases is often atypical. **(p. 151)**

A22. **False**
Pilar cysts show abrupt keratinization without a granular cell layer. Epidermal (epidermoid) cysts, in contrast, do retain a granular cell layer. **(p. 151)**

A23. **True**
These steatocystomas may be single or multiple (steatocystoma multiplex). Most cysts colloquially referred to as sebaceous cysts are in fact epidermoid cysts. Other rare types of cyst include cutaneous ciliated cysts, vellus hair cysts and 'bronchogenic' cysts. **(p. 152)**

A24. **True**
Also known as proliferating trichilemmal cysts, these tumors may simulate carcinoma histologically but have pushing borders and show trichilemmal keratinization. Their behavior is generally benign. **(p. 153)**

A25. **False**
Differentiation is toward the hair matrix and there is typically an admixture of basaloid cells and ghost (shadow) cells. A foreign body reaction and calcification are common. **(p. 153)**

A26. **False**
Although very typical and a great clue to the diagnosis of pilomatrixoma, ghost cells may occasionally be seen in other hair follicle tumors (e.g. trichoepithelioma) and rarely in basal cell carcinoma (showing matricial differentiation). **(p. 153)**

Melanocytes, their benign tumors and tumor-like conditions

A1. **False**
Differences result from changes in the amount of melanin in melanocytes, not in their number. Melanocytes are positive for melanin stains, tyrosinase, NSE and vimentin. **(p. 154)**

A2. **False**
The average number is much higher (20–30), most nevi becoming manifest before the age of 20 years. These clonal proliferations of neural crest-derived cells have been variably regarded as hamartomas or benign neoplasms. **(p. 155)**

A3. **True**
The melanocytic proliferation in junctional nevi is restricted to the basal portion of the epidermis. The common adult type of nevus is intradermal; the number of nevi that show a junctional component decreases with age. **(p. 155)**

A4. **True**
Vulvar or genital nevi in particular may show atypical histology (larger, irregular cell nests, lentiginous melanocytic hyperplasia etc.) and there is a risk of overdiagnosis of melanoma. **(p. 156)**

A5. True

The proliferations are usually ill-defined and accompanied by variable sclerosis and pigmentation. It is important to remember that these dendritic cells are HMB-45 positive. **(p. 156)**

A6. False

Extracutaneous blue nevi have been found in the cervix, breast, vagina and prostate. More importantly, the cellular blue nevus often extends into the subcutis. These cellular lesions may be difficult to distinguish from melanoma, but the pushing margin and biphasic growth pattern, together with the relative lack of atypia and mitoses, are helpful clues. **(p. 156)**

A7. True

Other elements of the Carney complex include cardiac myxoma, psammomatous melanotic schwannoma and endocrine overactivity. Epithelioid blue nevi may also occur outside this complex – a topic of recent renewed interest concerning the exact nature of these lesions. **(p. 157)**

A8. False

Although this is often the case, up to 20% of Spitz nevi are purely intradermal. Recognition of the classic spindle and epithelioid morphology of cells is important for the diagnosis. **(p. 157)**

A9. True

These amorphous eosinophilic structures at the dermoepidermal junction are believed to contain basement membrane material. They are often seen in Spitz nevi with an epidermal component (but not invariably), and are occasionally seen in melanoma. **(p. 158)**

A10. True

A rare variant of Spitz nevus, the pagetoid variant, can look worryingly like melanoma in situ. Recognition of the cell type, the sharp circumscription and the orderly ascension usually facilitate the diagnosis of Spitz nevus. **(p. 158)**

A11. False

Although many differences in staining patterns are described (e.g. for S100 and HMB-45), there is still too much overlap between Spitz nevus and melanoma. Some of the most useful features favoring Spitz nevus are in fact architectural: symmetry, sharp circumscription, orderly maturation with depth, and the presence of reactive changes. **(p. 159)**

A12. True

Unfortunately, this is true. There is undoubtedly a spectrum of clinical behavior as well as of histologic appearance. Many pathologists use the term 'atypical Spitz tumor' for worrying lesions that fall short of melanoma; this is not without its problems or critics. **(p. 159)**

A13. False

These lesions tend to be larger than acquired nevi, some reaching a very large size (giant congenital nevus); these giant nevi may rarely extend even into the placenta. **(p. 159)**

A14. True

There is a real risk of melanoma developing in giant congenital nevi; the risk in smaller congenital nevi is contentious. In giant congenital nevi associated with cerebral melanosis there is also a risk of melanoma of the CNS. Many advocate early surgical removal. **(p. 160)**

A15. False

This is a classic example of a halo nevus: a pigmented center with a surrounding oval area of depigmentation. This phenomenon represents a host immune response to nevus cells and is usually seen in young people. A similar appearance may sometimes occur in melanoma. **(p. 160)**

A16. True

Many cases will show abnormal architecture and an irregular junction component which, if severe, may mimic melanoma. It is important to be aware of this 'pseudomelanoma' phenomenon; sometimes it is worthwhile reviewing the original incomplete excision. **(p. 162)**

A17. True

These 'active' nevi may show increased cellularity and a more prominent junctional component. Pregnancy, contraceptive pill use and the presence of melanoma elsewhere in the body are said to produce similar effects. **(p. 162)**

A18. True

Although the dysplastic nevus is an intensely controversial entity, in its better-defined form it may be part of a genetically determined syndrome in families prone to develop malignant melanoma. Nevi are clinically atypical, with a large size (>5 mm), irregular outline and variegated appearance. **(p. 162–163)**

A19. False

Only a minority actually fulfill the microscopic criteria for dysplastic nevi. Some lesions prove to be pigmented basal cell carcinomas, seborrheic keratoses or adnexal tumors; others are specific melanocytic entities (e.g. combined nevi, Reed nevi, deep penetrating nevi) and others represent recurrent or traumatized nevi of usual type. **(p. 162)**

A20. False

Architectural atypia is very important in the diagnosis of dysplastic nevi: cell nests are irregularly shaped and sized, rete may be fused, the junctional component extends beyond the lateral margins of the dermal component, and there is a stromal response in the papillary dermis. Cytonuclear abnormalities are then added to these. **(p. 162)**

Malignant melanoma

A1. True

This is so, even when nevi are banal and not of dysplastic type. The association with dysplastic nevi is best illustrated in those families prone to familial melanoma. **(p. 164)**

A2. False

This large, asymmetric lesion with a notched border and irregular pigmentation is a good example of superficial spreading malignant melanoma. Nodular melanoma, lentigo maligna melanoma and acral lentiginous melanoma are the other major subtypes. **(p. 165)**

A3. True

Desmoplastic melanoma may simulate a hypertrophic scar or a fibrohistiocytic lesion. It may also be mistaken for another kind of malignancy, notably squamous cell carcinoma. Patchy inflammation, a fascicular growth pattern, infiltration around nerves and an overlying in-situ component are useful pointers to desmoplastic melanoma. **(p. 166)**

A4. True

No single feature can be relied upon alone, but the combination of poor circumscription, pagetoid upward extension of cells, lack of maturation in the deep dermis, cellular atypia, mitotic activity and a band-like inflammatory infiltrate are all pointers to malignancy. **(p. 168)**

A5. False

These markers are useful in the differential with non-melanocytic tumors, but the distinction between nevi and melanomas requires the integration of many architectural and cytological features (see Question 4). **(p. 169)**

A6. False

Desmoplastic melanomas are almost always negative for HMB-45 and Melan-A. Some non-desmoplastic melanomas are also negative for HMB-45, and it is important to remember that blue nevi and their variants are characteristically HMB-45 positive. **(p. 169)**

A7. True

This will stain many benign and malignant melanocytic tumors, but (like HMB-45) is often negative in desmoplastic melanoma. MiTF is not entirely lineage specific and has also been shown to stain some dermatofibromas and smooth muscle tumors. **(p. 169)**

A8. False

This is a dangerous pitfall, as some melanomas have been shown to express low molecular weight keratin (e.g. Cam 5.2) and not all melanomas stain with HMB-45, S100 or Melan-A. Hints on light microscopy as to the diagnosis of melanoma include nuclear pseudoinclusions, fascicular growth and a mixed epithelioid and spindle cell morphology. **(p. 169)**

A9. True

In particular, mutations affecting chromosome 9p21 have been described. This contains the p16 locus, a critical site for progression of the normal cell cycle. **(p. 170)**

A10. False

In 5–15% of cases of metastatic melanoma the primary tumor is never found. These cases are thought to represent regression in the primary melanoma, to the point where it is clinically no longer visible. **(p. 171)**

A11. True

These melanosomes are proof of melanocytic differentiation, and in the setting of an obviously malignant tumor confirm the diagnosis of melanoma. Although immunohistochemistry has largely replaced EM, it can still be very useful in such cases. **(p. 171)**

A12. False

Metastatic melanoma in the skin is often present deep in the dermis with no epidermal component, but some cases show epidermotropism, simulating primary melanoma at that site. In these cases the dermal component is often much wider than the epidermal one. **(p. 172)**

A13. False

One has to be very careful in interpreting S100 staining in sentinel node biopsies, as Langerhans' cells and other antigen-presenting cells in nodes may stain positively. Intracapsular nevi – a not uncommon finding – will also stain for S100; their bland cytology and typical location will help distinguish them from melanoma deposits. **(p. 173)**

A14. True

In one study, the 10-year survival rate was almost 70% for localized disease and less than 20% for metastatic disease. **(p. 174)**

A15. False

After tumor stage, the most powerful prognostic indicators are tumor *thickness* and ulceration. Thickness is measured according to Breslow's method from the top of the granular layer to the deepest tumor cell. Tumor *size* has no independent significance once correction has been made for tumor thickness; the same is largely true of tumor type. **(p. 174)**

A16. True

Females appear to have an improved survival, and the elderly generally have a worse prognosis. Certain anatomic sites, e.g. the scalp, upper trunk and subungual area, are also associated with a worse prognosis. **(p. 175)**

A17. False

This is a topic of much recent research. Lymphocytes that intermingle with tumor cells (tumor-infiltrating lymphocytes) have prognostic value in melanomas in the vertical growth phase; a brisk response is associated with a better prognosis than a 'non-brisk' or absent response. **(p. 175)**

A18. True

These satellites – defined as tumor groups larger than 50μ in diameter – show an association with regional lymph node metastases and therefore with prognosis. **(p. 176)**

Other tumors and tumor-like conditions

A1. False

These are dense-core neurosecretory granules from a case of Merkel cell carcinoma. They are rounder, smaller, and lack the lamellar appearance of melanosomes. **(p. 178)**

A2. False

These are very aggressive tumors that often recur locally and may spread to lymph nodes, lungs, liver and bone. Wide resection of the primary site is recommended. **(p. 179)**

A3. True

This dot-like positivity with keratin (notably CK20) is very characteristic of Merkel cell carcinomas. They also show staining with NSE and neurofilament in many cases, but importantly are TTF-1 negative (unlike small cell lung carcinomas). **(p. 179)**

A4. True

This is regarded as an abnormal pattern of dermal reaction to injury, producing characteristic thick, broad hyalinized collagen bundles. It differs somewhat histologically from hyperplastic scar, and is more likely to recur than the latter. **(p. 179)**

A5. False

Fibrous papule most often occurs as a solitary lesion on the nose or face of adult women, without any other association. Although it is true that 'adenoma sebaceum' of tuberous sclerosis also belongs to the group of lesions described as angiofibroma, the clinical appearance and setting are very different, and the histology also differs slightly. **(p. 180)**

A6. True

There are exceptions to every rule, but this is useful to remember in difficult cases. It is important also to remember that smooth muscle or myofibroblastic differentiation is not unusual in dermatofibromas – and they may then express SMA or other muscle markers. **(p. 182)**

A7. True

This is an aneurysmal fibrous histiocytoma and it may be mistaken clinically for a variety of vascular and nevoid neoplasms; it also looks worrisome microscopically. Close examination of the edge of the lesion usually discloses typical areas of dermatofibroma. **(p. 182)**

A8. True

This type often mimics a vascular or melanocytic neoplasm on H&E staining. It is usually strongly positive for factor XIIIa and negative for CD31 or S100. **(p. 181)**

A9. False

The nomenclature here is very confusing: there is a type of dermatofibroma with scattered atypical cells referred to as 'atypical fibrous histiocytoma' or 'dermatofibroma with monster cells.' Atypical fibroxanthoma is a cytologically malignant lesion of uncertain histogenesis, often occurring on the head and neck of the elderly, which usually has a very good prognosis. The two conditions are not believed to be related. **(p. 183)**

A10. False

The lesions are superficial and seem to 'push' structures to one side, rather than destroy them. Many authors would exclude lesions showing deep extension, vascular invasion or necrosis from the definition of atypical fibroxanthoma, diagnosing instead a superficial cutaneous sarcoma. Opinion is still divided on the matter of nomenclature. **(p. 183)**

A11. False

Malignant melanoma, squamous cell carcinoma and leiomyosarcoma may have a very similar histologic appearance. Immunohistochemical stains that include S100, keratin, EMA and desmin are mandatory. **(p. 183)**

A12. True

This 'boxing in' of individual adipocytes is characteristic of DFSP. Dermatofibromas may involve the superficial subcutis, but tend to do so in a pushing (not an infiltrating) fashion. **(p. 184)**

A13. False

These tumors have a very high tendency to local recurrence. Rare cases of metastasis may be associated with fibrosarcomatous transformation within DFSP, but metastasis is unusual in cases treated with adequate primary excision. **(p. 185)**

A14. True

Most cases of DFSP are strongly and diffusely positive with CD34 but there are exceptions – and CD34 positivity is not restricted to this tumor. DFSP shows supernumerary rings derived from chromosome 22 or a linear translocation in C22. **(p. 185)**

A15. True

This example of xanthoma tuberosum shows multiple periarticular nodules. There may be associated hyperlipidemia, diabetes, obstructive liver disease, hypothyroidism or a paraprotein. Histology shows many foamy dermal macrophages. **(p. 186)**

A16. False

The cells in juvenile xanthogranuloma are of non-Langerhans' type and are S100 negative. They usually show positivity with some histiocytic markers and factor XIIIa. **(p. 186)**

A17. True

Although most commonly seen in the skin, lesions may occur at almost any site (including the eye, skeletal muscle, CNS, bowel and testis). **(p. 186)**

A18. False

Primary dermal leiomyosarcomas almost never metastasize and are cured by adequate local excision. Subcutaneous and deeper leiomyosarcomas do carry a risk of metastasis. **(p. 187)**

A19. False

This is a difficult area. Neurothekeoma includes a spectrum of histologic appearances, from a myxoid spindled tumor (nerve sheath myxoma) to a more cellular tumor in fascicles or compact nests of small epithelioid cells. The myxoid variant is often S100 positive, but the cellular neurothekeoma is consistently negative for S100. **(p. 188)**

A20. True

These tumors show a wide spectrum of cytonuclear appearances (spindled or epithelioid) and are S100 negative. EMA positivity is an important clue to the diagnosis. **(p. 189)**

A21. True

This is an example of glomeruloid hemangioma – in this example the resemblance to renal glomeruli is striking. This is considered a cutaneous marker for multicentric Castleman's disease or POEMS syndrome. Rare sporadic cases are also described. **(p. 190)**

A22. False

Although epithelioid hemangioma is the most common epithelioid vascular tumor in the skin (and benign), epithelioid hemangioendothelioma and angiosarcoma also occur. **(p. 192)**

A23. True

Many consider this to be a distinctive form of organization and recanalization in a thrombus. It may occur in a normal vessel, hemangioma or vascular malformation. **(p. 191)**

A24. False

The Kaposi's sarcoma-associated virus is HHV-8, a γ-herpes virus related to EBV. It is also found in cases of primary effusion lymphoma and multicentric Castleman's disease. It seems the virus is necessary (but not sufficient) to cause Kaposi's sarcoma. **(p. 194)**

A25. False

Although typical – and a very helpful clue – these PAS-positive bodies probably represent degraded erythrocytes and may occasionally be seen in other vascular tumors. Spindle cells of Kaposi's sarcoma appear to differentiate toward (lymphatic) endothelium. **(p. 193)**

A26. False

Bacillary angiomatosis is an infectious condition caused by a rickettsia-like organism, *Bartonella henselae*. The infection may involve internal organs as well as the skin. **(p. 194)**

A27. False

Angiosarcoma of the skin – excluding those types related to lymphedema or radiation therapy – occurs almost exclusively on the head and neck of the elderly. Classic Kaposi's sarcoma typically affects the feet and lower legs, progressing slowly upwards. **(p. 195)**

A28. True

The characteristic dissecting growth pattern in angiosarcoma is very helpful. However, a similar pattern of dissecting growth may be seen in some benign processes (hobnail hemangioma and benign progressive lymphangioma). Cellular atypia, nuclear crowding and intraluminal papillary groups of atypical cells favor angiosarcoma. **(p. 196)**

A29. True

An admixture of T and B cells, prominent reactive blood vessels, polyclonal plasma cells and the absence of marginal zone cells favor a reactive condition. On a small biopsy it may be impossible to exclude lymphoma absolutely (even with PCR). **(p. 196)**

A30. True

This is a good example of epidermotropism of hyperchromatic T cells with lining up along the basal epidermis and the formation of small aggregates of haloed cells. Larger groups of these cells are called Pautrier microabscesses. Note the lack of spongiosis. **(p. 198)**

A31. False

Adnexal involvement is not uncommon in MF and there are subtypes that preferentially involve the hair follicle (follicular/pilotropic MF or MF-associated follicular mucinosis). A rare syringotropic variant is also described. **(p. 197)**

A32. False

Cerebriform cells are characteristic of MF, but may also be seen in some reactive conditions. The diagnosis of MF depends on the integration of all the clinical and histologic data, sometimes supported by TCR gene rearrangements on PCR. **(p. 198)**

A33. True

They are usually CD4 positive, but cases of CD8-positive MF are not rare. **(p. 198)**

A34. True

CD2, CD3, CD5 or CD7 may be lost – especially CD7. However, loss of CD7 has recently been described in some reactive conditions. **(p. 198)**

A35. True

Sometimes called Woringer–Kolopp disease, this condition often presents as a solitary erythematosquamous patch on an extremity. Histologically, the atypical cells are confined to the epidermis, which shows variable psoriasiform hyperplasia. **(p. 199)**

A36. False

This is lymphomatoid papulosis, the clue being the presence of multiple lesions in various stages of evolution, some ulcerating and others healing with a scar. Anaplastic large cell lymphoma typically presents as solitary or grouped lesions. The histology may sometimes be identical in both lymphomatoid papulosis and anaplastic large cell lymphoma. **(p. 199)**

A37. False

CD30 is an activation marker and may also be expressed in a variety of reactive conditions. Clinicopathologic correlation is essential in these circumstances in order not to overdiagnose lymphoma. **(p. 200)**

A38. False

These tumors used to be regarded as a systemic malignancy of vascular endothelium, but are in fact true lymphomas. Most are B-cell in origin. Cutaneous and neurologic manifestations dominate the clinical picture. **(p. 201)**

A39. True

This 'aleukemic leukemia cutis' may precede full-blown leukemia by some time. Myeloid or myelomonocytic forms often localize to the skin, but in theory almost any type may be seen. Some variants may mimic lobular breast carcinoma on biopsy. **(p. 201)**

A40. True

The combination of endometrial glands and stroma is very characteristic, but secondary hemorrhage and fibrosis may confuse the picture. There is a risk of overdiagnosing malignancy (e.g. metastatic carcinoma or sweat gland carcinoma). **(p. 202)**

A41. True

These sites are anatomically close to the sites of the major tumors (i.e. lung, breast, colon and ovary). The head and neck also seem to be involved more frequently than expected; involvement of the extremities is much less common. Melanoma may metastasize anywhere. **(p. 203)**

5 Oral cavity and oropharynx

Normal anatomy

Q1

The surface mucosa of the oropharynx consists primarily of stratified squamous epithelium.

Q2

The stratified squamous epithelium of the oropharynx contains remnants of hair follicles and sweat glands.

Q3

The presence of skeletal muscle in proximity to tonsillar tissue should be prominently mentioned in the diagnostic pathology report.

Congenital abnormalities

Q1

Despite being present at birth, dermoid cysts of the oropharynx may not be diagnosed until later in life.

Q2

All cysts of the alveolar ridge should be biopsied for definitive diagnosis.

Q3

White sponge nevus, a white plaque in the oral mucosa, is a sex-linked disorder.

Q4

Sebaceous glands never occur in the oral cavity.

Q5

Epithelial nests may be identified in intraoral sensory nerve endings and can be confused with perineural invasion by epidermoid carcinoma.

Inflammatory diseases

Q1

Inflammatory papillary hyperplasia of the oropharynx refers to a reactive process, typically secondary to chronic irritation.

Q2

Geographic tongue is a rare lesion associated with fungal infection and poor oral hygiene.

Q3

Inflammatory bowel disease may manifest itself within the oral cavity.

Q4

The triad of oral facial swelling, facial nerve paralysis and plicated tongue is known as Melkerson–Rosenthal syndrome.

Q5

Waldeyer's ring lymphoid hyperplasia is commonly associated with measles infection.

Other non-neoplastic lesions

Q1

Fibrous hyperplasia of the gingiva, typically secondary to dilantin therapy, can also be a consequence of ciclosporin A use.

Q2

Necrotizing sialometaplasia is a precursor to squamous cell carcinoma.

Q3

Plunging ranula is a variant of atypical histiocytic granuloma.

Q4

Common dermatologic disorders may also involve the oral cavity.

Tumors and tumor-like conditions of the surface epithelium

Q1

Leukoplakia is a well-defined histopathologic entity.

Q2

At the histopathologic level, keratosis, squamous hyperplasia, and verrucous hyperplasia are interchangeable.

Q3

Microscopic criteria for the diagnosis of dysplasia in the oral cavity and oropharynx are the same as those for other mucosal membranes.

Q4

The terminology encompassing oral intraepithelial neoplasia (OIN) is a well-accepted classification system.

Q5

Oral squamous dysplasia can be defined immunohistochemically by using the marker Ki-67.

Q6

There is a correlation between leukoplakia and squamous dysplasia if leukoplakia occurs on the floor of the mouth.

Q7

Changes in DNA ploidy of dysplastic squamous epithelium correlate directly with the incidence of developing carcinoma.

Q8

Heck's disease is sessile elevation of the buccal mucosa with balloon cells in the malpighian layer.

Q9

Verrucoid lesions of the oral cavity behave analogous to those located in the genital tract.

Q10

Hairy leukoplakia has been associated with HPV infection.

Squamous cell carcinoma

Q1

Oropharyngeal squamous carcinomas have been related to tobacco, alcohol, mechanical irritation and immunosuppression.

Q2

In terms of decreasing frequency of oropharyngeal squamous carcinoma, the correct geographic order is lip, tongue, and floor of mouth.

Q3

Oropharyngeal squamous cell carcinomas are typically keratinizing, well-differentiated lesions that are easily recognized by microscopic evaluation.

Q4

Intraoral squamous cell carcinomas typically exhibit cytokeratin 20.

Q5

The most common oncogene alteration in oral squamous cell carcinomas occurs in the P53 gene.

Q6

Distinguishing true dysplasia from radiation changes can be accomplished by employing well-defined cytologic criteria.

Q7

The pattern of spread of oropharyngeal carcinoma is dictated by the anatomic features of the primary site.

Q8

Carcinomas of the tongue base tend to metastasize to the posterior triangle lymph nodes.

Q9

Metastases from well-differentiated oropharyngeal squamous cell carcinomas may mimic a branchial cleft cyst with malignant transformation.

Q10

Chemotherapy is highly effective for oropharyngeal squamous carcinoma.

Q11

DNA ploidy is a significant independent prognostic factor in oropharyngeal squamous cell carcinomas.

Q12

Verrucous carcinoma is a well-differentiated variant of squamous cell carcinoma and is strongly associated with tobacco use.

Q13

Owing to its characteristic appearance, verrucous carcinoma is easily diagnosed by microscopic evaluation.

Q14

Radiation therapy is the treatment of choice for verrucous carcinoma.

Q15

Some forms of squamous cell carcinoma can mimic adenocarcinoma.

Q16

Basaloid squamous cell carcinoma of the oropharynx has a benign course, similar to basal cell carcinomas of the skin.

Q17

Oropharyngeal spindle cell carcinomas are a form of carcinosarcoma.

Tumors and other lesions of minor salivary glands

Q1

A microscopic focus of disorganized seromucinous glands mixed with sebaceous glands is known as a salivary gland choristoma.

Q2

Benign mixed tumors can occur in minor salivary gland tissue.

Q3

The most common malignant tumor of minor salivary gland tissue is the malignant mixed tumor.

Q4

Low-grade polymorphous adenocarcinomas are most common in elderly males with a history of smoking.

Q5

Cribriform adenocarcinoma of the tongue is a rare tumor that may be confused histologically with metastatic thyroid carcinoma.

Tumors of odontogenic epithelium

Q1

It is thought that peripheral ameloblastomas of the gingiva arise in remnants of dental lamina.

Tumors of melanocytes

Q1

Ephelis and lentigo typically present as pigmented patches on the upper gingiva.

Q2

Multiple pigmented macules of the lip may indicate the presence of small bowel polyps.

Q3

Melanocytic nevi are rare inside the oral cavity.

Q4

Malignant melanoma of the oral cavity is particularly common in caucasians of Scandinavian ancestry.

Q5

The spindle cell variant of oral malignant melanoma shows the usual immunohistochemical markers of S100 protein and HMB-45.

Tumors and tumor like conditions of lymphoid tissue

Q1

Prominent lymphoid proliferations of the buccal mucosa or hard palate are known as pseudolymphomas.

Q2

Malignant lymphoma of the oropharyngeal region commonly occurs in the palatine or lingual tonsil of children.

Q3

Malignant lymphoma of the oropharynx has its highest incidence in the Far East.

Q4

Most cases of oral pharyngeal lymphoma are of T-cell origin.

Q5

Epstein–Barr virus has been implicated in the etiology of oropharyngeal lymphomas.

Other tumors and tumor-like conditions

Q1

Peripheral giant cell granuloma (giant cell epulis) is most common in young males.

Q2

Congenital epulis is indistinguishable from granular cell tumor by light microscopy.

Q3

Both granular cell tumors and congenital epulis express S100 protein.

Q4

Pyogenic granuloma (lobular capillary hemangioma) and intravascular capillary endothelial hyperplasia (Masson's hemangioma) are two vasoformative processes that may mimic malignant neoplasms.

Q5

Kaposi's sarcoma of the oral cavity occurs most often in elderly males of Mediterranean descent.

Q6

Adult rhabdomyoma shows a predilection for the oral cavity and neck.

Q7

Malignant sarcomas are virtually absent from the oral cavity.

Q8

The oral cavity is resistant to metastatic disease.

Normal anatomy

A1. True

The oropharynx represents the upper portion of the digestive tract. The surface epithelium of this region is stratified squamous type. Keratinization occurs in areas exposed to mastication. **(p. 247)**

A2. False

The epithelium of the oropharynx lacks hair follicles and sweat glands. **(p. 247)**

A3. False

Skeletal muscle is typically present in close contact with the lymphoid tissue of this region. Its detection is not an indication of inappropriate surgical technique. **(p. 248)**

Congenital abnormalities

A1. True

These neoplasms may only become apparent when secondarily inflamed. They are typically lined by squamous epithelium and contain skin adnexal structures. This is an exception to the rule that the oropharynx contains no hair follicles. **(p. 248)**

A2. False

Minute cysts of odontogenic origin are commonly seen in the alveolar and palatal mucosa, especially in children. They need not be biopsied. **(p. 248)**

A3. False

A white sponge nevus is an autosomal dominant disorder. Grossly, large white plaques in the oral mucosa characterize this condition. Microscopically there is intracellular edema throughout the malpighian layer. **(p. 248)**

A4. False

The presence of normal sebaceous glands inside the oral cavity is common and is referred to as Fordyce's disease. Sometimes these glands are hyperplastic and appear as discrete nodules. **(p. 248)**

A5. True

These structures are known as the organ of Chievitz. The structures may lie deep in the internal pterygoid muscle and undergo nodular hyperplasia. They are associated with small branches from the buccal nerve. **(p. 248)**

Inflammatory diseases

A1. True

This is a chronic inflammatory lesion secondary to irritation from ill-fitting dentures, sharp teeth or poor dental hygiene. Removal of the offending agent results in regression. **(p. 249)**

A3. True

Crohn's disease can involve the oral cavity as the initial manifestation. The lesions consist of edema, mucosal ulcers, or polypoid epithelial hyperplasia. **(p. 250)**

A4. True

In addition, the entity known as cheilitis granulomatosa is probably an abortive variant. The etiology of this disease is not known. The microscopic appearance is that of granulomatous inflammation involving the stroma of the lip. **(p. 250)**

A5. False

This lymphoid hyperplasia is often a complication of HIV infection. **(p. 250)**

Other non-neoplastic lesions

A1. True

Also, cases can be genetically inherited or idiopathic. Extremely thickened gingiva necessitates surgical removal. **(p. 251)**

A2. False

This condition is a reactive process involving either minor or major salivary glands. The pathogenesis is probably ischemic. Some cases have been associated with systemic vasculitides. **(p. 251)**

A3. False

Plunging ranula is a consequence of extravasated mucus, extending into the neck above the hyoid bone. It is a subtype of mucocele. **(p. 251)**

A4. True

Bullous diseases such as pemphigus vulgaris, as well as lichen planus and lupus erythematosus, may affect the squamous mucosa of the oral cavity. **(p. 251)**

Tumors and tumor-like conditions of the surface epithelium

A1. False

Leukoplakia is a clinical term and represents a white patch or plaque. Typically the patch is not more than 5 mm in diameter. Its microscopic equivalent may represent a variety of pathologic disorders, including squamous hyperplasia and squamous dysplasia. **(p. 252)**

A2. True

Minor architectural differences may occur, prompting individual pathologist to specify one process over another. When dysplasia is present it is added to the diagnosis. **(p. 252)**

A3. True

Dysplasia is typically graded as mild, moderate, or severe. Full-thickness dysplasia warrants the diagnosis of carcinoma in situ. **(p. 252)**

A4. False

The use of the OIN terminology system is not well accepted and is not widespread. No matter what terminology is used, grading dysplasia is hampered by interobserver variability. **(p. 253)**

A5. True

The proliferation marker Ki-67 is a useful adjunct to the diagnosis of squamous dysplasia. Other markers, such as keratin 19 and epidermal growth factor expression, have not gained widespread use. **(p. 253)**

A6. True

White patches on the floor of the mouth have a higher probability of showing dysplastic features than patches occurring in other parts of the oral cavity. **(p. 253)**

A7. True

The incidence of carcinoma developing in diploid squamous lesions has been reported to be low, whereas tetraploid lesions show an increased incidence of neoplastic transformation. **(p. 254)**

A8. True

This disease process presents as a well-circumscribed patch on the buccal mucosa. It is common among Native Americans. **(p. 254)**

A9. True

Koilocytic changes are seen microscopically and an etiologic role for HPV has been suggested in the development of oral squamous cell carcinoma and its variants. HPV types 2, 4, 6, 11, 13, and 32 are statistically associated with benign lesions. Subtypes 16, 18, and 33 are associated with malignant lesions. **(p. 254)**

A10. False

It is now believed that hairy leukoplakia is related to Epstein–Barr virus infection. Microscopically, there is parakeratosis, dyskeratosis, and intranuclear inclusions. Some keratinocytes show ballooning or ground-glass cytoplasmic changes. Superinfection by *Candida* species is common. **(p. 254)**

Squamous cell carcinoma

A1. True

Additional etiologic factors include syphilis, oral sepsis, iron deficiency anemia and Fanconi's anemia. The role of HPV and oral squamous carcinomas is being actively investigated. **(p. 255)**

A2. True

Completing the descending order is buccal mucosa, lower gingiva, and, lastly, upper gingiva. **(p. 255)**

A3. False

Intraoral squamous carcinomas exhibit a wide range of histologic appearances and differentiation. Undifferentiated tumors with a solid growth pattern may be confused with large cell malignant lymphoma. **(p. 255)**

A4. False

These tumors typically express cytokeratins 8 and 19. Also, keratin 5/6 and keratin 13 are commonly expressed. **(p. 256)**

A5. **False**

The most common oncogene alteration involves p16. This may reflect an etiologic role for HPV infection. *p53* is the second most commonly altered gene, followed by changes in cyclin D1 and p63. **(p. 256)**

A6. **False**

It is often impossible to distinguish carcinoma in situ from radiation atypia. If there is a clinical history of prior radiation therapy, follow-up evaluation should wait a minimum of 6–8 weeks. **(p. 256)**

A7. **True**

Whereas carcinoma of the lip invades adjacent skin and the orbicular muscle, tumors of the floor of the mouth penetrate into the sublingual gland and midline muscles. Tumors of the oral tongue tend to remain localized for long periods. **(p. 256)**

A8. **False**

Carcinomas of the tongue base tend to metastasize to the deep retropharyngeal lymph nodes. Metastasis to the posterior triangle lymph nodes is relatively rare. **(p. 256)**

A9. **True**

Metastases from squamous cell carcinomas may undergo cystic degeneration and mimic a primary branchial cyst neoplasm. This is especially true in instances of undetected occult primary tumors. **(p. 256)**

A10. **False**

The pillars of therapy for oropharyngeal squamous carcinoma are surgery and radiation therapy. Advanced cases may benefit from the addition of adjuvant chemotherapy. **(p. 257)**

A11. **False**

DNA ploidy has not been shown to be an independent discriminator. To date, the important prognostic factors are stage, grade, location, *p21* gene overexpression, and amplification of the 3q26.3 locus. **(p. 257)**

A12. **True**

There is a close association between verrucous carcinoma and the use of tobacco, especially smokeless tobacco. **(p. 257)**

A13. **False**

The microscopic appearance of verrucous carcinoma may be difficult to differentiate because of its well-differentiated character. A superficial biopsy shows only hyperkeratosis and acanthosis. Deeper biopsies may demonstrate exaggerated rete pegs with a pushing margin but unconvincing stromal invasion. **(p. 257)**

A14. **False**

Radiation therapy may alter the biologic nature of this lesion. Surgical resection is the treatment of choice. **(p. 258)**

A15. **True**

Due to cellular necrosis and acantholysis, squamous carcinomas can exhibit a pseudoglandular or alveolar appearance. **(p. 258)**

A16. **False**

This is an aggressive form of squamous cell carcinoma and is akin to cloacogenic carcinoma of the anal canal. **(p. 258)**

A17. **False**

These neoplasms are a metaplastic form of squamous cell carcinoma. In some instances transformation from recognizable squamous elements is identifiable. Immunohistochemical stains for cytokeratin may be necessary to define the epithelial nature of this lesion. **(p. 259)**

Tumors and other lesions of minor salivary glands

A1. **True**

These lesions present as gingival nodules and are asymptomatic unless they are in areas of mechanical stress. **(p. 259)**

A2. **True**

The full spectrum of histologic patterns of mixed tumors may occur in the minor salivary glands. Benign mixed tumors account for approximately 50% of all palatal lesions, compared to a rate of 75% in the parotid gland. They may be overdiagnosed as cancer owing to their cellularity, nuclear atypia and prominent myoepithelial component. **(p. 260)**

A3. **False**

Adenoid cystic carcinoma, mucoepidermoid carcinoma and polymorphous low-grade adenocarcinoma comprise the majority of intraoral malignant salivary gland tumors. Rare cases of acinic cell carcinoma have been reported. **(p. 260)**

A4. False
Adult females are most commonly affected. This tumor is also known as low-grade papillary adenocarcinoma, terminal duct carcinoma or lobular carcinoma. Polymorphous low-grade adenocarcinoma is the second most common type of salivary gland carcinoma in minor salivary gland tissue (adenoid cystic carcinoma is the most common). **(p. 261)**

A5. True
This neoplasm resembles the solid and follicular variants of papillary thyroid carcinoma. However, thyroglobulin stains are consistently negative. **(p. 261)**

Tumors of odontogenic epithelium

A1. True
It is likely that these tumors arise from so-called 'rests of Serres.' Gingival ameloblastoma may be misdiagnosed as basal cell carcinoma. In this location they are usually cured by local excision. **(p. 262)**

Tumors of melanocytes

A1. False
These benign pigmented lesions are most common on the lower lip. They are more common in females and are characterized by hyperpigmentation of the basal layer on light microscopic evaluation. Often there is accompanying elongation of the rete ridges. **(p. 262)**

A2. True
Multiple pigmented macules are one component of the Peutz–Jeghers syndrome. **(p. 262)**

A3. True
The lips are the most common sites for oral nevi. **(p. 262)**

A4. False
Oral malignant melanoma is common in people of Japanese and black African origin. The palate and gingiva are the most common locations. Both pigmented and amelanotic varieties occur. **(p. 262)**

A5. False
Spindle cell melanomas are typically negative for HMB 45. **(p. 262)**

Tumors and tumor like conditions of lymphoid tissue

A1. True
These proliferations also may be called lymphoid polyps. When associated with glandular structures they may be designated lymphoepithelial cysts. **(p. 262)**

A2. False
Most patients affected by palatine or tonsillar lymphoma are in their sixth or seventh decades. **(p. 263)**

A3. False
The disease seems to be more common in Europe than in other parts of the world. **(p. 263)**

A4. False
These lesions are of B-cell type and follicular center in nature. **(p. 263)**

A5. False
In contrast to lymphomas of the nasopharyngeal region, those of tonsil and tongue are typically negative for Epstein–Barr virus. **(p. 263)**

Other tumors and tumor-like conditions

A1. False
This lesion is more common in females. There is no defined age preference. **(p. 263)**

A2. True
However, congenital epulis occurs in the gingiva of the newborn and is seen almost exclusively in females. This lesion behaves in a benign fashion. **(p. 263)**

A3. False
Congenital epulis generally does not stain for S100 protein. However, the adult form of this lesion will express the antigen. **(p. 263)**

A4. True
Both clinically and histologically, these lesions can simulate a malignant process. **(p. 264)**

A5. False
Kaposi's sarcoma in this region is typically associated with AIDS. The palate is the most common site and may be the first clinical manifestation of the disease. It is now known that these lesions will react with antisera to herpes VIII. **(p. 265)**

A6. True
Rhabdomyomas have a predilection for the oral cavity and neck. The floor of the mouth is the most common location, followed by the tongue. Both adult and fetal forms have been described. Tumors may be multiple and recur locally. **(p. 266)**

A7. False
Synovial sarcoma can occur as a primary tumor in the pharynx, tonsil, cheek, tongue or palate. Other reported sarcomas include alveolar soft part sarcoma, extraskeletal osteosarcoma, fibrosarcoma and liposarcoma. Rhabdomyosarcoma of the embryonal type has been described in the tongue of children. **(p. 267)**

A8. False
Many primary tumors can metastasize to the oral cavity. The gingiva is the classic location. Metastatic renal cell carcinoma has been reported to mimic pyogenic granuloma in this region. **(p. 267)**

6 Mandible and maxilla

Normal anatomy

Q1

The microscopic characteristics of the mandible and maxilla are significantly different from those of other bones in the body.

Q2

The odontogenic structures contain both ectodermal and mesodermal derivatives.

Q3

Ameloblasts are ectodermal in origin.

Q4

The dental papilla, a mesodermal derivative, gives rise to odontoblasts.

Q5

The major extracellular components of tooth are enamel, cementum, and collagen.

Q6

The presence of basophilic cementicles in the periodontal ligament is a sign of Paget's disease.

Q7

Nests of odontogenic epithelium located in the alveolar mucosa are referred to as nests of Serres.

Inflammatory diseases

Q1

Dental granulomas are typically symptomatic lesions measuring greater than 2.5 cm.

Q2

Osteomyelitis of the jaw usually arises from hematogenous bacterial seeding.

Simple bone cysts

Q1

Simple bone cysts of the jaw typically occur in the maxilla.

Q2

Morphologically, simple bone cysts are not lined by epithelium.

Q3

Simple bone cysts of the mandible typically recur despite thorough curettage.

QUESTIONS

Central giant cell granuloma and other giant cell-containing lesions

Q1

Lesions of the jaw that feature osteoclast-like giant cells include cherubism, hyperparathyroidism-associated tumors, and fibro-osseous lesions.

Q2

The most common giant cell lesion of the mandible is an osteoclastoma.

Q3

Cherubism is histologically indistinguishable from central giant cell granuloma.

Benign fibro-osseous lesions

Q1

Benign fibro-osseous lesions of the mandible and maxilla are clearly defined by their histologic patterns.

Q2

Both monostotic and polyostotic forms of fibrous dysplasia are associated with somatic mutations of the *GNAS1* gene.

Q3

Ossifying fibroma, cementifying fibroma and juvenile ossifying fibroma are all morphologic variants of benign fibro-osseous lesions.

Q4

Cementomas are rapidly expanding bone lesions that often require extensive surgical intervention.

Q5

Benign osteoblastomas contain irregular osteoid, proliferative fibrovascular connective tissue and plump osteoblasts.

Epithelial cysts

Q1

Odontogenic cysts and fissural cysts arise from the tooth-forming epithelium.

Q2

Dentigerous cysts are associated with erupted teeth in young adults.

Q3

Bohn's nodule is another name for a gingival cyst.

Q4

Lateral periodontal cysts are most common in the maxilla and are lined by multilayered odontogenic epithelium.

Q5

Keratinized ghost cells are a distinguishing feature when differentiating keratinizing odontogenic cyst from ameloblastoma.

Q6

Radicular cyst is the most frequently encountered cyst of the jaw and represents sequelae of inflammation.

Q7

The term Epstein's pearls refers to small nodules located at the junction of the hard and the soft palate in newborn infants.

Q8

Odontogenic keratocysts occur most frequently in association with the incisors.

Q9

Mutations in the human homologue of the Drosophila patched gene (PTC) may be involved in the pathogenesis of some keratocysts.

Odontogenic tumors

Q1

Adenomatoid odontogenic tumors of the maxilla are benign neoplasms that most commonly occur in adolescent males.

Q2

Calcifying epithelial odontogenic tumors commonly metastasize if incompletely excised.

Q3

Ameloblastic fibromas are commonly mistaken for ameloblastomas.

Q4

Odontomas are classified as ameloblastic, complex or compound.

Q5

Sheathlin, an enamel sheath protein, can be detected in odontomas.

Q6

Adenomatoid odontogenic tumors are benign neoplasms of odontogenic epithelium that are frequent in the second decade of life and occur more commonly in females.

Q7

Calcifying epithelial odontogenic tumors may contain an amyloid-like material that can secondarily calcify.

Q8

Squamous odontogenic tumors show islands of atypical squamous cells with moderate mitotic activity.

Q9

Ameloblastic fibroma is a benign tumor presenting in the fourth and fifth decades and is composed of cellular fibrous stroma enclosing thin strips of ameloblastic epithelium.

Q10

Compound odontomas can have the appearance of a misshapen tooth.

Q11

Myxomas of the jaw are derived from dental papilla and are generally classified as of tooth germ origin, specifically the dental papilla.

Q12

Odontogenic fibromas frequently contain epithelial rests and show a marked male predilection.

Q13

Ameloblastoma is the most common of the epithelial odontogenic tumors and typically arises in the maxilla.

Q14

Ameloblastoma typically occurs in late adolescence, coincident with the eruption of wisdom teeth.

Q15

Follicular, plexiform, acanthomatous, papilliferous–keratotic, granular cell, desmoplastic, vascular and dentoid are all microscopic subtypes of ameloblastoma.

Q16

The granular cell variant of ameloblastoma stains positive for S100 protein, similar to other granular cell tumors.

Q17

Ameloblastoma is an invasive tumor with a tendency to recur locally, but is classified as a borderline malignant tumor owing to its low propensity for metastasis.

Q18

Ameloblastic carcinoma is similar in microscopic appearance to ameloblastoma save for atypical cytologic features.

Q19

Clear cell odontogenic carcinoma is a rare malignant neoplasm that may be misdiagnosed as a metastatic salivary gland tumor.

Other tumors and tumor-like conditions

Q1

Paget's disease of the mandible and maxilla may be the dominant expression of a generalized systemic process.

Q2

Langerhans' cell histiocytosis is common in the upper airways but rarely involves the mandible.

Q3

Salivary gland tumors often involve the floor of the mouth but do not occur in the bones of the jaw.

Q4

Ectopic nests of arachnoidal cells may manifest themselves as interosseous meningiomas of the jaw.

Q5

The most common primary malignant bone tumor of the jaw is osteosarcoma.

Q6

Chondrosarcomas of the jaw show a predilection for the mandible.

Q7

The mandible and maxilla are privileged sites that are rarely affected by metastatic disease.

Diseases of the temporomandibular joint

Q1

Hypoplasia and hyperplasia of the mandibular condyle result in facial asymmetry and may be associated with other systemic abnormalities.

Q2

The microscopic finding of chondromyxoid tissue with atypical chondrocytes in the temporomandibular joint is pathognomonic for chondrosarcoma.

Normal anatomy

A1. False
There is no significant difference between these bones and other bones. However, they are in close proximity to the oral mucosa and enclose the odontogenic anlage. **(p. 279)**

A2. True
In addition, the mesodermal component has the added feature of originating from the neural crest. **(p. 279)**

A3. True
Ameloblasts develop along the inner aspect of the invaginated primitive dental lamina. **(p. 279)**

A4. True
These cells are responsible for the formation of the dentinal matrix. **(p. 279)**

A5. False
The extracellular tooth components are enamel, cementum and dentin. **(p. 280)**

A6. False
Basophilic cementicles are a normal feature in this region. **(p. 280)**

A7. True
The nests of Serres, resulting from the breakup of dental lamina, are normally found in the jaw. Epithelial nests embedded in the periodontium are known as rests of Malassez. **(p. 280)**

Inflammatory diseases

A1. False
Dental granulomas are typically asymptomatic and are detected by routine office X-ray. They rarely measure more than 1.5 cm in diameter. **(p. 280)**

A2. False
This inflammatory lesion typically represents an extension of dental or periodontal infection. *Staphylococcus aureus* is the organism most often cultured. **(p. 280)**

Simple bone cysts

A1. False
Simple cysts typically involve the mandible. They usually occur in young patients and are sharply demarcated and unilocular on X-ray. Simple cysts may involve the maxilla in older patients. **(p. 281)**

A2. True
Simple cysts contain surprisingly little at surgery. Morphologic examination may demonstrate a delicate fibrovascular lining if sections are taken from the periphery of the lesion. **(p. 281)**

A3. False
Recurrent is uncommon after adequate therapy. It has been reported that cysts with thickened walls and containing dysplastic bone may be more likely to recur. **(p. 281)**

Central giant cell granuloma and other giant cell-containing lesions

A1. True
In addition, giant cells can occur in central giant cell granuloma, osteoclastoma and aneurysmal bone cyst. **(p. 281)**

A2. False
Central giant cell granuloma is the most common lesion in this group. It is also known as reparative giant cell granuloma owing to the frequent history of antecedent trauma. **(p. 281)**

A3. True
Their microscopic appearance is identical. However, bilateral involvement in young individuals should alert one to this diagnosis. The mode of inheritance is autosomal dominant. The gene responsible has been mapped to chromosome 4p16.3 and identified as c-Abl-binding protein SH3BP2. **(p. 281)**

Benign fibro-osseous lesions

A1. False

This family of lesions shares many similar histologic features. The accurate diagnosis of fibro-osseous lesions depends upon the integration of microscopic appearance, medical and family history, radiographic appearance and intraoperative surgical findings. Furthermore, it is not uncommon to revise a primary diagnosis based on response to therapy and subsequent clinical course. **(p. 282)**

A2. True

The polyostotic form may be accompanied by pigmented skin lesions, endocrine dysfunction and other abnormalities (Albright's syndrome). Fibrous dysplasia confined to the jawbones is sometimes referred to as the craniofacial form of the disease. **(p. 282)**

A3. True

These conditions are linked due to their histologic resemblance. However, it is recognized that some may be odontogenic in origin. **(p. 282)**

A4. False

Cementomas are usually small lesions associated with the apices of teeth and are detected by radiologic examination. Typically they are asymptomatic and do not require treatment. **(p. 283)**

A5. True

In addition, these lesions may be heavily calcified. Osteoblastomas exhibiting a prominent epithelioid configuration of the osteoblasts are labeled aggressive osteoblastomas. Some authors regard these lesions as non-metastasizing osteosarcomas. **(p. 283)**

Epithelial cysts

A1. False

Whereas odontogenic cysts form from odontogenic epithelium, fissural cysts arise from epithelial inclusions that lack a tooth-forming lineage. **(p. 284)**

A2. False

These cysts typically surround unerupted teeth. They arise from altered enamel epithelium after enamel development, and are initially associated with the tooth crown. **(p. 285)**

A3. True

These lesions are seen in neonates and resolve spontaneously over a period of weeks. Microscopically they are lined by stratified squamous epithelium. **(p. 285)**

A4. False

Lateral periodontal cysts are more common in the mandible and are typically lined by thin epithelium, one or two cell layers thick. **(p. 285)**

A5. True

Keratinizing odontogenic cysts can be microscopically similar to an ameloblastoma. Ghost cells are a distinguishing feature of the keratinizing odontogenic cyst. **(p. 285)**

A6. True

These cysts are common in the third and fourth decades and are often seen in a periapical location. The cysts often contain a mixed inflammatory infiltrate, together with cholesterol crystals, foamy macrophages and multinucleated giant cells. **(p. 285)**

A7. True

The structures represent benign palatal cysts. Histologically, they are similar to gingival cysts. **(p. 286)**

A8. False

Keratocysts occur most frequently in the region of third molar of the mandible. The cysts are frequently multiloculated and have a high rate of recurrence. **(p. 286)**

A9. True

Keratocysts associated with the nevoid basal cell carcinoma syndrome are thought to be secondary to mutations in this molecular pathway. The syndrome is transmitted in an autosomal dominant manner with a high penetrance rate and variable expression. **(p. 286)**

Odontogenic tumors

A1. False
These tumors occur most frequently in females during the second decade of life. The anterior maxilla is the preferred site; this lesion is frequently associated with an unerupted canine tooth. **(p. 287)**

A2. False
These lesions tend to be less aggressive than ameloblastomas and rarely metastasize. Also known as Pindborg's tumor, most cases arise in the premolar region of the mandible. There is no sex predilection. The tumors can be invasive and recur locally. **(p. 288)**

A3. True
However, these tumors usually arise in younger patients and are rarely seen in those over 21 years of age. **(p. 289)**

A4. True
These lesions are odontogenic tumors characterized by the production of calcified parts of teeth. They usually occur in the alveolar ridge of the mandible or maxilla. **(p. 287)**

A5. True
This protein is expressed by odontomas and by other odontogenic tumors with dental hard tissue formation. **(p. 290)**

A6. True
These tumors are commonly found in the anterior maxilla and may be associated with an unerupted canine tooth. They appear cystic on X-ray and grow with an expanding but non-invasive border. **(p. 287)**

A7. True
This material appears eosinophilic and homogeneous by light microscopy. It has been shown to be amyloid or an amyloid-related substance. **(p. 288)**

A8. False
Typically this tumor is composed of nests of well-differentiated epithelium with no atypia and is devoid of mitotic activity. **(p. 289)**

A9. False
This benign neoplasm is rarely seen in individuals over 21 years of age. It is usually solid in appearance, but a cystic variety has been reported. The presence of a mesenchymal component distinguishes it from ameloblastoma. Simple curettage is adequate therapy. **(p. 289)**

A10. True
These lesions exhibit a high degree of differentiation and behave in a benign fashion. The degree of differentiation distinguishes this tumor from complex odontoma. Compound odontomas are frequently encountered in the anterior region of the jaws and maxilla. **(p. 289)**

A11. True
They are often associated with malformed and missing teeth. Most occur during the second and third decades of life. Approximately 60% occur in the second or third decades. These lesions are cystic on X-ray and may attain a large size, with resultant facial deformity. **(p. 290)**

A12. False
These tumors are more common in females. They are more cellular than myxomas and contain greater numbers of odontogenic epithelial rests. Tumors with a myxoid component are designated myxofibromas. **(p. 291)**

A13. False
Ameloblastoma is the most common of the epithelial odontogenic tumors, but over 80% of these neoplasms occur in the mandible and the majority of these occur in the molar–ramus area. **(p. 291)**

A14. False
These neoplasms appear in the third to fifth decades and show no sex or racial discrimination. **(p. 291)**

A15. True
Two more subtypes may occur in the same tumor. There is no evidence to suggest one subtype is clinically more aggressive than another. **(p. 291)**

A16. False
These neoplasms are keratin positive but do not express S-100. There is positive staining for CD68, indicating increased lysosomal structures within the granular cytoplasm. **(p. 292)**

A17. True
Only rare instances of metastatic disease have been reported. Of these cases, several rounds of local recurrence have preceded metastases. **(p. 293)**

A18. True
The malignant variant shows marked nuclear atypia and numerous mitotic figures. Some malignant variants show a marked degree of squamous change. **(p. 293)**

A19. True
Particular attention must be paid to the nesting arrangement of the clear cells surrounded by collagenous stroma. The cells are devoid of mucin but do contain glycogen. **(p. 294)**

Other tumors and tumor-like conditions

A1. True

Jaw involvement can also be a manifestation of localized disease in the monostotic form. **(p. 294)**

A2. False

So-called eosinophilic granulomas have a predilection for the jaw, especially the mandibular bone. **(p. 294)**

A3. False

Salivary gland tumors may present as primary intraosseous masses. In fact, mucoepidermoid carcinoma is a frequent tumor of the mandible. **(p. 295)**

A4. True

Alternatively, jaw meningiomas may arise from related perineural cells. **(p. 295)**

A5. True

The mandible is marginally more affected than the maxilla. Most cases arise de novo. However, some may represent complications of radiation therapy. The majority are of the intramedullary type. Rare parosteal forms have been reported. **(p. 295)**

A6. False

These neoplasms usually arise in the maxilla. Histologically, they may show conventional, mesenchymal or dedifferentiated features. **(p. 296)**

A7. False

Tumors from the breast, lung, bowel, prostate and kidney are all primary sites that metastasize to the bones of the jaw. In children, adrenal neuroblastoma, embryonal rhabdomyosarcoma and Wilms' tumor metastasize to the mandible and maxilla. **(p. 296)**

Diseases of the temporomandibular joint

A1. True

Changes may be either a unilateral or bilateral and may be associated with other cranial anomalies. These processes may be congenital or may be the result of acquired conditions such as fracture. **(p. 296)**

A2. False

These histologic features can be a result of pseudogout. The identification of birefringent crystals associated with a granulomatous reaction is the key to the diagnosis. **(p. 297)**

Respiratory tract 7

Nasal cavity, sinus and nasopharynx

Q1

Nasal inflammatory polyps are usually unilateral and frequently cause epistaxis.

Q2

Nasal inflammatory polyps are reactive, whereas choanal polyps are neoplastic.

Q3

Squamous metaplasia is a common finding in nasal inflammatory polyps.

Q4

The presence of eosinophils in the stroma of inflammatory nasal polyps is indicative of their allergic nature.

Q5

Hyperchromatic pleomorphic cells in the stroma of nasal inflammatory polyps are indicative of malignancy.

Q6

Nasal polyps are seen more frequently in persons who have cystic fibrosis (CF) than in the population at large.

Q7

Surgical removal of inflammatory nasal polyps is usually curative, with a low recurrence rate.

Q8

Chronic sinusitis is most commonly seen in the ethmoid sinus.

Q9

This nasal biopsy shows the typical features of myospherulosis.

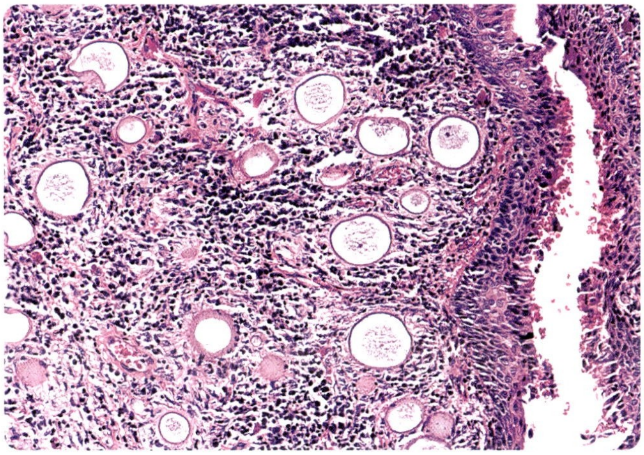

Fig. 7.1

Q10

Mycotic infection in patients with diabetic ketoacidosis in the upper respiratory tract is usually caused by *Aspergillus* species.

Q11

Rhinoscleroma is caused by *Klebsiella* sp., which may be visualized by the PAS stain.

Q12

The lesions of Wegener's granulomatosis are typically characterized by dense lymphoid infiltrates and vasculitis.

Q13

Eosinophilic angiocentric fibrosis is a fibroinflammatory disorder histologically similar to Wegener's disease.

Q14

Myospherulosis is a fungal disease of the paranasal sinuses with formation of granulomas.

Q15

Sinonasal papillomas as a group are more common in men than in women.

Q16

Everted (schneiderian) papillomas recur more frequently than do inverted papillomas.

Q17

This figure illustrates the typical features of an inverted squamous papilloma.

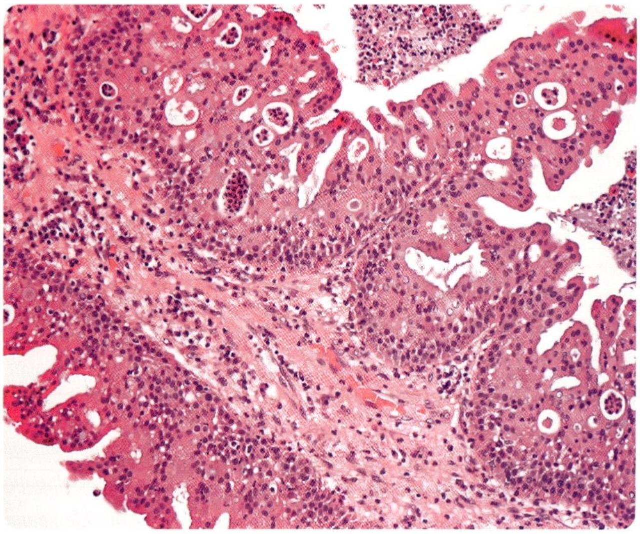

Fig. 7.2

Q18

Mucin-containing microcysts are a characteristic feature of all types of sinonasal (schneiderian) papillomas.

Q19

Although inverted papillomas may exhibit local destructive growth, true malignancy is never seen.

Q20

Human papillomavirus can be demonstrated in all types of sinonasal papilloma.

Q21

Sinonasal carcinomas usually arise from inverted papillomas.

Q22

Sinonasal carcinomas are most often of the transitional cell type.

Q23

Sinonasal adenocarcinomas of the tubulopapillary type most often originate from the subsurface mucous glands.

Q24

Nasopharyngeal carcinoma is a leading cause of death in southeast Asia.

Q25

This figure illustrates the typical microscopic features of an undifferentiated nasopharyngeal carcinoma, which may be confused with malignant lymphoma.

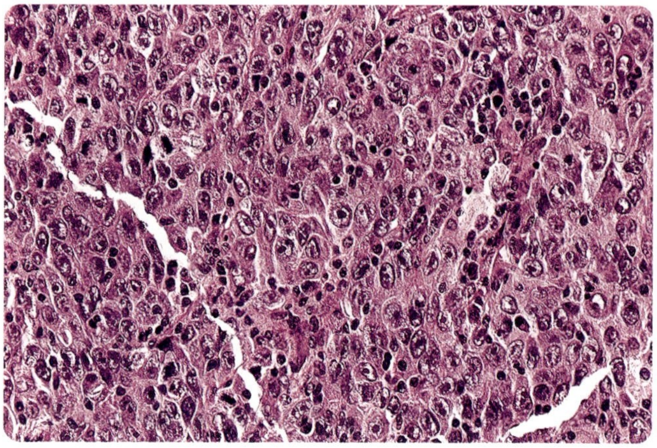

Fig. 7.3

Q26

Nasopharyngeal carcinomas may either be keratinizing or non-keratinizing.

Q27

Nasopharyngeal carcinomas usually present as a bulky mass and the diagnosis is clinically straightforward.

Q28

Surgery is the treatment of choice for nasopharyngeal carcinoma.

Q29

Salivary gland-type tumors of the paranasal sinuses are usually malignant.

Q30

Polymorphous low-grade carcinoma is the most frequent salivary gland tumor in the paranasal sinuses.

Q31

Nasal gliomas are tissue heterotopias related to developmental disorders rather than neoplasms.

Q32

Nasal gliomas usually present in the midline as a subcutaneous mass or as polyps in the nasal vestibule or paranasal sinuses.

Q33

Like conventional neuroblastoma, olfactory neuroblastoma (esthesioneuroblastoma) is a pediatric tumor.

Q34

Histologically, esthesioneuroblastoma often presents as a small blue round cell tumor.

Q35

Similar to peripheral neuroectodermal tumors (PNETs), esthesioneuroblastoma typically harbours a EWS/FLI gene translocation t(11; 22).

Q36

Early lymphatic metastasis is the rule in esthesioneuroblastoma.

Q37

Angiocentric lymphomas in the sinonasal region are immunophenotypically B-cell lymphomas.

Q38

Natural killer/T-cell lymphoma of the sinonasal region is an Epstein–Barr virus-associated lymphoma and may present with a hemophagocytic syndrome.

Q39

The most common type of non-Hodgkin lymphoma of the sinonasal region in the western world is diffuse large B-cell lymphoma.

Q40

Nasopharyngeal angiofibroma typically occurs in female adolescents and young adults.

Q41

Nasopharyngeal angiofibromas usually regress spontaneously after puberty.

Q42

This tumor removed from a 20-year-old woman represents a nasopharyngeal angiofibroma.

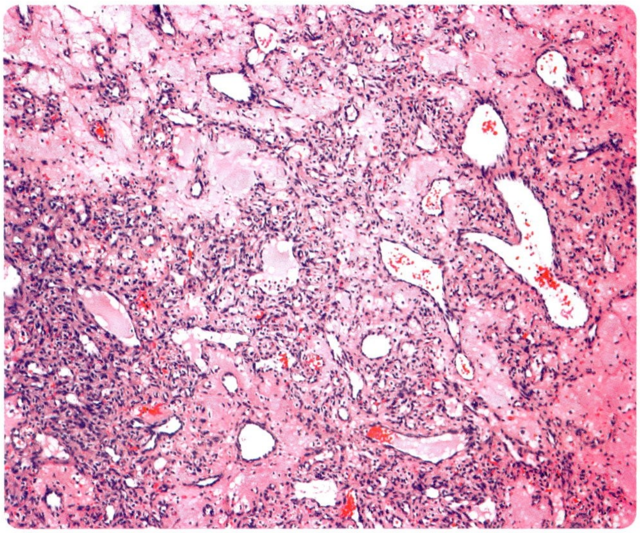

Fig. 7.4

Q43

Embryonal rhabdomyosarcoma, lymphoepithelioma (nasopharyngeal carcinoma) and non-Hodgkin lymphoma are the three most common pediatric malignancies of the sinonasal region.

Larynx and trachea

Q1

Saccular laryngeal cysts are distinguishing from laryngoceles by their contents.

Q2

Chronic laryngitis may be a consequence of chronic irritation by tobacco.

Q3

The advanced stage of a singer's nodule is called amyloid tumor of the vocal cords because of the extensive deposition of amyloid in the stroma.

Q4

Juvenile laryngeal papillomatosis is specifically related to human papillomavirus infection.

Q5

Excision of juvenile laryngeal papillomatosis is often followed by recurrence of lesions.

Q6

Voice misuse may cause singer's nodule or keratosis of the vocal cords.

Q7

Carcinoma in situ of the larynx may present as a papillary lesion.

Q8

This figure illustrates the typical features of severe dysplasia of the larynx.

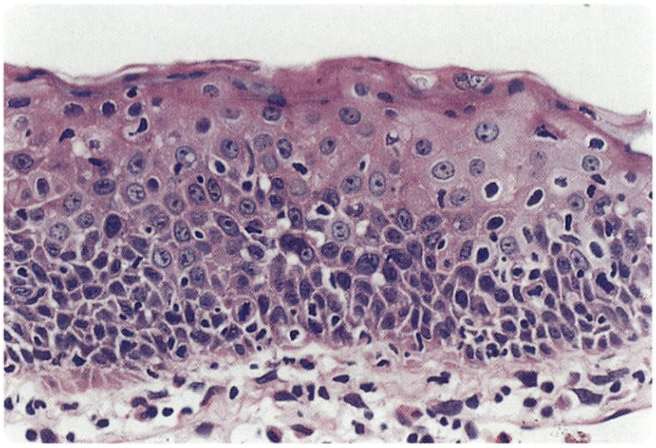

Fig. 7.5

Q9

Carcinoma of the larynx is more common in males than in females.

Q10

Smoking, alcohol use and human papillomavirus infection all predispose to laryngeal carcinoma.

Q11

Glottic carcinomas account for approximately two-thirds of all laryngeal carcinomas.

Q12

About 20–35% of laryngeal cancer patients thought to have no lymph node metastases during surgery are found to have metastases upon microscopic examination of lymph nodes.

Q13

Radiation treatment is contraindicated in verrucous carcinoma of the larynx.

Q14

Basaloid squamous carcinoma of the larynx is a low-grade malignancy.

Q15

Stage by stage, sarcomatoid carcinoma of the larynx has a much worse prognosis than the conventional squamous cell carcinoma.

Q16

Lymph node metastases are least common in glottic carcinomas, compared to supraglottic, transglottic and infraglottic carcinomas.

Q17

Mucoepidermoid carcinoma is the most common type of salivary gland tumor to arise in the larynx.

Q18

Similar to squamous cell carcinoma of the larynx, atypical carcinoid tumors and large cell neuroendocrine carcinoma of the larynx are strongly associated with smoking.

Q19

Paragangliomas of the larynx are most often supraglottic.

Q20

Cartilaginous tumors are the most common mesenchymal malignant tumors of the larynx.

Trachea

Q1

Papillomatosis may involve the trachea in the same way as it involves the larynx.

Q2

Squamous cell carcinoma is the most common tumor of the trachea and carries a poor prognosis.

Q3

Adenoid cystic carcinoma is the most common glandular tumor of the trachea.

Q4

Benign mixed tumor (pleomorphic adenoma) can occur in the trachea.

Pleura

Q1

Pleural disease in asbestos exposure is predominantly caused by fibers from the amphibole group.

Q2

Pleural plaques are found on the visceral aspect of the pleura and are rare on the diaphragm.

Q3

The interval between asbestos exposure and the development of mesothelioma is measured in decades.

Q4

Benign papillary mesothelioma is rare in the pleura.

Q5

Cough and shortness of breath are common presenting symptoms in malignant mesothelioma.

Q6

The main differential diagnosis of malignant mesothelioma is adenocarcinoma.

Q7

Positive immunostaining of a pleural-based tumor with antibodies to calretinin and WT1 strongly supports a diagnosis of malignant mesothelioma.

Q8

Cytokeratin expression is commonly lost in sarcomatoid and desmoplastic mesothelioma.

Q9

Solitary fibrous tumor of the pleura stains immunohistochemically with antibodies to cytokeratin but is negative for CD34.

Q10

Surgical excision is usually curative for solitary fibrous tumor.

Q11

Grossly, pleural angiosarcoma closely simulates malignant mesothelioma.

Q12

Pleural effusion in metastatic ovarian cancer is usually bilateral.

Q13

Pleural biopsy is more sensitive than cytological analysis of pleural effusion fluid in the analysis of suspected metastatic pleural malignancy.

Q14

In suspected tuberculous pleural effusion the finding of numerous mesothelial cells is supportive of a tuberculous cause.

Lungs

Q1

Congenital lobar emphysema and adult emphysema are both characterized by destruction of alveolar septa.

Q2

Extralobar bronchopulmonary sequestration is commonly left-sided.

Q3

Intra- and extralobar pulmonary sequestrations receive their blood supply from bronchial arteries.

Q4

Bronchiectasis is seen almost exclusively in the elderly.

Q5

Obstructive bronchiectasis usually regresses, whereas the non-obstructive bronchiectasis never regresses.

Q6

Most lung abscesses today develop after the aspiration of foreign material or result from secondary infection of lung carcinomas.

Q7

Surgical therapy has no place in the treatment of tuberculosis.

Q8

The Ghon focus in tuberculosis is synonymous with tuberculoma.

QUESTIONS

Q9

Transbronchial biopsy is a useful diagnostic technique in suspected sarcoidosis.

Q10

Limited Wegener's disease is characterized by lower respiratory tract and renal involvement but sparing of the upper respiratory tract.

Q11

The involvement of blood vessels outside areas of necrosis is a prerequisite for a certain diagnosis of Wegener's disease.

Q12

Multiple discrete nodular opacities are characteristic of bronchocentric granulomatosis.

Q13

The typical triad of allergic granulomatosis consists of eosinophilia, asthma and vasculitis.

Q14

Hemoptysis caused by an aspergilloma is caused by fungal invasion of the pulmonary blood vessels.

Q15

This slide impregnated with silver according to Grocott shows signs of pulmonary aspergillosis.

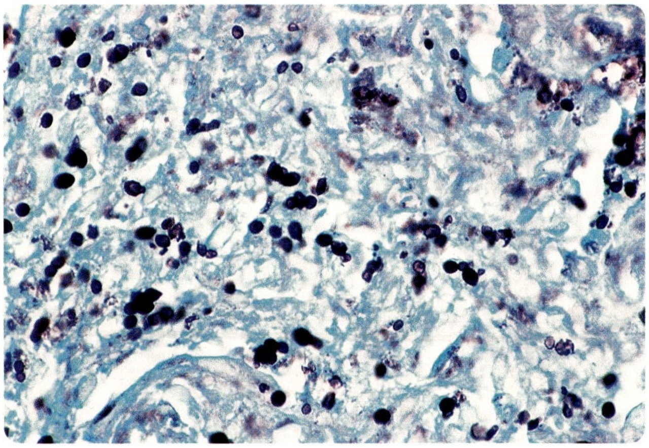

Fig. 7.6

Q16

The morphological changes in diffuse alveolar damage are non-specific in relation to the etiology.

Q17

The earliest morphological change seen in diffuse alveolar damage is the formation of hyaline membranes.

Q18

Hyperplasia, mitotic activity and atypia of type 2 pneumocytes do not signify malignant change in diffuse alveolar damage.

Q19

Histologically diffuse alveolar damage can be distinguished from acute interstitial pneumonia (Hamman–Rich syndrome) by the extensive fibroblast proliferation in the latter.

Q20

Bronchiolitis obliterans–organizing pneumonia (BOOP) – is characterized by irreversible diffuse fibrosis which is predominantly intraluminal in bronchioles and intra-alveolar.

Q21

Usual interstitial pneumonia (UIP) is typically morphologically heterogeneous, with both active inflammation and established fibrosis with distortion of lung architecture.

Q22

Honeycombing of lungs may be seen in any form of end-stage pulmonary fibrosis.

Q23

Desquamative interstitial pneumonia (DIP) results from sloughing-off of hyperplastic type 2 pneumocytes into the alveolar airspace.

Q24

Patients with Sjögren's syndrome are prone to developing follicular bronchiolitis.

Q25

Giant cell interstitial pneumonia is a granulomatous lung disease caused by exposure to beryllium.

Q26

Bronchial carcinoma may be complicated by lipoid pneumonia.

Q27

The diagnosis of eosinophilic pneumonia requires the presence of eosinophils in the lung and peripheral eosinophilia.

Q28

Pneumocystis carinii infection in the lung usually presents as a granulomatous disease.

Q29

The pneumonia of Legionnaires' disease is histologically generally similar to common bacterial pneumonias.

Q30

Although carbon deposition in the lung (anthracosis) is generally of little clinical significance it may result in progressive massive fibrosis.

Q31

Silicosis is characterized by a diffuse reticular fibrosis of the lungs.

Q32

Silo-filler's lung is set apart from other forms of hypersensitivity pneumonia because it has an immunological basis rather than a direct chemical toxic etiology.

Q33

The late stages of pulmonary Langerhans' cell histocytosis may lack diagnostic histological features.

Q34

In the differential diagnosis of pulmonary Langerhans' cell histiocytosis one should include reactive eosinophilic pleuritis.

Q35

Concentric laminar fibrosis in pulmonary arterial hypertension signifies irreversible changes of the pulmonary vascular bed and is a contraindication for surgery.

Q36

In addition to a diagnostic technique, lung lavage in alveolar proteinosis may also be used as a therapeutic procedure.

Q37

Goodpasture's syndrome is caused by antibodies reacting with mesangial proteins and pulmonary basement membrane constituents.

Q38

Pulmonary amyloidosis invariably presents as solitary or multiple nodular lesions.

Q39

Apical fibrotic caps in the superior parts of the lungs are usually sequelae of healed tuberculosis lesions.

Q40

Rounded atelectasis is frequently seen in persons exposed to asbestos.

Lung tumors

Q1

Anthracosilicosis is considered a risk factor for bronchial carcinoma.

Q2

In most lung tumors described as 'scar carcinomas' the scar is more likely a consequence of cancer than its cause.

Q3

Lung cancer is more common in males than in females.

Q4

Multicentric synchronous or metachronous lung cancers are most commonly related metastatic entities.

Q5

Pulmonary coin lesions prove to be carcinomas in a significant number of cases.

Q6

Hypercalcemia as a systemic effect of pulmonary carcinoma is particularly seen in squamous cell carcinoma.

Q7

TTF-1 (thyroid transcription factor-1) is a transcription factor that is detectable by immunohistochemistry in lung adenocarcinoma.

Q8

The basaloid variant of bronchial squamous cell carcinoma carries a favourable prognosis.

Q9

Central cavitation with necrosis is a characteristic feature of pulmonary squamous cell carcinoma and is uncommon in adenocarcinoma.

Q10

Mutations of *p53* are common in squamous cell carcinoma of the lung.

QUESTIONS

Q11

So-called scar cancers are most commonly adenocarcinomas, less frequently squamous cell carcinomas, and virtually never small cell carcinomas.

Q12

Pulmonary adenocarcinoma may closely simulate mesothelioma morphologically and can be distinguished by cytokeratin-7 staining.

Q13

Some adenocarcinomas of the lung are composed of cells that have the ultrastructural features of Clara cells.

Q14

Solid growth of tumor cells with mucin production, as evidenced by histochemical stains, without a ductal, tubular or papillary architecture is sufficient to classify a carcinoma as adenocarcinoma.

Q15

Mucinous bronchoalveolar carcinoma shows a gradual transition of tall mucinous tumour cells to cuboid cells and normal alveolar epithelium at the periphery of the tumor.

Q16

This specimen shows typical pulmonary small cell carcinoma.

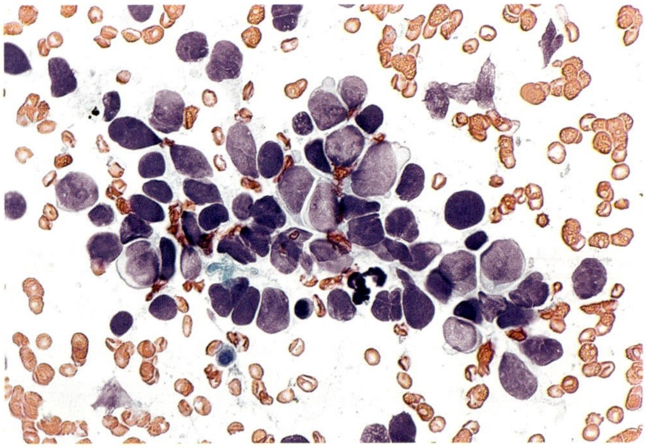

Fig. 7.7

Q17

Interstitial fibrosis in the sclerosing variant of non-mucinous bronchioloalveolar carcinoma does not indicate invasion.

Q18

Mucinous bronchioloalveolar carcinoma is frequently cytokeratin-20 and TTF-1 positive.

Q19

Pulmonary blastoma is a typical childhood tumor.

Q20

Small cell carcinoma is the most common type of lung cancer.

Q21

The so-called small cell appearance of small cell carcinoma is at least in part a biopsy artefact.

Q22

The diagnostic features of small cell carcinoma include small or non-detectable nucleoli and coarse nuclear chromatin.

Q23

Abnormalities of *p16* are common in small cell lung cancer.

Q24

The sensitivity of repeated sputum cytology in patients with carcinoma is approximately 80%.

Q25

Lung cancers tend to metastasize more often to the adrenals than to hilar or mediastinal lymph nodes.

Q26

Lung cancers as a group have a very poor 5-year prognosis.

Q27

Younger age (<40 years) is an adverse prognostic sign in lung cancer.

Q28

Adenocarcinoma is the most curable form of lung cancer.

Q29

Chondroid hamartomas most often present as polypoid lesions causing bronchial obstruction.

Q30

Regional lymph node metastases are seen in about 5% of typical carcinoid tumors.

Q31

Pulmonary carcinoid tumors do not express thyroid transcription factor-1 (TTF-1).

Q32

Dense-core secretory granules seen on electron microscopy are a distinctive feature of pulmonary carcinoids and may be a useful discriminating finding to separate these tumors from small cell carcinoma.

Q33

The cytomorphology of this carcinoid tumor suggests that it is of the peripheral rather than the central type.

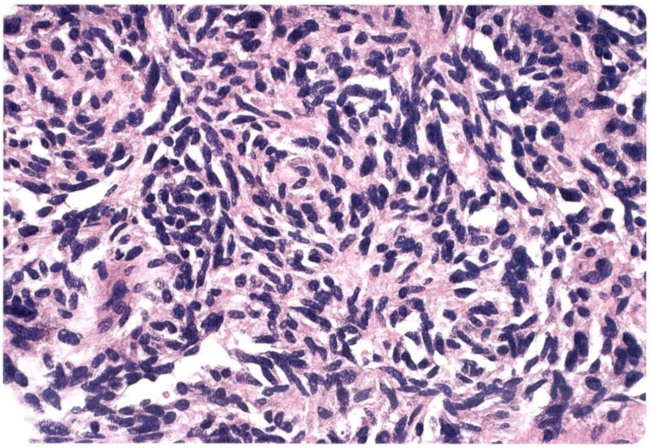

Fig. 7.8

Q34

Atypical carcinoid tumors are distinguished from typical carcinoid tumors by a higher mitotic rate and/or necrosis but maintenance of neuroendocrine architecture and staining characteristics.

Q35

The neuroendocrine architecture of large cell neuroendocrine carcinomas is not as clearly developed as in typical carcinoids. Nevertheless, their neuroendocrine properties can be recognized by ultrastructural and immunohistochemical studies.

Q36

Sclerosing hemangioma is a (involuting) benign vascular neoplasm restricted to the lung and considered to be the benign counterpart of epithelioid hemangioendothelioma (intra-vascular bronchioloalveolar tumor).

Q37

Rearrangements of the *ALK-1* gene are commonly seen in the inflammatory myofibroblastic tumor variant of inflammatory pseudotumors.

Q38

Pulmonary lymphangiomyomatosis, a proliferation that occurs almost exclusively in women, is composed of HMB-45-positive cells and shares other features that characterize tumors known as *pecomas* (perivascular endothelioid smooth muscle cell tumors).

Q39

Epithelioid hemangioendothelioma usually presents as multifocal pulmonary nodules with varying degrees of sclerosis and may be labeled immunohistochemically with anti-CD31 antibodies.

Q40

Lymphomatoid granulomatosis is an EBV-related T-cell lymphoma of the lung.

Q41

The most common type of salivary gland type tumor of the lung is mucoepidermoid carcinoma.

Q42

Renal cell carcinoma metastatic to the lungs can be distinguished from the sugar tumor of the lung by immunohistochemical detection of HMB-45 in the latter.

Q43

Leiomyoma of the lung may be easily confused with peripheral carcinoid tumor.

Q44

Pleuropulmonary blastoma and pulmonary blastoma are related entities distinguished by the presence of pleural involvement.

Q45

Immunohistochemistry is very useful for distinguishing primary from metastatic adenocarcinomas in the lung.

Q46

Pulmonary 'metastasectomy' in childhood sarcoma is primarily a symptomatic therapy with little impact on survival of the patient.

Nasal cavity, sinus and nasopharynx

A1. False
Nasal inflammatory polyps are usually bilateral and do not cause epistaxis. **(p. 305)**

A2. False
Choanal polyps that arise from the paranasal sinuses are morphologically similar to nasal polyps **(p. 305)**

A3. True
This adaptive change is quite common in polyps. **(p. 306)**

A4. False
Eosinophils may be present in all polyps but are usually more numerous in those that have a presumed allergic pathogenesis. **(p. 306)**

A5. False
Solitary pleomorphic cells are commonly seen in submucosal stroma and are not indicative of malignancy. **(p. 306)**

A6. True
Polyps are present in 6–10% of patients with CF. Their occurrence in children should prompt further investigation. **(p. 306)**

A7. False
Nasal polyps have a high recurrence rate, because the underlying immunological process remains active after removal. **(p. 306)**

A8. False
Chronic sinusitis most frequently affects the maxillary sinuses. **(p. 306)**

A9. False
This is rhinosporidiosis, an inflammatory disease endemic in India. Typical for this disease are thick-walled globular cysts surrounded by a chronic inflammatory infiltrate. **(p. 307)**

A10. False
Mucor (a zygomycete) is the most frequent causative fungus in patients with diabetic ketoacidosis and in immunocompromised patients. **(p. 306)**

A11. True
The Gram-negative rods of *Klebsiella rhinoscleromatis* are identified on PAS staining. **(p. 307)**

A12. False
Dense lymphoid infiltrates are not a typical feature of Wegener's disease; it is typified by leukocytoclastic vasculitis and a granulomatous reaction that contains scant lymphocytes. **(p. 307)**

A13. False
Eosinophilic angiocentric fibrosis differs from Wegener's granulomatosis and contains no foci of necrotizing granulomatous inflammation and vasculitis. It is characterized by perivascular 'onion-skin' fibrosis and a mixed inflammatory infiltrate rich in eosinophils. **(p. 307)**

A14. False
Myospherulosis is an iatrogenic condition caused by the use of oil-based hemostatic packing, with sharply demarcated tissue spaces with brown 'spherules' constituting changed erythrocytes. **(p. 307–308)**

A15. True
Men are affected twice as often as women. **(p. 308)**

A16. False
The inverted papillomas have a higher recurrence rate than everted papillomas. **(p. 309)**

A17. False
This is the oncocytic or cylindrical cell type everted sinonasal papilloma. **(p. 308)**

A18. True
Mucin-containing cells and mucinous microcysts are seen in all types of sinonasal papilloma. They are, however, not seen in squamous papillomas of the vestibule. **(p. 309)**

A19. False
Carcinoma arising in papilloma may occur at first presentation, or in recurrences. **(p. 309)**

A20. True
HPV can be demonstrated in all forms of sinonasal papilloma, although the detection rate varies considerably from one laboratory to another. The overall prevalence of HPV is much higher in everted than in inverted papillomas. **(p. 309)**

A21. False
Most sinonasal carcinomas arise de novo and there is usually no evidence of a pre-existing sinonasal papilloma. **(p. 309)**

A22. False
Squamous cell carcinoma is the most common microscopic type of sinonasal carcinoma. **(p. 310)**

A23. False
It is thought that most adenocarcinomas arise from the mucosal (lining) epithelium rather than the submucosal glands. Some tumors have the appearance of well differentiated tubulopapillary adenocarcinomas, whereas others resemble colorectal carcinomas. **(p. 310)**

A24. True
Nasopharyngeal carcinoma is a very common form of cancer in southeast Asia. The age-incidence curve is bimodal, with a peak occurring between 15 and 25 years and another between 60 and 69 years of age. Epstein–Barr virus, genetic predisposition and environmental factors play an important role in the pathogenesis of this cancer. **(p. 311)**

A25. True
This figure shows the typical features of an undifferentiated nasopharyngeal carcinoma, known as the 'Schmincke type' carcinoma. The nuclei are vesicular and contain prominent nucleoli. The cells grow diffusely without any distinct pattern. Scattered small lymphocytes can be seen between the tumor cells. **(p. 313)**

A26. True
The keratinizing type is less often EBV associated and is seen in older patients compared to the non-keratinizing type. **(p. 312)**

A27. False
Nasopharyngeal carcinomas are often clinically silent and detection and location can be problematic. Random ('blind') biopsies from the nasopharynx should be taken whenever the diagnosis is suspected, particularly from the fossa of Rosenmüller. **(p. 312)**

A28. False
Radiation is the treatment of choice for this tumor. **(p. 315)**

A29. True
This is in contrast to the nasal cavities, where benign mixed tumors are more common. **(p. 315)**

A30. False
Adenoid cystic carcinoma is the most frequent salivary gland tumor in this location. **(p. 315)**

A31. True
The term nasal glioma is commonly used for glial heterotopia or encephalocele. These developmental disorders should not be confused with true neoplasms of the brain, which are, however, also called gliomas. **(p. 315–316)**

A32. False
Glial heterotopias present either in the subcutaneous tissues at the base of the nose or as nasal polyps; they do not occur in the sinuses. **(p. 316)**

A33. False
Esthesioneuroblastoma has a wide age range distribution, but the median age is about 50 years of age. **(p. 316)**

A34. True
The differential diagnosis for this small blue cell tumor includes tumors of similar morphology, such as lymphoma, rhabdomyosarcoma and Ewing's sarcoma. **(p. 317)**

A35. False
The t(11;22) translocation, typical of PNETs, is also found in Ewing's sarcoma but is not found in esthesioneuroblastomas. **(p. 317)**

A36. False
The predominant problem in esthesioneuroblastoma is local invasion; distant metastases are seen in only 20% of patients. **(p. 317)**

A37. False
This is a natural killer/T-cell lymphoma with a distinct immunophenotype; it is positive for CD2 and CD56 and negative for surface CD3. **(p. 319)**

A38. True
Most cases of NK/T-cell lymphoma of nasal type are EBV related; the hemophagocytic syndrome is considered to be virus associated. **(p. 319)**

A39. True
In the western world B-cell lymphomas predominate, whereas in the Far East and Latin America NK/T-cell lymphoma is the most common type. **(p. 319)**

A40. False
Nasopharyngeal angiofibroma is seen almost exclusively in males. **(p. 320)**

A41. False
Although there are documented cases of regression, especially after incomplete surgical removal or radiation therapy, most angiofibromas do not regress spontaneously. **(p. 321)**

A42. False
This tumor is a lobular capillary hemangioma of the nasal cavity. It consists of numerous capillary lobules and should not be confused with angiofibroma. Furthermore, it should be noticed that angiofibromas occur almost exclusively in males. **(p. 321)**

A43. True
These three tumors represent the most common pediatric malignancies of the sinonasal region, but are rare in adults. **(p. 323)**

Larynx and trachea

A1. True

Laryngeal cysts contain mucus, laryngoceles contain air. **(p. 336)**

A2. True

Chronic laryngitis may be a consequence of chronic irritation by tobacco and alcohol, overuse of the voice or infection. **(p. 336)**

A3. False

The 'amyloid-like' material that may be seen in established laryngeal nodules is hyalinized collagen; the name is a misnomer. **(p. 337)**

A4. True

Juvenile laryngeal papillomatosis is typically associated with infection with HPV types 6 and 11. **(p. 338)**

A5. True

Multiple recurrences are common and the papillomas may extend into soft tissue. **(p. 338)**

A6. True

These are traumatic (singer's nodule) and adaptive phenomena to excessive or misuse of the voice. **(p. 337)**

A7. True

In such tumors true papillae with fibrovascular cores are covered with dysplastic squamous epithelium. **(p. 340)**

A8. True

The squamous epithelium shows a loss of maturation involving more than two-thirds of the epithelial thickness and prominent nuclear atypia, which are features of severe dysplasia. There is still surface maturation , which distinguishes this from carcinoma in-situ. **(p. 340)**

A9. True

Carcinoma of the larynx is more than five times as common in males than in females. **(p. 341)**

A10. False

HPV does not predispose to the development of laryngeal carcinoma, but cigarette smoking and alcohol use do. **(p. 341)**

A11. True

Approximately 60–65% of all laryngeal carcinomas are classified as glottic. Supraglottic tumors account for one-third of all cases. Infraglottic and transglottic tumors account for 5% of all laryngeal cancers. **(p. 343)**

A12. True

Gross examination of lymph nodes during surgery for the removal of laryngeal cancer is often misleading and 20–35% of patients will be found to harbour occult metastases on microscopic examination. **(p. 343)**

A13. True

Radiation treatment of verrucous carcinoma may cause anaplastic transformation, and for this reason is contraindicated for this subtype. **(p. 344)**

A14. False

Basaloid squamous carcinoma of the larynx is a highly malignant carcinoma composed of small crowded cells with scant cytoplasm, hyperchromatic nuclei showing peripheral palisading, and surrounding areas of necrosis. **(p. 345)**

A15. False

Stage by stage, sarcomatoid carcinoma of the larynx has the same prognosis as conventional squamous cell carcinoma. **(p. 346)**

A16. True

Rates for lymph node metastases in glottic (T2), supraglottic, transglottic and infraglottic tumors are 7, 40, 52 and 50%, respectively. **(p. 346)**

A17. False

Adenoid cystic carcinoma is the most common type of salivary gland tumor in the larynx. **(p. 346)**

A18. True

These tumors are most common in male smokers. **(p. 347)**

A19. True

Paragangliomas of the larynx are most often located in the supraglottic region, from where they often extend into the ipsilateral aryepiglottic fold. **(p. 347–348)**

A20. True

Cartilaginous tumors are the most common mesenchymal malignant tumors of the larynx and most of them are classified histologically as chondrosarcomas. **(p. 348)**

Trachea

A1. True
Solitary papillomas and papillomatosis occur in the trachea the same way as in the larynx. **(p. 349)**

A2. True
Most of these squamous cell carcinomas occur in the lower third of the trachea and have a poor prognosis. **(p. 350)**

A3. True
Adenoid cystic tumor is the most common glandular tumor and the second most common malignant tumor of the trachea. **(p. 380)**

A4. True
Benign mixed tumor (pleomorphic adenoma), like all other salivary gland tumors, can occur in the trachea, but not as often as adenoid cystic carcinoma. **(p. 350)**

Pleura

A1. True
Amosite and crocidolite from the amphibole group are most commonly implicated. **(p. 360)**

A2. False
The dome of the diaphragm is a very common site for pleural plaques in asbestos exposure. **(p. 361)**

A3. True
The interval between asbestos exposure and the development of mesothelioma is 20 years or more. **(p. 361)**

A4. True
This mesothelial proliferation is more commonly seen in the peritoneal cavity. **(p. 361)**

A5. False
The typical symptoms of mesothelioma are chest pain and effusion, which may cause shortness of breath. Cough is not a typical symptom of mesothelioma. **(p. 361)**

A6. True
Histologically mesothelioma and adenocarcinoma may be virtually indistinguishable without ancillary techniques. **(p. 362–363)**

A7. True
Calretinin, WT1 and cytokeratin 5/6 are considered to be positive markers for mesothelioma and are essentially negative in pulmonary adenocarcinoma. **(p. 363)**

A8. False
These types of mesothelioma retain their cytokeratin expression. **(p. 363)**

A9. False
Solitary fibrous tumor stains for CD34 but does not stain for cytokeratins. **(p. 365)**

A10. True
90% or more of patients are cured by complete excision. **(p. 366)**

A11. True
Pleural angiosarcoma can grow diffusely over the pleura, simulating mesothelioma. **(p. 366)**

A12. False
In 90% of cases the malignant pleural effusion is found on one side only and is typically ipsilateral with regard to the primary ovarian tumor. **(p. 366)**

A13. False
Cytological analysis of a pleural effusion has a greater sensitivity than pleural biopsy. **(p. 367)**

A14. False
Finding many mesothelial cells in a pleural aspirate virtually excludes tuberculosis. **(p. 367)**

Lungs

A1. False
In congenital lobar emphysema the air spaces are overdistended without tissue damage, in contrast to adult-type emphysema, which results from the destruction of alveolar septa. **(p. 368)**

A2. True
Approximately 90% of bronchopulmonary sequestrations are left-sided. **(p. 369)**

A3. False
The arterial blood supply of both intra- and extralobar pulmonary sequestrations is derived from the systemic circulation, usually the aorta or one of its branches. **(p. 369–370)**

A4. False
The majority of cases of bronchiectasis present in children and young adults. **(p. 370)**

A5. False
Established bronchiectasis is permanent, but in the early stages of obstructive bronchiectasis the lesion may regress if the cause of the obstruction is removed. **(p. 370)**

A6. True
In the preantibiotic era most lung abscesses followed tonsillectomies and other ENT operations. Currently most lung abscesses develop following the aspiration of foreign material or result from secondary infection of lung carcinomas. **(p. 371)**

A7. False
Surgical therapy in tuberculosis is reserved for patients with an incomplete response to antibiotic therapy. **(p. 372)**

A8. False
Tuberculomas result from reinfection; the Ghon focus is a primary manifestation of tuberculosis. **(p. 372)**

A9. True
The granulomas in sarcoidosis are frequently located around lymphatics adjacent to bronchioles. **(p. 373)**

A10. False
Limited Wegener's disease is restricted to the lungs, without renal involvement. **(p. 373)**

A11. True
Secondary inflammation of vessel walls in other granulomatous diseases is not uncommon, for instance tuberculosis and mycotic infection. **(p. 373)**

A12. False
The lesions of bronchocentric granulomatosis are usually solitary. **(p. 374)**

A13. True
Blood eosinophilia, systemic vasculitis and asthma form the classic triad of Churg–Strauss disease. **(p. 375)**

A14. False
Hemoptysis in aspergilloma is caused by damage to granulation-type tissue with fragile vessels around the aspergilloma, not by direct invasion of vessel walls. **(p. 375)**

A15. False
This figure illustrates the typical features of histoplasmosis. *Aspergillus* that forms branching hyphae is not seen in this silver-impregnated slide. **(p. 375)**

A16. True
Diffuse alveolar damage is a tissue reaction type, which may have many different causes. **(p. 376)**

A17. False
Edema and intra-alveolar haemorrhage are the earliest changes in diffuse alveolar damage. **(p. 376)**

A18. True
Atypia in regenerating type 2 pneumocytes should not be interpreted as malignant change. **(p. 376)**

A19. False
Acute interstitial pneumonia and diffuse alveolar damage have essentially similar microscopic features. **(p. 377)**

A20. False
The fibrosis and inflammation in BOOP is generally reversible and responsive to treatment with steroids. **(p. 377)**

A21. True
Spatial and temporal heterogeneity are characteristic features of UIP. **(p. 377)**

A22. True
Honeycombing is a non-specific end-stage remodeling of the airspaces in pulmonary fibrosis of any cause.

A23. False
DIP is a misnomer. The intra-alveolar cell accumulation is caused by excessive numbers of alveolar macrophages with an epithelioid appearance. **(p. 378)**

A24. False
Patients with Sjögren's syndrome are prone to developing lymphoid interstitial pneumonia, a diffuse infiltrate of lymphoid cells not necessarily bronchiolocentric. **(p. 379)**

A25. False
Giant cell interstitial pneumonia is caused by exposure to hard metals, tungsten in particular. Beryllium may cause granulomatous disease indistinguishable from sarcoidosis. **(p. 379)**

A26. True
Obstruction of the bronchus by tumor may cause stasis of secretions with associated endogenous lipoid pneumonia. **(p. 380)**

A27. False
Pulmonary eosinophilic infiltrates may or may not be associated with peripheral eosinophilia. Eosinophilia in blood is therefore not a diagnostic requirement for diagnosing eosinophilic pneumonia. **(p. 380)**

A28. False
The typical appearance of *Pneumocystis carinii* in the lung is foamy intra-alveolar exudates and interstitial lymphoplasmacytic infiltrates. The disease may occasionally present in other ways, including granulomatous inflammation. **(p. 381)**

A29. True

Histologically, Legionnaires' disease is similar to other bacterial pneumonias, although small-vessel leukocytoclastic vasculitis may be seen as well. **(p. 382)**

A30. True

Very large amounts of inhaled carbon (often admixed with other minerals) may lead to progressive massive fibrosis with pulmonary function compromise. **(p. 383)**

A31. False

Inhalation of silicates leads to nodular fibrotic lesions, which hyalinize over time and which may coalesce to form large masses; reticular fibrosis is not typical of silicosis. **(p. 383)**

A32. False

Silo-filler's lung is caused by the direct toxic effect of nitrogen dioxide (chemical pneumonitis); in contrast to extrinsic allergic alveolitis, it does not have an immunological basis. **(p. 383)**

A33. True

Later stages of Langerhans' cell histiocytosis consist of stellate scars with few or no Langerhans' cells. **(p. 383)**

A34. True

The combination of many eosinophils and mesothelial cells mimics Langerhans' cells in eosinophilic pleuritis. **(p. 384)**

A35. True

Plexiform lesions, fibrinoid necrosis of vessel walls and concentric laminar fibrosis are severe changes that are considered contraindications for surgery. **(p. 385)**

A36. True

'Washing-out' the exudate by lavage is curative in many cases. **(p. 386)**

A37. False

The disease is caused by circulating autoantibodies to type IV collagen in the glomerular basement membranes. **(p. 386)**

A38. False

Pulmonary amyloidosis may present as nodular parenchymal, nodular bronchial, vascular (wall) or diffuse alveolar septal deposits. **(p. 386)**

A39. False

These are not specific to tuberculosis and are probably ischemic in nature. **(p. 387)**

A40. True

Rounded atelectasis consists of collapsed lung parenchyma with fibrosis and retraction of the overlying pleura. It is often seen in patients with a history of asbestos exposure. **(p. 387)**

Lung tumors

A1. False

There is no evidence to support this supposition. **(p. 388)**

A2. True

There is no evidence that scars predispose to the formation of cancer in the lungs. **(p. 388)**

A3. True

The male to female ratio is currently 1.5:1. **(p. 388)**

A4. False

Molecular data show that over half of synchronous or metachronous lung cancers are distinct entities. **(p. 388)**

A5. True

Approximately 35–50% of coin lesions prove to be carcinomas. **(p. 388)**

A6. True

Although small cell carcinoma is renowned for the production of bioactive substances, parathyroid hormone-like polypeptide production causing hypercalcemia is seen mostly in association with squamous cell carcinoma. **(p. 389)**

A7. True

TTF-1 is expressed in most lung adenocarcinomas but is also found in thyroid tumors and normal thyroid epithelial cells. **(p. 390)**

A8. False

This subtype behaves aggressively and carries an unfavourable prognosis. **(p. 391)**

A9. True

Pulmonary squamous cell carcinoma usually shows central necrosis with cavitation. **(p. 391)**

A10. True

Mutations of *p53* are common and appear at an early stage of histogenesis in squamous cell carcinomas of the lung. **(p. 391)**

A11. True

In a series of 82 scar cancers 72% were adenocarcinomas and 18 were squamous cell carcinomas; there were no small cell carcinomas. **(p. 392)**

A12. False

Cytokeratin-7 is expressed in pulmonary epithelium and adenocarcinoma and in benign and malignant mesothelial cells. **(p. 393)**

A13. True

Actually, adenocarcinomas may contain cells that resemble not only Clara cells but also other major cells lining the bronchial tree: goblet cells, mucus cells, non-ciliated bronchial cells. **(p. 393)**

A14. True

Solid adenocarcinoma with mucin production is a subgroup of adenocarcinoma in the WHO classification. **(p. 393)**

A15. False

The transition of tall mucin-producing cells to normal epithelium is abrupt. **(p. 393)**

A16. True

Cytologically small cell carcinoma consists of cells with a high nuclear to cytoplasmic ratio and moulding of cell shape. **(p. 403)**

A17. True

Extensive fibrosis may be seen in non-mucinous bronchioloalveolar carcinoma and is referred to as the sclerosing variant; this does not imply invasion. **(p. 395)**

A18. True

CK20 staining is typically negative in conventional pulmonary adenocarcinoma but positive in mucinous bronchioloalveolar carcinoma; TTF-1 is expressed in conventional and bronchioloalveolar adenocarcinoma. α_1-Antitrypsin as a marker for Clara cells is positive in non-mucinous bronchioloalveolar carcinoma. **(p. 395)**

A19. False

This tumor is seen in adults, contrary to other 'blastomas', such as retinoblastoma or hepatoblastoma. **(p. 397)**

A20. False

Squamous cell carcinoma and adenocarcinoma are each more common than small cell carcinoma, which accounts for 10–20% of all lung cancers. **(p. 398)**

A21. True

The small cell size and high nuclear to cytoplasmic ratio of small cell carcinoma is in part a biopsy artefact, and in resection specimens the cells do not appear as small as in biopsies. **(p. 399)**

A22. True

The chromatin pattern and the nucleolar pattern are the two discriminating histological features of small cell carcinoma. **(p. 400)**

A23. False

Abnormalities of *p16* are highly uncommon in small cell carcinoma but frequently detected in non-small cell carcinoma. Mutations of *p53* and inactivation of the *Rb* gene are found in over 90% of small cell carcinomas. **(p. 401)**

A24. True

With repeated examination (five samples or more) the sensitivity of sputum cytology is approximately 80%. Sensitivity of single samples is in the range of 40–60%. **(p. 402)**

A25. False

Hilar lymph nodes are the most common site of metastasis of lung cancer. Distant metastases are most often found in the liver, adrenals, bones, central nervous system and kidneys. **(p. 404)**

A26. True

Recent figures show that the mean 5-year survival for all stages of lung cancer is approximately 12%. **(p. 404)**

A27. True

This is probably due to the advanced stage of the disease at the time of diagnosis. **(p. 405)**

A28. False

Squamous cell carcinoma is the most curable form of lung cancer. In series of long-term lung cancer survivors about half are patients who had squamous cell carcinoma. **(p. 405)**

A29. False

The usual location of chondroid hamartoma is the subpleural parenchyma. Such lesions are usually asymptomatic and are discovered accidentally as 'coin lesions' on routine X-ray examination. **(p. 406)**

A30. True

Regional lymph node metastases are seen in about 5% of typical carcinoid tumors, and distant metastases may be occasionally found. On the other hand, lymph node metastases are found in 70% of atypical carcinoids. **(p. 407)**

A31. False

Pulmonary carcinoids are consistently TTF-1 positive. Their usual keratin profiles are CK7+/CK20–. These immunohistochemical tests are important for distinguishing primary pulmonary carcinoids from metastastic lesions. **(p. 409)**

A32. False

Dense-core neurosecretory granules are found in carcinoid tumors but may also be seen in other neuroendocrine tumors, including small cell carcinoma. **(p. 409)**

A33. True

Spindle cell morphology is typical for peripheral carcinoids. **(p. 410)**

A34. True

Atypical carcinoids have 2–10 mitoses/10 high-power fields (hpf), in contrast to typical carcinoids, which have fewer than 2 mitoses/10 hpf. Atypical carcinoids also contain foci of 'spotty' necrosis, which are not seen in typical carcinoids. **(p. 411)**

A35. True

These tumors do not show the typical architectural features of neuroendocrine tumors, at most showing only some nesting and peripheral palisading and some rosette formation. Nevertheless, ultrastructurally and by immunohistochemistry they have the typical features of neuroendocrine tumors. **(p. 411)**

A36. False

Sclerosing hemangiomais is not derived from endothelial cells and is at least in part an epithelial neoplasm. **(p. 412–413)**

A37. True

ALK-1 aberrations may be detected by immunohistochemical staining or by molecular techniques. **(p. 414)**

A38. True

In pulmonary lymphangiomyomatosis cystic changes develop throughout the lungs and on CT scanning these changes resemble emphysema. The tumor is composed of HMB-45-positive cells, and together with tumors such as renal angiomyolipoma can be classified as a pecoma. **(p. 415–420)**

A39. True

This endothelial tumor, also known as intravascular bronchioloalveolar tumor (IV-BAT), typically presents as in the lung as multinodular disease. **(p. 415)**

A40. False

Lymphomatoid granulomatosis is an EBV-associated B-cell pulmonary lymphoma with an extensive admixture of T lymphocytes. Extrapulmonary involvement is found in 80% of cases. **(p. 418)**

A41. False

In the lungs, as well as in other parts of the respiratory tract, adenoid cystic carcinoma is the most common salivary gland tumor. **(p. 418)**

A42. True

Renal cell carcinoma is HMB-45 negative; sugar tumor (clear cell tumor) is HMB-45 positive. **(p. 419)**

A43. True

Peripheral carcinoid tumors are typically spindle cell type with a bland mesenchymal appearance and thus may be confused with a smooth muscle cell tumor. **(p. 420)**

A44. False

These tumors are not related entities: pleuropulmonary blastoma is a dysontogenetic pediatric tumor, whereas pulmonary blastoma occurs in adults. Pleuropulmonary blastoma is an aggressive tumor composed of primitive blastomatous and sarcomatous elements. The latter may exhibit signs of skeletal muscle and cartilaginous differentiation. The epithelial component is either lacking or present in the form of benign-looking, presumably entrapped, epithelium. Some tumors may be cystic. **(p. 421)**

A45. True

For example colorectal carcinomas are typically CDX2 (a marker of intestinal organogenesis) and CK20 (a low molecular weight keratin) positive and CK7 negative. Pulmonary adenocarcinomas very rarely stain positively for CDX2, and are CK7 positive and usually CK20 negative. **(p. 423)**

A46. False

This is essentially an intentionally curative procedure, which has been shown to improve survival rates. **(p. 424)**

8 Mediastinum

General

Q1

The superior vena cava syndrome occurs with equal frequency in both benign and malignant disease in the mediastinum.

Q2

Gastroenteric cysts are most commonly encountered in the posterior mediastinum.

Inflammatory diseases

Q1

Acute mediastinitis is usually idiopathic and its cause cannot be established.

Q2

Cryptococcus neoformans is the best-known cause of chronic (fibrosing) mediastinitis.

Q3

Phlebitis is a common finding in idiopathic fibrosing mediastinitis.

Q4

Hodgkin's disease should be included in the differential diagnosis of chronic fibrosing mediastinitis.

Cysts

Q1

Pericardial cysts are usually unilocular.

Q2

This figure shows the typical features of a pericardial cyst.

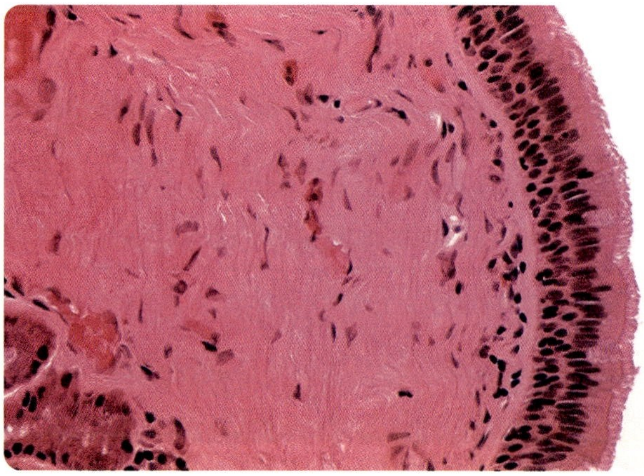

Fig. 8.1

Q3

Bronchial and esophageal cysts can be confidently distinguished one from another by their anatomic location and microscopic appearance.

Thyroid and parathyroid lesions

Q1

Mediastinal thyroid masses are excised primarily because of their propensity for malignant degeneration.

Q2

Parathyroid adenomas in the mediastinum on average are larger than cervical parathyroid adenomas.

Thymus

Q1

Hassall's corpuscles are remnants of apoptotic lymphoid cells.

Q2

In the complete form of DiGeorge syndrome it is the lymphocytic component of the thymus that fails to develop, whereas the rudimentary epithelial structures are preserved.

Q3

The presence of Hassall's corpuscles distinguishes acute thymic involution from thymic dysplasia.

Q4

Unilocular thymic cysts are developmental abnormalities, whereas multilocular thymic cysts are acquired.

Q5

True thymic hyperplasia and thymic follicular hyperplasia are conditions that are histologically dissimilar but are both characterized by increased gland size.

Q6

Thymomas are thymic tumors composed of neoplastic epithelial cells admixed with varying amounts of non-neoplastic lymphoid cells.

Q7

Myasthenia gravis is virtually always associated with thymoma.

Q8

Patients with myasthenia gravis most often have lymphocyte-rich thymomas.

Q9

The presence of myasthenia gravis is an adverse prognostic sign in patients with thymoma.

Q10

The muscle weakness of myasthenia gravis is also known as the Lambert–Eaton syndrome.

Q11

Although thymomas appear on X-ray as well circumscribed masses most of them are not encapsulated.

Q12

In the differential diagnosis of thymoma with cystic changes one should include multilocular thymic cysts, germ cell neoplasms and Hodgkin's disease.

Q13

The lymphocytic component of thymomas may show activation features with larger cell size, open chromatin, the presence of nucleoli, and frequent cleaved and convoluted nuclei.

Q14

Perivascular spaces with proteinaceous material are a characteristic finding in thymoma.

Q15

Most thymomas are benign tumors, which, however, may recur after excision.

Q16

Rosette-like structures with well-defined lumina are a common and characteristic feature of thymoma.

Q17

The presence of Hassall's corpuscles suggests thymic hyperplasia but does not rule out the diagnosis of thymoma.

Q18

The ultrastructural features of thymoma are typical of neoplastic lymphoid cells.

Q19

The lymphoid cells of thymoma have a CD3/CD1a/CD99 phenotype.

QUESTIONS

Q20

This figure illustrates the typical features of a cortical-type thymoma.

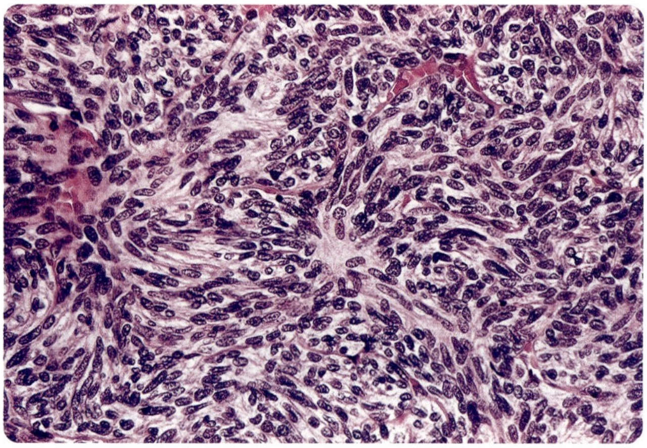

Fig. 8.2

Q21

Features favoring a diagnosis of thymic carcinoma over metastatic carcinoma to the mediastinum include lobulation and CD5 staining of the epithelial cells.

Q22

The immunoprofile of the lymphoid population in thymic carcinoma is identical to the lymphoid component of thymoma.

Q23

The sarcomatoid variant of thymic carcinoma may contain cartilage or striated muscle cell differentiation.

Q24

CD70 is a useful marker to separate thymic carcinoma from thymoma.

Q25

Medullary thymomas are characterized by plump epithelioid cells and small lymphoid cells.

Q26

The AB type of thymoma shows the greatest resemblance to the normal thymus gland.

Q27

Type C thymoma is a synonym for thymic carcinoma.

Q28

Microscopic subtype is the single most important prognostic determinant of thymoma.

Q29

In general, cortical thymomas have a worse prognosis than medullary thymomas.

Q30

The mucoepidermoid variant of thymic carcinoma has a better prognosis than the non-keratinizing epidermoid subtype.

Q31

Ectopic hamartomatous thymomas are supraclavicular–suprasternal lesions typically found in males and composed of spindle epithelial cells.

Q32

This figure illustrates the typical features of a spindle epithelial tumor with thymus-like elements (SETTLE), a lesion that is quite distinct from carcinoma with thymus-like elements (CASTLE).

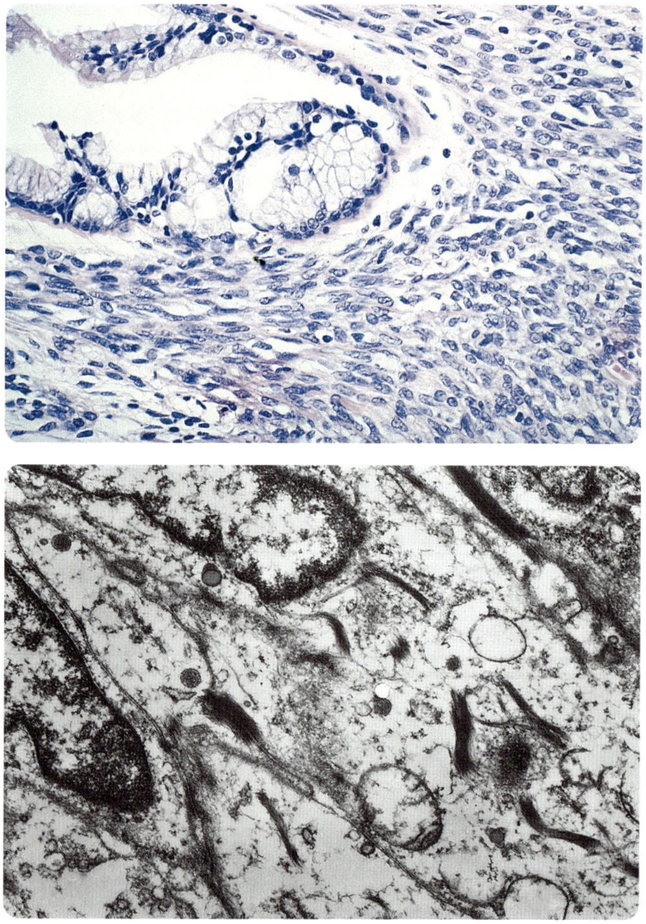

A

B

Fig. 8.3

Q33

Most thymic neuroendocrine tumors are classified as atypical carcinoids or neuroendocrine tumors of intermediate category.

Germ cell tumors

Q1

Mediastinal germ cell tumors are specifically related to the thymus.

Q2

Mediastinal germ cell tumors occur with the same frequency in both males and females.

Q3

Mediastinal germ cell tumors occur in increased frequency in patients with Turner syndrome.

Q4

In contrast to testicular seminomas mediastinal seminomas do not harbor c-*kit* mutations.

Q5

Embryonal carcinoma is the most common type of mediastinal germ cell tumor.

Q6

Chromosome 12p aberrations are common to both gonadal and mediastinal germ cell tumors.

Q7

Somatic malignancies, such as adenocarcinoma or sarcomas, arising in mediastinal germ cell tumors are ominous complications that have a poor prognosis.

Q8

Teratocarcinoma is a combined germ cell tumor consisting of teratoma and embryonal carcinoma.

Lymphoma

Q1

Mediastinal malignant lymphoma represents the most common primary neoplasm of the middle portion of the mediastinum.

Q2

The nodular sclerosing subtype is the most common form of Hodgkin's lymphoma in the mediastinum.

Q3

Mediastinal Hodgkin's disease may present as a multilocular thymic cyst.

Q4

Thymic Hodgkin's lymphoma carries a better prognosis than mediastinal lymph node Hodgkin's lymphoma.

Q5

Most mediastinal lymphoblastic lymphomas are of T-cell origin.

Q6

Like large B-cell lymphoma, lymphoblastic lymphoma has a strong female preponderance.

Q7

Mediastinal lymphoblastic lymphoma usually presents in children as disseminated disease with peripheral blood and bone marrow involvement.

Q8

Mediastinal lymphoblastic lymphoma typically presents as a medical emergency.

Q9

Mediastinal lymphoblastic lymphoma may histologically closely simulate the B3 subtype of thymoma.

Q10

Large cell lymphoma frequently presents as a medical emergency with superior vena cava syndrome.

Q11

Mediastinal large cell lymphoma is identical to its non-mediastinal counterpart on both the morphological and molecular levels.

Q12

CD30 expression is commonly observed in mediastinal large B-cell lymphoma.

Q13

Mediastinal large cell lymphoma may be of T-cell origin.

Q14

Marginal B-cell lymphoma of the mediastinum usually originates in the thyroid gland.

QUESTIONS

Q15

Similar to mediastinal large B-cell lymphoma, mediastinal marginal B-cell lymphoma shows a strong predilection for females.

Q16

Mediastinal marginal zone lymphoma usually expresses IgM, in keeping with MALT-type lymphoma elsewhere in the body.

Q17

Castleman's disease in the mediastinum is centered on the thymus.

Q18

Castleman's disease in the mediastinum is usually of the hyaline vascular type.

Neurogenic tumors

Q1

Within the mediastinum neuroblastoma is the most common type of neurogenic tumor in the pediatric age group.

Q2

Surgical excision is the treatment of choice for mediastinal ganglioneuroma.

Q3

Ganglioneuroblastoma and ganglioneuroma are located in the middle mediastinum.

Q4

Pleomorphism and mitotic activity in mediastinal schwannoma do not necessarily indicate malignant change in schwannoma in the mediastinum.

Q5

Neurofibromatosis type 2 (NF2) predisposes to malignant change in mediastinal neurofibroma

Other neurogenic tumors

Q1

Mediastinal paraganglioma is often functional ('mediastinal pheochromocytoma').

Q2

Paraganglioma in the mediastinum invariably behaves in a benign fashion.

Mesenchymal tumors

Q1

Mediastinal lymphangioma, lymphangiomyoma and lymphangiomyomatosis are exclusively seen in females in the pediatric age group.

Q2

Angiosarcoma is the most common malignant mesenchymal mediastinal tumor.

General

A1. False

The superior vena cava syndrome is seen predominantly in malignant disease and is most commonly caused by metastatic lung disease and lymphoma. **(p. 459)**

A2. True

Thymic cysts are seen in the anterior and superior mediastinum, bronchogenic and pericardial cysts are seen in the middle mediastinum. The gastroenteric cyst, however, is seen in the posterior mediastinum. **(p. 460)**

Inflammatory diseases

A1. False

Acute mediastinitis is usually the result of traumatic perforation of the esophagus or extension of infection in the soft tissues of the neck. It is typically located in the posterior mediastinum. **(p. 460)**

A2. False

Mycobacterium tuberculosis and *Histoplasma capsulatum* have been found to underlie a significant number of cases of chronic mediastinitis. *Cryptococcus* is not a common cause of chronic mediastinitis. In many cases a specific etiology cannot be demonstrated. **(p. 460)**

A3. True

Phlebitis is seen in addition to a fibrous reaction, and an inflammatory infiltrate with plasma cells and eosinophils. **(p. 460)**

A4. True

Hodgkin's disease in the mediastinum may present as a fibrotic lesion with a chronic inflammatory infiltrate similar to fibrosing mediastinitis. **(p. 460)**

Cysts

A1. True

Pericardial cysts contain clear fluid (unless infected) and are unilocular; they are developmental in origin. **(p. 460)**

A2. False

Pericardial cysts are lined by a single layer of mesothelial cells. This is a bronchial mediastinal cyst lined by ciliated epithelium. **(p. 461)**

A3. False

Bronchogenic cysts may be totally embedded within the wall of the esophagus and may show squamous metaplasis, thus resembling esophageal cysts. **(p. 461)**

Thyroid and parathyroid lesions

A1. False

Mediastinal thyroid masses may cause compression symptoms, necessitating surgical removal. **(p. 462)**

A2. True

Because there is less anatomic space restriction parathyroid adenomas can reach larger sizes in the mediastinum than in the neck. **(p. 462)**

Thymus

A1. False

Hassall's corpuscles are formed from the epithelial cells of the thymus. **(p. 462)**

A2. False

There is complete aplasia of all components of the gland. **(p. 464)**

A3. True

Hassall's corpuscles are not formed in thymic dysplasia but remain present in acute thymic involution. **(p. 464)**

A4. True

Unilocular thymic cysts are branchial pouch-derived developmental anomalies. Multilocular thymic cysts are in all likelihood acquired lesions. **(p. 464)**

A5. False

The thymus is increased in size in true thymic hyperplasia but is usually normal in thymic follicular hyperplasia. **(p. 465)**

A6. True

Thymomas are epithelial tumors usually containing a non-neoplastic lymphocytic component. **(p. 466)**

A7. False

Myasthenia gravis is most commonly associated with follicular hyperplasia (65% of cases) and less often with thymoma (10%). In the remaining 25% of patients no thymic abnormalities are found. **(p. 466)**

A8. False

There does not appear to be a relationship between the relative amounts of epithelial and lymphocytic cells in thymomas removed from patients with myasthenia gravis. **(p. 467)**

A9. False

Although this was true in the past, owing to improvements in treatment there is no difference in the survival of patients with thymoma with and without myasthenia. **(p. 468)**

A10. False

The Lambert–Eaton syndrome is a paraneoplastic syndrome seen in patients who have small cell lung carcinoma. **(p. 467)**

A11. False

80% of thymomas have a thick fibrous capsule. **(p. 468)**

A12. True

All these neoplasms may be partially cystic. Multilocular thymic cysts may require extensive sampling to uncover the true nature of the process and distinguish them from other cystic lesions of the anterior mediastinum. **(p. 468)**

A13. False

Cleaved and convoluted nuclei are not accepted as signs of lymphocyte activation. If they are present, the lesion needs to be further studied to exclude lymphoma. **(p. 468)**

A14. True

These perivascular spaces typically contain proteinaceous fluid and often lymphocytes, macrophages and red blood cells. **(p. 469)**

A15. False

All thymomas are essentially malignant tumors, which have the propensity to recur and metastasize. **(p. 471)**

A16. False

Rosette-like structures with well-defined lumina are not typical for thymoma and are highly suggestive of thymic carcinoid. **(p. 470)**

A17. True

Occasional Hassall's corpuscles may be observed in thymomas. **(p. 470)**

A18. False

Thymomas are epithelial tumors. Ultrastructurally, thymic tumor cells show signs of epithelial differentiation, including complex desmosomes and branching tonofilaments. **(p. 470)**

A19. True

The lymphocytes in thymoma have an immature T-cell phenotype and react with the antibodies to CD3/CD1a/CD99. They also express terminal deoxynucleotidyl transferrase (TdT). **(p. 471)**

A20. False

This thymoma is composed of spindle cells and is thus of the medullary type. **(p. 469)**

A21. True

Immunostaining with CD5 is seen in the epithelial cells of a significant proportion of thymic carcinomas. Lobulation as seen in thymoma favors a diagnosis of thymic carcinoma over metastatic carcinoma or direct ingrowth of a carcinoma from the lung. **(p. 473)**

A22. False

The lymphocytic infiltrate in thymic carcinoma, which may be extensive, is composed of mature rather than immature T lymphocytes. Occasionally the infiltrate is composed predominantly of B cells. **(p. 473)**

A23. True

Sarcomatoid thymomas may show cartilaginous and striated muscle cell differentiation and may be also called carcinosarcomas with heterologous differentiation. **(p. 474)**

A24. True

CD70 belongs to the tumor necrosis factor family of proteins that is frequently expressed in thymic carcinomas but not in other thymomas. **(p. 473)**

A25. False

Medullary thymoma (type A thymoma) is composed of spindle cells admixed with small lymphocytes. **(p. 477)**

A26. False

The AB type of thymoma is composed of spindle cells (medullary type or type A thymoma admixed with foci of rich in lymphocytes (B1 thymoma). The subtype B1 thymoma shows the most organoid pattern of growth and most closely resembles normal thymic tissue. **(p. 477)**

A27. True

In the WHO classification this thymic carcinoma is designated type C thymoma. However, type B3 thymoma is also known as well-differentiated thymic carcinoma. It is important to remember that all thymomas may behave in a malignant fashion. **(p. 477)**

A28. False

Stage is the most important factor that determines prognosis in thymoma. **(p. 479)**

A29. True

The relationship between microscopic type and prognosis with increasing aggressiveness is in the following order A<AB<B1<B2<B3<C. This corresponds to medullary<mixed medullary–cortical<increasing cortical epithelial component<thymic carcinoma. **(p. 479)**

A30. True

Non-keratinizing thymic carcinoma is an aggressive tumor; the mucoepidermoid has an indolent behavior. **(p. 480)**

A31. True

Ectopic hamartomatous thymoma is located in the supraclavicular and suprasternal regions. Most patients are males, in contrast to ectopic cervical thymomas, which occur in females. These lesions are composed of elongated fibroblast or Schwann-like spindled epithelial cells (which stain for cytokeratin) without atypia or necrosis. There is no mediastinal counterpart. The tumor behaves in a benign fashion.

A32. True

Both SETTLE and CASTLE are located in or around the thyroid gland. SETTLE is a biphasic tumor composed of spindle cells and mucin-producing cells. CASTLE is similar to thymic carcinoma in its appearance and may be regarded as the cervical (ectopic) variant of thymic carcinoma. **(p. 481)**

A33. True

Most thymic neuroendocrine tumors have the cytological features of carcinoid tumors but show increased mitotic activity and contain foci of necrosis. Accordingly they fall into the category of atypical carcinoid tumors or neuroendocrine tumors of intermediate category. **(p. 482)**

Germ cell tumors

A1. True

When germ cell tumors are encountered in the mediastinum they are always completely encased within the thymus. **(p. 485)**

A2. False

With the exception of mature cystic teratoma, which affects both sexes equally, there is a clear male predominance for all other germ cell tumors. Seminoma as a mediastinal tumor is seen exclusively in males. **(p. 485)**

A3. False

There is no predisposition for mediastinal germ cell tumors in patients with Turner syndrome. Mediastinal germ cell tumors are 30–40 times more common in patients with Klinefelter syndrome than in the general population. **(p. 485)**

A4. False

c-*kit* mutations are as commonly found in mediastinal seminomas as in testicular seminoma. Tumor cells accordingly react with antibodies to CD117. **(p. 486)**

A5. False

Mature cystic teratoma is the most common type of mediastinal germ cell tumor. **(p. 486)**

A6. True

Gain of chromosome 12p material in the form of isochromosome i (12) is found in a large percentage of germ cell tumors irrespective of their origin in the testis or mediastinum. **(p. 488)**

A7. True

Somatic malignancies arsing in germ cell tumors do not respond well to treatment protocols designed for germ cell tumors and are associated with a high mortality. **(p. 488)**

A8. True

The teratoma component may be mature or immature. **(p. 488)**

Lymphoma

A1. True
It may present there as a primary lesion or as part of a systemic process. The order of frequency of mediastinal lymphoma location is anterior, superior and middle mediastinum. **(p. 489)**

A2. True
When the primary is in the mediastinum nodular sclerosis is the most common subtype of Hodgkin's lymphoma. **(p. 489)**

A3. True
The gross appearance of mediastinal Hodgkin's lymphoma can be almost entirely cystic; adequate sampling may be required to uncover diagnostic features of these lymphomas. **(p. 489)**

A4. False
The prognosis is similar for mediastinal Hodgkin's lymphoma presenting primarily in the lymph nodes and for Hodgkin's lymphoma presenting in the thymus. **(p. 490)**

A5. True
Occasionally B-cell lymphoblastic lymphomas occur in the mediastinum, but the majority are T-precursor lymphoblastic lymphomas. **(p. 491)**

A6. False
Males are more frequently affected by mediastinal lymphoblastic lymphomas than are females. **(p. 491)**

A7. False
Although lymph nodes in the cervical, supraclavicular regions and axillae are often affected, peripheral blood and bone marrow involvement is unusual. **(p. 491)**

A8. True
Lymphoblastic lymphoma often forms a bulky mass in the mediastinum, with airway compression necessitating emergency intervention. **(p. 491)**

A9. False
Microscopically – and to a certain extent immunohistochemically – lymphoblastic lymphoma may simulate B1 thymoma, which is characterized by a dense lymphocytic component. **(p. 491)**

A10. True
Large cell lymphoma is an invasive tumor that often compresses vital structures in the mediastinum, requiring rapid treatment. **(p. 491)**

A11. False
The morphological and immunohistochemical features of mediastinal large cell lymphoma suggest that this is a distinct subtype of large cell lymphoma. **(p. 492)**

A12. True
CD30 staining is seen in approximately 70% of mediastinal large cell lymphomas. **(p. 492)**

A13. True
Most cases are of B-cell derivation but sparse cases are T-cell type. **(p. 492)**

A14. False
There is evidence that mediastinal marginal zone lymphomas originate in the thymus. **(p. 493)**

A15. True
Of the four most common types of mediastinal lymphoma Hodgkin's lymphoma, large cell lymphoma and marginal zone lymphoma are more common in females. Lymphoblastic lymphoma is more common in males. **(p. 493)**

A16. False
Marginal zone (MALT) lymphoma in the mediastinum usually expresses IgA, in contrast to MALT lymphoma elsewhere in which IgM expression is the norm. **(p. 493)**

A17. False
Castleman's disease in the mediastinum is centered on the lymph nodes and uncommonly is located in the thymus. **(p. 493)**

A18. True
The plasma cell type, which is essentially always multicentric, presents with generalized lymphadenopathy. **(p. 493 and 1908)**

Neurogenic tumors

A1. False
The most common neurogenic tumor in the mediastinum in the pediatric age group is ganglioneuroma. **(p. 494)**

A2. True
The ganglioneuromas are encapsulated tumors; complete surgical excision is curative. **(p. 494)**

A3. False
Neurogenic tumors, including tumors from the neuroblastoma–ganglioneuroblastoma and ganglioneuroma group, usually occur in the posterior mediastinum. **(p. 494)**

A4. True

'Ancient' or regressive changes, mitotic activity and increased cellularity do not indicate malignant change in mediastinal schwannoma. **(p. 495)**

A5. False

NF2 predisposes to the development of multiple schwannomas; these do not show malignant change. Neurofibromatosis type 1 does predispose individuals to develop malignant peripheral nerve sheath tumors (MPNST). **(p. 495)**

Other neurogenic tumors

A1. False

Most mediastinal paragangliomas are non-functional. Rarely, patients with mediastinal paraganglioma develop hypertension. **(p. 496)**

A2. False

Contrary to long-held beliefs mediastinal paragangliomas may well behave in an aggressive fashion. **(p. 496)**

Mesenchymal tumors

A1. False

Mediastinal lymphangioma does not show a sex predilection; lymphangiomyoma and lymphangiomyomatosis only occur in females. **(p. 496)**

A2. False

Liposarcoma is the most common malignant mesenchymal tumor. Angiosarcoma is less common and may arise as a somatic tumor in a germ cell neoplasm. **(p. 497)**

9 Thyroid gland

Normal anatomy

Q1

The thyroid *anlage* appears first in the embryo as a midline structure in the anterior neck.

Q2

Microscopically, the thyroid gland is made up of follicles lined by a single layer of follicular cells whose shape ranges from flattened to low columnar, depending on their degree of activity.

Q3

Thyroid transcription factor-1 (TTF-1) is a useful marker for thyroid follicular cells and thyroid tumors arising from these cells, but it is also expressed in the normal alveolar cells of the lungs and many lung tumors.

Q4

C cells are more common in the thyroid glands of adults than in those of elderly persons.

Q5

Solid cell nests (*rests*), found in most thyroids, are composed of polygonal or oval cells, often with central glandular lumina containing a mucinous secretion.

Congenital abnormalities

Q1

Thyroglossal duct cyst is typically located on the lateral side of the neck.

Q2

Tumors occasionally developing in thyroglossal cysts are most often follicular carcinomas.

Q3

Heterotopic thyroid tissue can be most frequently found at the base of the tongue.

Q4

Branchial cleft cyst are usually found on lateral sides of the neck and are lined by squamous epithelium.

Thyroiditis

Q1

Acute thyroiditis is usually caused by bacterial infection.

Q2

Granulomatous thyroiditis is characterized microscopically by the appearance of granulomas with multinucleated giant cells surrounding disrupted thyroid follicles.

Q3

Hashimoto's thyroiditis is an organ-specific inflammatory disorder mediated by both humoral and cellular immune reactions.

Q4

Hashimoto's thyroiditis typically presents as soft thyroid enlargement and severe hyperthyroidism in young postpubertal women.

Q5

Hashimoto's thyroiditis is characterized by lymphocytic infiltration of the stroma and oxyphilic change of the follicular epithelium.

Q6

The most common complication of Hashimoto's thyroiditis is medullary thyroid carcinoma.

Q7

Riedel's thyroiditis is the end-stage of Hashimoto's or granulomatous thyroiditis.

Q8

Dyshormonogentic goiter is a childhood disease characterized by prominent nuclear enlargement and atypia of thyroid follicular cells arranged into nodules.

Q9

Microscopically, the follicles in Graves' disease are lined by oxyphilic cells.

Q10

In Graves' disease there are aggregates of T-cell-rich lymphoid tissue with germinal center formation inside the stroma of the thyroid, but often also in the tissues around the thyroid.

Q11

Colloid goiter is typically composed of dilated follicles filled with colloid and lined uniformly by atrophic thyroid cells.

Q12

Secondary changes in colloid goiter are very common and include, among others, recent and old hemorrhage, granulomatous reaction to ruptured follicles, and fibrosis with calcification.

Q13

Follicular adenomas can be distinguished from so-called dominant nodules in colloid goiter, because the adenomas are tumors and thus monoclonal.

Tumors

Q1

The majority of clinically apparent thyroid neoplasms are primary and epithelial.

Q2

Follicular adenoma is a benign encapsulated tumor that shows evidence of follicular cell differentiation.

Q3

So-called hot thyroid nodules are usually but not always benign.

Q4

DNA aneuploidy is indicative of malignancy of thyroid nodules.

Q5

This thyroid tumor is malignant because it has large bizarre nuclei.

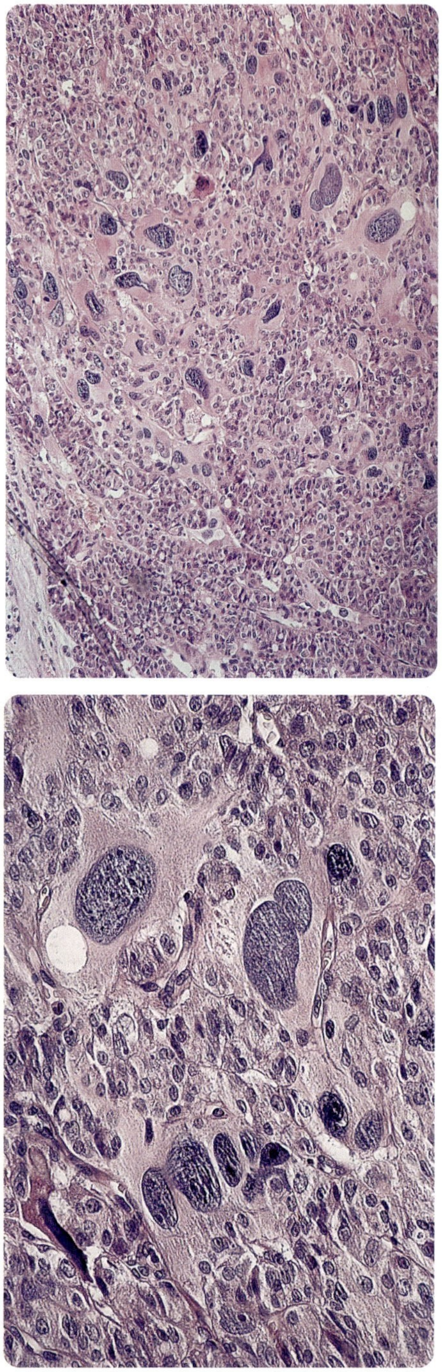

A

B

Fig. 9.1

Q6

Papillary carcinoma occurs more often in females than in males, and the mean age at the time of initial diagnosis is approximately 40 years.

Q7

The papillae of papillary carcinoma of the thyroid are usually complex, branching and randomly oriented, with a central fibrovascular core and a single or stratified lining of cuboidal cells.

Q8

The ground-glass nuclei typically found in papillary carcinoma of the thyroid are best seen in frozen sections or cytologic imprints.

Q9

Psammoma bodies are seen often on multinodular goiter and are of limited diagnostic significance.

Q10

Immunohistochemically, papillary carcinoma of the thyroid stains with antibodies to keratin CK7 and thyroid transcription factor-1 (TTF-1), but is unreactive with the antibodies to CK20.

Q11

Despite its name, the so-called encapsulated papillary carcinoma is rarely encapsulated and actually presents histologically as a stellate scar, measuring less than 1 cm in diameter.

Q12

Follicular variant of papillary carcinoma is a term used for papillary carcinomas showing a follicular pattern in at least 50% of all slides and almost all metastatic sites.

Q13

Tall cell variant of papillary carcinoma is composed of follicles lined by cuboidal or cylindrical cells with overlapping clear and grooved nuclei.

Q14

Approximately 50% of all patients with papillary carcinoma of the thyroid have distant metastases, usually in the lungs, at the time of diagnosis.

Q15

A history of previous irradiation and the young age of the patient adversely affect the prognosis of papillary carcinoma.

Q16

Minimally invasive follicular carcinoma is a grossly encapsulated tumor, often with a solid and fleshy cut surface.

Q17

The capsule of follicular carcinoma tends to be thicker and more irregular than that of adenoma.

Q18

Widely invasive follicular carcinoma is almost never encapsulated.

Q19

Oncocytic tumors are composed of cells that have well-developed eosinophilic granular cytoplasm, but also cells that may have a clear cytoplasm.

Q20

Oncocytic thyroid tumors have a tendency to undergo massive infarct-type necrosis, often following fine needle aspiration.

Q21

Unfavorable prognostic factors for Hürthle cell carcinomas are older patient age, large tumor size, extrathyroidal extension and metastases to local lymph nodes.

Q22

Clear cell carcinoma of the thyroid is a unique tumor that has a very poor prognosis.

Q23

Poorly differentiated invasive thyroid carcinomas composed of uniform small cells forming nests, solid sheets or microfollicular arrangement are classified as insular carcinomas.

Q24

Undifferentiated carcinomas almost invariably resemble spindle cell sarcomas.

Q25

Most, if not all, undifferentiated thyroid carcinomas arise as a result of anaplastic transformation of a pre-existing well-differentiated tumor.

Q26

Medullary carcinoma is a tumor composed of C (parafollicular) cells.

Q27

Most medullary carcinomas are composed of solid nests of round to polygonal cells that have an amphophilic cytoplasm and highly vascular, hyalinized or amyloid-rich stroma.

Q28

Medullary carcinomas are consistently positive for carcinoembryonic antigen (CEA).

Q29

Most medullary carcinomas occur in young persons under the age of 35 years.

Q30

Medullary carcinomas may be a component of multiple endocrine neoplasia type I.

Q31

Multiple nodules of the thyroid, especially in Hashimoto's thyroiditis, are more likely to be malignant than a solitary nodule.

Q32

Patients with papillary carcinoma of the thyroid usually have a normal or subnormal levels of thyroglobulin in serum.

Q33

Thyroid tissue found in the cervical lymph nodes in most cases represents metastases of a thyroid papillary carcinoma.

Q34

Most thyroid lymphomas are classified as diffuse large B-cell type.

Q35

Metastatic renal carcinoma clinically may simulate primary thyroid carcinoma.

Normal anatomy

A1. False

The thyroid *anlage* appears on the posterior tongue at the site corresponding to the foramen cecum. It gives rise to the thyroglossal duct, which in turn gives rise to the thyroid. **(p. 516)**

A2. True

The size and shape of cells lining the thyroid follicles varies depending on the degree of their activity. **(p. 516)**

A3. True

TTF-1 is a good marker for thyroid follicular cells and it does not react with C cells. Antibodies to TTF-1 react with pulmonary alveolar cells. These antibodies are useful for identifying thyroid and pulmonary tumors. **(p. 516)**

A4. False

The number of C cells varies according to age: they are more numerous in infancy and old age than in adults. In old age they even may form nodular aggregates. **(p. 516)**

A5. True

Solid nests are found in almost all thyroid glands and are thought to be remnants of the ultimobranchial body, which in turn is derived from the branchial cleft pouch complex IV–V. Such lumina contain mucin and may become cystically dilated. **(p. 516)**

Congenital abnormalities

A1. False

Thyroglossal duct cyst is typically located in the midline of the neck, in the region of the hyoid bone. It is a remnant of the thyroglossal duct, which normally involutes leaving no residues. **(p. 517)**

A2. False

As in the normal thyroid most malignant tumors developing in the thyroglossal cysts are papillary carcinomas. **(p. 517)**

A3. True

Heterotopic thyroid tissue can be found anywhere along the course of the thyroglossal duct. The most frequent location is the base of the tongue. **(p. 518)**

A4. True

The exact location of these cysts depends on their derivation, but generally they are found on the lateral sides of the neck. They are lined by squamous epithelium, but columnar ciliated epithelium is also common. Abundant lymphoid tissue, often with germinal centers, is observed beneath. Cysts located in the lower neck may also contain mucinous, seromucinous and sebaceous glands. **(p. 518)**

Thyroiditis

A1. True

It may be associated with acute infections of the upper aerodigestive tract, generalized sepsis, or major trauma to the neck with an open wound. It tends to affect the malnourished infant, the debilitated elderly, and the immunocompromised patient. **(p. 519)**

A2. True

Granulomatous thyroiditis, also known as de Quervain's or subacute thyroiditis, typically presents in middle-aged women with sore throat, painful deglutition, and marked tenderness on palpation. Microscopically, it presents with chronic inflammation and prominent granulomas that contain multinucleated giant cells surrounding disrupted thyroid follicles. **(p. 520)**

A3. True

Hashimoto's thyroiditis, also known as struma lymphomatosa, is a form of autoimmune thyroiditis characterized functionally by the production of autoantibodies to thyroid antigens. Cellular immune mechanisms also play a role in the destruction of the thyroid. **(p. 521)**

A4. False

Hashimoto's thyroiditis is predominantly a disease of women over 40 years of age. It presents as diffuse firm thyroid enlargement, initially accompanied by mild hyperthyroidism that subsequently evolves into hypothyroidism. In young women, enlargement of the thyroid that is soft on palpation is usually caused by colloid goiter. Severe hyperthyroidism at any age is most often caused by Graves' disease. **(p. 521)**

A5. True

The lymphoid tissue is distributed within and around the lobules, and it invariably exhibits large follicles with prominent germinal centers. The follicles are lined by oxyphilic Hürthle cells. These cells have eosinophilic cytoplasm filled with mitochondria. The nuclei of these cells may show enlargement and hyperchromasia or, conversely, an optically clear appearance and an overlapping quality reminiscent of that seen in papillary carcinoma. **(p. 521)**

A6. False

Medullary thyroid carcinoma rarely occurs in Hashimoto's thyroiditis, and if found it is usually a coincidental finding. Three most common complications are malignant lymphoma, papillary carcinoma and Hürthle cell neoplasms. As these complications evolve slowly it is often difficult to recognize them in the early stages of development. **(p. 523)**

A7. False

Riedel's thyroiditis, a very rare disease, is not pathogenetically related to Hashimoto's thyroiditis, which in turn is a very common disease. Instead, it is considered to be a form of *inflammatory fibrosclerosis* of unknown etiology and is probably pathogenetically related to mediastinal or retroperitoneal fibrosis, sclerosing cholangitis, or inflammatory pseudotumor of the orbit. Riedel's thyroiditis may coexist with these fibrosclerotic inflammatory diseases. **(p. 523–524)**

A8. False

Grossly, the thyroid glands of children with dyshormonogenetic goiter are enlarged and multinodular. Microscopically, the most hypercellular nodules exhibit a variety of architectural appearances, with a predominance of solid and microfollicular patterns. Fibrosis is a common finding. There is marked nuclear atypia and minimal amounts of colloid. A diagnostically important feature is the fact that the nuclear atypia (in the form of bizarre hyperchromatic nuclei) is present mainly in the tissue *between* the hyperplastic nodules rather than in the nodules themselves. Mitotic figures are often seen, presumably as a result of the continuous thyrotropin stimulation. **(p. 524)**

A9. False

The follicles in Graves' disease are hyperplastic and often show prominent papillary infolding that may cause confusion with papillary carcinoma. The lining epithelium is columnar, with basally located normochromatic or hyperchromatic nuclei and a clear, sometimes microvacuolated, cytoplasm. The colloid appears scalloped along the border with the epithelium. **(p. 525)**

A10. True

Lymphoid aggregates and follicles are common in Graves' disease. Hyperplastic lymphoid follicles may be seen inside and outside the thyroid gland, sometimes growing into the skeletal muscle of the neck. This may represent extrathyroid extension of the disease. Immunohistochemically, most of these lymphocytes are of the T-cell type, the cytotoxic–suppressor subtype predominating in the follicles and the helper-induced subtype in the interstitium. **(p. 525)**

A11. False

Some nodules are composed of huge follicles lined by flattened epithelium, others are extremely cellular and hyperplastic, and still others are composed predominantly or exclusively of Hürthle cells. Others have papillary projections facing the lumen of a cystic follicle, a feature that may lead to confusion with papillary carcinoma. **(p. 527–528)**

A12. True

Areas of fresh and old hemorrhage, coarse fibrous trabeculation, and foci of calcification are common. Rupture of follicles leads to a granulomatous reaction to the colloid, with the appearance of macrophages and foreign body-type giant cells. **(p. 528)**

A13. False

More recent studies have shown that a significant proportion of the 'dominant' nodules of nodular hyperplasia are monoclonal, whereas a smaller but still significant percentage of lesions morphologically consistent with follicular adenomas are polyclonal. Thus, the thyroid adenomas arising in multinodular goiters cannot be reliably distinguished from hyperplastic nodules. **(p. 528)**

Tumors

A1. True

Follicular adenomas arising from the follicular epithelium are the most common thyroid tumors. Primary malignant tumors are more common than metastases to the thyroid. **(p. 529)**

A2. True

Most follicular adenomas are well-encapsulated benign tumors composed of thyroid follicles. Usually they are hormonally inactive, or less active than the surrounding normal parenchyma. **(p. 529)**

A3. True

Thyroid adenomas typically present as a lump, which on scan is usually 'cold,' sometimes 'cool' or 'warm,' and only rarely 'hot.' Most hot nodules are benign, but of course there are exceptions. **(p. 529–530)**

A4. False

DNA aneuploidy is common in benign follicular adenomas and seems to be slightly more common in the cellular types. It is not an indicator of clinical malignancy, nor of an increased possibility of tumor recurrence. **(p. 530)**

A5. False

This is a thyroid adenoma with bizarre nuclei. Such nuclei occur usually in clusters, unaccompanied by other features of malignancy. This phenomenon is analogous to that seen in parathyroid adenomas and other endocrine neoplasms, and should not be considered a sign of malignancy. **(p. 530)**

A6. True

Females are affected by papillary carcinoma more often than males. It can present in any age group, the mean age at the time of initial diagnosis being approximately 40 years. Papillary carcinoma accounts for more than 90% of thyroid malignancies in children. **(p. 532)**

A7. True

The papillae of a classic papillary carcinoma are complex and branching and lined by a single layer of cuboidal cells. **(p. 533)**

A8. False

Ground-glass nuclei are best seen in sections obtained from paraffin-embedded material, regardless of the fixative used, but are less apparent or absent altogether in frozen sections or cytology material. **(p. 533)**

A9. False

Psammoma bodies are found almost exclusively in papillary carcinoma. They are found in approximately half of the cases. They may be located in the papillary stalk, in the fibrous stroma, or between tumor cells in solid foci. Their presence strongly suggests the diagnosis of papillary carcinoma, in as much as their occurrence in other thyroid lesions is exceptional. **(p. 534)**

A10. True

Papillary carcinoma of the thyroid is TTF-1+, and CK7+/CK20–. Of potentially greater diagnostic importance is the fact that the cells of this tumor stain for cytokeratin 19 and for the high molecular weight keratin demonstrated with 34βE12. **(p. 535)**

A11. False

Small thyroid tumors that present as a stellate scar are called papillary microcarcinoma or papillary microtumors. They may be completely encapsulated, but some of them are not. In contrast to these microcarcinomas, encapsulated papillary carcinomas are *totally* surrounded by a capsule. The cytoarchitectural (and particularly the nuclear) features of this variant are the same as for the conventional invasive type. **(p. 536)**

A12. False

This is a papillary carcinoma composed entirely or almost entirely of follicles. The diagnosis is based largely on the presence of the set of nuclear features classically associated with papillary carcinoma. Metastases typically show better-developed papillary structures. **(p. 537)**

A13. False

The *tall cell* variant is a type of papillary carcinoma characterized by papillae lined by a single layer of 'tall' cells (the height being at least twice the width) and an abundant acidophilic, quasi-oncocytic cytoplasm. These features should be present in at least half of the tumor for it to be placed in this category. The pattern of growth is usually highly papillary. The nuclei usually lack the optically clear appearance, grooves and pseudoinclusions seen in papillary carcinoma. **(p. 539)**

A14. False

Distant metastases may occur, but are uncommonly found at the time of diagnosis in the vast majority of patients. On the other hand, local extension into the neck structures and metastases to neck lymph nodes are found very often, particularly in young patients. **(p. 540)**

A15. False

Almost all patients who died of papillary carcinoma were over 40 years of age and the tumors of young women have a good prognosis. Despite previous statements to the contrary, the history of previous irradiation does not adversely affect the prognosis. **(p. 541)**

A16. True

Microscopically, the pattern of growth usually resembles that of an adenoma of embryonal, fetal or atypical type. The diagnosis of malignancy depends entirely on the demonstration of blood vessel and/or capsular invasion. **(p. 543)**

A17. True

This is a useful finding and should prompt the pathologist to sample adequately the border zones between the tumor and the normal thyroid to document the invasion. If the capsular invasion is questionable and the tumor shows no papillary carcinoma-type nuclear changes, it should be signed out as *follicular tumor of uncertain malignant potential*. If the nuclear changes are questionable, however, the tumor should be signed out as *well differentiated tumor of uncertain malignant potential*. **(p. 543)**

A18. False

Many widely invasive follicular carcinomas have a capsule, but it may be incomplete. Actually there are two categories of these tumors: the encapsulated tumors, in which one has to look for invasion; and the widely invasive tumors, in which one has a look for a capsule. **(p. 543)**

A19. True

Their cytoplasmic granularity is due to the accumulation of mitochondria. In H&E-stained sections the granularity should have a deeply eosinophilic quality. Secondary clearing is not uncommon, usually due to mitochondrial swelling. The term oncocytic tumor is reserved for tumors composed predominantly (over 75%) of oncocytes. **(p. 544)**

A20. True

This phenomenon, which is analogous to that seen in oncocytic tumors at other sites and which is probably the consequence of the great sensitivity of oncocytes to ischemia, can render the identification of the tumor difficult or impossible. **(p. 547)**

A21. True

Large, locally invasive Hürthle cell carcinomas, and especially those that have metastasized, have a poor prognosis. In contrast to papillary carcinoma the latter applies not only to distant metastases but also to regional lymph node involvement. **(p. 547)**

A22. False

Clear cell changes occur in many thyroid tumors and even in non-neoplastic follicular cells, especially in Hashimoto's thyroiditis and dyshormonogenetic goiter. These changes are due to the accumulation of glycogen, lipid, thyroglobulin or 'mucin.' The natural history of these tumors is determined by their basic nature rather than the presence of, degree of, or reason for cytoplasmic clearing in them. Therefore *clear cell carcinoma* should not be viewed as a specific tumor type. **(p. 547–548)**

A23. True

Insular carcinomas are tumors composed of relatively uniform small cells arranged into nests ('insular pattern of growth'). The nests may be solid or show a microfollicular arrangement. Fresh ischemic tumor necrosis may account for the peritheliomatous pattern, resulting from the preservation of tumor cells around the nutrient vessels and confluent necrosis at a distance from them. The insular pattern may result in a mistaken diagnosis of medullary carcinoma. **(p. 550)**

A24. False

Undifferentiated (anaplastic) carcinomas may be composed of spindle cells. These tumors are called *sarcomatoid* carcinomas. However, this is only one of several possible microscopic patterns recognized in these tumors. Some tumors show extreme anaplasia and are composed predominantly of giant cells. Still others, called *squamoid*, retain an unmistakable epithelioid appearance. In rare instances undifferentiated thyroid carcinomas resemble nasopharyngeal carcinomas and are referred to as *lymphoepithelioma-like* carcinomas. **(p. 552)**

A25. True

Most undifferentiated thyroid carcinoma arise from some other pre-existing thyroid tumor, usually papillary carcinoma, but also follicular carcinoma, Hürthle cell carcinoma and insular carcinoma. Residual parts of the existing tumor may be seen inside the predominantly undifferentiated carcinoma. In most instances the anaplastic transformation takes place in the primary tumor, but it can also occur in a metastatic focus. **(p. 553)**

A26. True

Like normal C cells, medullary carcinoma cells synthesize calcitonin. Medullary carcinomas contain stromal amyloid, which is derived from calcitonin. **(p. 554–556)**

A27. True

However, in addition to this most common growth pattern, several others are recognized, including carcinoid-like, paraganglioma-like, trabecular, glandular (tubular and follicular), or pseudopapillary. The stroma may be scanty, hemorrhagic, ossified or edematous. The amyloid deposition may be widespread, limited to small psammomatoid concretions, or altogether absent. Sometimes this amyloid elicits a florid foreign body-type giant cell reaction. True psammoma bodies may be present. **(p. 554)**

A28. True

Medullary carcinomas are consistently positive for CEA, but also stain with antibodies to calcitonin, TTF-1, cytokeratins and neuroendocrine markers such as synaptophysin and chromogranins. **(p. 555)**

A29. False

Medullary carcinomas are sporadic in 80% of cases and familial in 20%. Sporadic tumors occur most often in the fifth decade, the mean age at diagnosis being 45 years. Most familial tumors become clinically apparent before the age of 35 years. **(p. 556)**

A30. False

Together with pheochromocytoma, medullary carcinoma may be part of MEN II A or MEN IIB. In families with familial medullary carcinoma of MEN II there is a germline mutation of the tumor suppressor gene *RET* located on chromosome 10.q11.2. **(p. 556)**

A31. False

Solitary nodules are more likely to be malignant than multiple nodules. The likelihood of malignancy for nodules found in Hashimoto's thyroiditis is the same as for those found in the normal gland. **(p. 556)**

A32. False

Thyroglobulin is usually elevated in patients with either papillary or follicular carcinoma. Radioactive iodine can be used to scan the body for metastases of these thyroglobulin-producing tumors. Medullary carcinoma and undifferentiated carcinoma do not produce thyroglobulin. **(p. 560)**

A33. True

Thyroid tissue found in neck lymph nodes represents metastases from a papillary carcinoma of the thyroid. These microscopic foci usually show some or most cytoarchitectural features of papillary carcinoma. These metastases must be distinguished from occasional foci of ectopic thyroid tissue found in the lymph node capsule. These thyroid follicles lack the nuclear characteristics of papillary carcinoma. **(p. 562)**

A34. True

The majority of thyroid lymphomas are diffuse large B-cell lymphomas, followed by low-grade lymphomas composed of small or 'intermediate' lymphocytes having either a diffuse or a nodular (follicular) pattern of growth. **(p. 564)**

A35. True

Metastases to the thyroid may be found at autopsy in patients who have widespread terminal cancer, but rarely do such metastases present clinically in the differential diagnosis of thyroid masses. The only exception are renal cell carcinomas, which may present as a thyroid mass in the absence of renal symptoms, or years after the removal of the primary renal tumor. **(p. 568)**

Parathyroid glands 10

Normal anatomy and physiology

Q1
The parathyroid glands were the last major organ system to be recognized in humans.

Q2
Owing to embryologic considerations, humans invariably have four parathyroid glands, arranged in two pairs.

Q3
The upper and lower parathyroid glands arise from the fourth branchial cleft.

Q4
The location of paired parathyroid glands often reflects symmetrical mirror images.

Q5
The upper and lower parathyroid glands have independent blood supplies.

Q6
Abnormal migration of the glands during embryonic life may result in anomalous locations for the adult organs.

Q7
Current evidence suggests that the parathyroid gland is made up of one basic cell type, the chief cell.

Q8
The chief cell contains variable amounts of glycogen particles and secretory droplets.

Q9
Chief cells contain chromogranin A and B, as well as keratin and vimentin.

Q10
The oxyphil cell is a morphologic variant containing abundant mitochondria and few secretory granules.

Q11
The water-clear cell is defined by optically clear cytoplasm and sharply defined cell borders.

Q12
The chief cell and its morphologic variants are present in all parathyroid glands.

Q13
In the normal adult, the amount of fat in cells is approximately 60%.

Q14
Parathyroid tissue can be confused with thyroid tissue owing to the presence of microcysts and intracystic colloid-like material.

Q15
The endocrine function of parathyroid glands is mediated through the production of PTH, a polypeptide hormone whose activity resides in the first 34 amino acid residues.

Q16
The most important physiologic action of PTH is the mobilization of calcium from bone.

Parathyroid adenoma

Q1
Parathyroid adenomas occur most frequently in men than in women.

Q2
Adenomas can occur at any age, but are more common in the fourth decade.

Q3

Parathyroid adenomas occur only as single tumors.

Q4

The incidence of adenomas is evenly distributed among the four glands.

Q5

Microscopically, parathyroid adenomas consist of only one clonally expanded cell type.

Q6

A compressed rim of normal parathyroid tissue is necessary to make the diagnosis of adenoma.

Q7

Large, hyperchromatic nuclei are a sign of malignant transformation in adenomas.

Q8

In the typical clinical case, the presence of a microscopically normal second gland represents the best evidence that the index parathyroid lesion is an adenoma.

Q9

Parathyroid adenoma cells express neurofilament not normally found in normal parathyroid tissue.

Q10

Molecular alterations clearly distinguish adenomas from hyperplasia.

Q11

Oxyphilic adenomas usually present with hypercalcemia.

Q12

A lipoadenoma is defined as a parathyroid adenoma with abundant mature adipose tissue.

Q13

Overexpression of p53 is commonly found in parathyroid hyperplasia.

Parathyroid hyperplasia

Q1

Primary chief cell hyperplasia is a constant finding in MEN syndromes types I, IIa and IIb.

Q2

The finding of numerous microscopic foci of hyperplastic parathyroid tissue in the neck is known as parathyromatosis.

Q3

The distinction between primary and secondary chief cell hyperplasia cannot be made on morphologic grounds.

Q4

The degree of proliferative activity is an accurate way to distinguish between adenoma and chief cell hyperplasia.

Q5

Like chief cell hyperplasia, water-clear hyperplasia is associated with a familial incidence and occurs in multiple endocrine neoplasia syndromes.

Q6

The incidence of water-clear hyperplasia has been increasing in most surgical pathology laboratories.

Parathyroid carcinoma

Q1

Parathyroid carcinoma typically presents as a midline neck mass in patients with normal calcium levels.

Q2

Parathyroid glands that are hard and adherent to adjacent structures at the time of surgery are suspicious for carcinoma.

Q3

Microscopically, parathyroid carcinomas cannot be distinguished from adenomas.

Q4

Parathyroid carcinomas show an increase in the mean number of nuclear organizing regions (AgNOR).

Q5

Parathyroid carcinomas are characterized by increased Ki-67-positive cells and decreased cyclin-D1 expression.

Q6

Tumor size and lymph node status are significant prognostic factors in patients with parathyroid carcinoma.

Other lesions

Q1

Parathyroid cysts usually arise from the superior glands.

Q2

Systemic amyloidosis often involves the parathyroid glands.

Hyperparathyroidism

Q1

The pathologic changes in primary hyperthyroidism may be those of adenoma, hyperplasia or carcinoma.

Q2

The incidence of primary hyperparathyroidism is 2.5 per 1000 individuals and is restricted to the adult population.

Q3

The incidence of primary hyperparathyroidism is increased in patients who have had their necks irradiated.

Q4

Primary hyperparathyroidism can occur in patients with normal serum calcium levels.

Q5

Osteitis fibrosa cystica consists of bone cysts and brown tumors.

Q6

Brown tumors and giant cell granuloma of bone share similar radiographic features but are easily distinguished by microscopic examination.

Q7

Hereditary hyperparathyroidism and jaw tumors is a rare syndrome linked to the *HRPT2* gene at locus 1q21-23.

Q8

A symptom complex related to renal stones is a common clinical manifestation of hyperparathyroidism.

Q9

Intestinal malabsorption is the main cause of secondary hyperparathyroidism.

Q10

Circulating parathyroid hormone (PTH) levels are proportional to the severity of renal failure in secondary hyperthyroidism.

Q11

The bone changes of secondary hyperparathyroidism are distinct from those occurring in primary hyperthyroidism.

Q12

Cutaneous calciphylaxis is an uncommon skin disorder that is a cosmetic nuisance but of little clinical consequence.

Q13

Autonomous parathyroid stimulation characterizes tertiary hyperparathyroidism.

Q14

Morphometry has shown that nuclear size is greater in tertiary parathyroid disease than in secondary disease.

Q15

The differential diagnosis of primary hyperparathyroidism includes sarcoidosis, hyperthyroidism, multiple myeloma, milk-alkali syndrome, vitamin D overdose and vitamin A intoxication.

Q16

The cause of humoral hypercalcemia of malignancy is a nodular hyperplastic expansion of the parathyroid parenchyma.

Q17

The most common location of aberrant parathyroid glands in patients with persistent hyperparathyroidism after surgery is posterior to the thyroid gland.

Q18

Minimizing the disruption of the normal neck anatomy by the simple excision of a parathyroid adenoma is the preferred surgical approach to hyperparathyroidism.

Q19

An alternative approach to the treatment of primary or secondary hyperparathyroidism is the performance of a total parathyroidectomy with autotransplantation of parathyroid tissue into the forearm muscle.

Q20

Parathyroid carcinoma is best treated by excision of the tumor and associated soft tissues with ipsilateral lymph node dissection.

Frozen section

Q1

The main role of the pathologist at the time of frozen section is simply to determine whether a given nodule is in fact parathyroid tissue.

Q2

By careful cryostat sectioning and adherence to strict microscopic criteria, the pathologist can usually distinguish between parathyroid adenoma and parathyroid hyperplasia.

Q3

Staining with lipid stains such as oil red O greatly enhances diagnostic accuracy for distinguishing normal parathyroid glands from parathyroid hyperplasia and parathyroid adenoma.

Normal anatomy and physiology

A1. True

It was only in 1880 that Ivar Sandstrom, a Swedish medical student, discovered the parathyroid glands. **(p. 595)**

A2. False

In rare instances more than four glands are present. Studies have been reported in which there were five or six glands. **(p. 595)**

A3. False

Whereas the upper pair arises from the fourth branchial cleft, the lower pair arises from the third branchial cleft and descends into the neck with the thymus. **(p. 595)**

A4. True

When one parathyroid is located in one place, the opposite gland will be in the contralateral mirror image of that space. **(p. 595)**

A5. True

The vascular supply can be variable, but the superior thyroid artery typically feeds the upper glands and the blood supply for the lower parathyroid glands comes from branches of the inferior thyroid arteries. This fact may be helpful in locating abnormally placed glands during surgery. **(p. 595)**

A6. True

The upper glands may be located inside the carotid sheath or behind the cervical or thoracic esophagus. The lower glands may follow the thymus into the anterior portion of the mediastinum. They may also assume an intrathyroid location. **(p. 595)**

A7. True

It is now thought that all other cell types identified in the parathyroid gland represent chief cell variants, reflecting different physiologic activities. **(p. 596)**

A8. True

Ultrastructurally, both species are present in inverse proportions. **(p. 596)**

A9. False

These cells contain only chromogranin A and are typically negative for vimentin. **(p. 596)**

A10. True

Oxyphilic cells are often present in nodular collections and contain a high proportion of oxidative enzymes. **(p. 596)**

A11. True

There are also transitional water-clear cells that have an appearance intermediate between chief cells and water-clear cells. **(p. 596)**

A12. False

The adolescent gland typically is typically composed solely of chief cells. **(p. 596)**

A13. False

The average percentage of stromal fat in the adult parathyroid is closer to 40%. **(p. 596)**

A14. True

This distinction may be difficult on frozen section evaluation. The presence of birefringent calcium oxalate crystals favors thyroid. **(p. 596)**

A15. True

Under normal conditions serum calcium levels mediate the secretion of this hormone. **(p. 596)**

A16. False

PTH acts in multiple ways. In addition to mobilizing calcium from bone, it increases renal excretion of phosphate, increases renal reabsorption of calcium, and increases intestinal absorption of calcium. **(p. 596)**

Parathyroid adenoma

A1. False

Adenomas occur more frequently in women than in men, at a ratio of 3:1. **(p. 597)**

A2. True

However, adolescent cases have been reported. **(p. 597)**

A3. False

Although the vast majority of adenoma cases are single, cases of double or triple adenomas have been reported. **(p. 597)**

A4. False

75% of all adenomas of involve one of the inferior glands. **(p. 597)**

A5. False

An adenoma may be composed of a combination of any of the various cell types found in the normal parathyroid gland. **(p. 597)**

A6. False

A compressed rim of normal parathyroid tissue is only found in 60% of adenoma cases. **(p. 597)**

A7. False

The presence of these nuclei does not indicate malignancy. Paradoxically, atypical nuclei are seen more often in benign tumors. **(p. 597)**

A8. True
Owing to the vagaries in distinguishing parathyroid adenoma from parathyroid hyperplasia, the presence of a microscopically normal second gland militates for a diagnosis of adenoma. **(p. 598)**

A9. True
Immunoreactivity for this intermediate filament is typical of adenomatous transformation. **(p. 598)**

A10. False
To date, neither clonality studies nor specific genetic abnormalities definitely define parathyroid adenoma. **(p. 598)**

A11. False
Oxyphilic adenomas are typically non-functioning. **(p. 599)**

A12. True
Lipoadenoma is an unusual morphologic variant of parathyroid adenoma. Most cases are functioning. This entity has been reported as lipohyperplasia as well as parathyroid hamartoma. **(p. 599)**

A13. False
Although only some adenomas overexpress p53, it is practically never seen in secondary hyperplasias. **(p. 599)**

Parathyroid hyperplasia

A1. False
Patients with MEN IIb exhibit normal parathyroid histology during childhood and a minimal degree of chief cell hyperplasia in adulthood. **(p. 599)**

A2. True
This phenomenon may be responsible for some cases of recurrent hyperparathyroidism after technically successful surgery. **(p. 600)**

A3. True
In general, fibrous septation, acinar formation and giant nuclei occur more commonly in primary hyperplasia. Oxyphil cells tend to be more prominent in the secondary form. Usually the diagnosis is made using a combination of clinical information and laboratory test results. **(p. 601)**

A4. False
The presence of the rim of normal parenchyma around the mass and the identification of at least one normal parathyroid gland elsewhere are the only definitive criteria by which a diagnosis of adenoma can be made over chief cell hyperplasia. **(p. 601)**

A5. False
There is no familial incidence to chief cell hyperplasia, nor is there an association with multiple endocrine neoplasia syndromes. **(p. 601)**

A6. False
Water-clear hyperplasia is becoming increasingly rare. The reason for this is not known. **(p. 601)**

Parathyroid carcinoma

A1. False
Parathyroid carcinoma typically presents with hyperparathyroidism. In one series, skeletal disease was present in 73% of patients and renal disease was present in 26%. **(p. 602)**

A2. True
During surgical dissection parathyroid tumors that are hard, desmoplastic or infiltrative are most suspicious for being carcinoma. **(p. 602)**

A3. False
Although these entities may share histologic features, carcinomas typically grow in a trabecular arrangement, have dense fibrous bands, show a spindle cell morphology and have increased mitotic activity. Additionally, carcinomas tend to invade the glandular capsule and adjacent blood vessels. **(p. 602)**

A4. True
Compared to hyperplastic or adenomatous parathyroid glands, carcinomas show a statistically significant increased mean AgNOR number. **(p. 603)**

A5. False
Both markers are increased in parathyroid carcinoma. **(p. 603)**

A6. False
Neither tumor size nor nodal status was found to be a significant prognostic factor. **(p. 603)**

Other lesions

A1. False
Cysts usually arise from the inferior glands. **(p. 603)**

A2. True
Both AL amyloid and other systemic forms will affect the parathyroid glands. **(p. 603)**

Hyperparathyroidism

A1. True
Parathyroid carcinoma constitutes less than 4% of cases. Water-clear cell hyperplasia is rare. **(p. 603)**

A2. False
Although it usually occurs in adults, primary hyperparathyroidism can be found in children. **(p. 604)**

A3. True
Its incidence is also increased in patients with MEN syndromes. **(p. 604)**

A4. True
Although the typical findings include hypercalcemia, hypophosphatemia and hypercalcemia, well-documented instances of normocalcemic patients have been reported. **(p. 604)**

A5. True
This combination of findings should suggest the diagnosis of hyperparathyroidism. **(p. 604)**

A6. False
Their microscopic appearances are essentially identical. Laboratory findings are necessary to distinguish these two lesions. **(p. 605)**

A7. True
Patients with the syndrome may have Wilms' tumor or other renal abnormalities. **(p. 605)**

A8. True
Patients may also have associated hypertension, peptic ulcer and pancreatitis. Mental disturbances have been described. **(p. 605)**

A9. False
Chronic renal disease is the most common cause of secondary hyperthyroidism. **(p. 606)**

A10. True
Serum levels of PTH are higher in renal failure than in other forms of hyperparathyroidism. **(p. 606)**

A11. False
Bone changes are qualitatively similar. However, they are generally less severe. **(p. 606)**

A12. False
This disorder is potentially lethal. Microscopically there are vascular calcifications associated with skin ulcerations and calcifying septal panniculitis. **(p. 606)**

A13. True
This phenomenon also is referred to as non-suppressible or refractory hyperparathyroidism. It occurs despite the correction of the renal disease by hemodialysis or transplantation. **(p. 606)**

A14. True
Also, there is a greater tendency to histologic nodularity and a higher percentage of oxyphil cells in the non-suppressible state. **(p. 606)**

A15. True
Additional conditions include familial hypercalcemic hypocalciuria and humeral hypercalcemia of malignancy. **(p. 607)**

A16. False
In this syndrome the parathyroid glands appear morphologically normal or only minimally hyperplastic. Serum biochemical parameters indicate suppressed parathyroid function. The mechanism for hypercalcemia is the secretion of a peptide with partial homology to PTH. **(p. 607)**

A17. False
Most hidden glands are located in the posterosuperior portion of the mediastinum at the level of the thoracic inlet, or the anteroposterior portion of the mediastinum. **(p. 607)**

A18. False
Despite the complete excision of the presumed adenoma, it is generally recognized that additional tissue dissection with identification and biopsy of at least one other parathyroid gland is necessary to rule out hyperplasia. **(p. 607)**

A19. True
This approach avoids hypoparathyroidism. However, there may be a rapid growth of the transplanted tissue, leading to the recurrence of disease or the simulation of a malignant process. **(p. 608)**

A20. False
The indication for lymph node dissection remains controversial. **(p. 608)**

Frozen section

A1. True

In as much as it is very difficult to diagnose adenoma from hyperplasia, the identification of a small biopsy sample as normal parathyroid tissue becomes a significant issue. **(p. 608)**

A2. False

Given a single gland, it is usually not possible to distinguish between hyperplasia and adenoma. **(p. 608)**

A3. False

The rate of discordant results indicates caution for this technique. **(p. 608)**

Gastrointestinal tract 11

Esophagus

Q1

The normal lower esophageal sphincter is readily identified and has a fixed anatomic location.

Q2

Primary melanoma of the esophagus does not exist, as there are no melanocytes within the esophageal epithelium.

Q3

There is no muscularis mucosae within the esophagus.

Q4

The upper and lower thirds of the esophagus are drained into lymph node chains of disparate locations, from cervical to para-aortic and the celiac axis, respectively.

Q5

The complex embryologic development of the area accounts for varied congenital malformations.

Q6

Focal gastric-type epithelial lining only occurs in the lower esophagus secondary to reflux.

Q7

There are multiple possible mechanisms for diverticula/pseudodiverticula formation, but their clinical presentation and complications are similar.

Q8

Intraepithelial eosinophils are pathognomonic of reflux.

Q9

Various metaplasias, including goblet cells within the lower esophageal epithelium, are diagnostic of early uncomplicated reflux.

Q10

The gold standard of diagnosis for esophagitis in view of treatment is the microscopic appearance of the biopsy.

Q11

The gastroesophageal junction is 40 cm from the incisors, and biopsy demonstrating gastric epithelium will confirm this.

Q12

The so-called multilayered epithelium is a sign of early reflux disease and refers to thickening of the squamous epithelium.

Q13

For the microscopic diagnosis of Barrett's esophagus it should suffice to identify one or two goblet cells, particularly for the short segment variety.

Q14

Special stains are required for the diagnosis of Barrett's esophagus.

Q15

Because the metaplastic epithelium in Barrett's mucosa is by definition of the intestinal type, *Helicobacter pylori* is not expected to be adherent to mucus.

Q16

The mainstay of therapy in uncomplicated Barrett's esophagus is the prevention of acid reflux, the reflux being controlled by proton pump inhibitors.

Q17

Following the re-establishment of a lower esophageal sphincter function, including by surgical means, the metaplastic change is reversible; once the presence of a squamous epithelium is confirmed on a follow-up biopsy, the patient still needs regular follow-up.

Q18

Surface epithelial multilayering in a tufting pattern is a sign of low-grade dysplasia.

Q19

The dystrophic goblet cell refers to one with an enlarged nucleus and an irregular nuclear outline.

Q20

A biopsy with metaplastic epithelium and concurrent prominent inflammation can have cytoplasmic basophilia and anisonucleosis, and qualify for negative-for-dysplasia status.

Q21

The differential diagnosis between intramucosal carcinoma and invasive carcinoma in an esophageal biopsy is crucial to determine the right therapeutic approach.

Q22

The diagnosis of high-grade dysplasia relies on specific criteria separating it from in situ carcinoma.

Q23

Adenocarcinoma arising in a Barrett's mucosa is similar histologically and epidemiologically to gastric adenocarcinoma of the cardia, but differs in metastatic spread patterns.

Q24

Herpes simplex esophagitis is frequently found in autopsies from immunosuppressed hosts.

Q25

Multinucleated squamous cells in esophageal biopsies should prompt immunohistochemical evaluation for herpes simplex viral proteins.

Q26

Confirmed herpes esophagitis mandates a systematic evaluation to identify the underlying immunodeficiency state.

Q27

'Volcano ulcers' on endoscopy are suspicious for herpes or cytomegalovirus (CMV) disease.

Q28

Clinically significant esophagitis and dysmotility not uncommonly participate in systemic diseases, including scleroderma and hypersensitivity reactions.

Q29

Squamous cell carcinoma of the esophagus has a widely variable incidence around the world, with hot spots, most likely a function of lifestyle, dietary habits and environmental causes.

Q30

Oncogenic viral strains such as human papillomavirus (HPV) may have an important role in the etiology of esophageal cancer in some parts of the world.

Q31

Squamous cell carcinoma most commonly affects the middle and lower thirds of the esophagus.

Q32

A frozen section for margin evaluation is not justified during surgery for esophageal squamous cell carcinoma, as the surgeon has reliable clinical clues as far as free margins are concerned.

Q33

The diagnosis of squamous cell carcinoma of the esophagus relies heavily on the presence of squamous pearls, a constant and readily evident finding in biopsy material.

Q34

In situ carcinoma is increasingly recognized as the precursor lesion to invasive carcinoma in areas with a high incidence of esophageal cancer.

Q35

Superficial carcinoma and microinvasive carcinoma are terms that refer to the same entity regarding esophageal lesions.

Q36

Superficial spreading carcinoma is a synonym for intramucosal carcinoma.

Q37

So-called early carcinoma of the esophagus has an excellent prognosis.

Q38

Nodal metastasis is an early event in esophageal carcinoma and is often clinically silent at the time of initial therapy.

Q39

Diagnostic cytology, a low-tech approach to early diagnosis in terms of costs, is particularly well suited to mass screening in countries with a high incidence of carcinoma, such as China or South Africa.

Q40

Common stromal lesions include leiomyomas/smooth muscle hyperplasias, so-called gastrointestinal stromal tumors (GISTs) and granular cell tumors.

Stomach

Q1

The functional anatomy of the stomach is exactly superimposable on the regional anatomy, in that the cardia, fundic and antral-type mucosa always correspond to parts of the stomach with the same name.

Q2

The combined special stain for neutral and acidic mucins will typically be helpful in ruling out intestinal metaplasia in the normal stomach, as only neutral PAS-positive mucin should be present.

Q3

The relative ratio of length of pits (foveolae) versus that of glands is diagnostic of fundic and antral mucosa, respectively, under physiologic conditions.

Q4

The gastric neuroendocrine cell population is rich and varied, and the associated pathologies are subdivided according to the specific cell of origin, the basis for current classification.

Q5

The cardia and most of the lesser curve have a lymph node drainage into the hepatic and pyloric nodes at the head of the pancreas.

Q6

The anatomic pyloric sphincter corresponds to the inner circular layer of the muscularis externa at the gastroduodenal junction.

Q7

Based on the normal anatomy of gastric lymphatic drainage, a radiation oncologist will have to protect the left renal artery if the cancer involves the greater curvature and postoperative treatment is warranted.

Q8

The differential diagnosis of a gastric antral submucosal mass, sometimes ulcerated, includes heterotopic pancreas and adenomyoma.

Q9

Endocrine cells and even occasionally islets can be seen in both pancreatic heterotopia and metaplasia within the stomach.

Q10

Hypertrophic pyloric stenosis affects adults with long-standing peptic ulcer disease and attendant gastric outlet obstruction.

Q11

Gastric mass lesions are always malignant, and as the high incidence of false negative biopsies is well known, a gastrectomy is the most direct approach.

Q12

Chronic gastritis is defined for diagnostic purposes by the presence of inflammatory cells in the lamina propria.

Q13

Chronic antral gastritis is often associated with parietal cell antibodies.

Q14

The rather well defined variation in regional involvement by the inflammatory infiltrate within the stomach corresponds to different etiologic processes.

Q15

Complete or incomplete epithelial intestinal-type metaplastic changes may be part of the inflammatory process, involving surface or glandular epithelium or both.

Q16

In a surgical pathology report, description/identification of the type of mucosa seen is important, as a correctly identified gastric biopsy may have a totally convincing intestinal morphology.

Q17

There is excellent correlation of the endoscopic appearance and the morphology in gastritis.

Q18

Helicobacter pylori is a curved spirochete-like bacterium that is not readily seen on routine sections and needs electron microscopy for proper identification.

Q19

The presence of *Helicobacter pylori* is assumed in untreated so-called follicular gastritis.

Q20

The Sydney classification refers to the systematic reporting of gastritis in terms of clinically relevant features.

Q21

Severe acute illness and attendant stress, as well as anti-inflammatory medication (salicylates), have been implicated in hemorrhagic gastritis, which is uncommonly biopsied.

Q22

Lymphocytic gastritis refers to multiple lymphoid follicles within lamina propria with active germinal centers.

Q23

Eosinophilic gastroenteritis is a condition that has various etiologies, the presence of large numbers of tissue eosinophils being the common denominator.

Q24

The single cell drop-out (apoptosis) is the morphologic signature of graft-versus-host disease.

Q25

Peptic ulcers by definition occur as a result of acid bathing the mucosa, irrespective of site.

Q26

Because gastric acid is present in the normal stomach without causing ulcers, it is usually believed that a background of a disease process such as chronic gastritis is usually a predisposing factor in acid-mediated ulceration.

Q27

Chronic peptic ulcer occurs in the non-acid secreting (pyloric) portion of the stomach, mostly on the lesser curvature.

Q28

The endoscopic appearance of benign gastric ulcers is so typical that in the current cost-conscious era biopsy or brush cytology represent wasted medical resources and should be eliminated.

Q29

Clinical evidence of healing in a gastric ulcer under treatment is proof that it is benign.

Q30

A duodenal ulcer does not need to be biopsied, as it is always benign.

Q31

Biopsy interpretation of gastric ulcers is fraught with pitfalls, including cytologic features suspicious for malignancy.

Q32

Polyps of the stomach are very common lesions and are similar to those occurring in the colon, hence the same nomenclature.

Q33

The gastric hyperplastic polyp is the most common of the polypoid lesions, and has an unequivocal inflammatory component as well as a chronic inflammatory/atrophic context within adjacent mucosa.

Q34

Gastric hyperplastic polyps may be multiple and recur following polypectomy, without clinical implications unless a polyposis syndrome is operative or dysplasia is present.

Q35

Many polypoid lesions seen on endoscopy reveal inflammatory change and epithelial prominence, raising the possibility of a morphologic spectrum between simple inflammation, attendant polypoid hyperplasia and hyperplastic polyp.

Q36

Fundic gland polyps typically are multiple and consist of cystically dilated oxynthic glands with mostly unremarkable or subtle other features, but have different implications depending on the clinical context of the lesion.

Q37

The pathogenesis of certain types of gastric carcinoma is related to environmental factors, with a background of chronic atrophic gastritis, intestinal metaplasia and dysplasia.

Q38

The diffuse type signet ring cancer is less associated with environmental factors.

Q39

Epstein–Barr virus (EBV)-associated gastric cancers mainly present with a lymphoepithelioma-like morphology.

Q40

The diagnosis of gastric adenocarcinoma relies on a combination of a pathognomonic endoscopic picture and examination of two to three biopsy fragments.

Q41

Gastric xanthoma/xanthelasma is a diagnosis of exclusion.

Q42

Immunohistochemical evaluation for low molecular weight keratins may assist in the differentiation between epithelial characteristics (via epithelial type intermediary filaments) and phagocytes.

Q43

The mucin-specific antibodies are instrumental in diagnosing difficult cases.

Q44

The diffuse type of gastric cancer mainly affects an older age group.

Q45

Mutations of the e-cadherin gene are associated with the diffuse type signet ring carcinoma.

Q46

The involvement of the *APC* gene mutation in the adenoma carcinoma sequence is the same in the stomach as it is in the colon.

Q47

The presence of any neuroendocrine component in a gastric tumor implies an excellent prognosis.

Q48

The so-called neuroendocrine carcinomas (designation now modified to large cell NE carcinoma) have a particularly poor prognosis.

Q49

The lymphocyte-rich variant of gastric carcinoma is the morphologic type associated with EBV.

Q50

The prognosis of gastric carcinoma is in large part determined by stage, and is much better in the so-called early carcinoma.

Q51

The reported incidence of early gastric cancer depends on detection effort/success, which in turn depends on the magnitude of the public health issue/political will in a given country.

Q52

The different regions of the stomach, cardia, fundus/body and antrum, form a functional whole and their diseases, including malignancies, are clearly separate and different from those of the esophagus and small intestine.

Q53

The association between mutations in the e-cadherin gene and diffuse gastric carcinoma may be the explanation for the known clinical differences between the intestinal and diffuse types of carcinoma, particularly regarding modes of spread.

Q54

The prognosis of gastric carcinoma varies according to different reporting sources around the world.

Q55

In gastric neuroendocrine 'tumors,' neoplastic versus hyperplastic lesions are difficult or impossible to separate, as is sometimes the case at other neuroendocrine organ sites.

Q56

In well-differentiated neuroendocrine tumors of the stomach, prognosis is a function of metastatic nodal status.

Q57

Spindle cell lesions of the GI tract include smooth muscle tumors, nerve sheath tumors and undifferentiated tumors, but prognosis is unpredictable.

Q58

Reclassification of stromal tumors throughout the GI tract according to current genotypic criteria has clarified and simplified cell lineage/derivation issues, with both diagnostic and useful therapeutic implications.

Q59

The c-kit receptor is normally expressed on mast cells, the interstitial cells of Cajal and germ cells.

Q60

Based on elucidation of molecular mechanisms of tumorigenesis, the inhibitor of the tyrosine kinase receptor, imanitib mesylate (Gleevac), has been successfully used in the adjuvant therapeutic setting.

Q61

Conventional prognostic morphologic criteria are site dependent along the GI tract and are not always accurate predictors of GIST biologic behavior.

Q62

Long-term *Helicobacter pylori* infestation of the stomach results in a florid inflammatory reaction, including the presence of large lymphoid follicles – so-called follicular gastritis – currently thought to be the direct precursor/early stage of a low-grade lymphoma (= so-called MALToma or lymphoma of mucosa-associated lymphoid tissue).

Q63

The concept of a mucosa-associated lymphoid system has support from various physiologic and pathologic evidence, including homing recognition molecules for lymphocytes specific to the GI vasculature, and multiplicity, synchronously or sequentially, of low-grade lymphoma along this same axis.

Q64

The general classification of primary lymphomas had to be specially adapted to GI tract reality (modifed REAL classification), as the clinical situation and approach to diagnosis/treatment are different.

Q65

Low-grade lymphoma of the stomach is characterized by a long history of local involvement, and multiple, possibly synchronous (or not), involvement of other 'mucosal' lymphoid sites.

Q66

Gastric high-grade (large cell diffuse) lymphoma has a poor prognosis, worse than that of carcinoma.

Small bowel

Q1

The relative proportions of villi with about 20% crypt component is a foolproof identifier of normal small intestinal mucosa on a biopsy.

Q2

Human intestinal lacteals seem to have a unique transmembrane glycoprotein component, not present in other organ system lymphatics, recognized by the antibody CD38.

Q3

Normal lamina propria includes most of the conventional 'inflammatory cells,' and therefore chronic inflammation is always diagnosed in a biopsy.

Q4

Peyer's patch morphology in the normal specimen can be expected to remain constant throughout life.

Q5

The cellular complexity of the crypts of Lieberkuhn, made up of Paneth cells and a variety of neuroendocrine–paracrine cells, is ideal for 'sampling' of luminal contents and communicating the information.

Q6

The innervation of the small intestine includes the complex network of so-called interstitial cells scattered throughout the smooth muscle fibers of the wall.

Q7

The intercalated cells of Cajal are responsible for the pacemaking activity of the gastroenteric system.

Q8

The neural derivation of the cells of Cajal has been conclusively proved.

Q9

Some tumor-like conditions of the duodenum, such as adenomyoma and myoepithelial hamartoma, may in fact correspond to heterotopic pancreas.

Q10

When a duodenal biopsy from an endoscopic polypoid lesion shows perfectly 'good' fundic mucosa, you have to check the courier logs, all the day's requisitions, the daily histology worksheet and all the blocks of the day for an error of mixed-up specimens.

Q11

The architectural complexity of the duodenal/ampullary/choledochal carrefour makes any high-frequency diagnosis of duodenal duplication suspect.

Q12

Intestinal atresia is a discontinuity in the luminal flow resulting from embryologic malmigration or malassembly of segments of different derivations.

Q13

The evaluation of small intestinal biopsies has substantially changed as a function of the tissue procurement instrument and evolving general approaches to patient work-up.

Q14

Villous shape, height and regularity depend largely on the portion of the small bowel sampled.

Q15

Evaluation of duodenal biopsies for the rare celiac disease competes with the much more common pathology of peptic duodenitis in the differential diagnosis.

Q16

The histologic features of villous atrophy/crypt hyperplasia, loss of polarity of epithelium and intraepithelial lymphocytosis, are all reproducible by T-cell activation, so that one might argue that they are entirely nonspecific. The susceptible individuals (carriers of the class II antigen HLA DQ2) have an inappropriate T-cell activation response to gluten peptide moieties.

Q17

A simple increase in intraepithelial T lymphocytes can reliably differentiate celiac disease from all other small bowel conditions.

Q18

Celiac disease and dermatitis herpetiformis share the morphologic features of the small intestinal biopsy.

Q19

The morphologic hallmarks of gluten-sensitive enteropathy may be present at multiple levels of the gastrointestinal system.

Q20

Long-standing untreated celiac disease is devastating, mostly because of the metabolic consequences of malabsorption; even when responsive to gluten withdrawal initially, patients may become refractory so that gluten withdrawal is an exercise in futility and the whole issue can just be ignored.

Q21

Whipple disease is historically included in the small intestine chapter/malabsorption, as it is a good site to biopsy to establish the diagnosis. It is, however, a systemic infectious disease that presents with fever and weight loss, and a number of other sites might be the presenting problem.

Q22

The differential diagnosis of Whipple disease is mainly with *Mycobacterium avium intracellulare* (MAI) in patients with AIDS.

Q23

Duodenal peptic ulcer is currently understood to be part of the 'distal gastric unit' pathology, sharing the *Helicobacter* and hyperacidity etiopathogenesis.

Q24

Multiple and recurrent small bowel ulcers warrant evaluation for gastrin serum levels.

Q25

NSAIDs (non-steroidal anti-inflammatory agents) have a pathogenic role in gastroduodenal disease, including the ulcers.

Q26

Patients with anemia, abdominal pain, no radiologic evidence for any small intestinal pathology, and negative upper and lower endoscopies, were found to have small bowel ulcers during surgery for emergent perforation.

Q27

Crohn's disease is predominantly localized to the ileum.

Q28

Endoscopic biopsy of the terminal ileum is widely used for the diagnosis of Crohn's disease.

Q29

AIDS-related intestinal diseases always have an infectious etiologic agent.

Q30

Any luminal polypoid mass (lymphoid hyperplasia, lipoma, epithelial or stromal lesion) may cause intussusception.

Q31

Adenomas are extremely rare in the small intestine, with the exclusion of the ampulla of Vater.

Q32

Carcinoid tumors are rather uniform in their morphology as well as their biologic potential.

Q33

The carcinoid syndrome nearly always occurs after the tumor has metastasized to the liver.

Q34
B-cell lymphoma is far more prevalent in the small intestine than in the stomach.

Q35
B-cell immunoproliferative small intestinal disease (IPSID) is said to be reversible in the early stages by antibiotic treatment.

Q36
Post-transplant immunoproliferative disease prominently involves the small intestine.

Q37
Polypoid lymphoid hyperplasia has a variable disease association, ranging from reactive viral change to immunodeficient states.

Appendix

Q1
The variable morphology seen in appendectomy specimens is thought to be a function of patient age as a physiologic continuum.

Q2
The anatomic location of the appendix is highly variable and accounts for some of the difficulty in the clinical diagnosis of early acute appendicitis.

Q3
The exact etiology of acute appendicitis is poorly understood.

Q4
The clinical presentation of acute appendicitis is fraught with diagnostic problems because of the nonspecific features and the dire consequences of a missed diagnosis.

Q5
The morphologic criteria for the diagnosis of acute appendicitis are controversial in early lesions.

Q6
In the absence of mucosal pathology, isolated periappendicitis implies extra-appendiceal sources of pathology.

Q7
Granulomatous inflammation within an appendectomy specimen is almost invariably a sign of inflammatory bowel disease (IBD).

Q8
A morphology reminiscent of signet ring cells in an appendiceal lesion ought to trigger a neuroendocrine work-up for the lesion.

Q9
A grossly distended mucin-filled appendix may correspond to a number of different diagnostic entities.

Q10
There is an association between mucinous lesions of the appendix, other sites in the colon and mucinous lesions of the ovary.

Q11
Regardless of mucin 'dissecting' the appendiceal wall, and even presenting as a retroperitoneal mass, the prognosis of these lesions depends on the characteristics of the epithelial lining.

Q12
Pseudomyxoma peritonii is a condition with a poor prognosis resulting from widespread mucinous material and associated mucinous epithelium, which invests abdominal and eventually even thoracic cavities and all serosal surfaces.

Q13
Mucin is always an 'inactive' deposit, the only interesting component of these mucinous lesions anywhere in the GI tract being the epithelium.

Colon

Q1
In Hirschsprung's disease the dilated bowel segment is aganglionic and ought to be biopsied during surgery looking for a functional reanastomosis site.

Q2
Ulcerative colitis is said to have a two-peak incidence, at around ages 20–30 and another at 70–80 years of age.

Q3

Extraintestinal complications of ulcerative colitis may be found in the liver and several other organs.

Q4

If the rectal biopsy of an untreated patient with colitis is microscopically normal, the diagnosis of ulcerative colitis is unlikely.

Q5

A patient with suspected ulcerative colitis has a biopsy in order to make the diagnosis or rule it out, based on specific microscopic features.

Q6

In an established case of UC the inflammatory change on microscopy is the gold standard for diagnosis and indication for treatment.

Q7

Backwash ileitis occurs in most patients with ulcerative colitis and, like Crohn's disease, it is characterized by stenosis of the terminal ileum.

Q8

Pouchitis in the ileal (pelvic) reservoir occur preferentially in patients with total colectomy for complications of ulcerative colitis.

Q9

In ulcerative colitis carcinoma develops stepwise, including increasing degrees of dysplasia.

Q10

Carcinoma developing in long-standing UC has atypical endoscopic and other clinical characteristics.

Q11

The diagnostic morphologic criteria for dysplasia have been standardized.

Q12

Adenomatous polyps in the setting of UC have to be subdivided into those that are dysplastic versus those that are sporadic, as the immediate therapeutic decision-making processes are widely different.

Q13

Patients with long-standing ulcerative colitis are also at increased risk for lymphoma of the colon.

Q14

The diagnosis of Crohn's disease should be made only if granulomas are found in the colonic or ileal biopsies.

Q15

There is an increased risk for carcinoma in long-standing Crohn's disease.

Q16

Clinical and pathologic features of Crohn's disease include skip areas, fissuring, fistula formation and stricturing.

Q17

A similar morphology usually associated with ischemia can result either from a hemodynamic cause (including transient functional impairment), infectious agents (*Clostridium difficile*) or atherosclerosis.

Q18

The presence of a pseudomembrane separates so-called pseudomembranous colitis from all other ischemic lesions in the colon.

Q19

Microscopic lymphocytic colitis refers to increased lymphocytes in the lamina propria.

Q20

To make the diagnosis of collagenous colitis, one needs to measure the thickness of the subepithelial collagen plate on a Masson trichrome stain.

Q21

Pseudomembranes ought to be checked for trophozoites of amebae, as worldwide travel has redefined the scope of infectious disease.

Q22

The term mucosal prolapse syndrome refers to a family of lesions thought to result from abnormal segmental motility in the anorectum and may manifest itself as either ulcers or polyps.

Q23

All adenomatous lesions are not necessarily polypoid but still do correspond to a proliferative abnormality of crypt epithelium and attendant variable dysplasia in association with specific genetic alterations.

Q24

The surgical pathology diagnosis of colonic polyps is fairly straightforward, as the biopsies are readily subdivided into non-neoplastic (hyperplastic), adenomatous/villoglandular and inflammatory lesions.

Q25

The differential diagnosis between benign and malignant polyp (adenomatous/villoglandular lesion with adenocarcinoma) rests on the correct interpretation of glandular cross-sections within the stalk.

Q26

When an adenomatous/villoglandular lesion on a stalk has malignant well-differentiated elements within the stalk, well at a distance (more than 2 mm) from the cautery line, polypectomy is considered therapeutic.

Q27

Because hereditary non-polyposis colorectal cancer (HNPCC) detection cannot rely on the presence of endoscopic polyps it is regularly diagnosed at a later stage, and hence has a worse prognosis.

Q28

A low villous adenoma can go undetected on a rectal examination because of the soft consistency of the lesion.

Q29

When multiple biopsies from a villous lesion show benign features, it can be concluded that it is a villous adenoma.

Q30

Hyperplastic polyps in the right colon that have an adenomatous component are called serrated adenomas and may give rise to adenocarcinomas.

Q31

A number of left-sided polypoid lesions with features reminiscent of hyperplastic polyps are adjacent to diverticula, within prolapsed mucosa and at previous polypectomy sites within the scar, and further support the theory that they are possibly related to nonspecific reparative change.

Q32

Some polyposis syndromes never have associated cancers, and include those characterized by hyperplastic and metaplastic polyps.

Q33

Snared endoscopic polyps might correspond to benign and malignant stromal and other lesions on microscopy.

Q34

The highly variable geographic incidence of colorectal carcinoma implies an important environmental contribution to etiology.

Q35

'Acute appendicitis' in middle-aged/older individuals can not uncommonly be the presentation of cecal carcinoma.

Q36

The clinical presentation of colorectal carcinoma is non-specific and early symptoms are rarely a feature, so that strategies for detection include fecal occult blood tests, sigmoidoscopy and, increasingly, full colonoscopy.

Q37

Carcinoembryonic antigen (CEA) is glycocalix related, expressed at all levels of the GI tract and restricted to it; a serum assay is thus a reliable early diagnostic test for detection of carcinoma.

Q38

CEA has a reliable association with colon cancer and is stainable on routine sections.

Q39

DNA mismatch repair gene deficiencies, with resulting microsatellite instability (MSI), play an important role in the pathogenesis of hereditary non-polyposis colorectal carcinomas.

Q40

Mutations of tumor suppressor gene *p53* are usually found in right-sided colonic tumors that are polyploid.

Q41

Signet ring carcinoma is a rare form of colorectal malignancy usually found in young patients.

Q42

Small cell (oat cell-like) tumors, mostly located in the right colon, have a good prognosis based on their neuroendocrine derivation.

Q43

The gross appearance of colon cancer is so typical that biopsy and tissue diagnosis is mostly unnecessary.

Q44

A polypoid gross appearance in a carcinoma is proof that it arose in a benign polyp.

Q45

In rectal carcinoma, at the time of the gross examination proximal and distal free margins are the determinants of recurrence-free long-term prognosis, and need to be noted.

Q46

HNPCC-associated cancers have distinctive morphologic features and an overall better prognosis.

Q47

Vein invasion is controversial as a prognostic feature in colorectal carcinoma.

Q48

Despite a number of new classification schemes, we still rely on the basic premise of the Dukes classification for staging.

Q49

For rectal lesions, endorectal ultrasound has considerably improved staging and the planning of treatment strategies.

Q50

There has only recently been consensus on the definition of lymph node metastasis for the purpose of counting involved lymph nodes in the evaluation of colorectal specimens.

Q51

Lymph node dissection, and the attendant numbers of nodes found in colon cancer specimens, is the 'Holy Grail' of the relationship between colorectal surgeon and pathologist.

Q52

Genotypic subcategorization of colonic carcinoma may be helpful in predicting response to adjuvant treatment, and probably in general, to select tumors according to predicted biologic behavior rather than histology.

Anus

Q1

The anal canal is lined by columnar epithelium in the upper portion and by keratinized and non-keratinized squamous epithelium in its lower portion.

Q2

The lymphatic drainage of the anal canal is into the hypogastric, internal iliac and obturator nodes.

Q3

The area of the sphincters is extensively penetrated by anal glands and ducts.

Q4

The complex embryologic development of the anal canal explains the various potential congenital abnormalities of the region.

Q5

Microscopy of tissue from anal fistulae is rewarding from a diagnostic point of view, as some of these may be due to TB, Crohn's disease or ulcerative colitis.

Q6

In the current climate of cost containment, the 'gross only' evaluation of hemorrhoids is reasonable.

Q7

Although other associations do exist, a substantial portion of the premalignant and malignant tumors of this area are related to viral etiologies and sexually transmitted disease, including high-risk HPV strains such as HPV 16, 18 and others.

Q8

Tumors of this area show different morphologies depending on levels of derivation from anal canal and skin.

Q9

A presentation of low rectal polyp is not uncommon for an anal canal carcinoma (itself uncommon), where biopsy will be the initial procedure to establish the diagnosis.

Q10

Anal canal lesions are best treated with primary combination chemoradiation regimens, with surgery after the other treatment effects have been maximized.

Q11

Paget's disease refers to an epidermotropic malignant epithelial tumor that can have an exclusive or a predominantly intraepidermal location and presents as an ill-defined eczematous, red oozing or ulcerated plaque.

Q12

Malignant melanoma of the anal canal can present as a smooth polypoid mass in a patient with rectal bleeding, including within a hemorrhoidal sac.

Esophagus

A1. False

Theoretically at 40 cm from the incisors, it has considerable individual variation, complicating the evaluation of a major category of diseases. **(p. 615)**

A2. False

Melanocytes have been demonstrated within the basal layer of the squamous epithelium. **(p. 615)**

A3. False

Muscularis mucosae is well defined and prominent, particularly distally. **(p. 615)**

A4. True

The importance of this mapping cannot be underestimated for proper cancer staging. **(p. 615)**

A5. True

Atresia associated defects might include malformation of the heart and the respiratory tree. **(p. 616)**

A6. False

The so-called inlet patch is usually in the postcricoid region, and its pathogenesis is uncertain; some believe that it is reactive (metaplastic) and not heterotopic (congenital) in nature **(p. 616)**

A7. True

Whether abnormal motility is primary and etiologic or secondary, dysphagia will be part of the symptom complex and complications include bleeding, infection and rupture. **(p. 617)**

A8. False

The diagnostic significance depends on the number of eosinophils; a rare eosinophil is probably physiologic. Too many may represent other entities, such as idiopathic eosinophilic esophagitis. **(p. 619)**

A9. False

The early reflux related change is within squamous epithelium, with elongation of rete ridges and inflammatory cells within epithelium. **(p. 620)**

A10. True

Endoscopy at this site has a poor correlation to actual pathology, including the possible presence of an ulcer. The morphologic criteria for the establishment of inflammation include epithelial change, such as expansion of the basal compartment with elongation of the rete ridges. **(p. 619)**

A11. False

The determination of this site is fraught with controversy by all participating disciplines, including the endoscopist, those performing manometry, and the pathologist. **(p. 621)**

A12. False

The so-called multilayered epithelium refers to an early, intermediary stage in the metaplasia sequence from squamous to Barrett type. **(p. 621)**

A13. False

The diagnosis of Barrett's esophagus requires endoscopic correlation with metaplastic mucosa having been visualized; one or two goblet cells can be a normal component of epithelium. **(p. 615 and 621)**

A14. False

Microscopic identification of goblet cells *and* an endoscopic Barrett's mucosa are required for the diagnosis of Barrett's esophagus. Specifically, columnar 'blue cells' on the combined Alcian blue–PAS mucin stains (= partial metaplasia) or other special procedures without an actual goblet cell morphology do not fulfill diagnostic criteria. **(p. 621)**

A15. False

When *H. pylori* is present in the stomach it is possibly also expected in the refluxed contents, and can colonize gastric-type mucus coexistent with the metaplastic goblet cells of the Barrett epithelium. **(p. 621)**

A16. False

The treatment promotes gastric pH closer to neutral, reflux remaining to be dealt with, possibly surgically (fundoplication). The inhibitory effects of treatment on the secretory parietal cells will leave a morphologic footprint visible on subsequent biopsies. **(p. 620)**

A17. True

The reversal may be incomplete, with the possible – and even likely – presence of residual metaplastic epithelium tucked away in the glands, underneath a superficially reassuring squamous epithelium. Any residual metaplasias may enter the dysplastic neoplastic pathway. **(p. 622)**

A18. False

It is an acceptable reactive pattern in Barrett's esophagus, negative for dysplasia. **(p. 622)**

A19. False

It is a goblet cell with no luminal 'outlet' to discharge mucus, with the mucus droplet facing the basal membrane and the nucleus facing the luminal aspect of the cell. **(p. 622)**

A20. True

This is particularly so in the presence of erosion/ulceration. **(p. 622)**

A21. False

Usually this cannot be determined on a biopsy. Most biopsy specimens are not deep enough to rule out submucosal invasion. **(p. 622)**

A22. False
The two diagnoses cannot be separated reproducibly and are used together with a slash to emphasize this fact and the similar therapeutic implication. **(p. 622)**

A23. False
The esophagus has different lymphatic drainage, depending on upper/mid/lower location; the latter drains into the celiac periaortic nodes, similar to the gastric tumors of the cardia. **(p. 624 and 615)**

A24. True
Herpes simplex esophagitis is frequently found in immunosuppressed persons, but it can also present in immunocompetent hosts. The classic Cowdry type A inclusions are the hallmark of this disease but are not always identifiable. **(p. 624)**

A25. True
Despite being highly suggestive of herpes esophagitis, multinucleation can also be a nonspecific regenerative response to injury. **(p. 624)**

A26. False
Immunocompetent individuals can and do get herpes esophagitis. **(p. 624)**

A27. True
Herpes and cytomegalovirus are both pathogens on the increase; either brush cytology or biopsy material is suitable for diagnosis, supported by immunohistochemistry. **(p. 624)**

A28. True
The esophageal complaint may also be the presenting symptom. **(p. 625)**

A29. True
Smoking and alcohol are established risk factors, as are certain superinfected pickled foods (China), monotonous diets mostly lacking in (yet)-to-be-identified elements, chemical strictures (lye) and radiation. **(p. 625)**

A30. True
Studies have reported a variable prevalence of HPV in esophageal carcinomas in some parts of the world; HPV is not prevalent in North American cases. **(p. 625)**

A31. True
This is a statistical fact, but clinically, squamous cell carcinoma can occur anywhere in the esophagus. **(p. 625)**

A32. False
Squamous cell carcinoma can and does spread submucosally as well as intraepithelially quite widely beyond the visible mass lesion. **(p. 626)**

A33. False
Focal mucin-secreting, pseudoglandular (poorly cohesive squamoid) as well as non-keratinizing 'upper respiratory'-type morphologies are not uncommon, with additional possible variability within tumors and within the small superficial biopsies. **(p. 627)**

A34. True
Dysplasia and in situ carcinoma are used in strategies for cytologic early detection in high-incidence areas. **(p. 627)**

A35. True
They refer to invasive squamous cell carcinoma that does not penetrate beyond the submucosa. **(p. 627)**

A36. False
Superficial spreading – the two terms refer to entirely different parameters: carcinoma denotes lateral spread of at least 2 cm beyond an invasive component; intramucosal carcinoma remains confined to the lamina propria by definition. This substantial difference is further highlighted by the near-zero metastatic potential of intramucosal carcinoma, which rises to between 20% and 50% with the submucosal invasion of superficial spreading carcinoma. **(p. 627)**

A37. False
The prognosis is not universally good, as indicated by the 5-year survival of 50% for the superficial microinvasive/spreading carcinomas. The term 'early carcinoma of the esophagus' is confusing and should be abandoned. **(p. 628)**

A38. True
Unsuspected involvement of biopsied celiac nodes was documented in 40% in a study as the likely source of treatment failure. **(p. 628)**

A39. True
Positive cytologies can identify asymptomatic patients for treatment. **(p. 628)**

A40. True
These are submucosal lesions, usually presenting with a variably polypoid appearance, most commonly detected by endoscopy and treated during the procedure. Important potential pitfalls are pseudoepitheliomatous hyperplasia of overlying squamous epithelium and a false positive diagnosis of squamous cell carcinoma. For the same reasons, the differential diagnosis also includes squamous papilloma. **(p. 632)**

Stomach

A1. False

Even under physiologic conditions, there is a wide individual variability, with transitional areas in between. **(p. 648)**

A2. False

Normal mucous neck cells will produce some sulfo- and sialomucins, which will be positive with the Alcian blue component of the Alcian blue–PAS stain, but do not imply metaplasia. **(p. 648)**

A3. True

The ratio is one fourth of pits to glands in the body, whereas in the antrum it is two-thirds to one-third. **(p. 648)**

A4. False

Only two different lesional categories may be important and their exact morphologic separation is problematic, as is common in endocrine-type lesions: these are the hyperplasias versus the neoplasias, generic carcinoid tumors, the latter with invasive and metastatic capabilities. Other distinctions have scientific value but will not affect clinical considerations, except for G (gastrin-secreting) cell lesions (Zollinger–Ellison syndrome). **(p. 648)**

A5. False

The nodes, if involved by disease, are to be found within the left gastric group. **(p. 649)**

A6. True

The muscularis propria (externa) is composed of three layers: outer longitudinal, inner circular and innermost oblique, and will 'control' the sphincter. **(p. 648)**

A7. False

The potential site to be within the radiation field is the splenic hilum, with the pancreaticosplenic nodes. **(p. 649)**

A8. True

These lesions are benign, often found incidentally, and probably related in their pathogenesis. The (probably) hamartomatous tissue consists of ill-assembled ducts and other components with secondary change such as cystic dilation. **(p. 650)**

A9. True

However, in neither condition is the endocrine tissue necessary for the diagnosis. **(p. 649)**

A10. False

The condition of hypertrophic pyloric stenosis occurs in an (often) male baby, between 3 and 12 weeks of age, and has a currently poorly understood pathogenesis, but is decreasing in frequency. **(p. 650)**

A11. False

A wide range of conditions can present clinically as a gastric mass, from pyloric hypertrophy secondary to pyloric channel ulcers to antral gastritis, to diffuse adenocarcinoma (linitis plastica). **(p. 650)**

A12. False

The simple presence of a few inflammatory cells may represent the resident elements of the lamina propria. The diagnosis of chronic gastritis implies an epithelial involvement along the various stages of evolution of the lesion, the common pathway to end-stage disease being fibrosis; metaplasias and loss of secretory glandular parenchyma. **(p. 650)**

A13. False

It is involvement of the body (oxynthic mucosa) (type A gastritis) that has an autoimmune connotation with the α and β subunits of the proton pump as the molecular targets. In addition to the achlorhydria, intrinsic factor secretion is affected as well, resulting subsequently in pernicious anemia. **(p. 651)**

A14. True

The antral inflammation is mostly *Helicobacter* associated until proved otherwise, the association being so common. Antral sparing is typical of so-called autoimmune gastritis. **(p. 651)**

A15. True

It is probably a function of duration of disease and stage of atrophy. Other yet incompletely characterized factors may also play a role, including the host, as well as *Helicobacter pylori* genotypes. These organisms have complex interactions with gastric epithelial mucin-secreting cells, as well as the acid-secreting compartment. **(p. 650)**

A16. True

The metaplasia may be complete (type 1), including the villous architecture as well as the epithelial characteristics. **(p. 650)**

A17. False

A thinned translucent mucosa with prominent submucosal vessel patterns corresponds well only to loss of function/acid-secretory tests. Other hallmarks of endoscopy have poor correlation to histology or symptomatology. **(p. 651)**

A18. False

Although a number of special stains, a commercial monoclonal antibody, and now PCR techniques are available, the organism is readily seen on 'low-tech' routine H&E sections. **(p. 651)**

A19. True

In untreated patients such a morphology is always associated with *Helicobacter* gastritis. **(p. 681)**. The lymphoid follicles remain for a long time (months), present on several follow-up biopsies, with eventual regression. **(p. 651)**

A20. True

The reporting of gastritis needs to specify antral versus corpus, whether superficial, acute or chronic, and the presence or absence of metaplasias. In a summary comment, mention of *H. pylori* or other etiology (if known), as well as special morphologies, are featured. **(p. 652)**

A21. True

Prominent basophilia of the foveolar epithelium and interstitial hemorrhage with neutrophils are typical. **(p. 652)**

A22. False

Lymphocytic gastritis refers to intraepithelial lymphocytosis. The differential diagnosis includes celiac disease and *Helicobacter* infestation. **(p. 653)**

A23. True

Peripheral eosinophilia may coexist. This condition might involve other combinations of organ involvement (enterocolitis) and the presence of large numbers of mast cells as well, chemotactic for the eosinophils. The differential diagnosis includes parasitic infestation, collagen vascular diseases and medication-related hypersensitivities, with a large number of cases remaining as yet 'idiopathic.' **(p. 653)**

A24. True

In addition to the expected clinical settings of bone marrow transplantation, other unusual situations may exist, such as transfusion with chimera 'graft' formation, where the diagnosis is unexpected and based on morphology alone; CMV is not uncommonly a confounding factor both clinically and morphologically. **(p. 653)**

A25. True

Possible sites other than the stomach proper include Meckel's diverticulum with gastric fundic metaplasia/heterotopia, lower esophagus with reflux, the duodenum and gastrojejunostomy margin. **(p. 653)**

A26. True

Chronic gastritis is most commonly *Helicobacter* associated. **(p. 654)**

A27. True

Because there is near-universal chronic gastritis and associated pyloric metaplasia, which proceeds from distal to proximal, there could be peptic ulcers anywhere from distal to proximal in the stomach. **(p. 654)**

A28. False

Whereas the appearance of a benign ulcer is typical with a clean base and smooth edges, some malignant ulcers do not look dissimilar and the biopsy diagnosis of malignancy sometimes comes as a total surprise clinically. **(p. 654)**

A29. False

There is evidence for some healing in malignant ulcers. **(p. 654)**

A30. True

Adenocarcinoma of the duodenum is a rare disease (described later) but is not part of the differential diagnosis of a benign duodenal ulcer. **(p. 720)**

A31. True

The reasons include poorly cohesive degenerative and regenerative epithelium from the edges of the ulcer. Another scenario involves slipped/displaced catheters in celiac/hepatic arterial chemotherapy causing the resulting benign gastric ulcer to have the antimitotic effects of the chemotherapy agent, mimicking malignancy. **(p. 655)**

A32. False

The perception that this statement is true has plagued the diagnosis of gastric polyps, but nothing could be further from the truth! As the concept of obligate benign colonic hyperplastic polyp is currently undergoing significant re-evaluation, some aspects of the considerations regarding the stomach may well need revisiting. **(p. 657)**

A33. True

The constellation of foveolar elongation and tortuosity, cystic dilation of foveolae and pyloric (or occasionally fundic)-type glands with lamina propria changes is reminiscent of what is seen in inflammation, the reason for the other term, inflammatory polyp. **(p. 656)**

A34. True

Intestinal metaplasia or actual dysplasia within the polyp are the *only* markers indicating a need for follow-up, irrespective of multiplicity or recurrence. **(p. 657)**

A35. True

The reported reversal of some lesions following *Helicobacter pylori* eradication supports the possibility of evolution within the spectrum. However, not all hyperplastic polyps have a *Helicobacter* association. **(p. 657)**

A36. True

When looking at an H&E section of a fundic gland polyp, sporadic lesions cannot be differentiated from those associated with the adenomatous polyposis syndrome (APC gene related) in the absence of dysplasia. Some authors therefore recommend colonic screening in patients with fundic gland polyps; this, however, is quite an undertaking, as fundic gland polyps can also be associated with long-term proton pump inhibitor use (currently very large numbers of patients), as well as the Zollinger–Ellison syndrome (more manageably rare). **(p. 658)**

A37. True

Intestinal-type gastric cancers have a variable geographic incidence, with genetic susceptibility also probably playing a role. **(p. 661)**

A38. **True**

When incidences of gastric cancer are changing, they mainly affect the intestinal sub-type. **(p. 663)**

A39. **True**

There is a variable geographic distribution, and EBV is more significant in the US than in Europe or Japan. **(p. 662)**

A40. **False**

The diagnosis presents with an unacceptably high rate of false negatives unless seven to eight biopsy fragments are examined, with additional brush cytology to bring the diagnostic yield to 100%. In early lesions the endoscopic appearance is nonspecific and on occasion the examination is entirely negative. **(p. 664)**

A41. **True**

Foamy cytoplasm can be the deceptive common feature in a wide variety of conditions, including primary signet ring carcinoma, metastasis from lobular carcinoma (histiocytoid variant) of the breast, or benign but degenerative cells from the edge of an ulcer. **(p. 656)**

A42. **True**

In practice, the diagnosis remains very difficult both on biopsy and even on surgical specimens, as tumor cells may appear deceptively few among the massive stromal 'reactive' change. **(p. 664)**

A43. **False**

Immunohistochemistry and molecular/biochemical profiles of tumors are rather promising for selected therapeutic interventions, such as subdividing gastric cancers into three groups of intestinal, diffuse and EBV-associated lesions. Depending on what the tumors express, patients might benefit from attempts at interrupting the agonist–receptor cycle, such as EGF and/or EGFR, HER2, mutated e-cadherin. This approach is in its early stages in gastric cancer, but is a promising novel and possibly complementary avenue to current therapy. **(p. 665)**

A44. **False**

It is the most common histology, relatively speaking, in younger patients, age further lessening the clinical suspicion of malignancy and compounding the diagnostic difficulty. **(p. 664)**

A45. **True**

The germline mutation in the familial cases, necessitating prophylactic gastrectomy, showed multiple early, grossly unappreciated isolated 'microscopic' lesions. Somatic mutations in the e-cadherin gene are present in the sporadic form of signet ring carcinoma, but not in the intestinal type of gastric carcinoma. **(p. 665)**

A46. **False**

In the stomach other pathways are operative, as the high frequency of the mutation in gastric adenoma is not reflected in the low frequency of same in carcinoma, exactly opposite to the results in the colon (strict parallelism between the two lesions regarding APC). **(p. 665)**

A47. **False**

This is one of the most confusing concepts in surgical pathology. Pure neuroendocrine tumors span the entire spectrum of differentiation and prognosis will depend not only on location in the GI tract, but also on the degree of differentiation; prognosis is good only for the small, well-differentiated tumors (so-called carcinoids) and only at certain sites. There are also tumors of other predominant cell types with a neuroendocrine component, enhancing aggressive potential, which is also the case for tumors at other levels of the GI tract (colon) and in other organ systems. **(p. 666)**

A48. **True**

These tumors have the neuroendocrine growth pattern (ribbons, rosettes, trabeculae) but also mitoses, invasiveness, necrosis and early metastatic potential. **(p. 666 and also p. 131 of this manual; A42 Colon)**

A49. **False**

Tumors with conventional adenocarcinoma morphology also can be EBV associated, in addition to lymphoepithelial-like and gastric medullary carcinoma with lymphocytic infiltration. **(p. 667)**

A50. **True**

The assumption is misleading, however, and the two parts of the statement possibly unrelated. The so-called early carcinoma does have a better prognosis, but is not necessarily small or early. It is multicentric in a substantial number of cases. By definition, the deepest invasion is into submucosa, not breaching muscularis externa, independent of lymph node status. The intestinal type predominates. The 5-year survival is remarkably high even with lymph node involvement (80–95%), and raises the question of its being not simply a matter of stage but possibly of different biologic potential. **(p. 670)**

A51. **True**

For instance in Japan, where the high incidence of gastric cancer makes detection efforts a priority for early diagnosis, the endoscopic knowledge about subtle lesions in general is more advanced. This vast knowledge has of late also been applied to colonic lesions, with the discovery of lesions hitherto less recognized in the west. It was initially thought that these lesions were peculiar to the population in Japan, but it is now known that they exist and are important in the west as well, but have largely gone unrecognized. The reason for discussion of this topic is to point out that, not surprisingly, endoscopy competencies also impact 'the lesions most commonly seen'. **(p. 670)**

A52. **False**

Independent of their differing regional physiologies, their pathology tends to form 'functional' units, including types of malignancies and modes of spread: the cardia tends to cluster with the lower esophagus and esophagogastric junction versus the antrum/duodenum. **(p. 670)**

A53. True

The propensity of these tumors to spread more diffusely, and specifically more to peritoneal surfaces (including to ovaries – Krukenberg tumor), may be a function of their intercellular adhesion deficiency. There may also be some parallel between these lesions and lobular carcinoma of the breast, where the e-cadherin mutation is also operative and where a diffuse and 'unusual' tumor spread is the rule, also with clinical therapeutic and diagnostic implications. **(p. 670)**

A54. True

The differences could be the result of many factors, the diagnostic criteria separating high-grade dysplasia from carcinoma being potentially important. Others include screening efforts for early diagnosis, and possibly differences in both etiologic and susceptibility factors across geographic areas such as Japan, Europe and the US. **(p. 671)**

A55. True

Well-differentiated tumors have been reported to regress following antrectomy, presumably because the gastrin–trophic stimulatory loop is removed: this is suggestive of tumor-like hyperplasia rather than true (committed) neoplasia in these cells. **(p. 673)**

A56. False

Well differentiated neuroendocrine tumors grow very slowly and have a very long evolution even in the presence of widely metastatic disease (including liver), anecdotally, for several decades. **(p. 673)**

A57. False

The classification based on light microscopy phenotype cannot resolve the paradox of erratic immunohistochemical staining for apparently well-differentiated lesions, and the lack of expected electron microscopy features in parallel. **(p. 674)**

A58. True

Of 1869 gastric tumors previously diagnosed as of smooth muscle differentiation, over 90% had KIT expression, with either spindle or epitheloid cell morphology. The somatic mutation for CD117 (c-*kit*), a tyrosine kinase receptor, characterizes this more recently recognized set of stromal lesions. **(p. 676)**

A59. True

However, in the differential diagnosis of stromal tumors, demonstrating the mutation either by the protein product (IHC membranous reaction product) or by genetic analysis is conclusive for the entity of gastrointestinal stromal tumors (GIST). The differential diagnosis includes, in addition to the foregoing, solitary fibrous tumor, inflammatory fibrous tumor, glomus tumor and fibromatosis, none expected to be reactive for c-*kit*, but rather for CD34 in variable proportions. **(p. 678)**

A60. True

Although the primary treatment is surgery, tumors with the CD117 mutation respond in a spectacular manner to Gleevac treatment, until additional mutations confer acquired resistance. **(p. 678)**

A61. True

In the stomach, tumors smaller than 10 cm with fewer than 5 mitoses/50 hpf rarely metastasize (2–3%). Of those that are larger and more mitotically active, 86% have metastatic lesions. An intermediate category of metastatic potential includes larger tumors with fewer mitoses and smaller tumors with more mitoses (11–15%). **(p. 678)**

A62 True with qualifiers

The stomach does not physiologically have a lymphoid compartment organized into germinal centers. The formation of these is accomplished through a B cell-dependent organizing principle triggered by certain genetic types of *Helicobacter*, and may be clonally restricted. Whether it is stage related in the process (when early) or depends on other yet unknown factors, the monoclonal lymphoid infiltrates are still responsive to antigen drive and may sometimes resolve with antibiotic therapy. **(p. 680)**

A63. True

The implication is that primary GI lymphomas can either be the low-grade (small cell) MALTomas or the high-grade (large cell) lymphomas, possibly evolving from low-grade tumors. 'Local' lymph node involvement may ultimately occur in both. **(p. 681)**

A64. True

The diagnostic hallmarks of gastric MALT lymphoma are its B-cell lineage, its ability to recapitulate centrocyte-like features, such as invest epithelium (lymphoepithelial complexes), infiltrate germinal centers, and its reactivity to CD20, CD21 and CD35. It may be low or high grade. Low-grade lesions are given a therapeutic trial with antibiotics and follow-up biopsy; if ineffective, a chemotherapy regimen is initiated. **(p. 681)**

A65. True

Lymph node involvement is rare at diagnosis, but the lesion is often multifocal in the stomach despite a dominant mass, and the extent of involvement is only appreciated on microscopy. Hence, if surgery is contemplated and is short of gastrectomy, preoperative biopsy mapping is warranted. Most cases will, however, be treated medically. **(p. 684)**

A66. False

The stage at presentation may be more advanced than in the low-grade variety and the prognosis might go from 91% 5-year survival to 56%, but is far better than that of carcinoma. The therapy of high-grade lymphoma typically involves combined modalities. **(p. 684)**

Small bowel

A1. False
Villus length and attendant villus–crypt proportions as well as architectural regularity depend entirely on the level of the biopsy throughout the length of the small bowel: irregular and chubby in the duodenum, tall and slender in the jejunum, and less tall but still regular in the ileum. Rules for normalcy are different again for biopsies from the area of the ileocecal valve. **(p. 712)**

A2. True
The intestinal compartment is involved in specific (round trip) immunologic priming through adhesion and specific signaling at that address (addressins). **(p. 712)**

A3. False
'Resident' lamina propria cells come in different constellations, different levels of activation and numbers, and different physiologic and pathologic relationships to epithelium, so that their presence per se does not inflammation make. **(p. 712)**

A4. False
There is substantial physiologic change within the lymphoid compartment during life, and biopsy interpretation of whether this is physiologic or pathologic will ultimately depend mostly on patient age. **(p. 712)**

A5. True
The complex environment also includes bacterial and archaea commensals for best mutual adaptive results. **(p. 712)**

A6. False
These cells are not of neural crest origin and their development is under the control of the c-*kit* receptor pathway. They play a similar role all along the GI tract. **(p. 713)**

A7. True
This network of cells and their elaborate processes are intercalated between ganglion cells and effector smooth muscle cells. **(p. 713)**

A8. False
The names interstitial and intercalated cell of Cajal refer to the same cell, originating from the same mesodermal precursor as the smooth muscle cells of the wall and not from the neural crest, even though Cajal first visualized them with silver stains (in his time implying a neural origin). **(p. 713)**

A9. True
Heterotopic pancreas most often consists of ductal elements with or without acinar and rarely an endocrine component. These may become degenerated (?inflamed), cystically dilated and correspond to the 'misplaced' pancreatic tissue consisting of the ductal component only. **(p. 713)**

A10. False
It is fairly common for heterotopic gastric mucosa to masquerade as a duodenal polyp, and *Helicobacter* organisms may be present if surface epithelium is the gastric type as well. **(p. 713)**

A11. True
Duplication in the area of the duodenum is very rare, and other lesions need to be ruled out first, such as choledochal cyst/choledochocele. **(p. 713)**

A12. False
This conventional dogma has been challenged recently, to include probable intrauterine causes such as maternal infection, mechanical injury, and chemical agents with attendant (multi)segmental secondary luminal resorption. **(p. 713)**

A13. True
Endoscopic biopsies have long replaced capsule biopsies, and diagnostic criteria can no longer rely on the well-oriented villi from large biopsies, except for experimental/investigational purposes. Two levels/sites, including variable distance into the duodenum and terminal ileum (at the time of colonoscopy), are the most commonly sampled and have their specific 'physiologic' appearance for one to be familiar with. **(p. 716)**

A14. True
For instance, duodenal mucosa 'physiologically' presents some villous irregularity, and interpretation of blunting and villous shortening needs to take this into consideration. **(p. 716)**

A15. True for the differential diagnosis. Not true for the statement of celiac disease currently believed to be rare
Previously, this diagnosis was entertained only for full-blown clinical malabsorption in the appropriate ethnic/genetic background. Currently, it is increasingly appreciated that beyond the now relatively rare classic presentation, there are patients with anemia and minimal malabsorption, in whom the hallmark of complete or partial villous atrophy is rarely present. **(p. 717)**

A16. True
This condition was thought to be uncommon, except for specific ethnic backgrounds (Irish). With more specific antibody tests (below) there is now an evolving definition of the condition; it may also be present in a 'form fruste' in much larger numbers of patients, and in the family members of patients with the full-blown symptomatology. **(p. 717)**

A17. False

It is the high point of the differential diagnosis in flat mucosa. When there is preservation of a near-normal villous architecture with intraepithelial lymphocytosis, serum assay of tissue transglutaminase and endomysial antibodies is needed to confirm a diagnosis of celiac sprue. Antral *Helicobacter* and a broad array of other causes (enteric infection, autoimmune disease, therapeutic drugs) need to be ruled out. **(p. 716)**

A18. True

The morphologic features alone are indistinguishable. **(p. 716)**

A19. True

There may be lymphocytic gastritis as well as lymphocytic colitis in these patients. In contrast, a subset of patients with lymphocytic colitis alone, have gluten sensitivity responsive to gluten withdrawal; any patient with lymphocytic colitis might therefore benefit from exploration of small intestinal status. **(p. 717)**

A20. False

There is an increased risk for T-cell lymphoma (enteropathy associated, probably including also the so-called chronic nonspecific ulcerative duodenojejunitis) as well as carcinoma in untreated patients; newly developed refractoriness in a patient is a possible sign of the onset of the complication, and has a poor prognosis. **(p. 717)**

A21. True

Tropheryma whippelii is the bacilliform offending agent identified, present in interepithelial spaces between enterocytes and within sheets of macrophages as a 'space-occupying' infiltrate within lamina propria of the villous core, deforming the villi. The hallmark is PAS-positive/diastase-resistant non-acid-fast organisms. The breakdown cell wall product remains for a very long time as a membranous content in macrophage lysosomes, making the diagnosis impossible in suspected reactivation after antibiotic therapy. Electron microscopy can demonstrate whole intact, presumably active, organisms. There may well be an abnormal immune response in these patients. **(p. 718)**

A22. True

With similar features on routine histology and the nonspecific presentation of malabsorption, acid fastness will differentiate the two conditions. **(p. 718)**.

A23. True

This understanding currently directs the treatment strategy of *Helicobacter pylori* eradication, with also a decrease in the recurrence rate of ulcers. The rather uncommon surgical specimens for ulcer (complications) often do not contain the actual ulcer, which just gets sewn over. **(p. 720)**

A24. True

The Zollinger–Ellison syndrome needs to be ruled out; the source of the excess gastrin may be from a minute pancreatic tumor or a duodenal lesion masquerading as a 'polyp.' **(p. 720)**

A25. True

NSAIDs have also been additionally implicated in the formation of webs/strictures more distally in the small intestine, as well as reactivation of Crohn's disease in remission. **(p. 721)**

A26. True

Non-invasive exploration of the small intestine had to await the newer capsule endoscopy techniques, with their unique potential to explore the so-called idiopathic lesions; the interpretation is driven by subsequent computer-assisted analysis of thousands of endoscopy frames. **(p. 721)**

A27. False

Studies from the 1970s report that about two-thirds of all cases have involvement restricted to the small intestine, whereas currently this is closer to one-third. The remainder tend to show some combination of colonic involvement together with the small intestine. **(p. 721)**

A28. True

After the exclusion of TB and *Yersinia*, a prominently edematous, congested villous architecture with acute crypt/pericrypt polymorphonuclear involvement and granuloma formation is highly suggestive of the diagnosis, particularly when the biopsy is from the so-called endoscopic aphthous ulcer/lesion. Backwash ileitis, biopsied in the clinical setting of ulcerative colitis, might have crypt abscess formation, congestion and chronic inflammation, but will be in continuity with a florid pancolitis and a patent distended ileocecal valve. **(p. 723)**

A29. False

Both usual and unusual infectious agents are often causal and need to first be ruled out, including the need for special culture techniques or PCR. The immunodeficiency per se can result in loss of trophic cytokines, a shared feature with other etiologies of immunodeficiency. Neoplastic lesions, including Kaposi's sarcoma, malignant lymphoma and stromal tumors, must also be considered. **(p. 724)**

A30. True

Any luminal polypoid mass may cause intussusception. In young patients, a barium enema might be used early as a therapeutic maneuver. Hamartomatous polyps in the Peutz–Jeghers syndrome commonly and repeatedly intussuscept, with all the traction possibly contributing to enteritis cystica profunda. **(p. 727)**

A31. **False**

With the increasing use of endoscopy, adenomatous lesions are found much more commonly and often show the morphology of a villoglandular polyp. The small intestinal lesions may also be 'participatory' in the so-called colonic polyposis syndromes, or represent the evolution to neoplastic change, including in the hamartomatous lesions of the Peutz–Jeghers syndrome. **(p. 728)**

A32. **False**

The morphology, the biologic potential and the secretory products are all variable, depending on the level of the tumor within the GI tract. For investigational purposes, electron microscopy of neurosecretory granule morphology parallels the level of origin within the GI tract. Granule morphology also has some predictive value as to secretory product, which is best identified by immunohistochemistry with antibodies to the array of polypeptide hormones. Ileal carcinoids mostly present with the insular morphology, are not uncommonly multiple, are always deeply invasive, and metastatize early. **(p. 730)**

A33. **True**

An array of vasoactive substances is responsible for the symptoms. In addition, there is a fibrosing principle elaborated that is responsible for local and distant deposition of fibrous tissue, including at valvular and vascular sites. **(p. 733)**

A34. **False**

Lymphoma in general is more common in the small intestine, and both B- and T-cell types occur. T-cell lymphoma may or may not be enteropathy associated. B-cell lymphoma can be the MALT type or IPSID, mostly a function of the geographic location. Other associations include the immunodeficiency-related lymphoma, the post-transplant lymphoproliferative diseases and the Burkitt type lymphoma. **(p. 735)**

A35. **True**

This is reminiscent of features of *Helicobacter pylori*-related MALToma in the stomach. **(p. 735)**

A36. **True**

This EBV-driven lymphoid proliferation, which is polyclonal in its early stages, is responsive to restoration of immune function. Monoclonality signals pending transformation to a high-grade lymphoma. **(p. 735)**

A37. **True**

Some of these lesions probably belong to a low-grade follicular lymphoma category. **(p. 737)**

Appendix

A1. **True**

The exact nature of the change, however, is somewhat uncertain, whether the result of multiple bouts of inflammation/scarring, or physiologic involution of the lymphoid component, or a combination. The end result is fibrous obliteration of the lumen, with nerve hyperplasia and variable prominence of a neuroendocrine component. This process may involve the distal tip or the entire appendix. **(p. 757)**

A2. **True**

The appendix may be located in front or behind the cecum and/or terminal ileum, as well as in aberrant sites such as the subhepatic region. **(p. 757)**

A3. **True**

It is predominantly a disease of the western world; luminal obstruction seems to play some role, including possibly the reactive lymphoid hyperplasia in viral disease. **(p. 758)**

A4. **True**

There is the additional complexity of the wide range of pathologies, depending on the age of the patient, that may present as an acute appendicitis. This includes viral etiologies in children, carcinoid tumors and adenocarcinoma in the older age group, possibly also of the cecum. **(p. 758)**

A5. **True**

The dusky surface and transmural necrosis stages are 'easy' to correlate to 'acute abdomen' symptomatology. The relevance of mucosal collections of polymorphonuclears versus those in the lumen are not universally agreed upon, with or without attendant ulceration. **(p. 758)**

A6. **True**

Not uncommonly this would be adnexal in female patients and highly relevant to further clinical work-up. **(p. 759)**

A7. **False**

Granulomatous appendicitis may be part of Crohn's disease but may also be an isolated phenomenon. Only follow-up will determine the true potential of the lesion. **(p. 761)**

A8. True

Signet ring carcinoma is an extremely rare occurrence at this site and more common relatively is the so-called goblet cell carcinoid, which has a neuroendocrine component in addition to the cells that have a well-differentiated signet ring appearance, singly or in clusters. There is wide variation of the extent of the neuroendocrine component. This highly characteristic morphology presents substantial difficulty in predicting prognosis, as some of these have proved to be extremely bad actors. **(p. 767)**

A9. True

The main differential diagnosis is between the flattened and 'inactive' mucosal lining due to some degree of obstruction, with stasis versus the so-called borderline proliferative mucinous lesions (previously mucinous tumors of uncertain biologic potential). **(p. 762)**

A10. True

Synchronous and metachronous colonic lesions, as well as a strikingly similar morphology in ovarian lesions are well recognized but the pathogenesis is poorly understood. Whether the ovarian lesion corresponds to implants originating from the appendix is unresolved, but is a possibility. **(p. 762)**

A11. True

Whether appendectomy suffices or whether right hemicolectomy is to be the treatment depends on the atypicality and the invasiveness of the epithelial lesion. Invasion through the wall, and cellular association to the extra-appendiceal mucin deposits, are the diagnostic hallmarks of cystadenocarcinoma. **(p. 763)**

A12. True

Sometimes the diagnosis is made on an involved hernia sac, excised during a herniorrhaphy. **(p. 764)**

A13. False

Antibodies to the different mucins were instrumental in our understanding of their possible contributions: for instance, gel-forming activity in MUC2 mucins with strong stromal bonds and also altered cell polarity may have additional roles in tumor progression. **(p. 765)**

Colon

A1. False

The dilated segment of bowel is proximal to the aganglionic bowel which appears grossly normal in caliber. The large, 'irregularly proliferated' submucosal plexus does coexist with absent ganglion cells and is a helpful diagnostic hint. **(p. 777)**

A2. True

Beyond the theoretical knowledge UC can present at any age, including childhood, and age will not help in ruling this diagnosis in or out. **(p. 782)**

A3. True

The extraintestinal organ involvement in UC includes the liver, the biliary tract (sclerosing cholangitis), carcinoma arising on this background, arthritis, uveitis, pyoderma gangrenosum etc. **(p. 785)**

A4. True

Ulcerative colitis typically involves the rectum, but one should remember that the inflammation may be mild, particularly in children. Patients treated with steroid or 5-aminosalicylic acid enemas also show atypical features. **(p. 784)**

A5. False

Reasons to biopsy such a patient include documenting actual inflammation, with multiple biopsies delineating the extent and pattern of involvement, to rule out special types of colitis, and to follow the evolution/spontaneous resolution, all correlated with endoscopic findings. **(p. 786)**

A6. False

Biopsies during treatment and/or clinical remission can have scattered clinically asymptomatic crypt abscesses without the need to ramp up therapy. On the other hand, microscopic evidence of significant active inflammation with crypt epithelial destruction can precede a clinical flare. So the role of the biopsy findings is to better frame the clinical impression, and in cases of long-standing disease carry out surveillance for dysplasia/carcinoma. **(p. 786)**

A7. False

Backwash ileitis occurs in only one-third of ulcerative colitis patients. The involved terminal ileum is dilated, rather than stenosed as in Crohn's disease. **(p. 784)**

A8. True

This operation, also performed in familial adenomatosis patients, has no such complication. The diagnosis relies heavily on clinical pathologic correlation and UC-like endoscopic changes within the mucosa. **(p. 784)**

A9. True

The initial concept of dysplasia included the assumption – since proven – that carcinoma in longstanding inflammatory conditions develops through a series of 'steps' that include increasing degrees of dysplasia. The hope of instituting early/preventative surgical therapy spawned the practice of surveillance biopsies, tested for the last 30 or so years. Some of the concepts have evolved since then, specifically the use of rectal biopsies to indicate patients at risk for dysplasia or carcinoma, currently replaced by total colonoscopy and multiple biopsies. However, other features of the dysplasia premise still drive the care of UC patients, even though we now know that high grade dysplasia is not an obligate step, i.e. all steps may not be necessary in the sequence to carcinoma. **(p. 786)**

A10. True

The complicated patterns of recurrent ulcerating lesions, irregular repair/loss of architectural hallmarks/scarring, adenoma formation and carcinoma are a difficult terrain to navigate for the endoscopist. The area of malignancy can simply be a raised thickened plaque or, more rarely, a polypoid or stricturing (as in scarring) mass (DALM = dysplasia-associated mass). Improved recognition of these features has allowed for targeted biopsies and hence better diagnosis. **(p. 786)**

A11. True

In current surgical pathology practice the original classification has been substantially simplified, both to improve interobserver variability and to make it more user friendly for follow-up strategies for clinicians. The result is a category of negative for dysplasia, indeterminate (with possibly but not necessarily a comment), and positive for dysplasia, low or high grade. **(p. 787)**

A12. False

The theoretical implications are different, but in practice the two types of lesions cannot be reliably separated; accordingly, treatment is currently the same and consists of polypectomy. Surveillance biopsies from adjacent mucosa will establish the presence or absence of dysplasia and take the patient into those algorithms for follow-up decision-making. **(p. 787)**

A13. True

This complication is less common than adenocarcinoma. Duration and extent of disease are factors in the development of mostly B-cell lymphoma. **(p. 822)**

A14. False

The finding of granulomas is not critical for the diagnosis of Crohn's disease. In fact, although it is also known as granulomatous colitis, the term is a misnomer for this systemic disease. It presents with fever, weight loss, and can involve multiple levels of the GI tract, small intestine and or colon as well as extraintestinal sites. When the predominant site of involvement is the colon, it is in the differential diagnosis of ulcerative colitis. Granulomas are found in less than 50% of cases. Some poorly formed granulomas may well be secondary to a ruptured or destroyed crypt in UC! **(p. 788)**

A15. True

There is a surveillance protocol in these patients with similar criteria of disease duration for the detection of dysplasia, using the same diagnostic categories with identical implications. **(p. 789)**

A16. True

These findings are important for distinguishing Crohn's disease from ulcerative colitis. **(p. 789)**

A17. True

In addition to these varied etiologies, rate of onset/duration will change the morphologic picture, as well as time of biopsy after the episode. The affected segment sampled on an endoscopic biopsy is often low-left-sided rather than splenic flexure, as would be expected from anatomy alone (watershed zone). **(p. 790)**

A18. False

So-called pseudomembranous colitis refers to *C. difficile*-associated colitis, often – but not necessarily – following antibiotic therapy; short of demonstrating the toxin in stool or culturing the organism, the pseudomembrane could simply be due to atherosclerotic ischemic colitis; clinical history and laboratory data are other more helpful criteria to separate the two entities. **(p. 790)**

A19. False

Microscopic colitis refers to the clinical constellation of a patient with watery diarrhea, a normal colonoscopy and an abnormal biopsy (lesion only seen on biopsy/microscopy). This may consist of intraepithelial lymphocytosis (in some cases as part of a known or unsuspected celiac disease complex) and variable degrees of stromal hyalinization; depending on the predominance of either feature, the entity is designated lymphocytic or collagenous colitis. **(p. 791)**

A20. False

There are pitfalls of measurement, including a tangential cutting incidence. The distinctive clinical context and the presence of inflammatory cells within and adjacent to the thickened collagen are more diagnostically useful than thickness per se, and special stains are not necessary for the diagnosis despite being esthetically pleasing. **(p. 791)**

A21. True for the wrong reasons

There are so-called commensal (non-hemolytic) entameba species that are pathogenic in immunosuppressed individuals, including AIDS patients. They can be present in a biopsy of a rectal ulcer and are readily seen on the routine section. **(p. 793)**

A22. True

There is a pre-ulcer polypoid stage, previously in a separate diagnostic category of so-called inflammatory cloacogenic polyp. The ulcerative stage, so-called solitary rectal ulcer, is often multiple and may not be ulcerated; moreover, the diagnostic change of fibrous obliteration of the lamina propria is in the mucosa adjacent to ulcers, with inflammation not usually part of the picture. Localized colitis cystica profunda may also be part of this family of lesions. **(p. 798)**

A23. True

Increasingly recognized is the entire gross/endoscopic spectrum of adenomatous change, from simple patches of reddened granular mucosa that have 'advanced' dysplastic change on biopsy – the so-called flat adenoma – to the pedunculated or sessile adenoma with various additional villous change. **(p. 799)**

A24. False

With the advent of the 'routine' colonoscopy screening procedure as a cancer prevention strategy, the lesions removed are ever smaller and incipient, and often highlight the spectrum of changes present within the same lesion that are separated only artificially into rigidly distinct categories. The insight into the complexities keeps evolving: the hyperplastic polyp currently being subdivided into four types is just an example. This is not only an academic exercise, as the right-sided sessile serrated adenoma is possibly an entry point into the serrated carcinoma pathway. **(p. 805)**

A25. True

The term pseudoinvasion refers to herniated crypts within the stalk with a range of degenerative and inflammatory changes, recognizable by the presence of hemosiderin-laden macrophages, irregularly splayed smooth muscle strands, bland nuclei within epithelium, and polymorphs within ruptured mucin-filled lumina. The differential diagnosis to rule out carcinoma invasive into stalk can, however, be fiendishly difficult. **(p. 800)**

A26. True

The further clinical implication of these lesions depends most importantly on whether they are sporadic (including possibly multiple) or part of some polyposis syndrome, of which novel constellations are increasingly recognized. Because the morphology is identical in the sporadic and familial forms, either clinical history or the age of the patient ought to trigger the further inquiry: for instance a 35–40-year-old patient with a large/'advanced' adenoma. **(p. 809)**

A27. False

Polyps are the hallmarks of this familial polyposis syndrome and serve as index lesions in prevention/detection efforts. **(p. 813)**

A28. True

These lesions are soft to palpation and may be so low that the endoscope goes past them, unless viewed again in retroflexion. **(p. 803)**

A29. False

The lesion is typically sessile, the fronds presenting only superficial aspects for biopsy, where the changes are possibly not representative of the lesion; indeed, high-grade dysplasia/carcinoma in situ within the superficial/papillary fronds would not be actionable in and of itself. It is the base that harbors the significant pathology, not uncommonly infiltrating carcinoma, not readily accessible to biopsy. Therefore, the complete removal of the lesion, increasingly endomucosally, is the diagnostic manoeuver and, if the lesion is benign, therapeutic. Such a specimen can be inked to help with deep 'margin' evaluation, fixed flat and sectioned in an optimal plane for best results. **(p. 803)**

A30. True

Hyperplastic polyps are currently subdivided into small left-sided ones that might well represent reactive change to a number of local inflammatory or other stimuli, responding with deranged maturation. The right-sided lesions, which can and often do have an adenomatous component, now called serrated adenoma, or sessile serrated adenoma may operate through the microsatellite instability genetic pathway and may be precursors to right-sided sporadic cancers, as well as, in the event of a germline mutation, familial non-polypoid colorectal cancer syndrome. **(p. 813)**

A31. True

These lesions have as yet no defined associated genetic change. **(p. 804)**

A32. False

Although cancer develops at a much lower incidence in the Peutz–Jeghers as well as the hyperplastic polyposis syndromes, when compared to familial polyposis/GARDNER syndrome, there is always a potential risk justifying surveillance. Focal adenomatous proliferation in these can trigger the adenoma carcinoma, the microsatellite instability, or yet another pathway leading to malignancy. **(p. 807)**

A33. True

Ganglioneuroma (sporadic or part of ganglioneuromatosis), perineurioma, neurofibroma, schwannoma and Kaposi sarcoma can all present as sporadic colonic polyps, correctly identifiable only on microscopy. Refer to the GIST concept as well. **(p. 824)**

A34. True

The exact nature of this is not entirely elucidated, but low-residue/high-fat western diets have been implicated. **(p. 810)**

A35. True

The mass interferes with luminal continuity. More rarely, perforation may also occur and be the presenting symptom. **(p. 765)**

A36. True

The various screening tests, the political will to reduce the incidence of this disease (Medicare reimbursement for screening colonoscopy) and improved understanding of the genotypic 'susceptibility' factors in familial and sporadic carcinoma aided in a 33% reduction of 13-year cumulative mortality in one study. **(p. 810)**

A37. False

It is a useful test to monitor tumor recurrence and metastatic status after surgery for colonic carcinoma, when previously elevated levels should return to and stay low. CEA also occurs in carcinoma of other extra-GI sites, such as the prostate, but in specific clinical settings it is a useful test for follow-up. **(p. 811)**

A38. True

In the differential diagnosis of a metastatic lesion of unknown primary, absence of staining for CEA tends to make a colonic lesion unlikely. **(p. 811)**

A39. True

DNA mismatch repair gene deficiencies play an important role in hereditary non-polyposis colorectal carcinomas. These tumors tend to be mucinous or poorly differentiated, with a prominent host immune response and a circumscribed growth pattern, and are usually located on the right side. **(p. 813)**

A40. False

p53 mutations are found in the majority of colonic carcinomas. The tumors expressing p53 do not seem to differ from others in terms of site, differentiation or DNA ploidy. **(p. 813)**

A41. True

Signet ring carcinomas tend to occur in the young. These tumors have a propensity for peritoneal dissemination and have a poor prognosis. **(p. 815)**

A42. False

Neuroendocrine tumors have a negative impact on survival in general, contrary to long-held views. The small cell variety in particular, similar to its pulmonary counterpart, has early metastasis to liver and a poor prognosis. GABA and other neurotransmitters produced by tumor cells have recently been found to activate signaling and metastatic pathways that are particularly aggressive. Not uncommonly small cell neuroendocrine carcinoma is associated with a villous adenoma. Adjuvant strategies such as chemotherapy, effective in pulmonary oat cell tumors, may be applicable if the diagnosis is considered. **(p. 816)**

A43. False

Although overall there is a good correlation between endoscopic impression and biopsy results, some inflammatory lesions have a malignant appearance with fixation to adjacent structures, and only the morphology clarifies the nature of the lesion. The contrary is also true, in that some diffuse, poorly differentiated lesions have a deceptively benign appearance. Moreover, cases of malignant melanoma have been seen masquerading in a 'congested' hemorrhoid, or in a cecal 'polyp' as well. **(p. 823)**

A44. False

Colon carcinoma has multiple possible growth patterns, probably determined by the molecular mechanisms that drive tumor formation, and polypid growth is one such possible pattern. Flat or depressed lesions have a tendency for deeper penetration into wall (more advanced stage). **(p. 811)**

A45. False

Radial margin (= adventitial soft tissue margin of non-peritonealized surface) determination by inking is paramount and will determine subsequent adjuvant therapies and prognosis. In cancer of the rectum, more than at any other site, local recurrence has no good options of 'rescue.' **(p. 819)**

A46. True

They are right-sided and mucinous, with a prominent 'Crohn-like' inflammatory infiltrate. **(p. 813)**

A47. False

The old debate centered on the caliber of the permeated vein as to prognostic relevance; any invasion, whether in biopsies, the submucosa/specimen or grossly in the mesentery, is significant. The extramural veins are the most predictive. **(p. 819)**

A48. True

The classification, proposed in 1937 by Cuthbert Dukes for rectal cancers, is still the organizing principle of the current TNM staging. The only significant refinement is within the group of stage C tumors. **(p. 817)**

A49. True

Depending on the depth of involvement and suspicion of positive nodes a number of pre-/postoperative radiation and adjuvant chemotherapy protocols now supplement the surgical approach. **(p. 818)**

A50. True

Prognosis and apportioning patients to new protocols now stratifies the number of nodes involved, and necessarily defines the minimum number of nodes to be harvested for meaningful evaluation in the standardization of treatment protocols. So-called *pericolonic tumor deposits* (PTDs) are recognized as a separate phenomenon, not to be 'counted' as a metastatic node. **(p. 818)**

A51. True

Although the number of nodes in the specimen is partially a function of site (rectum versus other sites), it is now an integral part of the data needed in multidisciplinary approach to colon carcinoma that involves radiation and medical oncology. A minimum of 14–15 nodes evaluated is the current standard for adequacy in the determination of nodal status. The pattern of node involvement is counterintuitive, in that the 'easy' large node is not uncommonly reactive and the metastasis is in some 1–2 mm node! The number of involved nodes *and* their distribution are highly predictive of prognosis. **(p. 820)**

A52. True

Microsatellite stable or near-stable tumors benefit from treatment with fluorouracil compounds, whereas microsatellite highly unstable cancers do not; patients who will not benefit can then be spared the toxic effects and expense of this treatment. **(p. 820)**

Anus

A1. True

Proximal to the dentate (pectinate) line the epithelium is columnar, and distally it is squamous keratinizing and non-keratinizing. The dentate line interface is lined by transitional epithelium, also known as cloacogenic epithelium. Microscopically it resembles bladder epithelium, but differs from it ultrastructurally. Immunohistochemically it expresses keratins 7 and 19, but not keratin 20. **(p. 856)**

A2. False

The upper portion drains into the wide field of hypogastric, obturator and internal iliac nodes, whereas the lower half drains into the superficial inguinal chain. **(p. 857)**

A3. True

Inflammatory change involving these epithelia, including in IBD, can invest and not uncommonly destroy sphincter function. **(p. 858)**

A4. True

These are broadly divided into supralevator, with a poor prognosis, and infralevator, easier to repair surgically because of normal innervation. **(p. 857)**

A5. False

Although it is true that the above may be etiologic in fistula formation, the most common histology is nonspecific granulation tissue formation, and the eventual presence of a granuloma can be entirely nonspecific as well. **(p. 858)**

A6. False, emphatically so

The vast majority of these specimens consist of thrombosed vessels at various stages of recanalization, with secondary stromal/epithelial change. On occasion, however, and entirely unsuspected clinically, malignant tumors are present, not grossly recognizable because of hemorrhage/induration, including melanoma, squamous cell carcinoma and others. **(p. 859)**

A7. True

The entire spectrum of benign squamous cell lesions dysplasia, intraepithelial neoplasia within adjacent mucosa, as well as the infiltrating tumor itself, is positive for these viral markers. HPV subtyping and IHC for proliferative markers (p16,ki67) are helpful in therapeutic decision making. Patients with HIV are particularly prone to this complication. **(p. 860)**

A8. False

This concept was replaced by the recognition that a variably differentiated squamous cell cancer is the unifying lesion, similar to upper digestive carcinoma. This allows for the inclusion of tumors with keratinization, basaloid, and some glandular features. **(p. 862)**

A9. True

In addition, in a female patient a recommendation for a pelvic examination is in order, as these are also associated with separate squamous cell carcinoma of the cervix and lower genital area. **(p. 860)**

A10. True

The best results are obtained with combined modalities. **(p. 863)**

A11. True

The differential diagnosis includes malignant melanoma and intraepithelial squamous cell carcinoma (Bowen's disease) and rests on the presence of intracytoplasmic acid mucosubstances, positive staining with antibodies to CEA and EMA, and the absence of melanoma markers. The prognosis depends on whether there is an associated invasive adenocarcinoma and/or lymph node involvement. **(p. 863)**

A12. True

A not uncommon lesion, primary melanoma with a junctional component can masquerade as an anorectal tumor. It has a poor prognosis. **(p. 859, 865)**

12 Major and minor salivary glands

Normal anatomy

Q1

The major duct of the parotid gland is known as Warthin's duct.

Q2

The parotid gland consists of superficial, intermediate and deep lobes.

Q3

The ratio of serous to mucinous components of the major salivary glands is constant.

Q4

The distribution of the facial nerve is in proximity to the parotid gland.

Q5

Under normal conditions sebaceous gland elements are never found associated with the major salivary glands.

Q6

Reserve cells of intercalated ducts are the source of stem cells for the regeneration of acinar tissue.

Q7

The myoepithelial cell component of the major salivary glands shows a consistent phenotype.

Q8

Salivary gland duct epithelium shows immunoreactivity for prostate-specific antigen.

Non-neoplastic lesions

Q1

The most common location of heterotopic salivary gland tissue is the mylohyoid muscle.

Q2

Mucoepidermoid carcinoma is the most frequent neoplasm affecting heterotopic salivary gland tissue.

Q3

Calculi are found most frequently in the major ducts of the parotid gland.

Q4

The composition of salivary gland stones is a mix of sodium and magnesium salts.

Q5

Acute inflammation of the salivary gland can be either a local or a systemic process.

Q6

Chronic sialadenitis may be secondary to either mixed connective tissue disorders or local obstructive processes.

Q7

Mycobacterial infection is the primary cause of granulomatous sialadenitis.

Q8

Multiloculated cysts of the parotid gland, lined by glandular or squamous epithelium and surrounded by florid lymphoid hyperplasia, is characteristic of a low-grade B-cell lymphoma.

Q9

Lymphoepithelial lesions of the salivary glands showing numerous interfollicular CD8+ cells have been associated with HIV infection.

Q10

Bilateral parotid enlargement, with the microscopic identification of epimyoepithelial islands and a brisk lymphoid infiltrate, is characteristic of Mikulicz's disease.

Q11

Mikulicz's disease may be localized to the salivary gland. When it is associated with a generalized symptom complex, it is known as Sjögren's syndrome.

Q12

The etiology of Mikulicz's disease and Sjögren's syndrome has been causally linked to Epstein–Barr virus.

Q13

The clonal expansion of lymphocytes in Mikulicz's disease and Sjögren's syndrome often gives rise to T-cell lymphomas.

Q14

Atypical cytologic changes and squamous elements in irradiated salivary glands usually represent either neoplastic transformation or metastatic disease.

Q15

Lymphoid hyperplasia of the salivary gland may be mistaken for a primary salivary gland tumor.

Q16

Epithelial hyperplasia of the salivary gland may be either ductal or acinar.

Tumors

Q1

Benign mixed tumor is most commonly seen in the submaxillary gland of middle-aged men.

Q2

Benign mixed tumor can be mistaken for carcinoma due to cytologic atypia and its propensity for capsular penetration.

Q3

The mucin present in benign mixed tumor consists of neutral glycoproteins.

Q4

Extremely cellular benign mixed tumors with cytologic atypia have a propensity for malignant transformation.

Q5

The keratins most frequently expressed by the ductal epithelial cells of benign mixed tumors are CK19 and CK14.

Q6

The expression of glial markers such as glial fibrillary acid protein and astroprotein in benign mixed tumors supports a neural crest origin for these lesions.

Q7

Benign mixed tumors may show a normal karyotype, rearrangement of 8q12, or rearrangements of 12q14-15.

Q8

The recurrence rate of benign mixed tumor is dependent on the type of chromosomal rearrangement.

Q9

Benign mixed tumors do not metastasize.

Q10

The transformation of a benign mixed tumor to a malignant form is often heralded by the onset of local clinical symptoms in a previously asymptomatic nodule.

Q11

Benign mixed tumors of the parotid gland are more likely to undergo malignant transformation than are tumors of the other major salivary glands.

Q12

Malignant transformation in benign mixed tumors can occur in either the epithelial or the stromal component.

Q13

Immunoreactivity for p53 is more common in malignant tumors than in benign mixed tumors.

Q14

The majority of oxyphilic adenomas occur in the submaxillary gland.

Q15

Oxyphilic change in benign salivary gland tumors is increased in those patients with a history of radiation exposure.

Q16

Malignant change in oxyphilic adenomas occurs at the same rate as malignant transformation of benign mixed tumors.

Q17

Warthin's tumors most commonly occur in the parotid gland.

Q18

The lymphocytic component of Warthin's tumors is typically composed of T cells and dendritic cells.

Q19

The epithelial component of Warthin's tumor may undergo malignant transformation.

Q20

Basal cell adenoma usually occurs in the parotid gland.

Q21

Basal cell adenomas may have a varied histologic appearance.

Q22

Canalicular adenoma is a variant of basal cell adenoma.

Q23

A major differential diagnosis of basal cell adenoma is adenoid cystic carcinoma.

Q24

Basal cell adenocarcinoma shows an identical immunohistochemical profile to basal cell adenoma.

Q25

Sebaceous differentiation may occur in Warthin's tumor but is not seen in mucoepidermoid carcinoma or adenoid cystic carcinoma.

Q26

Tumors with predominant sebaceous differentiation are restricted to cutaneous neoplasms and are not found in major salivary glands.

Q27

Salivary gland tumors showing a myoepithelial cell type – so-called myoepitheliomas – may occur in a variety of morphologic forms.

Q28

The collagenous crystalloids occurring in myoepitheliomas are composed of laminin and type IV collagen.

Q29

The clear cell type of myoepithelioma contains cytoplasmic mucin and fat.

Q30

As the name implies, myoepitheliomas show strong immunoreactivity for smooth muscle actin.

Q31

All clear cell myoepitheliomas should be regarded as potentially malignant.

Q32

Hyalinizing clear cell carcinoma refers to a heterogeneous group of neoplasms occurring in the oral cavity without a specific form of clear cell differentiation.

Q33

Mucoepidermoid carcinoma represents the most common malignant salivary gland tumor in children.

Q34

Mucoepidermoid carcinoma consists of two major cell types, mucin producing and keratinizing.

Q35

Low-grade mucoepidermoid carcinoma consists of well-differentiated squamous elements.

Q36

Inflammatory reactions to mucin and keratin can obscure the diagnosis of mucoepidermoid carcinoma.

Q37

The prognosis of mucoepidermoid carcinoma is dependent on grade.

Q38

Most acinic cell carcinomas occur in older women and are located in the minor salivary glands.

Q39

Acinic cell carcinomas show a uniform histology composed of polygonal cells with basophilic granules and a solid growth pattern.

Q40

Acinic cell carcinomas may undergo dedifferentiation.

Q41

Adenoid cystic carcinomas also are known as cylindromas.

Q42

Adenoid cystic carcinoma contains PAS-positive material.

Q43

Perineural invasion is rarely found in adenoid cystic carcinoma.

Q44

There are no consistent chromosomal abnormalities associated with adenoid cystic carcinoma.

Q45

Immunohistochemical staining is crucial in distinguishing benign mixed tumor from adenoid cystic carcinoma.

Q46

Polymorphous low-grade carcinoma may be confused with adenoid cystic carcinoma.

Q47

Solid forms of adenoid cystic carcinoma show a worse prognosis than tubular patterns.

Q48

Adenoid cystic carcinomas frequently metastasize to the liver.

Q49

Salivary duct carcinoma resembles microscopically ductal carcinoma of the breast.

Q50

Biomarkers are helpful in predicting the outcome of salivary duct carcinoma.

Q51

Polymorphous low-grade adenocarcinoma is synonymous with terminal duct carcinoma.

Q52

Papillary adenocarcinomas of the parotid gland show mucinous and squamous differentiation.

Q53

Most squamous cell carcinomas the parotid region represent either a metastasis or over-represented squamous differentiation in a mucoepidermoid carcinoma.

Q54

Neuroendocrine neoplasms of the salivary gland do not express the usual immunohistochemical markers associated with similar neoplasms in other organ systems.

Q55

Lymphoepithelioma-like carcinoma represents an undifferentiated carcinoma.

Q56

BK polyoma virus is commonly found in lymphoepithelioma-like carcinoma.

Q57

Most salivary gland lymphomas are composed of small cells and belong to the group of lesions known as MALT/marginal zone lymphoma.

Q58

Salivary gland lymphomas may present as chronic sclerosing sialadenitis.

Q59

The most common benign salivary gland tumor in infants and children is pleomorphic adenoma.

Q60

True spindle cell sarcomas do not occur in the major salivary glands.

Q61

Most metastatic tumors to major salivary glands actually occur in the closely associated intraglandular or periglandular lymph nodes.

Q62

Salivary gland tumors occur more often in the oral cavity and submaxillary region than elsewhere.

Q63

The incidence of malignant primary salivary gland tumor is highest in the parotid gland.

Q64

The most common malignant tumor of the submaxillary gland is a mucoepidermoid carcinoma.

Q65

Whether benign or malignant, primary salivary gland tumors are almost invariably unilateral.

Q66

Little is known about the etiology of most salivary gland neoplasms.

Q67

Fine needle aspiration and core needle biopsy of salivary gland tumors is contraindicated owing to the risk of tumor implantation along the needle track.

Q68

The most common diagnostic error on frozen section evaluation of salivary gland tumors is under-diagnosis of mucoepidermoid carcinoma.

Q69

Low-dose radiation therapy is an acceptable mode of primary therapy for localized benign mixed tumors.

Q70

The prognosis of salivary gland tumors is dependent on histologic type, clinical stage and location.

Normal anatomy

A1. False

The major parotid gland duct is Stensen's duct. Warthin's duct is found in the submaxillary gland and Bartholin's duct is associated with the sublingual gland. **(p. 873)**

A2. False

The parotid gland consists of superficial and deep lobes only. Running between the two lobes is the facial nerve. **(p. 873)**

A3. False

The parotid gland is exclusively serous. The submaxillary gland is mixed seromucinous. The sublingual gland shows a mucinous predominance. **(p. 873)**

A4. True

This nerve usually is situated between the superficial and deep lobes. Anatomic variations occur. **(p. 873)**

A5. False

Sebaceous glands are often annexed to the duct system in the parotid and submaxillary glands. **(p. 874)**

A6. True

Additionally, the reserve cells are thought to be the progenitors of most of the common epithelial cell tumors. **(p. 874)**

A7. False

Myoepithelial cells of the parotid will express calponin and h-caldesmon. Those of the submaxillary gland also express smooth muscle actin, and in the minor salivary glands these cells will express smooth muscle myosin heavy chain. **(p. 874)**

A8. True

This is a peculiar feature of salivary duct epithelium. Interestingly, some tumors arising from these structures also will express PSA. **(p. 874)**

Non-neoplastic lesions

A1. False

Most displaced salivary gland tissue occurs in regional lymph nodes. **(p. 874)**

A2. False

Warthin's tumor is the most frequently diagnosed neoplasm. **(p. 874)**

A3. False

The major ducts of the submaxillary gland are most often affected. **(p. 874)**

A4. False

Salivary gland calculi are typically composed of calcium salts. **(p. 874)**

A5. True

Sialadenitis may be a local infection or secondary to a systemic process such as mumps (paramyxovirus). **(p. 875)**

A6. True

Although the majority of infiltrating lymphocytes in chronic sialadenitis are of B-cell origin, the underlying process is thought to be a T cell-mediated response against antigens expressed by the duct epithelium. **(p. 875)**

A7. False

Granulomatous inflammation may be seen in sarcoidosis, but may also be secondary to duct obstruction or infection with fungi such as *Histoplasma capsulatum*. **(p. 875)**

A8. False

This process represents a benign lymphoepithelial cyst and most likely represents an acquired process secondary to the proliferation of branchial patch-derived epithelium and the recruitment of benign lymphocytes. **(p. 875)**

A9. True

The combination of lymphoepithelial cysts and solid lymphoepithelial islands strongly suggests HIV-induced salivary gland disease. **(p. 876)**

A10. True

The lymphoid tissue typically contains well-formed germinal centers and shows a mixed population of B and T cells. **(p. 876)**

A11. True

The symptom complex of keratoconjunctivitis, xerostomia, rheumatoid arthritis and hypergammaglobulinemia is known as Sjögren's syndrome. **(p. 876)**

A12. False

The etiology of these diseases remains unknown. The association with Epstein–Barr virus is casual rather than causal. The incidence of these diseases is increased in HIV-infected patients and in patients with hepatitis C-related chronic liver disease. **(p. 877)**

A13. False

T-cell lymphomas occur but are rare. Most cases of salivary gland lymphomas are B cell in origin, either large B-cell lymphomas or small lymphocytic lymphomas with or without plasmacytoid features. **(p. 877)**

A14. False

These changes are metaplastic and represent collateral damage in irradiated fields. Over-diagnosing such changes as either primary or metastatic tumor can result in unnecessary radical surgery. **(p. 878)**

A15. True

Clinically, lymphoid hyperplasia presents as a mass lesion. These changes are usually nonspecific but may be secondary to infection, such as cat scratch disease. **(p. 878)**

A16. True

Adenomatoid acinar hyperplasia is found predominantly in the intraoral salivary glands. Ductal hyperplasia is seen in the major glands and may be a precursor to epithelial tumors. **(p. 878)**

Tumors

A1. False

These benign tumors are most frequent in women in the fourth decade and are 10 times more common in the parotid than in the submaxillary gland. **(p. 879)**

A2. True

Microscopic examination frequently shows a cellular lesion with scattered bizarre tumor cells and areas of capsular penetration. Furthermore, tumor cells can be found occupying vascular lumina. An understanding of the pleomorphic nature of this neoplasm and the presence of a mixed cell population in a chondroid matrix are aids in avoiding a diagnosis of malignancy. **(p. 879)**

A3. False

Benign mixed tumor contains two types of mucin. The epithelial mucin has a high content of neutral glycoproteins. The connective tissue type of mucin contains both sulfated and non-sulfated glycosaminoglycans. **(p. 880)**

A4. False

Follow-up studies have shown that cellular variants with scattered hyperchromatic cells do not behave differently from the usual form of benign mixed tumor. The absence of significant mitotic activity and cellular necrosis helps differentiate benign from malignant tumors. **(p. 880)**

A5. True

A shortlist of antigens expressed by this epithelium includes EMA, type IV collagen, laminin, secretory component, CEA, lysozyme, α-antitrypsin, and α-antichymotrypsin. It should be noted that the myoepithelial component of these tumors is immunoreactive for keratin, actin, myosin, other smooth muscle-specific proteins, and S-100 protein. **(p. 880)**

A6. False

The expression of glial markers in benign mixed tumors is difficult to explain. The phenomenon may be secondary to cross-reactivity with intermediate filaments of similar structure. Expression may be related to the capacity for cartilaginous differentiation. These antigens may be exploited in differentiating benign mixed tumors from adenoid cystic carcinoma and basal cell adenoma. **(p. 880)**

A7. True

The above rearrangements have been reported in benign mixed tumors. Interestingly, there is no overexpression of p53. **(p. 881)**

A8. False

The recurrence rate of benign mixed tumors depends upon the adequacy of primary excision. Inapparent satellite nodules may be present surrounding the main mass. These tumor nodules are not addressed by simple enucleation. **(p. 881)**

A9. False

Rarely, a benign mixed tumor of ordinary microscopic appearance will metastasize. This has been reported in immunocompromised patients. A good number of the reported metastases have presented as isolated renal masses. **(p. 881)**

A10. True

This complication occurs in approximately 10% of cases. Clinical symptoms include pain, rapid growth, and facial nerve paralysis. **(p. 881)**

A11. False

Tumors of the submandibular gland show a greater propensity to malignant transformation. **(p. 882)**

A12. True

The malignant component of these tumors is usually epithelial and assumes the appearance of one of the well-recognized variants of salivary gland carcinoma, such as mucoepidermoid or adenoid cystic carcinoma. However, transformation can occur in the mesenchymal elements, typically in the form of chondrosarcoma. **(p. 882)**

A13. True

Malignant areas often react with antibody B72.3 and also overexpress p53 and c-erbB-2 as well. **(p. 882)**

A14. False

The majority of benign tumors with oncocytic change occur in the parotid gland. **(p. 882)**

A15. True
Patients with either therapeutic radiation exposure or long-term low-dose occupational exposure show a higher incidence of oxyphilic adenomas. **(p. 882)**

A16. False
Malignant transformation in oxyphilic adenomas is vanishingly rare. **(p. 883)**

A17. True
Cases involving the submaxillary gland have been reported but are usually secondary to the mandibular extension of the parotid gland. **(p. 883)**

A18. False
The lymphoid stroma is predominantly of B-cell origin, with fewer T cells, mast cells and dendritic cells. Interestingly, there is a predominance of IgA-producing B cells. **(p. 884)**

A19. True
The epithelial component may involve into adenocarcinoma, mucoepidermoid carcinoma or squamous cell carcinoma. Cases of oncocytic carcinoma and Merkel cell carcinoma have been reported. In addition, the lymphocytic component of Warthin's tumor may undergo transformation to lymphoma. **(p. 884)**

A20. True
Additionally, these benign neoplasms usually arise in adults and show a slight female preponderance. **(p. 885)**

A21. True
These neoplasms may be cystic or solid. The pattern of growth may be either tubular or trabecular. Some variants show abundant basal laminar material around epithelial nests, identical to cutaneous eccrine dermal cylindroma. **(p. 886)**

A22. True
However, these tumors show a tendency to arise from minor salivary glands and grow in loose stroma in the form of bilayered strands and ribbons. **(p. 886)**

A23. True
Distinguishing points include encapsulation, lack of stromal invasion, and no perineural invasion. **(p. 886)**

A24. False
Although the immunohistochemical profiles are similar, malignant tumors tend to express p53, bcl-2 and EGFR. **(p. 886)**

A25. False
Sebaceous differentiation may occur in benign or malignant salivary gland tumors, including benign mixed tumors. **(p. 887)**

A26. False
Benign and malignant tumors with a predominant sebaceous component occur in the salivary gland. Additionally, sebaceous differentiation can accompany tumors with a lymphoid stroma. **(p. 888)**

A27. True
Myoepitheliomas may occur in a spindle cell, hyaline (plasmacytoid) or clear cell type. Mixed cell types are seen. **(p. 888)**

A28. False
These crystalloids are composed of actin and keratin. **(p. 888)**

A29. False
The clear cells contain variable amounts of glycogen but no fat or mucin. **(p. 889)**

A30. False
Myoepithelioma cells show reactivity for keratin and S-100 protein, but many are negative for smooth muscle actin. There is variable staining for vimentin. **(p. 889)**

A31. True
Series have been published that show increased rates of recurrence, nodal metastasis, distant metastasis and tumor-related deaths. **(p. 890)**

A32. True
There is a group of neoplasms without a homogeneous or specific cell type and which cannot be placed into a specific descriptive category. Most show a prominent fibrohyaline stroma and are given a descriptive designation. **(p. 890)**

A33. True
These carcinomas are most commonly found in the parotid gland in children. **(p. 890)**

A34. False
These tumors consist of four cell types, mucin-producing cells, squamous cells, intermediate cells and clear cells. Also, they are divided into low- and high-grade malignancies. **(p. 890)**

A35. False
Low-grade variants show well-differentiated mucinous cells with cystic areas. High-grade lesions are more solid and display an infiltrative pattern, with intermediate and clear cells dominate over mucin-producing cells. **(p. 890)**

A36. True
Fibrosis and dense inflammation can hide the presence of mucoepidermoid carcinoma. Extensive sampling is necessary to ensure the proper diagnosis. **(p. 891)**

A37. True
Patients who have low-grade lesions do well. Some authors suggest a point system that includes histology, cytologic atypia, invasion, necrosis and mitotic activity. Interestingly, young patients do better than old patients, females do better than males, and parotid lesions do better than submandibular tumors. **(p. 891)**

A38. False
There is a male preponderance, with a peak incidence of the third decade of life. Most tumors occur in the parotid gland. **(p. 891)**

A39. False

These tumors may be solid, microcystic, papillary–cystic or follicular. Additionally, there is variability in cell types, designated as intercalated, clear or vacuolated. A neuroendocrine component may be identified both histologically and by immunoreactivity for vasoactive intestinal peptide. **(p. 891)**

A40. True

This is a poor prognostic sign. The cells are associated with aneuploidy and helioid inclusions at the ultrastructural level. **(p. 892)**

A41. True

These tumors are generally slow growing but relentless in their recurrences. They are the most common malignant tumor of minor salivary gland tissue. **(p. 892)**

A42. True

These tumors classically have a cribriform pattern with nests of tumor cells arranged around PAS-positive pseudocysts. Both pseudocysts and true glandular lumina must be identified for the proper diagnosis of adenoid cystic carcinoma. **(p. 892)**

A43. False

If the tissue is adequately sampled, perineural invasion is invariably identified. The diagnosis should be questioned if numerous samples from the periphery of the tumor do not exhibit this feature. **(p. 892)**

A44. False

There is a high incidence of loss of heterozygosity (LOH) at 6q23-35. **(p. 893)**

A45. False

There is similar histogenesis (intercalated duct cells) between these neoplasms and staining panels are not useful. There is a greater representation of non-sulfated glycosaminoglycans in benign mixed tumors. **(p. 893)**

A46. True

However, adenoid cystic carcinoma usually shows strong immunoreactivity for CD-117, whereas polymorphous low-grade carcinoma is negative or shows only weak staining. **(p. 894)**

A47. True

Growth patterns are used in some grading systems. The classic cribriform growth pattern has an intermediate prognosis. **(p. 894)**

A48. False

These neoplasms frequently metastasize to the lung. Metastases are clinically silent and are usually multiple. **(p. 894)**

A49. True

This malignant neoplasm exhibits a similar range of histologic appearances as seen in mammary carcinoma, with comedo, solid, cribriform, papillary and mucinous varieties. It is a tumor of elderly men, affecting both the parotid gland and the submaxillary gland. **(p. 894)**

A50. True

Data concerning Her2/neu expression, p53 expression and DNA content mirror those obtained from the study of mammary carcinomas. **(p. 894)**

A51. True

Some authors also describe these lesions as lobular carcinoma. They usually occur in the minor salivary glands of the oral cavity. In the differential diagnosis one should consider adenoid cystic carcinoma and benign mixed tumor. **(p. 895)**

A52. False

These neoplasms have well defined papillary structures and generally produce mucin. Typically there are no squamous or intermediate components. **(p. 895)**

A53. True

Primary squamous cell carcinoma in the parotid region is rare. **(p. 895)**

A54. False

As in the lung, these tumors contain dense core granules on electron microscopy and immunohistochemically stain with antibodies to typical neuroendocrine markers such as NSE, chromogranin, synaptophysin and Leu7. Keratins and EMA are regularly expressed. **(p. 895)**

A55. True

Lymphoepithelioma-like carcinoma is an important subtype of undifferentiated carcinoma. It is particularly frequent among Chinese, in whom it may show familial clustering. Regional lymph node metastases are very common, but the overall outcome in the better-documented cases seems to be overall relatively good. **(p. 896)**

A56. False

Patients with this tumor typically have clinical evidence of Epstein–Barr virus infection. EBV DNA can be demonstrated in these tumors by in situ hybridization or polymerase chain reaction. **(p. 896)**

A57. True

These lymphomas are characterized by slow clinical evolution and an excellent long-term prognosis. **(p. 896)**

A58. True

These neoplasms have been reported to cause obstructive symptoms, with a resultant hard fibrotic mass (Kuttner's tumor). **(p. 896)**

A59. False

Capillary hemangioma of the benign hemangioendothelioma type is the most common salivary gland tumor in children. Typically it involves the parotid gland and forms a diffuse soft mass without fixation. **(p. 897)**

A60. False

Fibrosarcoma, synovial sarcoma and angiosarcoma have been reported arising in association with salivary gland tissue. Additionally, malignant nerve sheath tumors can present within the parotid gland. In children, embryonal rhabdomyosarcoma can arise in the parotid region and secondarily invade the gland. **(p. 897)**

A61. True

As the metastatic tumor grows, it can mimic a primary neoplasm in the salivary gland. Importantly, the most common tumor of the submaxillary region is a metastasis rather than a primary salivary gland neoplasm. **(p. 897)**

A62. False

Most primary tumors arise in the parotid gland. Further, most primary tumors are not malignant and fall into the category of benign mixed tumor. **(p. 898)**

A63. False

The incidence of malignancy is highest in tumors of the sublingual gland. **(p. 898)**

A64. False

Most malignant submaxillary gland tumors are adenoid cystic carcinomas. Mucoepidermoid carcinomas are more common in the parotid gland. **(p. 898)**

A65. False

Although most salivary tumors are usually unilateral, Warthin's tumors are commonly bilateral. **(p. 898)**

A66. True

Save for the association of Epstein–Barr virus with lymphoepithelioma-like carcinoma, there are few etiologic data. An increased incidence has been reported in atomic bomb survivors and in children with a history of regional radiation therapy. **(p. 898)**

A67. False

Tumor implantation is theoretically possible with core needle biopsy. However, fine needle aspiration has proved to be a successful clinical procedure. In some instances the aspiration procedure can induce inflammatory and reparative changes that complicate the subsequent histopathologic evaluation, although these rarely compromise the final diagnosis. **(p. 899)**

A68. True

The accuracy of intraoperative frozen sections is dependent on the expertise of the pathologist. A common error is diagnosing mucoepidermoid carcinoma as a benign tumor. **(p. 899)**

A69. False

The preferred treatment of benign or malignant salivary gland tumors is complete surgical removal. Radiation therapy has been used as the primary modality in inoperable tumors. It is also used as an adjunct for incomplete resections or recurrent lesions. **(p. 900)**

A70. True

Low-stage tumors that are easily excised in their entirety do well. This is especially true if located in a superficial lobe of parotid gland. For adenoid cystic carcinoma the prognosis is best when located in the palate, and worse when they are located in the submaxillary gland. Histologic type will dictate long-term survival as an independent prognostic indicator. Well differentiated mucoepidermoid carcinomas tend to do well. High-grade carcinoma in pleomorphic adenoma does poorly. **(p. 900)**

13 Liver

Normal anatomy

Q1

The hepatic lobule is centered on the centrilobular vein and surrounded at its periphery by approximately six portal tracts.

Q2

The space of Disse is located between the sinusoidal (apical) cell surface of hepatocytes and the sinusoidal lining cells.

Q3

Each portal tract contains a 'triad' comprising a single branch of the hepatic artery and portal vein and only one bile duct.

Q4

Hepatocytes contain abundant cytoplasmic glycogen, but intranuclear glycogen is seen only in pathological conditions, such as diabetes and Wilson disease.

Q5

Normal liver plates are two cells thick in both children and adults.

Biopsy

Q1

There are four primary methods to obtain a liver biopsy, based on a transcutaneous, peritoneoscopic, open surgical or transvenous approach.

Q2

Foci of necrosis surrounded by neutrophils are common in liver tissue obtained by surgical incisional biopsy at the end of long operations.

Q3

The liver biopsy is still the best approach to the diagnosis of acute viral hepatitis.

Q4

The liver biopsy is still the gold standard for the diagnosis of liver transplant rejection.

Q5

Perls' stain for iron is the best histochemical method for the diagnosis of α_1-antitrypsin deficiency.

QUESTIONS

Viral hepatitis

Q1

In the classic form, acute viral hepatitis caused by one of the five major hepatotropic viruses is best described as lobular hepatitis with spotty necrosis.

Q2

This liver biopsy shows the typical features of acute viral hepatitis. The round eosinophilic structures in the center of the field represent apoptotic bodies.

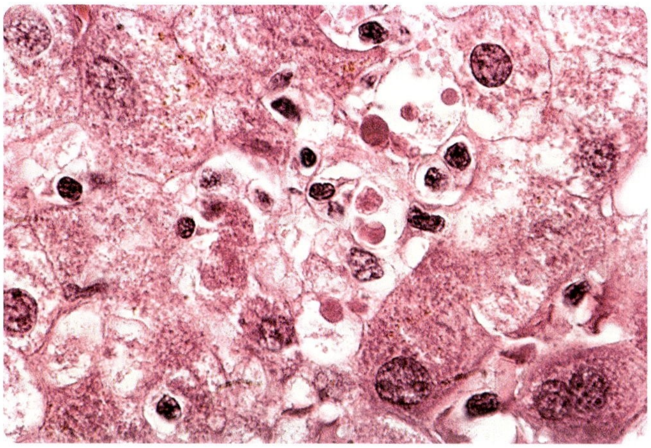

Fig. 13.1

Q3

'Lobular disarray' seen in viral hepatitis results from the inability of the hepatocytes to regenerate and thus repair the virus-induced damage.

Q4

Inflammatory infiltrates inside the lobules affected by one of the major five hepatitis viruses consist predominantly of neutrophils (polymorphonuclear leukocytes).

Q5

In acute viral hepatitis the inflammation is intralobular and the portal tracts are not inflamed.

Q6

'Piecemeal necrosis,' i.e. interface hepatitis blurring the outlines of portal tracts, is diagnostic of chronic hepatitis and does not occur in acute viral hepatitis.

Q7

Severe viral hepatitis may cause extensive necrosis that is most prominent in the centrilobular zone.

Q8

Submassive liver necrosis caused by hepatitis viruses is typically panlobular and multilobular, but may still be missed on liver biopsy.

Q9

Submassive liver necrosis is almost invariably caused by viruses or toxins.

Q10

Viral hepatitis A may present as mild cholestatic hepatitis, especially in adults.

Q11

Liver cell injury in viral hepatitis B is caused by viruses that are typically located in the liver cell nuclei.

Q12

Viral antigens are readily demonstrable immunohistochemically in hepatocytes during acute viral hepatitis B.

Q13

Acute viral hepatitis C may cause the same pathologic changes as HAV or HBV, but may also cause prominent steatosis, bile duct injury, and induce the formation of lymphoid aggregates in portal tracts.

Q14

Acute viral hepatitis can be histologically indistinguishable from drug-induced hepatitis.

Q15

The elementary lesions of chronic hepatitis include necroinflammatory intralobular lesions, portal inflammation, interface hepatitis and fibrosis.

Q16

The etiologic diagnosis of chronic hepatitis cannot be made on the basis of histologic findings alone, but requires correlation of histology with serologic and clinical data.

Q17

Histologic grading of chronic hepatitis is based on the extent of fibrosis.

Q18

Ground-glass hepatocytes develop only in the course of chronic viral hepatitis B and are diagnostic of that disease.

Q19

Portal tract lymphoid follicles with germinal centers are diagnostic of chronic viral hepatitis C.

Q20

Large cell dysplasia that develops in the course of chronic viral hepatitis B or C is composed of atypical cells that are the direct precursors of liver cell carcinoma.

Q21

Bilirubin stasis occurs much more frequently in chronic than in acute hepatitis.

Cirrhosis

Q1

Cirrhosis is the end stage of many liver diseases and is characterized by a loss of normal liver architecture and replacement of normal liver parenchyma by nodules and diffuse internodular fibrosis.

Q2

Fragmentation of the needle liver biopsy specimen is often indicative of cirrhosis.

Q3

Incomplete septal cirrhosis may be hard to diagnose by needle biopsy.

Q4

In biliary cirrhosis the liver nodules are composed of small dark-brown hepatocytes and are surrounded by almost completely round strands of fibrous tissue.

Q5

Deposits of copper in liver cells, demonstrable by rhodanine staining, are diagnostic of Wilson disease.

Q6

Inactive cirrhosis is characterized by an almost complete absence of necroinflammatory lesions and a sharp delineation between the liver cell nodules and the fibrous septa, which contain few inflammatory cells.

Q7

Coagulation necrosis of the entire hepatocellular nodules in cirrhosis is usually a consequence of hypoperfusion.

Q8

Focal nodular hyperplasia consists histologically of nodules and fibrous septa and may thus resemble cirrhosis.

Drug-induced and toxic liver injury

Q1

The same drug may cause different patterns of liver injury in different patients.

Q2

The drug reactions can be classified as predictable, which are dose dependent, or unpredictable, which are caused by hypersensitivity, a host-dependent reaction, or simply idiosyncratic.

Q3

Drug-induced changes show zonal distribution inside the liver lobule.

Q4

Macrovesical steatosis is typically caused by tetracycline, and in children it is seen in Reye's syndrome related to treatment with acetyl salicylate (aspirin).

Q5

Cholestatic drug injury is the most common hepatic side effect of drugs.

Q6

Mushroom poisoning with *Amanita phalloides* causes centrilobular hepatic necrosis.

Q7

Intravenous illicit drug abuse is often associated with an accumulation of talc particles in liver cells.

Q8

Hepatic adverse drug reaction may present in the form of granulomas.

Q9

Drugs may cause bile ductular injury, which may progress to ductopenic cholestasis.

Q10

Veno-occlusive disease found after bone marrow transplantation involves the main hepatic vein and results clinically in Budd–Chiari syndrome.

Q11

A drug reaction should be suspected if the liver biopsy shows signs of viral hepatitis with a disproportionately severe degree of parenchymal necrosis in relation to the patient's clinical condition, or coincidental other lesions such as steatosis, bile ductular injury, eosinophils or granulomas.

Steatosis and steatohepatitis

Q1

Steatosis is a nonspecific sign of reversible liver cell injury.

Q2

In AIDS, steatosis is predominantly centrilobular.

Q3

Lipogranulomas represent a focal reaction of macrophages and lymphocytes to ruptured lipid-laden hepatocytes.

Q4

All patients with steatosis of the liver ultimately develop fibrosis, which may lead to cirrhosis.

Q5

Alcoholic steatohepatitis involves predominantly the periportal zone.

Q6

Alcoholic cirrhosis is typically macronodular.

Q7

Hepatocellular siderosis occurs in some alcoholics and may be difficult to distinguish from genetic hemochromatosis.

Q8

Fibrosis restricted to portal areas and accompanied by cholestasis in a person known for alcohol abuse should arouse the suspicion of alcohol-induced chronic pancreatitis and chronic biliary obstruction.

Q9

Non-alcoholic steatohepatitis (NASH) has most often a multifactorial etiology.

Q10

Liver biopsy is the most reliable approach to distinguishing alcoholic from non-alcoholic steatohepatitis.

Cholestasis and biliary diseases

Q1

Cholestasis results from disturbances in bile secretion or bile flow.

Q2

Cholestasis may be intrahepatic or extrahepatic, complete or incomplete, acute or chronic.

Q3

The first histologic signs of acute complete cholestasis are bile canalicular bilirubin plugs in the periportal zone.

Q4

Kupffer cell bilirubin stasis occurs only a few days after the onset of acute complete cholestasis.

Q5

Bilirubin is birefringent under polarized light and thus can be distinguished from other brown pigments, such as hemosiderin.

Q6

Cholate stasis is a feature of chronic cholestasis.

Q7

Cholestatic liver cell rosettes are a sign of liver cell regeneration in chronic cholestasis.

Q8

Bile infarcts are usually a consequence of long-standing cholestasis caused by large bile duct obstruction.

Q9

Parenchymal multinucleated giant cells are diagnostic of chronic cholestasis in infants.

Q10

Extramedullary hematopoiesis is diagnostic of extrahepatic biliary obstruction in infancy.

Q11

Ductular reaction is a constant feature of chronic incomplete cholestasis but may be absent in some conditions, such as Alagille syndrome, primary sclerosing cholangitis and chronic transplant rejection.

Q12

Chronic cholestasis-induced ductular changes, portal fibrosis and the architectural changes in the liver parenchyma may be graded on a scale from 1 to 4.

Q13

Progressive familial intrahepatic cholestasis (PFIC) is not a single disease but includes several entities, each of which is related to a specific genetic mutation.

Q14

Ductular bilirubin stasis is diagnostic of septicemia and endotoxic shock.

Q15

Approximately 70–80% of portal tract arteries are accompanied by a bile duct, and so-called 'widowed' arteries unaccompanied by bile ducts signal a missing bile duct.

Q16

Congenital biliary atresia is limited to the extrahepatic bile ducts.

Q17

Primary biliary cirrhosis (PBC) is a chronic non-suppurative, destructive cholangitis that in more than 90% of patients is associated with antimitochondrial antibodies.

Q18

This figure illustrates the typical features of the florid bile duct lesions characteristically found in primary biliary cirrhosis.

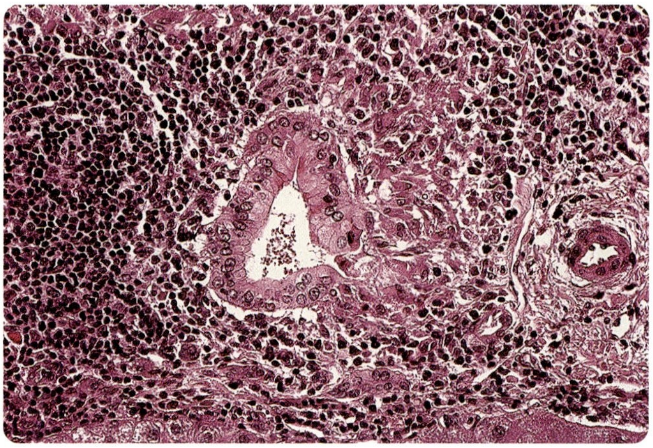

Fig. 13.2

Q19

Immune cholangitis is a term used for a disease that is pathologically indistinguishable from primary biliary cirrhosis but not accompanied by the antimitochondrial antibodies.

Q20

Primary sclerosing cholangitis (PSC) is more common in women than in men.

Q21

Most patients with PSC have only large bile duct involvement.

Q22

Concentric periductal fibrosis is diagnostic of primary sclerosing cholangitis.

Q23

Infiltrates of neutrophils in portal tracts are found in both aseptic biliary obstruction and ascending bacterial cholangitis.

Childhood disorders and disorders of metabolism

Q1

Neonatal cholestasis may be caused by a variety of genetic, developmental or infectious diseases.

Q2

In Gilbert's syndrome the liver shows no pathologic histologic changes.

Q3

α_1-Antitrypsin deficiency is a lysosomal storage disease.

Q4

α_1-Antitrypsin deficiency can be recognized on liver biopsy in the immediate postnatal period.

Q5

In neonates and young children α_1-antitrypsin deficiency may cause pathologic changes that are indistinguishable from those of bile duct atresia.

Q6

Indian childhood cirrhosis, characterized by an accumulation of copper and copper-binding protein in liver cells, occurs only in India.

Disorders of copper and iron metabolism

Q1

Wilson disease is an autosomal dominant recessive genetic disease resulting in iron overload that causes symptoms in infancy and early childhood.

Q2

Wilson disease is characterized by steatosis, glycogenated nuclei, ballooning of hepatocytes, Mallory bodies and interface lymphocytic hepatitis.

Q3

Acute liver failure and massive necrosis may be the first signs of Wilson disease.

Q4

For the definitive diagnosis of Wilson disease one must perform copper measurements on fresh unfixed tissue frozen immediately after biopsy.

Q5

Hemosiderosis of the liver may occur in genetic hemochromatosis as well as being due to secondary iron accumulation after blood transfusions, hemolytic anemia, or in chronic renal failure.

Q6

Perls' iron stain can demonstrate only iron that is present inside the liver cells in form of hemosiderin.

Q7

Hepatic iron index can be measured in slides stained with Perls' iron stain.

Q8

Genetic hemochromatosis is an autosomal recessive disordered cause by a missense mutation of the *HFE* gene encoding a regulatory protein that limits the iron absorption in the small intestine.

Q9

In genetic hemochromatosis the deposition of iron is always most prominent in the centrilobular hepatocytes.

Q10

Fibrosis that develops in genetic hemochromatosis usually affects the centrilobular area.

Q11

Excessive alcohol intake in persons who have genetic hemochromatosis may shift hemosiderin from hepatocytes to Kupffer cells and macrophages in fibrous septa.

Q12

Liver cell cancers develop in about 15% of patients who have cirrhosis caused by genetic hemochromatosis, and the incidence of tumors is not reduced by the removal of iron.

Q13

Phlebotomies can be used to remove excess iron, which stays the longest in the encrusted portal collagen.

Fibropolycystic diseases

Q1

Fibropolycystic liver diseases result from the abnormal development of ductal system and the persistence of the embryonic ductal plate.

Q2

Caroli's disease corresponds to the congenital dilatation of larger intrahepatic bile ducts.

Q3

von Meyenburg complexes may present in form of 1–2 mm nodules on the surface of the liver and during surgery may be mistaken for metastatic carcinomas.

Q4

Grossly visible multiple liver cysts are most often found in persons who have autosomal dominant polycystic kidney disease.

Vascular disorders

Q1

Hepatoportal sclerosis is a term used to describe portal changes in cirrhosis.

Q2

The hallmarks of hepatoportal sclerosis are thrombi and sclerosis of hepatic vein branches, but these changes may not be evident in liver biopsies.

Q3

Nodular regenerative hyperplasia may be found to some degree in most patients with hepatoportal sclerosis.

Q4

Sinusoidal dilatation occurs most often in the periportal parts of the lobule.

Q5

Periportal sinusoidal dilatation and thrombosis is a feature of eclampsia.

Q6

Treatment with steroid hormones may produce peliosis hepatis.

Q7

Acute venous outflow obstruction is associated with dilatation of sinusoids, predominantly in the periportal areas.

Q8

Centrilobular fibrosis is a consequence of chronic venous outflow obstruction.

Liver cell tumors and tumor-like conditions

Q1

Focal nodular hyperplasia can occur in age group, but is always more common in women than in men.

Q2

Focal nodular hyperplasia is asymptomatic in most instances and is discovered incidentally as a solitary nodule in the liver.

Q3

On gross examination the nodule of focal nodular hyperplasia typically has a central stellate scar, and microscopically such nodules contain all the components of the liver lobule.

Q4

Liver cell adenomas are more common in women than in men and are pathogenetically related to the use of oral contraceptives.

Q5

Liver cell adenomas consist predominantly of liver cells, but also contain portal triads and central veins.

Q6

Predictions are that the incidence of liver cell carcinoma will increase in the United States.

Q7

Serial determinations of serum α-fetoprotein (AFP) offer a good clue to early detection of hepatocellular carcinoma in populations at risk.

Q8

Viral hepatitis B and C are the leading risk factors for liver cell carcinoma worldwide.

Q9

Large cell dysplasia is found only in livers that also contain liver cell carcinoma.

Q10

Macroregenerative nodules (also known as adenomatous hyperplasia) have a greater predisposition to the development of malignancy than the smaller nodules of cirrhotic livers.

Q11

Livers with cirrhosis tend to develop liver cell carcinoma presenting as a large solitary mass.

Q12

This hepatocellular carcinoma show a typical growth pattern that is best described as tubular.

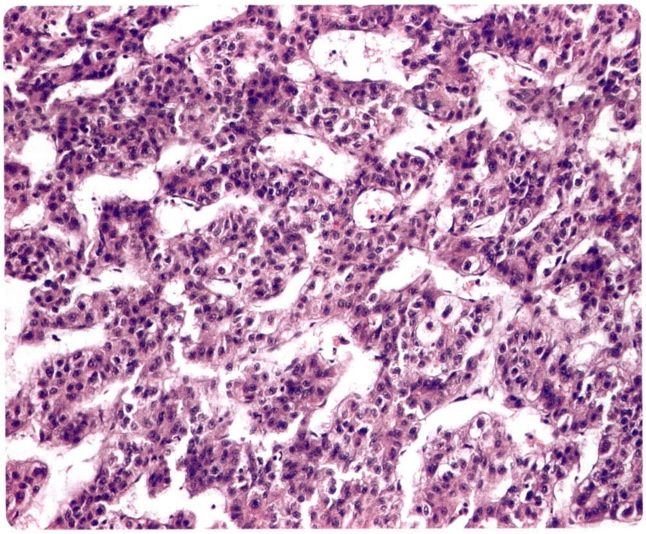

Fig. 13.3

Q13

AFP is a very sensitive and highly specific immunohistochemical marker of hepatocellular carcinoma.

Q14

Monoclonal antibodies that recognize keratin-8, such as Cam 5.2 and 35βH11, react with normal liver cells and hepatocellular carcinoma as well.

Q15

Some malignant liver tumors may combine features of liver cell carcinoma and bile ductular carcinoma and are best classified as mixed hepatocarcinoma–cholangiocarcinoma.

Q16

Fibrolamellar carcinoma is a tumor that develops in cirrhotic livers of older persons and has a worse prognosis than classic hepatocellular carcinoma.

Q17

Most hepatocellular carcinomas invade bile duct and have a tendency to spread through the biliary system.

Q18

Liver carcinoma is an absolute contraindication for liver transplantation.

Q19

Portal vein involvement by hepatocellular carcinoma is an important prognostic sign.

Q20

Hepatoblastoma is a childhood tumor that may be associated with a variety of congenital anomalies and even other tumors, such as Wilms' tumor.

Q21

Most hepatoblastomas are composed of spindle cells arranged into rosettes.

Q22

Approximately 25% of all hepatoblastomas contain not only immature liver cells but also mesenchymal components, such as bone or cartilage.

Q23

Bile duct adenomas do not express carcinoembryonic antigen and thus differ from bile duct hamartomas (von Meyenburg complexes).

Q24

Biliary cystadenomas are multilocular benign tumors composed of cuboidal or columnar mucin-secreting cells, which in women are surrounded by ovarian-like stroma.

Q25

Bile duct carcinomas typically occur as solitary nodules in cirrhotic liver.

Q26

Heterogeneity of epithelial tumor cells within a single neoplastic gland is a unique feature of intrahepatic bile duct carcinomas.

Q27

Bile duct carcinomas typically produce bile.

Q28

Hemangioma is the most common tumor of the liver.

Q29

Benign (infantile) hemangioendothelioma is typically found in infants and children younger than 6 months.

Q30

In epithelioid hemangioendothelioma the neoplastic endothelial cells infiltrate sinusoids and veins and form intravascular tuft-like structures.

Normal anatomy

A1. True

The hepatic lobule is a roughly hexagonal histologic structure centered on a centrilobular or central vein containing on average six portal tracts at its periphery. Following the blood as it enters the lobule through the portal tract one can subdivide the lobule into three zones: periportal, midzonal and centrilobular. **(p. 918)**

A2. True

The space of Disse is a virtual cleft between the hepatocytes and the sinusoidal lining cells. The sinusoids are lined by fenestrated endothelial lining cells and Kupffer cells, i.e. resident phagocytes. Inside the space of Disse one may also find scattered hepatic stellate cells (Ito cells) and 'pit cells' corresponding to resident hepatic lymphocytes. The space of Disse is not visible in biopsy specimens but is often dilated in livers removed at autopsy. **(p. 918)**

A3. False

'Idealized' portal triads comprising one branch of the hepatic artery and vein and a single bile duct are typically found in the hilar and central parts of the liver. However, as the portal tracts become smaller and smaller toward the periphery of the liver they often contain dyads, i.e. only two of the three components of the typical triad. On the other hand, many portal tracts contain two or more branches of the hepatic artery, the portal vein or the bile ducts. All portal tracts also contain lymphatics. **(p. 919)**

A4. False

Normal hepatocytes contain glycogen, the amount of which varies depending on nutritional status. This glycogen can be demonstrated by the PAS reaction in the cytoplasm and can be removed with diastase pretreatment. Some glycogen can be also found inside the nuclei, especially in children. Glycogenated nuclei appear optically clear and are most prominent in the periportal zone. Nuclear accumulation of glycogen is very prominent in diabetes and Wilson disease, but this finding is of limited diagnostic significance. **(p. 919)**

A5. False

The hepatic plates of neonates and children are normally two cells thick, but in adults they are only one cell thick. Two cell plates are indicative of regeneration and are typically often found inside the hepatocellular nodules of cirrhosis. **(p. 919)**

Biopsy

A1. True

These four approaches are most commonly used for obtaining liver biopsies. The choice of technique will depend on the clinical situation and the type of the lesion to be sampled. **(p. 919)**

A2. True

Foci of so-called 'surgical necrosis' are common artifacts in surgically obtained liver biopsies. In order to minimize the occurrence of such foci the surgeon should biopsy the liver immediately upon entering the abdominal cavity. **(p. 919)**

A3. False

Serologic techniques have replaced liver biopsy as the method of choice for diagnosing acute viral hepatitis. Liver biopsy may be used, however, to confirm the diagnosis, to assess the severity and evolution of the disease, and to exclude concomitant disease such as alcohol-induced liver damage. **(p. 921)**

A4. True

Liver biopsy is widely used in monitoring the results of liver transplantation and it remains the gold standard for assessing acute and chronic transplant rejection or recurrence of viral hepatitis C in allografts. **(p. 920)**

A5. False

Perls' stain for iron is very useful for demonstrating hemosiderin accumulation in hemochromatosis, but it does help in the diagnosis of α_1-antitrypsin deficiency. Cytoplasmic inclusions of α_1-antitrypsin, typically found in that disease, are best demonstrated by PAS reaction preceded by diastase treatment to remove glycogen from hepatocytes. **(p. 920)**

Viral hepatitis

A1. True

Acute viral hepatitis caused by one of the five major hepatotropic viruses (HAV, HBV, HCV, HDV, HEV) is a panlobular disease that may be mild, moderate, severe or fatal. Most often it presents as lobular hepatitis with spotty necrosis. **(p. 921)**

A2. True

The round eosinophilic structures represent apoptotic bodies, which are commonly found in all forms of acute viral hepatitis. Dead fragmented hepatocytes have attracted mononuclear cells, which will ultimately phagocytose the apoptotic bodies and remove them from the liver parenchyma. **(p. 922)**

A3. False

Lobular disarray results from virus-induced changes in the hepatocytes, which vary in size and shape and show signs of shrinkage, swelling or apoptosis. The surviving hepatocytes regenerate and contribute to the 'lobular disarray,' which is a diagnostically useful feature typically found in viral hepatitis. **(p. 922)**

A4. False

Neutrophils do not play a prominent role in the intralobular inflammatory response to the infection with the major hepatotropic viruses. The intralobular inflammatory infiltrate consists rather of lymphocytes and macrophages or plasma cells. **(p. 922)**

A5. False

Portal tracts are usually affected as well and contain infiltrates of lymphocytes, admixed with a few plasma cells. Eosinophils and neutrophils may be also found. Pigment-laden macrophages are common in protracted inflammation. **(p. 922)**

A6. False

'Piecemeal necrosis' is a typical feature of chronic hepatitis, but it can occur, usually in a milder form, in acute viral hepatitis as well. Accordingly, it is not always possible to differentiate acute from chronic hepatitis on morphologic grounds alone. **(p. 922)**

A7. True

Confluent necroses begin in the centrilobular area but may spread toward the periphery of the lobules, leading to portal–central bridging necrosis. **(p. 923)**

A8. True

Submassive liver necrosis caused by hepatitis viruses is typically panlobular (i.e. involves almost the entire liver lobule) and multilobular (i.e. involves many lobules). It may still be missed on liver biopsy because the areas of confluent necrosis are distributed at random and intermixed with apparently normal or less-affected liver parenchyma. **(p. 923)**

A9. False

Submassive liver necrosis may be caused by major hepatotropic viruses, toxins, drugs taken in large amounts, adverse drug reactions, and also by autoimmune hepatitis and Wilson disease. **(p. 924)**

A10. True

Viral hepatitis A may present in adults with mild cholestasis that may be mistaken for drug-induced cholestasis. Immunohistochemically, the viral antigen can be demonstrated in the cytoplasm of hepatocytes and Kupffer cells. **(p. 924)**

A11. False

Liver cell injury is caused by T cells and antibodies. T lymphocytes attacking the liver cells show peripolesis (close contact with hepatocytes) or emperipolesis (invagination into the cytoplasm of hepatocytes). **(p. 924)**

A12. False

During acute viral hepatitis B very little viral antigen can be demonstrated by standard immunohistochemistry using antibodies to the core (HbcAg) or surface antigen (HsAg). This is in keeping with the notion that acute viral hepatitis B is an 'elimination-type' disease, resulting in the eradication of the virus and a self-limited course of the infection. **(p. 924)**

A13. True

Acute viral hepatitis C may cause essentially the same pathologic changes as HAV or HBV. Fatty change of hepatocytes (steatosis), bile duct injury and lymphoid aggregates in portal tracts, i.e. the histologic changes that are often seen in chronic HCV, may be also found in acute HCV. **(p. 924)**

A14. True

Drug-induced hepatitis may present in the so-called 'viral hepatitis-like form,' which is indistinguishable from acute or chronic viral hepatitis. Histologic findings favoring the diagnosis of drug-induced hepatitis are sharply delineated centrilobular necrosis, infiltrates of eosinophils, and granulomas, but in many instances such lesions are not evident. **(p. 925)**

A15. True

The term 'necroinflammatory hepatic lesions' includes various forms of liver cell necrosis accompanied by an inflammatory reaction. These lesions are signs of ongoing liver cell injury and persistent inflammation. The chronic inflammation is not limited to the lobules but involves the portal tracts, and is best seen along the limiting plate as interface hepatitis. Portal tract inflammation is accompanied by bile duct injury and regeneration and prominent fibrosis that extends into the lobules. Ultimately this fibrosis will lead to cirrhosis. **(p. 925–926)**

A16. True

The histologic changes caused by one hepatitis virus may be indistinguishable from those caused by other viruses, drugs, or even some metabolic and autoimmune diseases. Serologic and clinical data are therefore essential for the proper etiologic diagnosis of chronic hepatitis. **(p. 927)**

A17. False

Grading of chronic hepatitis is based on estimating the disease activity. Staging is based on the extent of hepatic fibrosis. The disease activity can be estimated by evaluating the extent of interface hepatitis, confluent necrosis, foci of (spotty) lytic necrosis and focal inflammation inside the lobule, and portal inflammation. **(p. 927–928)**

A18. False

'Ground-glass hepatocytes' are typically found in chronic viral hepatitis B but are not diagnostic of the disease. Similarly, the finely granular pale appearance of the liver cell cytoplasm may be caused by drug-induced hypertrophy and hyperplasia of smooth endoplasmic reticulum in liver cells. Similar cytoplasmic changes occur in some congenital diseases, such as congenital hypofibrinogenemia, Lafora's disease (myoclonus epilepsy) and glycogenosis type IV. Antibodies to HBsAg are used to identify the HBV-infected ground-glass hepatocytes and distinguish them from other similar cells. **(p. 928–929)**

A19. False

Portal tract lymphoid follicles with germinal centers are often prominent in livers infected with HCV, but are not diagnostic of that viral disease. Similar lymphoid follicles can be seen in the course of viral hepatitis B, autoimmune hepatitis and primary biliary cirrhosis. **(p. 931)**

A20. False

Large cell dysplasia is not a direct precursor of hepatocellular carcinoma. These changes are considered as warning signs and have proved to be an independent risk factor for liver cell carcinoma. Small cell dysplasia is considered by some authors as a better predictor of cancer. **(p. 933)**

A21. False

Bilirubin stasis occurs much more frequently in acute than chronic hepatitis. **(p. 933)**

Cirrhosis

A1. True

Cirrhosis is the end stage of many liver diseases. Three principal features of cirrhosis are loss of normal architecture, regeneratory nodules and diffuse internodular fibrosis. **(p. 934)**

A2. True

Cirrhotic liver tissue tends to fragment during the biopsy procedure. This happens because the fibrous tissue presents more resistance to the cutting edge of the biopsy tool than the nodules composed of liver cells. The nodular tissue also tends to adhere to fibrous strands and hence cleave irregularly under pressure. Several other findings that are helpful for the diagnosis of cirrhosis are listed on page 934 of *Surgical Pathology*. **(p. 934)**

A3. True

Incomplete septal cirrhosis is a condition that is borderline between fully established cirrhosis and other non-cirrhotic forms of portal hypertension. As such it has some but not all the typical features of cirrhosis, and may be difficult to diagnose in needle biopsy specimens. The diagnosis is much easier in surgically obtained specimens. **(p. 935)**

A4. False

The nodules in biliary cirrhosis tend to be garland shaped and are surrounded by fibrous septa that resemble arcades on a bridge. The peripheral parts of the nodules are composed of swollen hepatocytes that show cholate stasis and have clear cytoplasm or contain Mallory-like cytoplasmic bodies. The septa may contain an increased number of bile ducts or show ductopenia, as in primary biliary cirrhosis or primary sclerosing cholangitis. **(p. 935)**

A5. False

Deposits of copper in liver cells can be demonstrated by rhodanine staining in many forms of cirrhosis. Perinodal deposits involving the hepatocytes bordering on fibrous septa are most indicative of biliary obstruction. In Wilson disease the deposits of copper may be abundant in some nodules and practically invisible in others. **(p. 935)**

A6. True

Inactive cirrhosis lacks histologic signs of 'activity,' i.e. shows no necroinflammatory lesions, no or minimal interface hepatitis and no septal inflammation. **(p. 935)**

A7. True

Necrosis of the entire hepatocellular nodules is most often caused by hypoperfusion, which occurs during surgery owing to blood loss or any other hypovolemic shock. **(p. 935)**

A8. True

Histologically, focal nodular hyperplasia may be indistinguishable from cirrhosis. However, it is typically a localized tumor-like lesion, whereas cirrhosis is diffuse and involves the entire liver. **(p. 935)**

Drug-induced and toxic liver injury

A1. True

Drug-induced liver injury may be quite variable, and even the same drug may have different effects on different people. **(p. 936)**

A2. True

Predictable reactions are dose dependent and occur in all exposed individuals. For example, acetaminophen overdose is invariably associated with liver necrosis. Unpredictable drug reactions occur in a small number of patients and are hard to explain in most instances. **(p. 936)**

A3. True

The distribution of drug-induced changes depends on the concentration of various enzymes involved in the metabolism of drugs. For example, the centrilobular hepatocytes contain more microsomal biotransformation enzymes than the cells of the peripheral zone, and so some drug reactions are more prominent in the centrilobular zone. For example, acetaminophen poisoning is characterized by centrilobular necrosis. **(p. 936–937)**

A4. False

Tetracycline treatment and Reye's syndrome are associated with microvesicular steatosis. Macrovesicular steatosis is typically seen in carbon tetrachloride toxicity and methotrexate treatment. Ethanol may cause both micro- and macrovesicular fatty change. **(p. 937)**

A5. True

Simple cholestasis is the most common hepatic adverse drug reaction. Typically it may be induced by anabolic or contraceptive steroids, but it also occurs in the course of treatment with many other drugs. **(p. 937)**

A6. True

Amanita phalloides causes centrilobular hepatic necrosis. Most hepatotoxic drugs, such as chloroform, also cause centrilobular necrosis. On the other hand, intoxication with ferrous sulfate and the yellow form of inorganic phosphorus is accompanied by periportal liver cell necrosis. **(p. 937)**

A7. False

Intravenous drug abuse is associated with an accumulation of talc in phagocytic Kupffer cells. **(p. 937)**

A8. True

More than 60 drugs have been incriminated in the production of granulomas in the liver. The reasons for the granuloma formation are not known. **(p. 937)**

A9. True

Several drugs have been linked to bile ductular injury, which may result from direct toxicity or an immunoallergic reaction, leading over time to bile duct destruction and ductopenic cholestasis. This condition is similar to the vanishing bile duct disease in chronic liver allograft rejection and several other diseases affecting the bile ductules listed on page 948. **(p. 938)**

A10. False

Veno-occlusive hepatic disease induced by drugs used during bone marrow transplantation represents a non-thrombotic narrowing of centrilobular veins. Budd–Chiari syndrome is a consequence of thrombosis of the hepatic vein or its major tributaries. **(p. 938)**

A11. True

Drug-induced liver injury should always be considered in the differential diagnosis of acute as well as chronic liver diseases. The suspicion should be even higher if the histopathologic findings are complex and discordant with the clinical findings. **(p. 938)**

Steatosis and steatohepatitis

A1. True

The accumulation of triglycerides, leading to macrovesicular or microvesicular steatosis, is a very common sign of reversible liver cell injury. **(p. 938)**

A2. False

Steatosis in AIDS, like that in protein–energy malnutrition (kwashiorkor) or total parenteral nutrition, is predominantly periportal. However, exceptions to this rule are common and therefore it is not possible to define the etiology of steatosis on the pattern of lipid distribution inside the lobule. **(p. 939)**

A3. True

Lipogranulomas are aggregates of macrophages, lymphocytes and occasional eosinophils or giant cells around a lipid droplet, derived from a ruptured hepatocyte. They are especially common in alcohol-induced steatosis. Lipogranulomas are replaced by fibrous scars without great significance. **(p. 940)**

A4. False

Many patients who have steatosis of the liver have no clinical symptoms and never develop significant liver disease. It is not known why steatosis in some patients will be accompanied by fibrosis and will progress to steatohepatitis. It is thought that progression to steatohepatitis is a 'two-hit' process and that, in addition to fatty change of hepatocytes, an additional injury is required for this progression to occur in both alcoholic and non-alcoholic steatosis. **(p. 940)**

A5. False

Alcoholic steatohepatitis involves predominantly the centrilobular zone. Liver cells in this area show apoptosis or ballooning with or without Mallory body formation, and are surrounded by neutrophils and pericellular fibrosis ('chicken-wire fibrosis'). **(p. 940)**

A6. False

Alcoholic cirrhosis is in most instances micronodular, but if the patient stops drinking and the regeneration improves it may become mixed micronodular and macronodular. Histologic findings favoring alcoholic etiology are steatosis, ongoing steatohepatitis, occlusion of central veins, and fibrous blurring of the edges of the liver cell nodules. **(p. 940)**

A7. True

Hemosiderin accumulates in the liver of some alcoholics and may occasionally be very prominent. In such cases one must perform quantitative iron determination and genetic studies to exclude genetic hemochromatosis, which is a rather common disease and may be coincidental with alcohol abuse. **(p. 941)**

A8. True

Alcohol abuse is a common cause of chronic pancreatitis, which may cause bile duct obstruction, cholestasis, and cholangitis accompanied by periportal fibrosis. On the other hand, predominantly centrilobular fibrosis in an alcoholic could be a sign of alcoholic cardiomyopathy causing chronic venous congestion in the liver. **(p. 941)**

A9. True

NASH is most often related to the metabolic syndrome or syndrome X, including obesity, type 2 diabetes and hypertriglyceridemia. Other well documented causes of NASH are jejunoileal bypass surgery and other interventions aimed at rapid weight loss in obese persons, total parenteral nutrition, and various drugs and hormones. **(p. 942)**

A10. False

There are no qualitative histologic differences between ASH and NASH that would allow one to clearly separate these two forms of liver disease in each liver biopsy. In general terms NASH is associated with more fat accumulation and nuclear glycogen, but less hepatocellular damage, inflammation and fibrosis and fewer Mallory bodies than ASH. However, both conditions can progress to cirrhosis and the histopathologic findings should be interpreted in the context of other clinical data. **(p. 942)**

Cholestasis and biliary diseases

A1. True

Cholestasis may be a consequence of hepatocellular disturbances involving the secretion of bile or an obstruction at any level of the biliary excretory system. **(p. 942)**

A2. True

Intrahepatic cholestasis results from a disturbance of hepatocellular bile secretion or obstruction of bile flow inside the liver; extrahepatic cholestasis refers to the obstruction of major extrahepatic bile ducts. In either case cholestasis can be complete or incomplete, acute or chronic. In some diseases, such as primary biliary cirrhosis, there is both intra- and extrahepatic cholestasis. **(p. 942–943)**

A3. False

The first histologic signs of acute complete cholestasis are intracytoplasmic granules in hepatocytes (hepatocellular bilirubin stasis) and bilirubin-stained brown plugs in the intercellular canaliculi in the centrilobular zone (canalicular bilirubin stasis). **(p. 943)**

A4. True

Bile retained inside the hepatocytes has a detergent action leading to cell rupture and the death of hepatocytes. Bilirubin released from damaged and dead hepatocytes is taken up a few days later by Kupffer cells. **(p. 943)**

A5. False

Bilirubin is not birefringent under polarized light. Black pigment that may resemble bilirubin but which is birefringent under polarized light is protoporphyrin. Protoporphyrin accumulates in liver cells, bile ductular cells and Kupffer cells in erythropoietic protoporphyria. Hemosiderin can be distinguished from bilirubin because the former stains blue with Perls' iron reaction. **(p. 943)**

A6. True

Cholate stasis presents as a lesion of periportal hepatocytes. Hepatocytes damaged by the retained bile acids appear swollen, pale, and have a coarsely granular cytoplasm. They contain lysosomes rich in copper and metallothionine, which can be demonstrated histochemically with rhodanine or orcein, respectively. These hepatocytes also react with the antibodies to keratin CK-7, which is normally not found in liver cells; it is, however, normally expressed in bile ductular cells. **(p. 944)**

A7. False

Cholestatic liver cell rosettes are a hallmark of chronic cholestasis, but they do not represent signs of liver cell regeneration. The liver cells forming such rosettes are arranged around a clear space that may still contain bile. The hepatocytes show signs of feathery degeneration and react with the antibodies to CK-7, suggesting a transition to a bile-ductular cell phenotype. **(p. 945)**

A8. True

Bile infarcts usually result from large bile duct obstruction, but are not diagnostic of this condition and may be found in other forms of chronic cholestasis. **(p. 945)**

A9. False

Parenchymal multinucleated giant cells are often found in biliary obstruction of infancy and childhood, but can also occur in other liver diseases as well. They seem to be more specific to young age than to disease. Occasionally large multinucleated hepatocytes may be seen even in adults. **(p. 945)**

A10. False

Extramedullary hematopoiesis is not diagnostic of extrahepatic biliary obstruction in infancy. It may be found in many other liver diseases of infancy and early childhood. **(p. 946)**

A11. True

Ductular reaction, involving an increased number of bile ducts, usually accompanied by inflammation, is found in most cases of chronic biliary obstruction. Its extension into the periportal hepatic parenchyma leads to 'biliary piecemeal necrosis,' portal-to-portal fibrosis, and ultimately to biliary cirrhosis. For some unknown reason ductal reaction is not evident in Alagille syndrome, primary sclerosing cholangitis and chronic transplant rejection. **(p. 946)**

A12. True

The extent and severity of hepatic changes induced by chronic cholestasis can be graded as follows: stage 1 portal; stage 2 periportal; stage 3 septal; stage 4 cirrhosis. **(p. 946)**

A13. True

PFIC is a term used for a group of genetic disorders, each of which has been linked to a mutation of a specific gene. For example, PFIC-1 (also known as Byler disease) is caused by a mutation of the *ATP8B1* gene, an ATPase that may be involved bile salt excretion or enterohepatic recirculation. The histopathologic changes in PFIC-1 differ from those in PFIC-2 and PFIC-3. **(p. 946–947)**

A14. False

Septicemia and endotoxic shock may be the most common causes of ductular bilirubin stasis, but this pathologic change may be also seen in other conditions, such as massive liver necrosis, extrahepatic biliary atresia, mucoviscidosis and total parenteral nutrition. **(p. 947)**

A15. True

If more than one-third of all portal tracts have 'widowed' arteries this should be taken as evidence of ductopenia. A more accurate estimate can be obtained by measuring the ratio of interlobular ducts to the number of portal tracts. In normal adults this ratio is 0.9 to 1.8, and a ratio of 0.5 or less is a sign of ductopenia. It is important to note that in neonates, and especially in premature infants, the normal ration is below 0.9. Furthermore, the diagnosis of ductopenia can be made even if the ratio is above 0.5 if there is evidence that many bile ducts are in the process of being destroyed. **(p. 949)**

A16. False

Biliary atresia, also known as extrahepatic biliary atresia, is a panbiliary disease affecting both extrahepatic and intrahepatic bile ducts. The disease may start in utero or in the perinatal period. **(p. 949)**

A17. True

PBC is an autoimmune disease characterized by non-suppurative destructive cholangitis. The vast majority of patients (90%) have antimitochondrial antibodies. **(p. 950)**

A18. True

At the site of rupture of this interlobular bile duct there is an epithelioid granuloma. The portal tissue adjacent to the bile duct contains infiltrates of lymphocytes and plasma cells and a lymphoid aggregate. These findings are typical of primary biliary cirrhosis. **(p. 950)**

A19. True

Immune cholangitis or autoimmune cholangiopathy represents antimitochondrial antibody-negative PBC. **(p. 951)**

A20. False

PSC is more common in men than in women: 75% of all patients are male. In 70% of all cases PSC is associated with inflammatory bowel disease. **(p. 951)**

A21. False

Most patients suffering from PSC have both small and large bile duct disease. Both the extrahepatic and the intrahepatic bile ducts are affected, and so the liver biopsy and cholangiography provide complementary data essential for the diagnosis and staging of the disease. **(p. 951)**

A22. False

Concentric periductal fibrosis is not diagnostic of primary sclerosing cholangitis and similar changes can be seen in other bile duct diseases. It is found in only 40% of biopsies of PSC patients, but is nevertheless a helpful finding for the final diagnosis of that disease. **(p. 952)**

A23. True

Infiltrates of neutrophils are present in cholestasis as well as in bacterial infection of bile ducts. In general, infection is accompanied by more prominent infiltrates of neutrophils. Rupture of pus-filled bile ducts and periductal abscesses are also more typical of infection. **(p. 953)**

Childhood disorders and disorders of metabolism

A1. True

The list of the diseases that could cause neonatal cholestasis is very long and includes genetic, developmental and infectious diseases. **(p. 953)**

A2. True

Gilbert's syndrome is a very common form of familial unconjugated hyperbilirubinemia. The liver biopsy shows no pathologic changes. **(p. 953)**

A3. False

α_1-Antitrypsin deficiency is characterized by the accumulation of α_1-antitrypsin inside the rough endoplasmic reticulum and not in lysosomes. **(p. 954)**

A4. False

PAS-positive cytoplasmic globules typical of α_1-antitrypsin deficiency are difficult to find before the age of 3 months. **(p. 954)**

A5. True

Because the changes caused by α_1-antitrypsin deficiency may be indistinguishable from those of biliary atresia, theses children should be tested genetically before major surgery is undertaken. **(p. 954)**

A6. False

Indian childhood cirrhosis is a disease of unknown origin that sometimes appears to be familial. It was described in India but can affect caucasians as well. It is characterized by an accumulation of copper and copper-binding proteins in liver cells and a high mortality. Other histologic findings include ballooning of hepatocytes, the accumulation of Mallory bodies and liver cell necrosis. In contrast to alcoholic liver disease, there is no fatty change. **(p. 954)**

Disorders of copper and iron metabolism

A1. False

Wilson disease is an autosomal recessive genetic disease resulting in an overload of copper at very young age, but the clinical symptoms do not develop before the age of 5 years. Iron may accumulate in Kupffer cells, because of frequent hemolytic crises that occur in this disease. **(p. 955)**

A2. True

These changes are nonspecific and do not occur all at the same time. Nevertheless, these findings are important, especially in young non-obese patients who have no history of alcoholism and no other reasons to develop steatohepatitis. While examining a liver biopsy with such nonspecific changes one should develop a habit of suspecting Wilson disease at all ages, but especially in young persons. **(p. 955)**

A3. True

Wilson disease may present with acute liver failure and submassive liver necrosis. **(p. 955)**

A4. False

Copper measurements are important for the diagnosis of Wilson disease in liver biopsy, but such measurements can be performed on formalin-fixed and paraffin-embedded tissue. **(p. 955)**

A5. True

Hepatic hemosiderosis or siderosis is a term used to denote the presence of stainable iron in the liver. Hence it includes a variety of diseases, including genetic hemochromatosis and many secondary hemosideroses due to iron overload. **(p. 955)**

A6. False

Perls' iron stain will stain granular hemosiderin inside the siderosomes but will also react and form a bluish tinge with the finely dispersed ferritin particle in the cytoplasm of liver cells. In genetic hemochromatosis it will also stain the deposits of hemosiderin in Kupffer cells, bile ductular cells and connective tissue cells forming the septa of cirrhosis. **(p. 956)**

A7. False

Hepatic iron index (HII) is expressed as the amount of iron determined chemically in the liver tissue per gram of dry weight of liver tissue, divided by the age of the patient. HII is useful for differentiating genetic hemochromatosis from secondary hemosiderosis. **(p. 956)**

A8. True

The mutation of the *HFE* gene, located on chromosome 6, is the underlying cause of genetic hemochromatosis. In homozygous persons this mutation results in abnormal iron absorption in the intestines and iron overload, affecting the liver, many endocrine glands, the skin and the heart. **(p. 956)**

A9. False

Deposits of iron in genetic hemochromatosis are always more pronounced in periportal hepatocytes. The finding of hemosiderin in periportal hepatocytes could be actually the first sign of genetic hemochromatosis. **(p. 956)**

A10. False

Fibrosis in genetic hemochromatosis usually develops in and around the portal tracts, conferring a spiked appearance to them. Fibrosis forms portal-to-portal septa, which may resemble the changes that occur in biliary cirrhosis. **(p. 957)**

A11. True

Alcohol abuse may cause the accumulation of hemosiderin in many cells, including the endothelial cells of the liver, and it seems that the same mechanism plays a role in shifting the hemosiderin from hepatocytes to other cells in those who both have genetic hemochromatosis and suffer from alcohol abuse. **(p. 957)**

A12. True

However, the reasons for tumor development are not known. **(p. 957)**

A13. True

The iron is removed first from the centrilobular hepatocytes, and periportal hepatocytes remain hemosiderin laden the longest. The most resistant to removal is the hemosiderin in the encrusted collagen in the portal tracts of fibrous septa of cirrhosis. **(p. 957)**

Fibropolycystic diseases

A1. True

Cysts, and portal fibrosis forming around them, result from abnormal development of the fetal ductal system and the persistence of embryonic ductal plate. **(p. 958)**

A2. True

Dilatation may be isolated or associated with congenital hepatic fibrosis (Caroli's syndrome). The ectatic parts of the ductal system predispose to recurrent cholangitis. Complications include intrahepatic cholelithiasis and cholangiocarcinoma. **(p. 958)**

A3. True

von Meyenburg complexes are small developmental malformations of the ductal plate consisting of dilated bile ducts and fibrous tissue. They may present as small white nodules, which may be mistaken by the unwary for metastatic carcinoma. **(p. 959)**

A4. True

Liver cysts are found in most patients with ADPKD, a disease that affects 1 in 400 to 1 in 1000 persons. The liver contains numerous cysts, which increase with age. Cysts are lined by biliary epithelium. They are associated with fibrosis that contains numerous von Meyenburg complexes. **(p. 959)**

Vascular disorders

A1. False

Hepatoportal sclerosis is fibrous intimal thickening of the portal vein in patients who have portal hypertension without evidence of cirrhosis. The cause of this pathologic change is in most instances unknown. The disease is a major cause of portal hypertension in Japan and India. **(p. 959)**

A2. False

Thrombi and sclerosis involve the branches of the portal vein and are often associated with the formation of aberrant blood vessels. Abnormal vessels called periportal megasinusoids, periportal angiomatosis and cavernous transformation of recanalized portal vein branches may be found histologically. **(p. 959)**

A3. True

Nodular regenerative hyperplasia and hepatoportal sclerosis represent lesions that are probably pathogenetically related, and thus it is not surprising that the two conditions could coexist. Both conditions are classified under the heading of non-cirrhotic causes of portal hypertension. **(p. 959)**

A4. False

Sinusoidal dilatation occurs most often in the centrilobular zone, which is the integral part of the venous outflow system and is often dilated in chronic passive congestion. **(p. 960)**

A5. True

Dilatation of periportal sinusoids is a feature of pre-eclampsia and eclampsia and may be related to long-term oral contraceptive use. In pre-eclampsia and eclampsia it may be associated with thrombosis leading to periportal liver cell necrosis. **(p. 960)**

A6. True

Peliosis hepatis, a condition marked by the formation of cystic blood-filled spaces in the liver parenchyma, may be caused by steroid hormone treatment. However, it may have many other causes and is found during many wasting diseases, in patients receiving chemotherapy, following liver or kidney transplantation etc. The blood accumulates inside cystically dilated sinusoids, which may otherwise be normal or lack normal endothelial lining. **(p. 960)**

A7. False

Acute venous outflow obstruction, often included under the confusing term of Budd–Chiari syndrome, is accompanied by pooling of venous blood, predominantly in the centrilobular veins and adjacent sinusoids. **(p. 960)**

A8. True

Chronic venous outflow obstruction results in centrilobular fibrosis of variable extent. Ultimately it may lead to central–central bridging fibrosis that encircles normal portal tracts and the periportal parenchyma ('reversed lobulation').Cardiac cirrhosis is found in advanced cases. **(p. 960)**

Liver cell tumors and tumor-like conditions

A1. True

Even though FNP has a peak incidence in the third to fifth decades of life, it may occur in any age group. In all age groups the lesion is more common in women. **(p. 992)**

A2. True

FNH is asymptomatic in approximately 80% of cases. Most lesions present as solitary nodules, but in 20% of cases the nodules may be multiple. **(p. 992)**

A3. True

The central fibrous scar is a typical feature of FNH. Fibrous tissue may radiate towards the periphery and divide the parenchyma into nodules similar to those in cirrhosis. All cellular components of the normal liver are present histologically, and there is usually evidence of chronic inflammation. **(p. 992)**

A4. True

Liver cell adenomas occur at increased incidence in people taking anabolic–androgenic steroids as well, and in some genetic diseases affecting the liver, such as glycogen storage diseases. **(p. 993)**

A5. False

Liver cell adenomas are composed of liver cells arranged in nodules that do not contain portal tracts, or fibrous scars typical of FNH. **(p. 993–994)**

A6. True

Liver cell carcinoma is a relatively rare tumor in the United States, in contrast to some parts of Africa and Asia, where it is quite common. Predictions are that the incidence of this tumor increased in the US, mostly because of the high prevalence of viral hepatitis C in the population at large. **(p. 994)**

A7. True

AFP is elevated in serum of 40–60% of patients who have hepatocellular carcinoma in Europe and the United States, and in over 70% of patients in endemic areas. Increases over 100 times normal are almost diagnostic of liver cell carcinoma. Serial determinations of AFP in serum are a good approach to monitoring these patients who are at risk. **(p. 994)**

A8. True

Viral hepatitis caused by HBV and HCV are the leading risk factors for hepatocellular carcinoma worldwide. Serologic evidence of HBV or HCV infection can be found in over 90% of patients diagnosed with hepatocellular carcinoma. **(p. 995)**

A9. False

Large cell dysplasia is indeed found in 64.5% of patients who have cirrhosis and liver cell carcinoma, but also in 20.3% of livers with cirrhosis and no evidence of cancer, and in 1% of normal livers without cirrhosis. **(p. 996)**

A10. False

Macroregenerative nodules are not thought to predispose more to cancer than the usual small nodules in the cirrhotic liver. **(p. 996)**

A11. False

Liver cell carcinoma developing in cirrhotic liver is usually multinodular in type. Other forms of tumor, i.e. solitary, diffuse or massive hepatocellular carcinomas, are less common. **(p. 997)**

A12. False

This figure illustrates the typical trabecular growth pattern of a hepatocellular carcinoma. Trabeculae several cells thick are surrounded by sinusoids, some of which are lined by tumor cells. Other growth patterns are described as solid or tubular. The latter is known also as pseudoglandular or acinar, and may give rise to papillary structures similar to those in bile duct carcinomas. **(p. 998)**

A13. False

AFP is a relatively specific but rather insensitive marker of hepatocellular carcinoma. Overall there are no specific immunohistochemical markers of hepatocellular carcinoma, but a battery of judiciously chosen tests could help in the differential diagnosis. **(p. 998)**

A14. True

These antibodies, especially if used in combination with other antibodies to cytokeratins that are not expressed in normal liver cells, are useful for distinguishing liver cell carcinoma from bile duct and metastatic adenocarcinomas. Bile duct carcinomas typically express CK7, which may be useful for distinguishing this tumor from hepatocellular carcinomas. Caution should be used, however, as CK7 may be expressed focally in some hepatocellular carcinomas. Furthermore, there are many otherwise typical hepatocellular carcinomas expressing other cytokeratins that are not found in normal liver cells. **(p. 999)**

A15. True

Mixed hepatocarcinoma–cholangiocarcinoma is a well recognized entity, reflecting the fact that these tumors most likely originate from common precursor cells capable of differentiating into hepatocytes and bile duct cells. **(p. 1001)**

A16. False

Fibrolamellar carcinoma, also known as polygonal cell hepatocellular carcinoma with fibrous stroma, is a tumor that occurs most often in patients younger than 35 years. These patients typically do not have cirrhosis. This tumor has a cure rate of 50% and hence a better prognosis than classic hepatocellular carcinoma. **(p. 1001)**

A17. False

Most hepatocellular carcinomas invade sinusoids and have a tendency for hematogenous spread. Metastases to the lungs are common. Gross invasion of the biliary tree by tumor is less common, but it does occur in some cases. **(p. 1002)**

A18. False

Many patients with hepatocellular carcinoma have been treated with hepatectomy and liver transplantation, and this approach is widely used for treatment of liver cancer. Good results have been reported in most centers with solitary small tumors (less than 5 cm in diameter), but some authors have not found that the size of the tumor per se is important for the prognosis, the stage of the tumor being the most important prognostic determinant. **(p. 1003)**

A19. True

Tumors that invade the portal vein have a poor prognosis. **(p. 1003)**

A20. True

Hepatoblastoma is primarily a tumor of infants and children and is only rarely found in adults. It may be associated with congenital anomalies, most notably hemihypertrophy and Wilms' tumor. **(p. 1003)**

A21. False

Hepatoblastomas show several growth patterns, known as pure hepatoblastic or epithelial, fetal, embryonal, macrotrabecular. Pure hepatoblastic tumors composed of immature hepatocytes predominate and are typically associated with high serum AFP. **(p. 1003)**

A22. True

Such tumors containing stromal elements differentiating into bone, cartilage and other mesenchymal components are also called mixed hepatoblastomas. **(p. 1004)**

A23. False

Bile duct adenomas and bile duct hamartomas cannot be readily distinguished from one another histologically or immunohistochemically, and some authors group them together as benign bile duct proliferations. **(p. 1006)**

A24. True

Biliary cystadenomas in women have an ovarian-like stroma. Such tumors have an indolent course, in contrast to tumors in males, which lack ovarian-like stroma and may be more aggressive. **(p. 1006)**

A25. False

Most bile duct carcinomas develop in non-cirrhotic livers. Multicentricity of tumors is common. **(p. 1007)**

A26. False

Heterogeneity of epithelial cells within a single neoplastic gland is a common and diagnostically important feature of bile duct carcinomas. However, the same phenomenon is seen in adenocarcinoma of the entire biliary–pancreatic system, and cannot be used to distinguish primary intrahepatic bile duct tumors from tumors of the extrahepatic biliary ducts, gallbladder or pancreas. **(p. 1007)**

A27. False

Bile duct carcinomas do not produce bile, which may, however, be found in hepatocellular carcinomas. **(p. 1008)**

A28. True

Most tumors are, however, small and rarely require treatment. **(p. 1008)**

A29. True

They may be solitary or multiple. Multiple hemangioendotheliomas may be associated with hemangiomas in other sites, and may also be part of congenital syndromes such as Beckwith–Wiedemann syndrome. **(p. 1008)**

A30. True

In epithelioid hemangioendothelioma the neoplastic endothelial cells infiltrate sinusoids and veins, forming intravascular tuft-like structures lined by plump tumor cells that are often acidophilic and vacuolated and express typical immunohistochemical endothelial cell markers. **(p. 1009)**

14 Gallbladder and extrahepatic bile ducts

Normal anatomy

Q1

The surface of the gallbladder is entirely covered by serosa, which is then continuous with that on the hepatic surface.

Q2

Hartmann's pouch is a bulge in the fundus of the gallbladder.

Q3

The gallbladder is supplied by the cystic artery, which is usually a branch of the right hepatic artery.

Q4

The submucosa of the gallbladder contains mucous glands, which produce sulfated acid-type mucin.

Q5

The mucosa of the gallbladder is lined by a single layer of columnar cells with basally located nuclei, pale cytoplasm and occasional small apical vacuoles, and also by smaller, darkly staining columnar, so-called 'pencil-like' cells.

Q6

In the normal gallbladder, scattered neuroendocrine cells can be found only in the mucous glands of the neck.

Q7

In the gallbladder, ganglion cells are found only in the minute paraganglia of the subserosal region.

Q8

The lining of the cystic bile duct is the same as that of hepatic and common bile ducts.

Q9

Sacculi of Beale are pits of epithelium that penetrate into the stroma of the extrahepatic ducts.

Q10

The lining epithelium of the extrahepatic bile ducts is similar to that of the gallbladder.

Congenital abnormalities

Q1

In biliary atresia the hepatic and extrahepatic bile ducts are damaged and the hepatic artery and its branches commonly show hypertrophic and hyperplastic changes.

Q2

Biliary atresia is a relatively benign condition, as the gallbladder is not necessary for survival.

Q3

Most cases of biliary atresia are 'non-correctable.'

Q4

'Correctable biliary atresia' is corrected by biliary–enteric anastomosis.

Q5

The so-called Kasai operation is curative in 'non-correctable' biliary atresia.

Q6

Choledochal cyst is the most common cause of obstructive jaundice in young infants.

Q7

Choledochal cyst is not really a cyst but rather a cystic dilatation of the common bile duct, distal to which the bile duct is narrowed.

Q8

In choledochal cyst, histological changes are directly related to the age of the patient.

Q9

In adult patients choledochal cysts can contain tumors.

Q10

Agenesis of the gallbladder is usually a solitary congenital anomaly, but may be part of trisomy 18 (Edwards) syndrome.

Q11

The histological finding of intestinal and gastric mucosa in the gallbladder indicates intestinal and gastric metaplasia.

Q12

This large cystic structure attached to the gallbladder (to the left) is most likely a choledochal cyst.

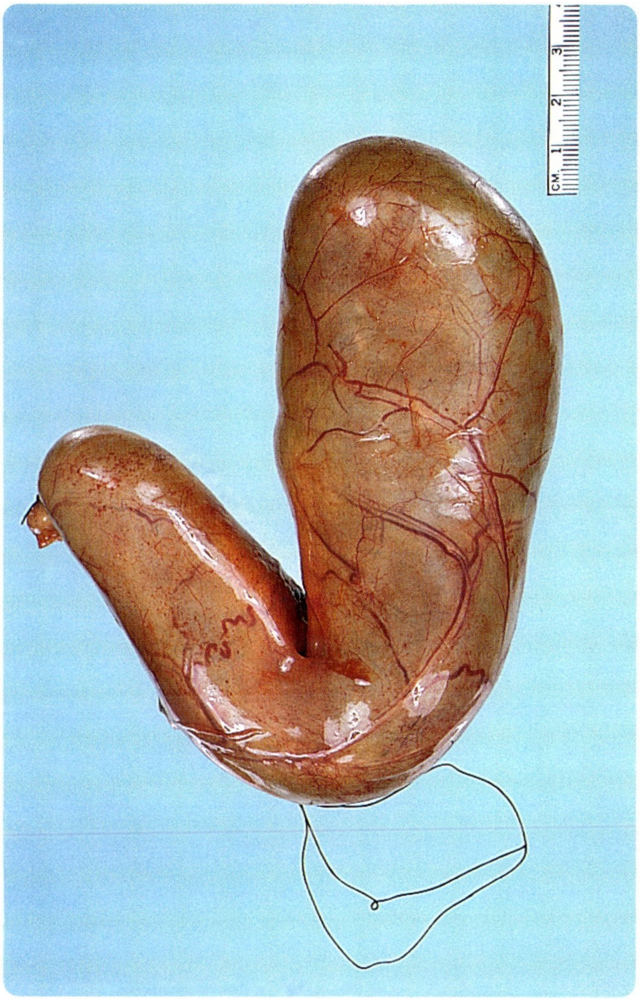

Fig. 14.1

Cholelithiasis

Q1

Supersaturation with cholesterol, crystallization and the growth of stones are the three steps in gallstone formation.

Q2

The majority of gallstones contain sufficient calcium to be detectable on X-ray.

Q3

In the United States 10–15% of adults have gallstones.

Q4

Gallstones are much more frequent in females.

Q5

Gallstones can be divided into pure, mixed and combined types.

Q6

Pure gallstones can be divided into pure cholesterol stones, calcium bilirubinate stones and calcium carbonate stones.

QUESTIONS

QUESTIONS

Q7

Pigmented stones are synonymous with pure calcium bilirubinate stones.

Q8

Only brown pigmented stones (so-called 'mixed stones,' which comprise about 80% of all stones) have a clearly infectious etiology.

Q9

Pure cholesterol stones consist only of cholesterol and are more frequent in people with high cholesterol levels.

Q10

The majority of 'hard' gallstones are 'calcified stones.'

Q11

Combined gallstones consist of a pure nucleus and a mixed shell (or the reverse) and are characteristically large and single, just like pure cholesterol stones.

Q12

Choledocholithiasis, with or without obstruction, is almost always associated with cholelithiasis.

Q13

Most patients with cholelithiasis are symptomatic.

Q14

Variations in the anatomy of the gallbladder may predispose to the development of gallstones.

Q15

In cholelithiasis, complications are most common in patients with a single large stone.

Q16

This dilated gallbladder contains four mixed stones, which are predominantly composed of calcium carbonate, having a characteristic jet black color.

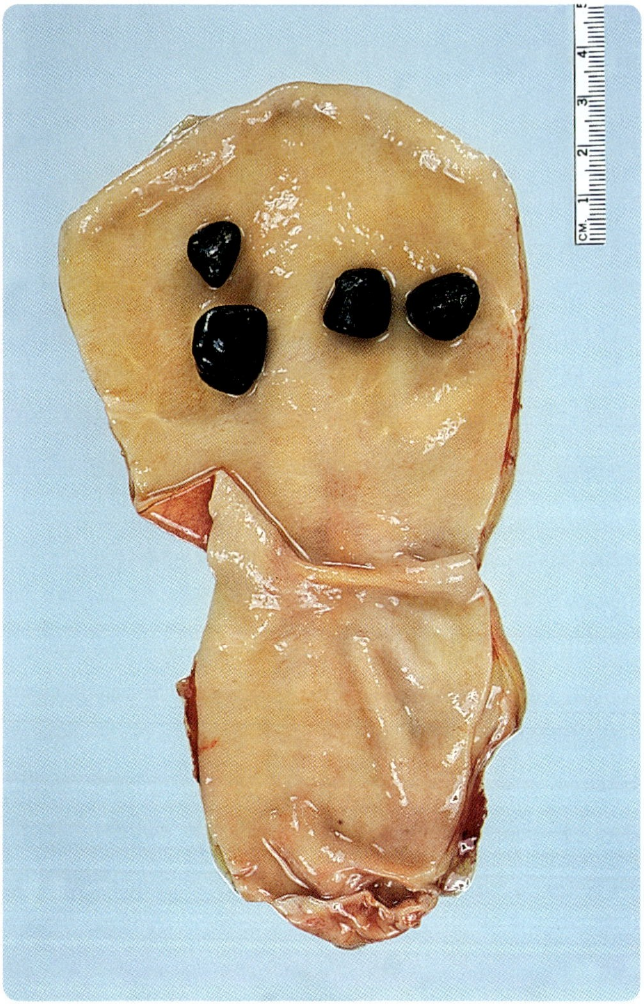

Fig. 14.2

Q17

Impaction of the stone in the cystic duct may lead to cystic dilatation of the gallbladder (hydrops; see below), which is also know as 'Mirizzi's syndrome.'

Cholesterolosis

Q1

Cholesterolosis is a condition in which foamy macrophages containing triglycerides and cholesterol esters accumulate in the lamina propria of the gallbladder wall.

Q2

Cholesterolosis is frequently associated with advanced chronic cholecystitis.

Q3

In cholesterolosis the bile is unusually dark and thick and shows a very high concentration of cholesterol.

Q4

Cholesterolosis is associated with cholelithiasis.

Acute cholecystitis

Q1

Acute cholecystitis may have a diverse etiology, but acute calculous cholecystitis is by far the most common.

Q2

Microscopically, acute inflammation of the gallbladder is characterized by an abundant polymorphonuclear infiltrate, as in most other organs in the body.

Q3

Reactive cytologic atypia of the mucosal epithelium as well as the stromal cells is a common histological finding and should not be confused with malignancy.

Q4

Acute calculous cholecystitis is caused by secondary infection of the obstructed gallbladder.

Q5

Acute calculous cholecystitis is not related to chronic cholecystitis.

Q6

Emphysematous cholecystitis is most common in multiparous women.

Q7

Emphysematous cholecystitis is associated with gallstones.

Q8

Acalculous cholecystitis, like calculous cholecystitis, appears to be related to bile stasis.

Q9

Gangrene complicates about 20% of acute calculous cholecystitis cases.

Q10

Acute vascular thrombosis and fibrinoid necrosis of the muscular arteries in the wall of the gallbladder may be seen in acute cholecystitis.

Chronic cholecystitis and cholangitis

Q1

Chronic cholecystitis is rarely seen in the absence of cholelithiasis.

Q2

Chronic cholecystitis results from repeated attacks of mild acute cholecystitis.

Q3

'Porcelain gallbladder' is a form of chronic cholecystitis in which the wall of the gallbladder is markedly thickened by fibrosis and calcification.

Q4

Thickening of the gallbladder wall is not typical of usual chronic cholecystitis.

Q5

The epithelium of the gallbladder is most often atrophied in chronic cholecystitis.

Q6

Microscopically, the outpouchings of the mucosa through the muscle of the gallbladder wall (Rokitansky–Aschoff sinuses) are a diagnostic feature of chronic cholecystitis.

Q7

The incidence of metaplastic change in chronic cholecystitis increases steadily with age.

Q8

Metaplastic epithelium in the gallbladder contains acid mucin just as do normal glands in the gallbladder neck.

Q9

Adenomyomatosis is a common tumor-like lesion of the gallbladder with no malignant potential and may involve the gallbladder in a focal, segmental or diffuse form.

Q10

Follicular cholecystitis is a form of chronic cholecystitis.

Q11

Diffuse lymphoplasmacytic cholecystitis is a marker of sclerosing cholangitis.

Q12

Eosinophilic cholecystitis is usually acalculous.

Q13

Xanthogranulomatous cholecystitis is synonymous with cholecystic granuloma, ceroid granuloma and malakoplakia.

Q14

Cholelithiasis may cause internal biliary fistulas, but these are clinically silent.

Q15

Strictures of the common duct are usually caused by chronic inflammation.

Q16

Sclerosing cholangitis is strongly associated with HLA-DRw52a antigen.

Q17

Sclerosing cholangitis is associated with HIV infection.

Q18

The most typical microscopic changes of sclerosing cholangitis are present in the extrahepatic bile ducts.

Q19

This image illustrates Kulchitsky's cell hyperplasia (cells with red cytoplasmic granulation), which can occur in chronic cholecystitis.

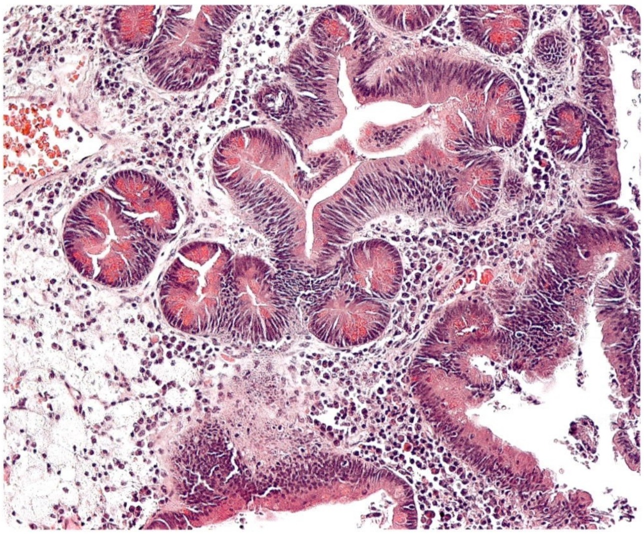

Fig. 14.3

Tumors

Q1

Cholesterol polyps represent mucosal hyperplasia associated with pure cholesterol gallstones.

Q2

Inflammatory polyps occur in association with CMV cholecystitis.

Q3

Adenomatous hyperplasia or adenomyomatous hyperplasia are reactive mucosal changes seen in association with chronic cholecystitis or lithiasis.

Q4

Villous papilloma of the gallbladder is a precancerous condition.

Q5

Adenomas of the gallbladder are a common precursor of gallbladder adenocarcinoma.

Q6

Adenomas of the gallbladder may be tubular, tubulovillous, or villous with varying degrees of dysplasia.

Q7

Cystadenomas of the extrahepatic bile ducts resemble those of the pancreas.

Q8

Papillomatosis of the extrahepatic bile ducts is difficult to treat owing to the high recurrence rate, but malignant transformation has not been described in this condition.

Q9

As in other sites, granular cell tumor of the gallbladder is associated with hyperplasia and pseudocarcinomatous change in the overlying epithelium.

Q10

Carcinoma of the gallbladder is four times more common in women than in men.

Q11

Adenocarcinoma of the gallbladder is most common in white people of European origin.

Q12

Adenocarcinoma of the gallbladder is a common complication of cholelithiasis.

Q13

Gardner's syndrome is associated with an increased risk of gallbladder carcinoma.

Q14

Porcelain gallbladder is associated with adenocarcinoma of the gallbladder.

Q15

Most carcinomas of the gallbladder are polypoid or fungating tumors.

Q16

Most carcinomas of the gallbladder are adenocarcinomas with a papillary growth pattern.

Q17

Intestinal differentiation is common in adenocarcinoma of the gallbladder.

Q18

As does the epithelium of the normal, inflamed or obstructed gallbladder, adenocarcinomas of the gallbladder produce sulfomucins.

Q19

Adenocarcinomas of the extrahepatic bile duct are immunohistochemically identical to intrahepatic bile duct adenocarcinomas.

Q20

No specific molecular abnormalities are found in adenocarcinoma of the gallbladder.

Q21

Gallstones are a risk factor for cholangiocarcinoma.

Q22

Squamous cell carcinoma is a common histological type of carcinoma of the gallbladder.

Q23

Signet-ring is a rare variant of adenocarcinoma of the gallbladder.

Q24

Lymphoepithelial carcinoma of the gallbladder is associated with EBV.

Q25

As in the colorectum, most cases of gallbladder adenocarcinoma are preceded by adenomas.

Q26

The mucin phenotypes of dysplastic mucosa and invasive adenocarcinoma of the gallbladder are basically the same and are of gastric type.

Q27

Gallbladder carcinoma invades the liver directly and, to a lesser extent, the stomach and duodenum.

Q28

The most important prognostic factor in gallbladder carcinoma is the grade of the tumor.

Q29

Well-differentiated adenocarcinoma of the gallbladder, as shown in this image, can be correctly diagnosed because of the presence of clear-cut invasion into the muscular layer.

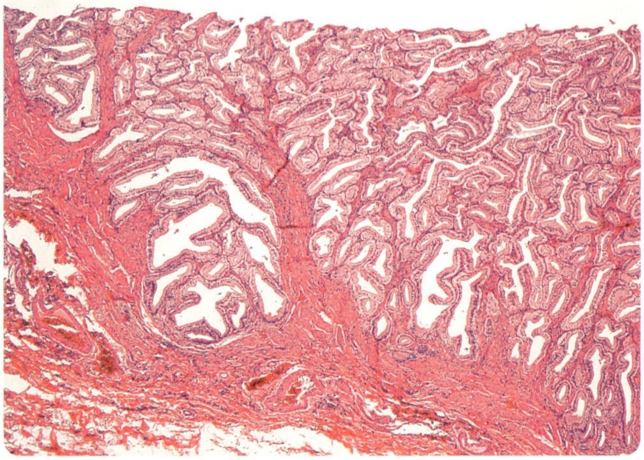

Fig. 14.4

Q30

Even in well-differentiated adenocarcinoma of the gallbladder it is common to observe high-grade cytologic features.

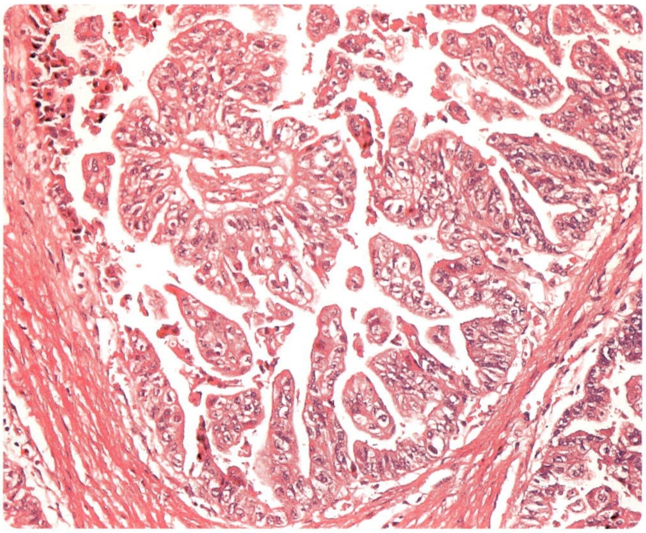

Fig. 14.5

Carcinoma of the extrahepatic bile ducts

Q1

As in the gallbladder, bile duct carcinoma occurs more frequently in women.

Q2

Bile duct carcinoma usually presents with painless jaundice.

Q3

Predisposing factors for bile duct carcinoma include ulcerative colitis and sclerosing cholangitis.

Q4

Cholangiocarcinomas can be classified anatomically into intrahepatic, perihilar and distal extrahepatic.

Q5

Cytological procedures are not recommended in the diagnostic evaluation of bile duct carcinoma owing to their low sensitivity.

Q6

Grossly, most bile duct carcinomas are polypoid and superficial.

Q7

Histologically, bile duct carcinomas are most often well-differentiated, mucin-secreting adenocarcinomas.

Q8

Extrahepatic bile duct carcinoma resembles gallbladder carcinoma morphologically, histochemically and immunohistochemically.

Q9

Overexpression of p53 is present in most bile duct adenocarcinomas.

Q10

No specific molecular changes are described in bile duct carcinoma.

Q11

Primary malignant melanoma of the gallbladder or extrahepatic bile ducts has been described.

Q12

Botryoid rhabdomyosarcoma is the most common malignant tumor of extrahepatic bile ducts in children.

Q13

Carcinoid tumors can arise in the gallbladder or extrahepatic bile ducts.

Q14

Mesenchymal tumors of the gallbladder and extrahepatic bile ducts include GIST, leiomyosarcoma, angiosarcoma and malignant fibrous histiocytoma.

Q15

Metastatic lung carcinoma to the gallbladder is more common than primary tumors.

Normal anatomy

A1. False
Only free surface of the gallbladder is covered by the serosa. **(p. 1035)**

A2. False
Hartmann's pouch is a bulge in the infundibulum, a part of the neck of the gallbladder. Anomaly in the fundus of the gallbladder is known as a Phrygian cap, which develops secondary to angulation or kinking of the gallbladder fundus. **(p. 1035)**

A3. True
There are several anomalous arrangements of the cystic artery, of which caudad origin is the most frequent. **(p. 1036)**

A4. False
First, there is no submucosa or muscularis mucosae in the gallbladder. Second, true glands are present only in the neck region. They are mucous (tubuloalveolar type) and they produce sulfated acid-type mucin just like lining cells of the mucosa. **(p. 1035)**

A5. True
Just like other simple epithelia, these epithelial cells express EMA and low molecular weight cytokeratins. Interestingly, both of these cell types are recapitulated in well-differentiated adenocarcinoma of the gallbladder. **(p. 1035)**

A6. True
Normal mucosal lining does not contain any neuroendocrine cells. However, they appear also in the mucosa of the gallbladder in intestinal metaplasia. **(p. 1035)**

A7. False
In the gallbladder, ganglion cells are found both in the minute subserosal paraganglia and anywhere in the wall of the gallbladder. **(p. 1035)**

A8. False
Although their general organization is similar, the lining of the cystic duct is pleated, with large oblique folds containing smooth muscle (spiral valve of Heister). The cystic duct wall contains smooth muscle throughout, and bursts of spikes moving peristaltically towards the common duct have been recorded electromyographically from the region. Note that the cystic duct is the only 'two-way' duct and therefore needs a special anatomical organization for the transportation of bile both ways. **(p. 1036)**

A9. True
They are surrounded by small glands, which are embedded in dense stroma and may mimic well-differentiated carcinoma. Their lobular architecture argues against the diagnosis of malignancy. **(p. 1036)**

A10. True
The similarities are noted ultrastructurally, histochemically and immunohistochemically. **(p. 1036)**

Congenital abnormalities

A1. True
The damage to the bile ducts is caused by abnormal bile flow (stasis), but primary (viral?) damage to the biliary system cannot be fully excluded and some postulate that it may even be the cause of the biliary atresia. **(p. 1037)**

A2. False
This is a condition of the extrahepatic ducts with or without agenesis of the gallbladder. Therefore, the varying degrees of biliary stasis will cause liver damage. This will ultimately cause cirrhosis of the liver and death of the patient. Watching a young infant suffer from biliary atresia is a devastating experience. **(p. 1037)**

A3. True
About 90% of cases have no patent portion of the extrahepatic bile system that communicates with the intrahepatic portion. **(p. 1037)**

A4. True
These patients have a patent proximal bile duct system. **(p. 1037)**

A5. False
The Kasai operation (a portoenterostomy is created whereby the porta hepatis is connected directly to the jejunum or gallbladder when present) is primarily a palliative procedure. Liver transplant is primarily curative. **(p. 1037)**

A6. False
It is the most common cause of obstructive jaundice in children beyond infancy, and may even present in adulthood. However, this may present dramatically even in young infants. **(p. 1037)**

A7. True
However, this is true only of type I choledochal cysts. Todani further classified choledochal cysts as follows: a diverticulum of the common bile duct (type II), arising in the intraduodenal portion of the duct (type III, also known as choledochocele), may consist of multiple dilatations of the intrahepatic and extrahepatic bile ducts (type IVA and IVB and type V). **(p. 1037)**

A8. True

The amount of inflammation and the degree of the damage to the epithelial lining increase with the age of the patient. **(p. 1037)**

A9. True

In addition to metaplasia related to the prolonged exposure to chronic inflammation, papillomas, adenocarcinomas, carcinoid tumor and embryonal rhabdomyosarcoma have also been described. **(p. 1037)**

A10. False

It is true that agenesis of the gallbladder may be seen in trisomy 18, but in other patients it is often seen in biliary atresia and sometimes associated with duodenal atresia. **(p. 1037)**

A11. True

However, in patients without chronic cholecystitis these tissues may also indicate heterotopia. They differ from metaplastic tissue because they are found in small, well-defined intramural nodules. Other heterotopic tissues in the gallbladder include pancreas, liver, adrenal and thyroid. **(p. 1038)**

A12. True

This is a choledochal cyst. The term is misleading because this is actually a focal spherical dilatation of the common bile duct which is connected through the cystic duct to the gallbladder. Choledochal cysts have a fibrous wall and may contain up to 2L of bile. **(p. 1037)**

Cholelithiasis

A1. True

Crystallization is secondary to the precipitation of cholesterol monohydrate crystals, which seems to occur in the mucous gel on the epithelial surface. However, this pathophysiology only accounts for cholesterol stones, which comprise about 80% of gallstones. About 20% are pigmented and their pathophysiology is less well understood. **(p. 1038)**

A2. False

Only 15–20% of stones are visible on plain radiographs. Therefore, ultrasonography is the method of choice for the detection of cholelithiasis. However, even ultrasonography will not reliably detect biliary microlithiasis, which refers to the presence of gallbladder calculi smaller than 2mm, which are too small to be detected by current imaging techniques. **(p. 1038)**

A3. True

The Framingham study found that 11% of the general population has gallstones. The incidence was thought to be highest in Sweden, where 50% of the people have gallstones by the age of 70, but it was found that by age 30 70% of female Pima Indians have gallstones and 70% of male Pima Indians are affected by age 60. Gallstones are rare in inhabitants of sub-Saharan Africa and in the Inuit. **(p. 1038)**

A4. False

This depends on the age group. Although it is generally true that in the adult population cholesterol gallstones are roughly three to four times more common in women than in men, among children gallstones are more frequent in boys than in girls. In adults, this is due to the effect of estrogen on cholesterol metabolism. **(p. 1038)**

A5. True

Generally speaking, pure gallstones are not associated with cholecystitis if there is no obstruction of the bile flow. **(p. 1038)**

A6. True

Black pigmented stones are due to precipitation of calcium bilirubinate, whereas calcium carbonate stones appear chalky, amorphous, and grayish white in color. **(p. 1038)**

A7. False

Brown pigmented stones are composed of unconjugated bilirubin monomers as well as cholesterol, calcium bilirubinate, calcium carbonate, and fatty acids, and are therefore mixed stones. Black pigmented stones are pure calcium bilirubinate. **(p. 1038)**

A8. False

This was traditionally thought to be true. However, today we know that most (72%) pigmented stones, both brown and black, contain bacteria. However, the majority of pigmented stones are brown, and not black as traditionally thought. **(p. 1038)**

A9. False

They contain >90% cholesterol. They are usually single, spheroidal, and translucent bluish white in color. They are more common in multiparous women. No correlation with cholesterol levels in the blood is found. **(p. 1038)**

A10. False

The majority of 'hard' gallstones are hard due to a high protein (mucoprotein) content. Some hard stones contain high levels of calcium carbonate. **(p. 1038)**

A11. True

This is in contrast to 'mixed stones,' which are characteristically variable in size, multiple, faceted and laminated. **(p. 1038)**

A12. True

The stones in choledocholithiasis originate most often in the gallbladder. However, they can also form outside the gallbladder. **(p. 1039)**

A13. False

Only 1–4% of patients are symptomatic. Both symptomatic and asymptomatic patients develop complications of cholelithiasis at a similar rate of about 2% per year. **(p. 1039)**

A14. True

Anything that can disturb bile flow increases the risk of cholelithiasis. This may include a diverticulum, Hartmann's pouch, Phrygian cap, mucosal septation, or variations in the cystic duct. **(p. 1039)**

A15. False

Complications are most common in patients with multiple smaller stones (which is the case with the most frequent type of gallstone, mixed gallstones). **(p. 1039)**

A16. False

Calcium carbonate stones are usually white, whereas the jet black color is typical of calcium bilirubinate stones. **(p. 1038)**

A17. False

Mirizzi's syndrome is caused by an impacted cystic duct stone, but the term does not refer to hydrops, rather to secondary compression of the adjacent common hepatic duct. This is more common in gallbladders with Hartmann's pouch. **(p. 1039)**

Cholesterolosis

A1. True

The gross appearance is characteristic: linear yellow streaks are seen in the prominence of the ridges, surrounded by a congested mucosa ('strawberry gallbladder'). **(p. 1039)**

A2. False

For unknown reasons, cholesterolosis is rarely present in advanced chronic inflammation. **(p. 1039)**

A3. True

As with pure cholesterol gallstones, this condition is most frequent in multiparous women. **(p. 1039)**

A4. False

Cholesterolosis has no clinical significance and is not associated with any symptoms. **(p. 1040)**

Acute cholecystitis

A1. True

About 95% of cases are associated with cholelithiasis. The inflammatory process begins with a calculous obstruction of the cystic duct or gallbladder neck. **(p. 1040)**

A2. False

Whereas other components of acute inflammation are readily found (edema, hyperemia, extravasation of red cells), acute cholecystitis is less likely to show an abundant neutrophilic infiltrate. However, fibroblastic proliferation is frequently seen and small collections of neutrophils may be found in the mucosa. **(p. 1040)**

A3. True

Occasionally it is difficult to distinguish between reactive atypia and carcinoma in situ. Some authors recommend immunostaining for detection of p53 protein. If p53 is very strongly expressed in all atypical cells, the diagnosis of carcinoma is favored. **(p. 1040)**

A4. False

There is experimental evidence that acute calculous (obstructive) cholecystitis is of chemical, rather than infectious, etiology. Unconjugated bile salts, trypsin from pancreatic juice, and phospholipid lysolecithin may play a role. However, secondary bacterial infection is very common. **(p. 1040)**

A5. False

The great majority of cases are superimposed on chronic cholecystitis. This reflects the fact that both are caused by gallstones. **(p. 1040)**

A6. False

Emphysematous cholecystitis has been associated with diabetes mellitus (30–50% of patients have diabetes mellitus), with a male-to-female ratio of 5:1. **(p. 1041)**

A7. True

However, gallstones are not present in about 30–50% patients. Mortality in this type of acute cholecystitis is about 15%, which is much higher than in usual calculous acute cholecystitis. **(p. 1041)**

A8. **True**
However, it occurs in a totally different clinical setting: it is more frequent in males (usually children), and in those older than 65 years. **(p. 1041)**

A9. **True**
However, this complication rate is significantly higher in acute acalculous cholecytistis and emphysematous cholecystitis, which accounts for the mortality rates of the latter two. **(p. 1041)**

A10. **True**
These should not be confused with the changes seen in primary systemic vascular disorders. However, vasculitides may very rarely be associated with acute cholecystitis. **(p. 1041)**

Chronic cholecystitis and cholangitis

A1. **True**
Most often the stones are of mixed type. Chronic bile stasis is thought to cause the chronic inflammation. **(p. 1041)**

A2. **True**
However, the pathogenesis of chronic cholecystitis is not well understood. **(p. 1041)**

A3. **True**
For unknown reasons, this form of chronic cholecystitis is more commonly associated with the development of adenocarcinoma than are other forms of cholecystitis. **(p. 1041)**

A4. **False**
The wall is often thickened twice or three times its normal size. **(p. 1041)**

A5. **False**
Whereas atrophy of the epithelium may be present in some cases of chronic cholecystitis, the epithelium may also be normal, hyperplastic or metaplastic. **(p. 1041)**

A6. **False**
Rokitansky–Aschoff sinuses are characteristic, but not diagnostic of chronic cholecystitis. Macrophages, lymphocytes and plasma cells are also found in varying degrees. **(p. 1042)**

A7. **True**
Intestinal and antral (pyloric/gastric) metaplasia may be found. **(p. 1041)**

A8. **True**
However, metaplastic glands contain non-sulfated acid mucin and also neutral mucin, whereas normal glands in the gallbladder neck contain only sulfated acid mucin. **(p. 1041)**

A9. **True**
It is most commonly located in the fundus. Some consider adenomyomatosis to represent an exaggerated form of Rokitansky–Aschoff sinuses. **(p. 1042)**

A10. **True**
Lymphoid follicles with germinal centers are present throughout the wall of the gallbladder. The presence of reactive follicles does not exclude malignant lymphoma because primary marginal zone lymphoma may be associated with numerous benign follicles. **(p. 1042)**

A11. **False**
Although diffuse lymphoplasmacytic cholecystitis may be associated with sclerosing cholangitis, this association is not very strong or specific. **(p. 1042)**

A12. **True**
It is characterized by massive eosinophilic infiltration. **(p. 1042)**

A13. **False**
Xanthogranulomatous cholecystitis is synonymous with cholecystic granuloma and ceroid granuloma, and refers to nodular collections of macrophages with neutral fat and lipofuscin (ceroid) pigment. Malakoplakia also occurs in the gallbladder, but is a different disorder characterized by the presence of calcium- and iron-positive Michaelis–Gutmann bodies in the cytoplasm of the histiocytes. **(p. 1042)**

A14. **False**
Whereas biliary fistulas may be clinically silent, cholecystocolic fistulas are associated with severe infection. Treatment involves cholecystectomy and repair of the involved portion of bowel. **(p. 1043)**

A15. **False**
These are most commonly the result of surgical trauma, in which the duct is inadvertently injured or ligated. **(p. 1043)**

A16. **True**
In one series this association was 100%, whereas it occurs in only 35% of the general population. **(p. 1043)**

A17. **True**
It has been also associated with Riedel's thyroiditis, retroperitoneal or mediastinal fibrosis, orbital pseudotumor, Crohn's disease, sclerosing pancreatitis, and, in particular, ulcerative colitis. **(p. 1043)**

A18. False

The most characteristic changes are present in the intrahepatic bile ducts and may be observed in the liver biopsy. Duct segments are chronically inflamed and are eventually replaced by fibrous tissue. **(p. 1043)**

A19. False

The red granules containing the bacteriocidal lysozymes are characteristic of Paneth cells. This is a nice example of complete intestinal metaplasia in the gallbladder with chronic cholecystitis. Kulchitsky's cells also have red cytoplasmic granulation, but the granules are much smaller, less refractive, and the nuclei are oriented towards the lumina of the glands, not towards the basement membrane as in Paneth cells. **(p. 1042)**

Tumors

A1. False

Cholesterol polyps are an exaggerated form of cholesterolosis. **(p. 1043)**

A2. False

Inflammatory polyps are always associated with chronic cholecystitis. **(p. 1043)**

A3. True

Adenomyoma (when focal) and adenomyomatosis (when diffuse) are synonyms. **(p. 1044)**

A4. False

Villous papilloma is associated with metachromatic leukodystrophy and may result in massive hemobilia. It should not be confused with villous adenoma, which is a precancerous lesion. **(p. 1044)**

A5. False

In contrast to adenomas of the colon, in the gallbladder adenomas are rare and are not significant precursors of adenocarcinoma. **(p. 1044)**

A6. True

They also may be sessile or pedunculated. Interestingly, tubular adenomas are usually composed of pyloric-type glands, whereas the glands of tubulovillous and villous adenoma more closely resemble those of the colorectum. **(p. 1044)**

A7. True

As in the pancreas, they are surrounded by ovarian-type stroma. **(p. 1044)**

A8. False

Patients with papillomatosis have a high risk of malignant transformation. Overall, however, this is a rare condition and therefore a rare cause of cholangiocarcinoma. **(p. 1044)**

A9. True

The cells of the granular cell tumor may be inconspicuous and overlooked if not specifically sought in the biopsy specimen. **(p. 1044)**

A10. True

Over 90% of patients are 50 years of age or older. **(p. 1044)**

A11. False

It is most common in American Indians, relatively infrequent in whites of European origin, and very rare in blacks. **(p. 1044)**

A12. False

Only 0.3% of patients with lithiasis develop adenocarcinoma. **(p. 1045)**

A13. True

Gardner's syndrome, a variant of familial adenomatous polyposis (FAP), is an autosomal dominant disease characterized by gastrointestinal polyps, multiple osteomas, and skin and soft tissue tumors. As in usual FAP, an association with gallbladder carcinomas has also been described. **(p. 1045)**

A14. True

Some other conditions associated with adenocarcinoma of the gallbladder include cholecystoenteric fistula, ulcerative colitis, adenomyomatosis, and anomalous connection between the common bile duct and the pancreatic duct. **(p. 1045)**

A15. False

Most carcinomas of the gallbladder are diffuse and may be difficult to distinguish grossly from chronic or even acute cholecystitis. This is why microscopic examination is always indicated in cholecystectomy specimens. Extensive sampling may be needed in an acutely inflamed gallbladder. **(p. 1045)**

A16. True

Typically these are well differentiated architecturally, but the nuclear features are those of high-grade tumors. **(p. 1046)**

A17. True

Foci of intestinal differentiation are commonly found in otherwise typical well-differentiated adenocarcinomas of the gallbladder. Occasionally the entire tumor shows intestinal differentiation on morphologic, histochemical and immunohistochemical grounds. **(p. 1046)**

A18. False

Adenocarcinomas typically produce sialomucins. However, both sialomucins and sulfomucins are acid mucins. Both stain blue with the Alcian blue (AB at pH 2.5) histochemical stain, but can be distinguished by using high-iron diamine–Alcian blue (HID-AB at pH 2.5) staining (blue sialomucin and black sulfomucin). **(p. 1046)**

A19. False

According to some authors, intrahepatic adenocarcinomas are usually CK7+ and CK20–, whereas adenocarcinomas of the extrahepatic bile ducts and gallbladder are usually CK7+ and CK20+. This was not the case in all studies. **(p. 1046)**

A20. True

Most common are *p53* mutations and K-*ras* mutations, which lack any specificity. **(p. 1046)**

A21. False

However, hepatolithiasis, a condition common in East Asia, is strongly associated with cholangiocarcinoma. **(p. 1045)**

A22. False

Although squamous metaplasia occurs frequently in adenocarcinoma of this region, pure squamous cell carcinoma is very rare. **(p. 1046)**

A23. True

In some reports these tumors showed expression of CDX-2 and CK20, which may indicate intestinal differentiation. **(p. 1046)**

A24. True

As in other sites, most lymphoepithelial carcinomas show an association with EBV, which may be demonstrated by EBER in situ hybridization or by immunohistochemical detection of EBNA 1 (type 1 latency). **(p. 1046)**

A25. False

As in the stomach, most cases of gallbladder adenocarcinoma are preceded by a sequence of intestinal metaplasia, dysplasia and carcinoma in situ. **(p. 1045)**

A26. False

In dysplastic mucosa both intestinal and gastric-type mucins are found, whereas in adenocarcinoma the gastric type predominates. **(p. 1048)**

A27. True

It also gives rise to liver metastases through the portal tract as well as to the regional lymph nodes. **(p. 1048)**

A28. False

The most important factor is the stage. However, other important prognostic factors include a status of surgical margins and histological grade. **(p. 1049)**

A29. False

This is an example of adenomyoma, which should not be mistaken for well-differentiated adenocarcinoma. When the process is diffuse the term adenomyosis can be used instead. **(p. 1042)**

A30. True

A well-formed gland with wide lumina lined by one or a few rows of highly atypical cuboidal cells is a common feature in carcinomas of the pancreatobiliary region. **(p. 1046)**

Carcinoma of the extrahepatic bile ducts

A1. False

Bile duct carcinoma has equal frequency in both sexes. **(p. 1049)**

A2. True

The average age of presentation is 60 years. Patients with predisposing factors are usually one decade younger. **(p. 1049)**

A3. True

Infection with liver flukes, choledochal cysts and hepatolithiasis are also predisposing factors. **(p. 1049)**

A4. True

The disease is further classified according to the Bismuth–Corlette classification system, in which type I lesions are confined to the common hepatic duct and type II lesions involve the bifurcation of the hepatic duct. Types III and IV lesions involve the secondary hepatic ducts, with IIIa involving the right side, IIIb the left, and type IV both sides. **(p. 1049)**

A5. False

Diagnostic material is obtained in about 70% of cases by using fine needle aspiration, brushing, or bile aspiration techniques. **(p. 1049)**

A6. False

Most bile duct carcinomas are nodular or sclerosing, with deep penetration into the wall. **(p. 1049)**

A7. True

The papillary variant of bile duct adenocarcinoma was, in some reports, associated with the best prognosis. **(p. 1050)**

A8. True

The primary site of these carcinomas needs to be established clinically. **(p. 1050)**

A9. True

This may be a helpful feature in distinction from sclerosing cholangitis, which is occasionally difficult to distinguish from adenocarcinoma, and so far has not been shown to overexpress p53. **(p. 1050)**

A10. True

Overexpression of p53 has been associated with mass-forming tumors, whereas k-ras overexpression correlates with extensive periductal extension. Overexpression of COX-2, c-erb-B-2, and ets-1 has also been described in extrahepatic cholangiocarcinoma. **(p. 1050)**

A11. True

Some of the cases were associated with dysplastic nevus syndrome. **(p. 1051)**

A12. True

However, few cases have been described in adults. **(p. 1051)**

A13. True

They may be insular or tubular in type. Signet ring cell and clear cell variants have been described. **(p. 1050)**

A14. True

However, before the diagnosis of any sarcoma is made in this location, the diagnosis of carcinosarcoma should be considered. **(p. 1051)**

A15. False

Metastatic carcinomas are exceptionally rare in the gallbladder. Most reported cases were melanomas, renal cell carcinomas and breast carcinomas. **(p. 1052)**

Pancreas and ampullary region 15

Normal anatomy

Q1
The pancreas forms from two separate buds or *Anlagen*, which later rotate and fuse.

Q2
The exocrine pancreas is composed basically of acinar cells and duct cells.

Q3
The main pancreatic duct (duct of Wirsung) and accessory duct (duct of Santorini) are the two principal ducts of the pancreas and in the normal pancreas are not connected.

Q4
All pancreatic ducts are lined by the same type of simple columnar epithelium.

Q5
Centroacinar cells are a transitional type of cell between acinar and ductal epithelium, the function of which is not known.

Q6
Langerhans' islets contain four types of endocrine cell: B cells, A cells, C cells and D cells.

Q7
Langerhans' islets larger than 400 μm should be regarded as too large.

Q8
Insulin is secreted by B cells, which constitute about 30% of the Langerhans' islet population.

Q9
A cells secrete glucagons and are located in the center of the Langerhans' islet.

Q10
D cells are scattered throughout the islets.

Q11
Endocrine cells of the pancreas are of neural crest derivation.

Q12
Langerhans' islets are histologically the same throughout the pancreas.

Q13
In the pancreas, scattered endocrine cells can also be found associated with ducts and acini.

Q14
Nesidioblastosis refers to hyperplasia of Langerhans' islets and may be associated with neonatal hypoglycemia.

Congenital abnormalities

Q1
Annular pancreas is associated with Down syndrome.

Q2
Heterotopia of pancreatic tissue is most common in the duodenum, stomach and jejunum.

Q3
Radiographically, central umbilication of the submucosal ectopic pancreatic tissue is a useful diagnostic clue.

Q4
Heterotopic pancreas can contain all components of the normal pancreatic tissues.

Q5

This image illustrates submucosal ectopic pancreas in the wall of the duodenum.

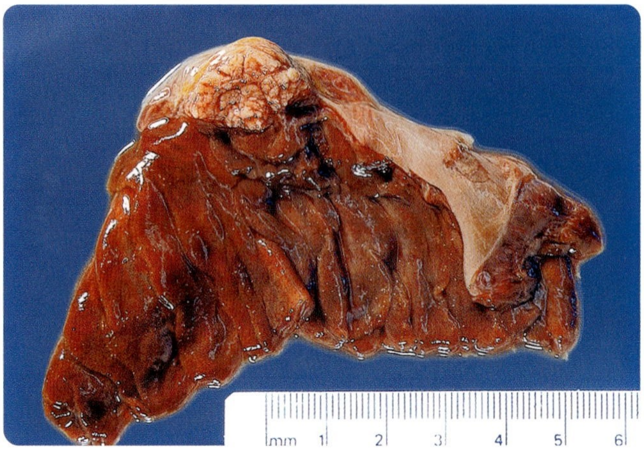

Fig. 15.1

Pancreatitis

Q1

The etiology of acute pancreatitis is not fully understood, but many cases are associated with cholelithiasis and alcoholism.

Q2

Fat necrosis is a characteristic finding in pancreatitis.

Q3

Foci of fat necrosis are rich in neutrophils in the early stages of acute pancreatitis.

Q4

Acute interstitial pancreatitis, characterized only by edema and fat necrosis, is the mildest form of acute pancreatitis.

Q5

The majority of cases of chronic pancreatitis are preceded by an acute pancreatitis.

Q6

Acute pancreatitis is a severe disease with an overall mortality of 20%. One such case is illustrated in this figure.

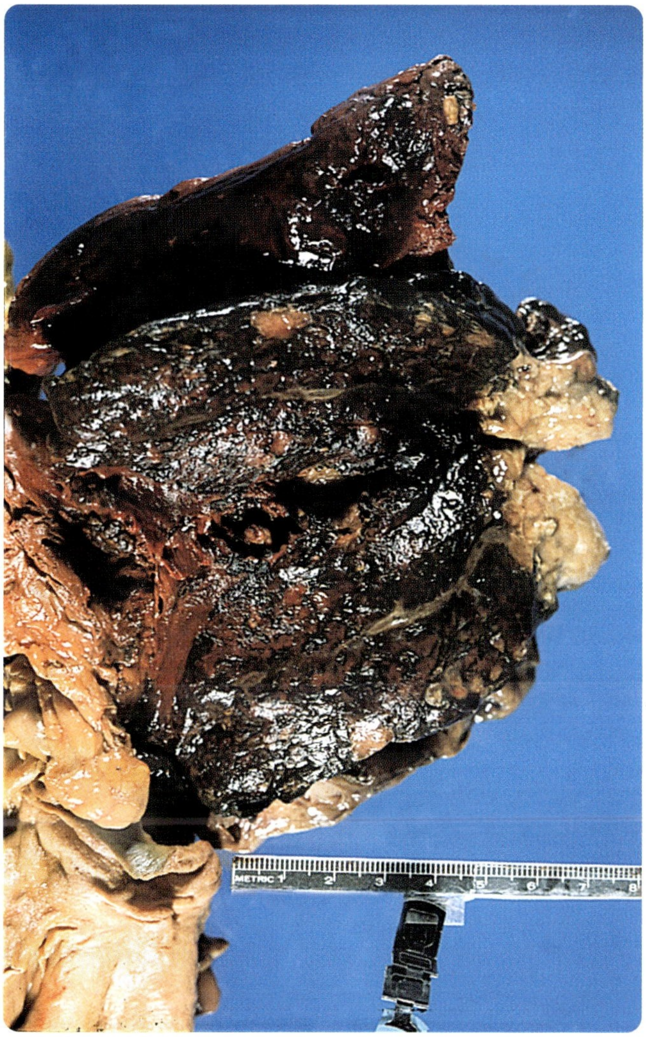

Fig. 15.2

Q7

Chronic pancreatitis causes loss of pancreatic parenchyma, which is replaced by fibrosis. The patient suffers from variable pain and symptoms of pancreatic insufficiency, including diabetes and malabsorption.

Q8

Alcoholism and obstruction of the pancreatic ducts by gallstones or tumors are the most frequent causes of chronic pancreatitis.

Q9

There is no clear association between genetic factors and chronic pancreatitis.

Q10

Non-alcoholic tropical pancreatitis develops as a result of repeated gastrointestinal infections.

Q11

K-*ras* mutations can be found in chronic pancreatitis.

Q12

Lymphoplasmacytic sclerosing pancreatitis is the most common form of chronic pancreatitis.

Q13

Eosinophilic pancreatitis is a form of chronic pancreatitis associated with chronic infestation by a nematode.

Q14

The term groove pancreatitis designates a condition in which scar develops between the head of the pancreas and the duodenum.

Q15

Chronic pancreatitis can generally be classified into three categories: chronic calcifying pancreatitis, chronic obstructive pancreatitis, and chronic inflammatory pancreatitis.

Q16

Chronic calcifying pancreatitis starts with precipitation of proteinaceous material in the pancreatic ducts to form protein plugs that subsequently calcify. The ductal epithelium undergoes atrophy, hyperplasia and metaplasia at the site of the protein plugs.

Q17

In chronic calcifying pancreatitis, peripancreatic fibrosis is usually a late finding that involves the portal and/or splenic veins.

Q18

In chronic obstructive pancreatitis the prominent histologic changes are periductal fibrosis and subsequent ductal dilatation.

Q19

Cholelithiasis is a major cause of chronic obstructive pancreatitis.

Q20

Chronic inflammatory pancreatitis is a rare form of chronic pancreatitis and affects young people with autoimmune diseases.

Q21

The most common cause of chronic pancreatitis in children is a familial hereditary pancreatitis.

Q22

Hyperplasia of Brunner's glands in the duodenum is a common finding in chronic pancreatitis.

Q23

Metastatic fat necrosis occurs in pancreatic tumors, which produce lipase.

Q24

In pancreatic transplantation, graft survival is poor due to 'graft pancreatitis' and acute and chronic rejection.

Q25

Pancreatic abscess and infected necrosis of the pancreas are basically the same process.

Q26

Pseudocysts have a ragged inner surface and no epithelial lining.

Q27

External drainage of a pseudocyst is the treatment of choice for this lesion.

Q28

True cysts of the pancreas could be considered cystadenomas.

Q29

Lymphoepithelial cysts of the pancreas are associated with HIV infection.

Q30

Lymphoepithelial cysts of the pancreas are located in the pancreatic tail.

Q31

Mucinous non-neoplastic cyst is similar to mucinous cystadenoma.

Q32

Ductal adenocarcinoma is the most common malignancy of the pancreas.

Q33

Peripheral venous thrombosis occurs in most patients with advanced pancreatic carcinoma.

Q34

Pancreatic carcinomas frequently show familial aggregation, which is consistent with genetic susceptibility.

Q35

Pancreatic carcinoma occurs more frequently in patients having familial breast carcinoma with mutation of the *BRCA2* gene.

Q36

Pancreatic ductal adenocarcinoma originates in the head of the pancreas in the majority of cases.

Q37

Disparity between the high degree of cytologic atypia and the low level of architectural atypia is typical of tumors of the pancreaticobiliary region.

Q38

Identification of glands in the perineural space in the pancreas is diagnostic of malignancy.

Q39

In almost all patients with invasive ductal adenocarcinoma of the pancreas one can also find carcinoma in situ.

Q40

'Insular pancreas' refers to secondary hyperplasia of the endocrine pancreas.

Q41

Pancreatic ductal adenocarcinomas produce small and large intestinal mucins.

Q42

Immunohistochemically, pancreatic ductal adenocarcinoma has the immunophenotype of simple epithelium.

Q43

Cytokeratin typing is useful in pancreatic adenocarcinoma.

Q44

CK17 is frequently expressed by pancreaticobiliary adenocarcinoma, but not by other non-mucinous adenocarcinomas.

Q45

The expression of MUC2 and CDX2 is restricted to the intestinal, mucinous and signet ring cell-type adenocarcinomas of duodenal papillary origin and not pancreatic ductal carcinoma.

Q46

The finding of inactivated *Smad-4* (*DPC4*) is useful in the diagnostic work-up of pancreatic adenocarcinoma.

Q47

KOC (K homology domain containing protein overexpressed in cancer) is a novel oncofetal RNA-binding protein highly expressed in pancreatic carcinomas.

Q48

CA19-9 is an oncofetal antigen expressed by several different cancers, but especially by carcinomas of the gastrointestinal tract, including pancreatic adenocarcinoma.

Q49

The most frequent molecular abnormalities in pancreatic ductal adenocarcinoma are mutations of the *TP53* and K-*ras* genes.

Q50

Medullary carcinoma of the pancreas is strongly associated with microsatellite instability.

Q51

No recurrent cytogenetic aberrations are found in ductal adenocarcinoma of the pancreas.

Q52

Mucoepidermoid carcinoma and adenoacanthoma of the pancreas are synonymous.

Q53

Mucinous (colloid) carcinoma is a variant of mucinous cystadenocarcinoma.

Q54

Pancreatic ductal adenocarcinoma tends to metastasize to the liver first.

Q55

Duodenal secretions are the most suitable cytologic material for diagnosis of pancreatic ductal adenocarcinoma.

Q56

Anaplastic carcinoma of the pancreas has features of an undifferentiated tumor with various morphologic appearances, but it is correctly diagnosed owing to its constant expression of epithelial markers such as EMA, keratin and CEA.

Q57

Giant cell tumor of the pancreas refers to the same lesion as anaplastic carcinoma of the pancreas.

Q58

Microcystic cystadenoma is usually a large lesion at presentation and grossly shows multiple small cysts filled with serous fluid.

Q59

The cystic spaces in microcystic cystadenoma are lined by optically clear mucin-rich cuboidal epithelium without cytologic atypia.

Q60

Microcystic cystadenoma is a tumor of centroacinar cells.

Q61

Microcystic cystadenoma has several distinct features: there is no mucin production, Langerhans' islets can be found between the cysts, the tumor is highly vascular, and the epithelial lining of the microcysts demonstrates a myoepithelial layer.

Q62

Solid serous adenoma and serous (or microcystic) adenocarcinoma are synonymous.

Q63

Mucinous cystic tumors of the pancreas are seen in patients older than those with microcystic cystadenoma.

Q64

As in pancreatic ductal adenocarcinoma, mucinous cystic neoplasms occur most frequently in the head of the pancreas.

Q65

Mucinous cystic neoplasms typically have 'ovarian-like' stroma.

Q66

Mucinous cystadenoma and cystadenocarcinoma are lined by simple columnar epithelium rich in mucin.

Q67

The *DPC4* gene is inactivated in about half of mucinous cystic neoplasms of the pancreas.

Q68

Mucinous cystic neoplasms of the pancreas usually lack MUC1 expression, except when they become invasive.

Q69

Mucinous cystic neoplasms of the pancreas do express MUC2.

Q70

All mucinous cystic tumors of the pancreas should be regarded as mucinous cystadenocarcinomas of low-grade malignant potential.

Q71

Some microscopic characteristics of mucinous cystic neoplasm include 'mural nodules' (with features of giant cell tumor, MFH or anaplastic carcinoma), endocrine cells often scattered among columnar lining cells, and calcification.

Q72

In contrast to mucinous cystic neoplasms, which occur in the body and tail of the pancreas and are more common in women, intraductal papillary mucinous neoplasms (IPMN) occur most often in the head of the pancreas and are more common in men.

Q73

Intraductal papillary mucinous neoplasms (IPMN) are in most cases associated with an invasive carcinoma.

Q74

IPMN histologically show complex papillary fronds of mucin-producing epithelial cells, ductal fibrosis, and no evidence of ovarian-type stroma.

Q75

The intestinal type of IPMN may be associated with colloid carcinoma.

Q76

PanIN (pancreatic intraepithelial lesions) are epithelial proliferative lesions of small ducts, most of which are not visible grossly or radiologically.

Q77

Reactive changes may mimic PanINs.

Q78

PanINs are positive for MUC1 and negative for MUC2.

Q79

Classification of PanIN into grades 1A, 1B, 2 and 3 is based on the degree of nuclear atypia and architectural complexity.

Q80

The differential diagnosis of a PanIN lesion includes cancerization of the ducts by adenocarcinoma and intraductal papillary mucinous neoplasms.

Q81

Acinar cell hyperplasia may be confused with hyperplastic islets.

Q82

Acinar cell adenoma is a precursor of acinar cell carcinoma.

Q83

Acinar cell carcinoma may occur in children.

Q84

Acinar cell carcinoma needs to be ruled out in patients with metastatic fat necrosis and arthralgia.

Q85

Acinar cell carcinoma shows a prominent intraductal growth pattern.

Q86

Well-differentiated acinar cell tumors may histologically mimic normal pancreas.

Q87

In most acinar cell carcinomas the cytoplasm is abundant, eosinophilic, granular, and PAS-positive, diastase-resistant cytoplasmic granules are common.

Q88

At the molecular genetic level acinar cell carcinoma is very similar to pancreatic duct carcinoma.

Q89

'Mixed acinar–endocrine tumor' displays an even admixture of acinar and endocrine cells.

Q90

Acinar cell cystadenocarcinoma is cystic and grossly may mimic the appearance of mucinous cystic adenocarcinoma.

Q91

Solid-pseudopapillary tumor of the pancreas is a low-grade tumor of young women (mean 30–35 years), often non-white, and is cured by resection in 95% of cases.

Q92

The differential diagnosis of solid-pseudopapillary tumor of the pancreas includes pancreatic endocrine tumor and adrenal cortical tumors.

Q93

Pancreatoblastoma is the most common pancreatic tumor in children.

Q94

Pancreatoblastoma has been associated with von Hippel–Lindau disease.

Q95

Pancreatoblastoma occurs in children with a mean age of 5 years.

Q96

Histologically, pancreatoblastoma consists of solid sheets and nests of uniform epithelial cells admixed with well-formed acinar structures and occasional dilated ductules.

Q97

α-Fetoprotein may be expressed in pancreatoblastomas.

Q98

The prognosis of pancreatoblastoma is more favorable in adults than in children.

Q99

Like pancreatic ductal adenocarcinoma, pancreatic endocrine neoplasms are most frequent in the head of the pancreas.

Q100

Occasionally, endocrine neoplasm of the pancreas has a cystic appearance.

Q101

The solid pattern of growth in endocrine tumors of the pancreas is strongly associated with the β-cell type.

Q102

Amyloid is found most often in pancreatic neuroendocrine tumors, which secrete glucagon.

Q103

Clear cell change in pancreatic neuroendocrine tumors may be seen in patients with von Hippel–Lindau disease.

Q104

80% of pancreatic neuroendocrine tumors occur in MEN I patients.

Q105

Most pancreatic neuroendocrine tumors are non-functional.

Q106

Pancreatic neuroendocrine tumors are either syndromic or not. Non-syndromic tumors are also known as 'non-functional.'

Q107

Pancreatic neuroendocrine tumors are high grade if they show more than 10 mitotic figures per 50 hpf.

Q108

Secretion of the α or β subunit of hCG is more frequent in more aggressive pancreatic neuroendocrine tumors.

Q109

Pancreatic neuroendocrine tumors, like other neuroendocrine tumors, show expression of epithelial and neural markers.

Q110

Sporadic pancreatic neuroendocrine tumors do not show recurrent molecular or cytogenetic abnormalities.

Q111

Insulinomas are β-cell tumors and occur most often in patients with MEN I.

Q112

The great majority of insulinomas are solitary lesions.

Q113

Insulinomas show strong expression of chromogranin.

Q114

The majority of β-cell tumors are malignant.

Q115

Solitary fibrous tumor is an extrapancreatic tumor that clinically can mimic insulinoma.

Q116

Glucagonomas associated with glucagonoma syndrome are dissimilar to syndromic insulinomas because these tumors are usually large and have a high incidence of malignancy.

Q117

Syndromic glucagonomas occur most often in adult females.

Q118

Gastrinomas (G-cell tumors) produce Zollinger–Ellison syndrome.

Q119

Sporadic syndromic G-cell tumors are solitary tumors of the pancreas or duodenal wall and are often benign.

Q120

Diarrheogenic syndrome is caused by VIP-producing tumors.

Q121

VIPomas are morphologically indistinguishable from G-cell tumors.

Q122

δ-Cell tumors are usually clinically silent.

Q123

Psammoma bodies are a characteristic microscopic finding in carcinoid tumors.

Q124

PP-secreting pancreatic neuroendocrine tumors are rare.

Q125

Carcinoid tumors are frequent in the pancreas.

Q126

In children, a tumor that looks like high-grade neuroendocrine tumor of the pancreas is more likely to be a primitive neuroectodermal tumor (PNET) than small cell carcinoma.

Q127

Pancreatic neuroendocrine tumors are classified into three groups by WHO.

Q128

MEN I may involve the anterior pituitary gland (adenomas), parathyroid glands (chief cell hyperplasia) and pancreas (gastrinomas > insulinomas > VIPomas > glucagonomas).

Q129

Germline mutation of the *MEN I* gene may be associated with carcinoid tumors and soft tissue tumors.

Q130

MEN type II is caused by germline mutation of the *MEN II* gene.

Q131

Inherited as an autosomal dominant disorder, MEN II has two distinct subtypes: MEN IIA and MEN IIB.

Q132

Familial medullary thyroid carcinoma-only (FMTC-only) is a subtype of MEN II syndrome in which more than one family member has medullary carcinoma of the thyroid, but the other features of MEN II are not present.

Q133

Medullary thyroid carcinoma and primary hyperparathyroidism are more frequent in MEN IIA than in MEN IIB, whereas the opposite is true for pheochromocytoma.

Q134

MEN IIA patients have a less virulent form of medullary thyroid carcinoma than MEN IIB patients.

Q135

Pancreatic involvement by malignant lymphoma is rare and is usually secondary to spread from regional lymph nodes or systemic disease.

Q136

Benign mesenchymal tumors of the pancreas are relatively common compared to other acinar-type glands.

Q137

Sarcoma of the pancreas is more common than anaplastic carcinoma with sarcomatous appearance.

Q138

Metastatic tumors to the pancreas most often originate in the colon or kidney.

Q139

Small cords of epithelial cells embedded in fibrous stroma indicate the invasive nature of the lesion and are a valuable diagnostic feature during frozen section.

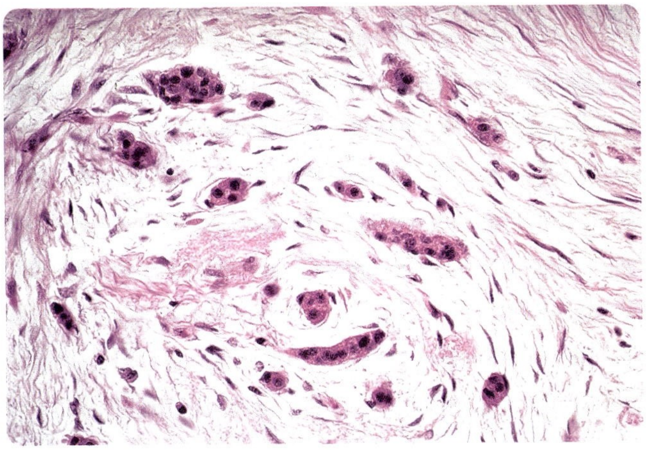

Fig. 15.3

Q140

The presence of epithelial cells in the perineural space is a sure sign of malignancy in pancreatic tissue.

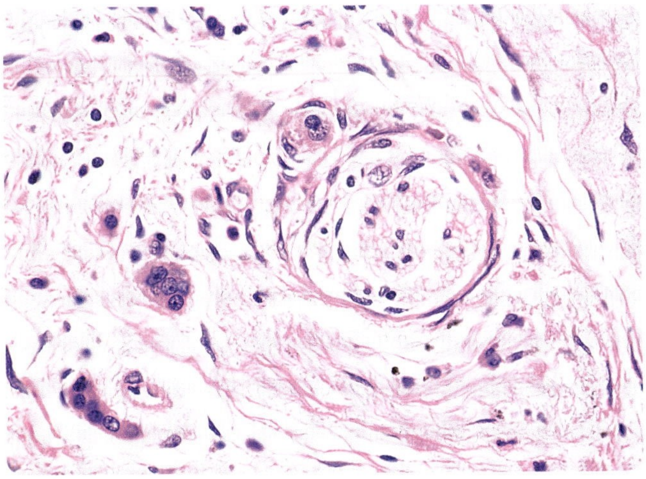

Fig. 15.4

Q141

When both sarcomatoid and carcinomatous elements are found in the tumor of the pancreas, the best diagnosis is sarcomatoid carcinoma.

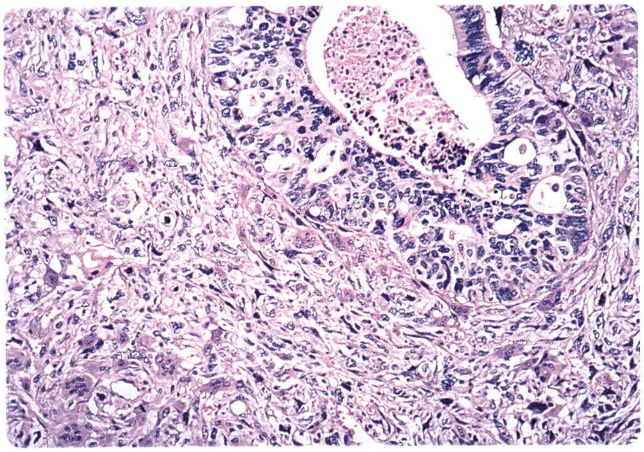

Fig. 15.5

Q142

This is the typical appearance of a mucinous cystic neoplasm.

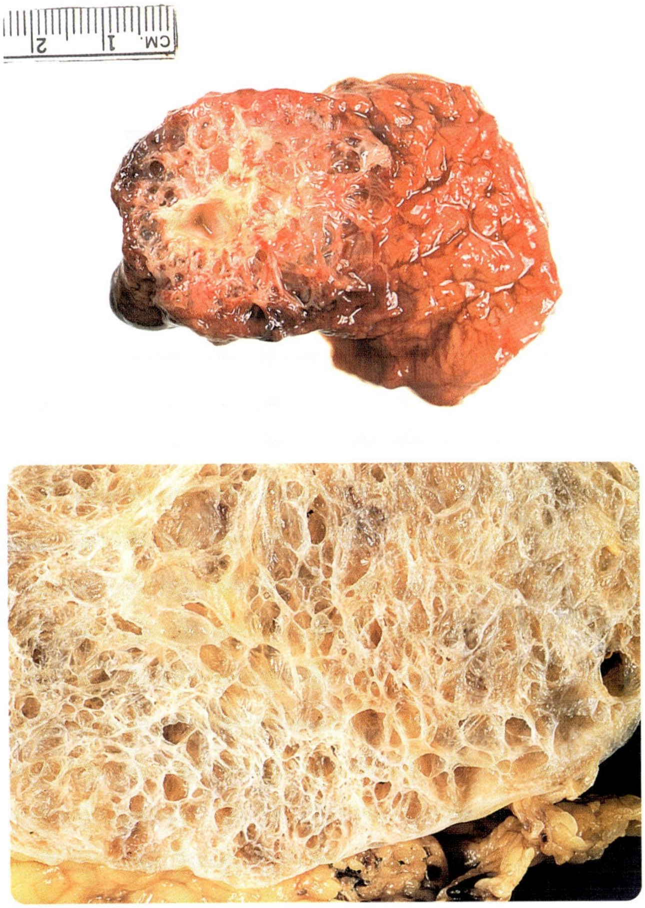

A

B

Fig. 15.6

Q143

Some mucinous cystadenomas of the pancreas show focal papillary growth, as shown in this figure.

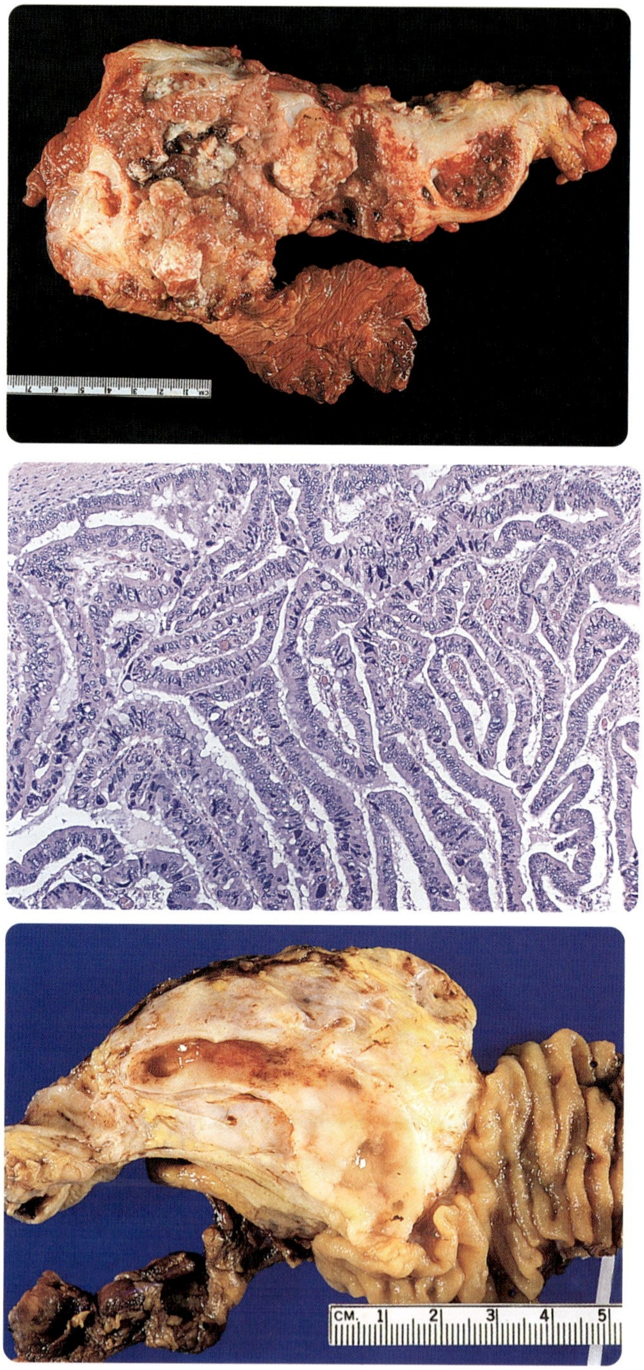

A

B

C

Fig. 15.7

Q144

The histology of acinar cell carcinoma may resemble normal pancreas, as shown here.

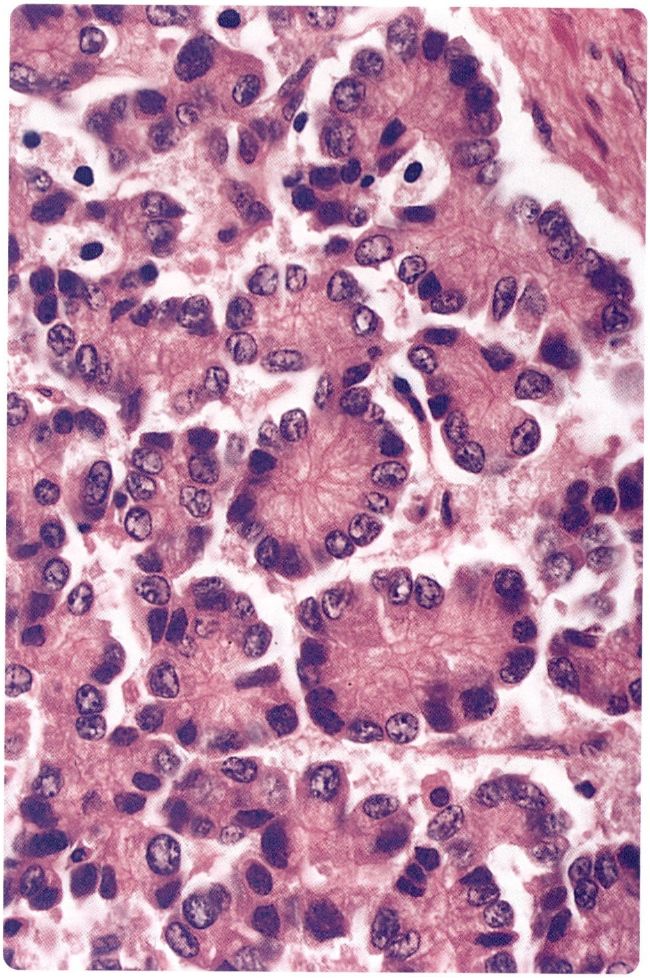

Fig. 15.8

Q145

A solid pattern of growth in combination with small rosette-like glandular formations is characteristic of neuroendocrine tumors of the pancreas.

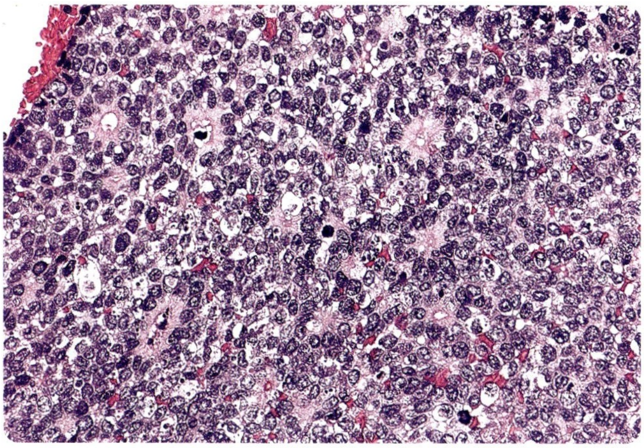

Fig. 15.9

Ampullary region

Q1

Ampullary carcinoma usually represents pancreatic ductal carcinoma arising in this region.

Q2

When no in situ lesion is present, it is most appropriate to designate a tumor of the ampullary region as 'carcinoma of the pancreaticobiliary–ampullary region.'

Q3

Intra-ampullary carcinoma and periampullary carcinoma are the two patterns of spread of ampullary carcinoma.

Q4

It appears that at least some cases of ampullary adenocarcinoma are preceded by a villous adenoma or villoglandular polyp.

Q5

Signet ring carcinoma is a common histological type of ampullary adenocarcinoma.

Q6

As in pancreatic duct carcinoma, ampullary adenocarcinoma frequently shows loss of *DPC4* gene expression and K-*ras* mutations.

Q7

Ampullary carcinoma is most common in elderly men.

Q8

The prognosis of ampullary carcinoma is similar to that of pancreatic and bile duct adenocarcinoma, and therefore the distinction between these entities is only of academic importance.

Q9

Grading differentiation of ampullary adenocarcinoma is based on the percentage of glands present.

Q10

Frozen section diagnosis of ampullary adenocarcinoma may be very difficult.

Q11

Primary ampullary adenocarcinoma of small intestinal mucosal origin has the same immunophenotype as primary pancreatic ductal adenocarcinoma.

Q12

Adenomyoma, adenomyomatous hyperplasia, and inflammatory polyp are benign lesions that may cause obstruction of the ampulla of Vater.

QUESTIONS

Q13

Carcinoid tumor of the ampulla of Vater is always benign in this location.

Q14

Well-differentiated papillary proliferation in the ampulla with morphologic features analogous to those of villous adenoma of the large bowel could occasionally be associated with adenocarcinoma of the ampulla of Vater.

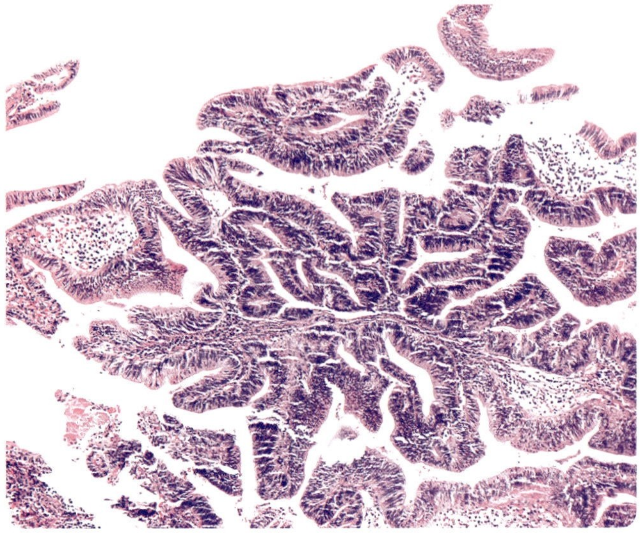

Fig. 15.10

Normal anatomy

A1. True

Abnormalities of the Anlagen (primordia) fusion are the basis for formation of annular pancreas. **(p. 1061)**

A2. False

Although acinar cells and duct cells are most prominent, there is also a population of 'centroacinar cells' that are found in the center of the acinus. They have pale cytoplasm and oval nuclei, and blend with the cells of the intercalated duct, which drains the acinus. **(p. 1061)**

A3. False

Usually these two ducts are joined by numerous anastomotic connections. This is not the case in 10% of individuals, however, in whom the duct of Santorini constitutes the principal drainage for the organ, and *pancreas divisum* results. **(p. 1061)**

A4. False

Intercalated ducts and intralobular ducts are lined by small cuboidal cells with pale cytoplasm, whereas interlobular ducts are also lined by mucin-producing columnar cells. The major ducts of Wirsung and Santorini are similar to interlobular ducts but have more goblet cells. **(p. 1062)**

A5. False

Centroacinar cells secrete bicarbonate-rich fluid to neutralize acid in the duodenum. **(p. 1062)**

A6. False

They do contain B cells, A cells and D cells, but not C cells. Instead, they contain PP cells, which are pancreatic polypeptide-secreting cells. These cells are very rare and are typically located at the periphery of the islets. **(p. 1062)**

A7. True

In general, islets are more numerous and larger in small children. However, 400 μm is too large for any age. **(p. 1062)**

A8. False

Although B cells do secrete insulin and islet cell amyloid polypeptide (IAPP), they represent the most numerous cell type and constitute about 60–75% of the total population. **(p. 1062)**

A9. False

A cells do secrete glucagons, but like PP cells are located at the periphery of the islets. **(p. 1062)**

A10. True

These somatostatin-secreting cells are randomly distributed in the islets. **(p. 1062)**

A11. False

Like the exocrine pancreas, the endocrine pancreas is endodermal in origin. Expression of Ngn3 (a key component of the Notch pathway) in pancreatic precursor cells designates the beginning of endocrine differentiation. **(p. 1062)**

A12. False

Langerhans' islets in the head of the pancreas (which are derived from the ventral bud) have highly irregular outlines, a trabecular arrangement and a very high content of PP cells. **(p. 1062)**

A13. True

Most of these are of Kultschitsky (which produce serotonin) and PP type. **(p. 1062)**

A14. False

Nesidioblastosis may cause neonatal hypoglycemia, but it refers to the formation of so-called 'ductuloinsular complexes,' an intimate association of islets with ducts, which may or may not be associated with hyperplasia of Langerhans' islets. **(p. 1062)**

Congenital abnormalities

A1. True

Annular pancreas is also associated with pancreatitis, pancreatic duct obstruction and peptic ulcer. Because it encircles the duodenum, it may also lead to constriction of the duodenal lumen. **(p. 1062)**

A2. True

It also occurs in the ileum, Meckel's diverticulum, gastric and intestinal diverticula, gallbladder, bile ducts and other organs. **(p. 1063)**

A3. True

The umbilication corresponds to a central duct that opens into the lumen. **(p. 1063)**

A4. True

However, endocrine pancreas is present in only 30% of cases. The composition of the endocrine pancreas also varies greatly from case to case. **(p. 1063)**

A5. True

Note that ectopic pancreas has a gross appearance identical to that of this organ in its normal anatomic location. **(p. 1063)**

ANSWERS

Pancreatitis

A1. True

Experimental evidence suggests that the most frequent etiology is a 'common channel between common bile duct and main pancreatic duct' due to a migrating gallstone, biliary sludge, or spasm of the sphincter of Oddi. **(p. 1063)**

A2. True

This feature is recognized grossly as yellow plaques and nodules in the pancreas and throughout the mesenteric and peritoneal fat. Fat necrosis is also frequently seen in mastectomy specimens, in the tissues surrounding a breast biopsy excision site, and in traumatized lipoma. **(p. 1063)**

A3. True

Later this population changes to foamy histiocytes and lymphocytes, and calcification is prominent. **(p. 1063)**

A4. True

More severe forms include acute necrotizing pancreatitis, hemorrhagic pancreatitis and infected pancreatic necrosis. **(p. 1065)**

A5. False

Although acute pancreatitis can in some cases evolve into chronic pancreatitis, chronic pancreatitis is generally not preceded by an acute phase. **(p. 1065)**

A6. False

The overall mortality of acute pancreatitis is 20%. However, the mortality of more severe forms (hemorrhagic/necrotizing), illustrated here, is about 50%. The late sequelae of acute pancreatitis in some cases include diabetes mellitus. **(p. 1064)**

A7. True

Chronic pancreatitis may simulate or coexist with pancreatic carcinoma. **(p. 1065)**

A8. True

Other important conditions that predispose to chronic pancreatitis include hypercalcemia, hyperparathyroidism, hyperlipoproteinemia, and some infections and autoimmune disorders. **(p. 1065)**

A9. False

Two forms of chronic pancreatitis are genetically related. *Familial hereditary pancreatitis* is inherited in an autosomal dominant manner, and results from mutation of the trypsinogen gene that causes persistent trypsin activation. Patients with mutations of the *cystic fibrosis* gene also frequently suffer from chronic pancreatitis. **(p. 1065)**

A10. False

It is due to protein–calorie malnutrition. **(p. 1065)**

A11. True

This is an important observation indicating that molecular abnormalities occur in non-neoplastic disease and are not per se sufficient to define the neoplasia. **(p. 1065)**

A12. False

The most common form is chronic calcifying pancreatitis (95% of cases). Lymphoplasmacytic sclerosing pancreatitis is an unusual form of chronic pancreatitis that resembles primary sclerosing cholangitis involving the pancreas. **(p. 1065)**

A13. False

It is a very rare form of chronic pancreatitis and may be part of hypereosinophilic syndrome. However, all other causes of eosinophilia need to be excluded, particularly parasitic infections and leukemia. **(p. 1065)**

A14. True

Groove pancreatitis is a rare form of segmental chronic pancreatitis that involves the anatomic space between the head of the pancreas, the duodenum and the common bile duct. In a comparison with non-segmental chronic pancreatitis, no differences were observed in age and sex distribution or in alcohol consumption. Clinically, in contrast, prior diseases of the biliary system, peptic ulcers and gastric resections were more frequently identified in groove pancreatitis. **(p. 1065)**

A15. True

The most common cause of chronic pancreatitis is excessive alcohol consumption, which is associated with chronic calcifying pancreatitis. **(p. 1065)**

A16. True

Furthermore, many of the small ductules dilate, whereas others are obliterated by fibrosis (producing typical alternating stenosis and dilatation). **(p. 1065)**

A17. True

Peripancreatic fibrosis causes stenosis or occlusion of retroperitoneal lymph channels. In 1–2% of patients ascites may complicate chronic calcific pancreatitis as a result of portal hypertension or lymphatic obstruction. **(p. 1065)**

A18. True

These changes are much more focal than those in the other forms, and in most patients the changes involve only the portion of the pancreas in which ductal drainage is impaired. Protein inspissation may occur, but histologic changes in the ductal mucosa are less common and calcification is unusual. **(p. 1065)**

A19. False

A variety of factors are implicated in chronic obstructive pancreatitis; etiology is idiopathic in as many as 40% of cases. Known associations include cholelithiasis in about 20% of patients, ductal obstruction due to ampullary stenosis, inflammatory or neoplastic causes, surgical ductal ligation, and fibrosis due to a pseudocyst as a complication of acute pancreatitis. **(p. 1065)**

A20. False

Most patients are elderly. Chronic inflammatory pancreatitis is a rare disease and includes idiopathic duct-destructive pancreatitis and lymphoplasmacytic pancreatitis. The latter may be associated with an autoimmune etiology (autoimmune pancreatitis). **(p. 1065)**

A21. False

The most common causes in children include trauma followed by cystic fibrosis. **(p. 1065)**

A22. True

Hyperplasia of Brunner's glands is probably an adaptive response to the exocrine insufficiency of the pancreas or the changes in gastric function (hyperacidity, accelerated emptying of the stomach) caused by chronic pancreatitis. It develops in about 75% of patients. **(p. 1066)**

A23. True

In more than half of affected patients, metastatic fat necrosis (distant sites of fat necrosis cause by released lipase) is caused by acinar cell carcinoma of the pancreas. However, in other patients, lipase originates from a pancreas damaged by both acute and chronic pancreatitis. These released enzymes may also cause erythema nodosum-like lesions, polyarthropathy and avascular bone necrosis. **(p. 1067)**

A24. False

Graft survival is about 80–90% at 1 year. About 85% of pancreas transplants are performed with a kidney transplant in diabetic patients. **(p. 1067)**

A25. False

A pancreatic abscess is a collection of pus resulting from tissue necrosis, liquefaction and infection. Infected necrosis refers to bacterial contamination of necrotic pancreatic tissue in the absence of abscess formation. Pancreatic abscess formation is a late complication of acute necrotizing pancreatitis (ANP), occurring more than 4 weeks after the initial attack. The mortality rate associated with pancreatic abscess is generally less than that of infected necrosis. **(p. 1067)**

A26. True

Pseudocysts are associated with pancreatitis, trauma and neoplastic obstruction of large ducts, and are multiple in 15% cases. **(p. 1067)**

A27. True

Most cases are treated by external drainage, but this type of treatment is contraindicated if the pseudocyst communicates with the ductal system. **(p. 1068)**

A28. False

True cysts of the pancreas are lined by non-neoplastic epithelium and are often associated with similar cysts of other viscera, such as the liver or kidney. **(p. 1068)**

A29. False

This multilocular cyst lined by squamous epithelium is a dysembryoplastic lesion, which is not associated with HIV or other infections and is not associated with the clinical syndromes that are seen with their analogues in the salivary glands. Interestingly, it has been documented almost exclusively in males having a mean age of 56 years. **(p. 1068)**

A30. True

At the same time, the pancreatic tail is the most frequent location of most cystic pancreatic neoplasms. **(p. 1068)**

A31. True

However, it is considered to be non-neoplastic, is located in the head of the pancreas, has no sex predilection, is lined by a single layer of cuboidal epithelium, does not recur, and does not undergo neoplastic transformation. This is in contrast to mucinous cystadenoma, which is more common in women, is localized to the body and tail of the pancreas, and is lined by tall columnar epithelium. **(p. 1068)**

A32. True

It constitutes the fourth most common cause of death from cancer in the United States. **(p. 1068)**

A33. False

Although the association between pancreatic carcinoma and peripheral venous thrombosis (so-called migratory thrombophlebitis) is well known, it occurs in only 25% of patients. Other clinical associations include pancreatitis, hypoglycemia, hypercalcemia, endocarditis and diabetes mellitus. **(p. 1069)**

A34. False

Only 10% of cases show familial aggregation. **(p. 1068)**

A35. True

It is also more frequent in patients with familial atypical multiple mole melanoma syndrome, Peutz–Jeghers' syndrome, hereditary non-polyposis colorectal cancer and hereditary pancreatitis. **(p. 1068)**

A36. True

Only one-third originate in the body or tail of the pancreas. **(p. 1069)**

A37. True

In some cases of well-differentiated adenocarcinoma of the pancreas the correct diagnosis can be made only by close attention to cytologic features. **(p. 1069)**

A38. False
As in the prostate, benign epithelial inclusions have been observed around pancreatic nerves. Therefore, other features of malignancy should be looked for to confirm the diagnosis of malignancy. **(p. 1070)**

A39. False
Only about one-third of patients also have carcinoma in situ, and about one-third show papillary hyperplasia of the ducts. **(p. 1070)**

A40. False
It refers to atrophy of the exocrine pancreas due to pancreatic duct obstruction that selectively spares Langerhans' islets, which may or may not be hyperplastic. **(p. 1070)**

A41. False
They produce small intestinal and gastric mucins. **(p. 1071)**

A42. True
For practical purposes, this means that it will always be positive for CK8 (or other low molecular weight cytokeratins such as CAM5.2). Also, it is regularly positive for EMA. **(p. 1071)**

A43. True
However, it is of very limited value. These tumors are typically CK7+ and also CK20+, which is the same as/similar to tumors of the gallbladder and extrahepatic bile ducts. Primary hepatic cholangiocarcinoma is usually negative for CK20. **(p. 1071)**

A44. True
However, it does not help distinguish between the different sites of origin in the pancreaticobiliary group. **(p. 1071)**

A45. True
MUC2 is very rarely expressed in pancreatic ductal carcinoma. It is also negative in ampullary carcinoma of pancreaticobiliary origin and in intrahepatic cholangiocarcinoma. **(p. 1071)**

A46. True
It is inactivated in about 50% of pancreatic ductal adenocarcinomas, but never in benign tissues. **(p. 1071)**

A47. True
A recent study found that it may differentiate between benign/reactive and malignant (invasive adenocarcinoma and adenocarcinoma in situ) lesions of the pancreas. **(p. 1071)**

A48. True
However, it is quite nonspecific and is also present in cancers of the liver, lung, breast, uterus and ovary (mucinous). **(p. 1071)**

A49. True
Also frequent are amplification of Her2/*neu* and inactivation of *DPC4* and p16. **(p. 1071)**

A50. False
Only about one-fifth of cases are MSI+. These tumors usually have K-*ras* wildtype genes (in contrast to usual pancreatic ductal adenocarcinoma) and are associated with inherited susceptibility for cancer in first-degree relatives. A minority of these are associated with EBV infection, and these cases are accompanied by an intense lymphoid infiltration (as in lymphoepithelial carcinomas of other sites). **(p. 1072)**

A51. False
Relatively frequent are structural rearrangements with loss of the genes located on 1p, 3p, 6p, 8p and 17p. **(p. 1071)**

A52. True
However, the preferred terminology for this distinct histologic variant is 'adenosquamous carcinoma.' Pure squamous cell carcinoma of the pancreas probably represents one end of the spectrum of adenosquamous carcinoma. **(p. 1072)**

A53. False
Mucinous (colloid) carcinoma is associated with a significantly better prognosis than ordinary ductal adenocarcinoma. It may cause pseudomyxoma peritonei and is not related to mucinous cystadenocarcinoma. **(p. 1072)**

A54. False
The earliest metastases are present in regional lymph nodes. However, the most common sites of distant metastases are liver, peritoneum, lung, adrenal, bone and other. Curiously, lymph node metastases in the supraclavicular region may be the first manifestation of pancreatic carcinoma. **(p. 1072)**

A55. False
The overall sensitivity is only 66%. The most sensitive methods are CT-guided percutaneous fine needle aspiration and intraoperative fine needle aspiration, which have a sensitivity of >90%. **(p. 1072)**

A56. False
These tumors may have a sarcomatoid appearance and frequently fail to express epithelial markers, which are usually found in the obvious epithelial component. Therefore, it may not always be possible to rule out primary sarcoma of the pancreas on the small biopsy specimen. **(p. 1074)**

A57. False
Two populations characterize this tumor: smaller tumor cells, which may be spindled or rounded, and giant cells of the osteoclast type (both morphologically and immunohistochemically). These tumors have a better prognosis than anaplastic carcinoma. **(p. 1074)**

A58. True
The cut surface may show a central scar and the lesion is usually solitary. **(p. 1075)**

A59. False
The optically clear cuboidal epithelium contains glycogen, not mucin. Therefore, the luminal content will not show positivity for CEA. **(p. 1076)**

A60. True
Ultrastructural studies show features of normal centroacinar cells. **(p. 1075)**

A61. True
Some cases are part of von Hippel–Lindau disease and sporadic cases show allelic deletions and mutation of the von Hippel–Lindau tumor suppressor gene. **(p. 1076)**

A62. False
Solid serous adenoma is a solid variant of benign microcystic cystadenoma. Microcystic adenocarcinoma is a biologically malignant tumor that often shows nuclear atypia, but which is otherwise morphologically very similar to microcystic cystadenoma. **(p. 1076)**

A63. False
Mucinous cystic tumors typically occur in younger patients than microcystic cystadenoma, and more often in women than in men, whereas in microcystic cystadenoma there is no sex predilection. **(p. 1076)**

A64. False
Mucinous cystic neoplasms occur most often in the body and the tail of the pancreas. In contrast, colloid carcinoma and mucinous non-neoplastic cysts are most often found in the head of the pancreas. **(p. 1077)**

A65. True
The resemblance is both morphological and immunohistochemical (the stromal cells show expression of estrogen and progesterone receptors and inhibin). This type of stroma recapitulates fetal pancreatic mesenchyme around ducts. **(p. 1077)**

A66. True
The mucin produced by these cells, similar to pancreatic ductal adenocarcinoma and intraductal papillary mucinous neoplasms, shows positivity for MUC5AC. **(p. 1078)**

A67. True
However, some recent reports have not confirmed these findings. **(p. 1078)**

A68. True
MUC1 expression was found only in the invasive component of these tumors. Similarly, p53 overexpression is seen only in advanced, aggressive lesions. **(p. 1078)**

A69. True
However, MUC2 is found only in goblet cells and not in columnar cells. Goblet cells are found to be more numerous in borderline and frankly malignant lesions than in clearly benign cystadenoma. **(p. 1078)**

A70. False
These tumors are classified based on the degree of cytologic atypia and the degree of architectural complexity as benign, borderline or malignant. **(p. 1077)**

A71. True
Extensive sampling is needed so as not to miss small nodules with invasive carcinoma. **(p. 1078)**

A72. True
This disease is characterized by the production of excess mucus, which can be seen oozing from the ampulla of Vater, and dilatation of the pancreatic ducts. **(p. 1078)**

A73. False
About 30% of cases are associated with adenocarcinoma, and these are usually of the colloid type. **(p. 1078)**

A74. True
Based on the differentiation of the papillae, this entity is classified into intestinal type (MUC1–, MUC2+), pancreaticobiliary type (MUC1+, MUC2–/focal), and oncocytic type (MUC1+, MUC2+). **(p. 1078)**

A75. True
Similarly, pancreaticobiliary-type IPMN may be associated with usual ductal adenocarcinoma. **(p. 1078)**

A76. True
Most of these are premalignant lesions (except for PanIN-1A). Lesions of the larger ducts belong to the IPMN spectrum. **(p. 1078)**

A77. True
The presence of numerous inflammatory cells, particular polymorphonuclear leukocytes, should raise the possibility of reactive changes. **(p. 1079)**

A78. True
Normal pancreatic ductal epithelium is negative for MUC1. **(p. 1079)**

A79. True
PanIN 3 represents carcinoma in situ. **(p. 1079)**

A80. True
Mucinous cystic neoplasms should also be considered, but these are usually much larger and have no connection to the duct system. **(p. 1079)**

A81. True
They are paler in color and somewhat smaller than the surrounding acinar cells. These foci may represent precursors of acinar cell carcinoma. **(p. 1080)**

A82. False
It is not clear whether 'acinar cell adenoma' represents a distinct entity. Most cases in adults were misdiagnosed well-differentiated acinar cell carcinomas and, in children, pancreatoblastomas. **(p. 1080)**

A83. True
However, the great majority of cases occur in adults. **(p. 1080)**

A84. True
In some cases the same presentation is found in patients with acute or chronic pancreatitis. **(p. 1080)**

A85. False
The great majority of the tumors form a well-circumscribed mass and only exceptionally may they grow intraductally. **(p. 1080)**

A86. True
This pattern of growth is referred to as 'normal acinar.' Other patterns include solid, trabecular and glandular. **(p. 1080)**

A87. True
In the solid variant the cytoplasm may be scant. Immunohistochemically, the cytoplasm shows reactivity for trypsin, lipase, and less often for chymotrypsin and amylase. **(p. 1080)**

A88. False
Acinar cell carcinomas show a high frequency of allelic loss of 11p and mutations in the APC/β catenin pathway, which is similar to pancreatoblastoma and distinct from pancreatic ductal adenocarcinoma. **(p. 1080)**

A89. True
However, one-third of usual acinar cell tumors also show scattered neuroendocrine cells or small groups of neuroendocrine cells mimicking islets, which is best demonstrated by chromogranin immunostaining. Also noteworthy is the fact that some mixed tumors may show a component with ductal differentiation. **(p. 1081)**

A90. False
These tumors usually have a microcystic appearance and no mucin production, and therefore mimic microcystic adenoma. **(p. 1081)**

A91. True
In contrast to its non-aggressive biology, the gross appearance of this lesion may be ominous. It is usually a large, encapsulated tumor, and cross-sections often contain areas of hemorrhage and necrosis. **(p. 1082)**

A92. True
CD10 and progesterone receptor are typically expressed by solid-pseudopapillary tumors, but neuroendocrine markers are less helpful because of the frequent neuroendocrine differentiation (which, however, is usually focal rather than diffuse). The finding of hyaline globules that are PAS+ (for α_1-antitrypsin) is very helpful. **(p. 1082)**

A93. True
However, it has also been described in adults. There is no sex predilection. **(p. 1083)**

A94. False
Pancreatoblastoma has been associated with Beckwith–Wiedemann syndrome and familial adenomatous polyposis. **(p. 1083)**

A95. False
Pancreatoblastoma characteristically has a bimodal age distribution, with peaks at 2.4 and 33 years. **(p. 1083)**

A96. True
Most characteristically these tumors show 'squamoid corpuscules,' which contain cells with optically clear nuclei (due to their biotin content). **(p. 1083)**

A97. True
In addition, pancreatoblastoma shows immunoreactivity for acinar, endocrine and duct differentiation markers. **(p. 1083)**

A98. False
Almost half of children are cured by resection, whereas only one-quarter of adult patients survive. **(p. 1083)**

A99. False
Pancreatic endocrine neoplasms are most frequent in the body and tail of the pancreas, corresponding with a greater concentration of islets in these areas. **(p. 1083)**

A100. True
This should not be confused with solid-pseudopapillary tumor with partial endocrine differentiation, or with mucinous cystic neoplasm, in which neuroendocrine tumors may rarely arise. **(p. 1084)**

A101. False
A solid pattern of growth may be associated with any cell type. However, predominantly gyriform tumors are often of β- or α-cell type, whereas glandular tumors are often of G (gastrin)- or VIP-cell type. **(p. 1084)**

A102. False
Amyloid is most commonly found in insulin-secreting tumors. **(p. 1084)**

A103. True
Owing to their high vascularity neuroendocrine pancreatic tumors with clear cell change may mimic renal cell carcinoma. **(p. 1084)**

A104. True
Usually the age of presentation is 50–60 years. In MEN I patients these tumors are associated with nesidioblastosis in 30% of cases. **(p. 1085)**

A105. False
Most tumors are functional and secrete multiple hormones. **(p. 1084)**

A106. False
Non-syndromic tumors may also be functional. **(p. 1084)**

A107. False

There are no definitional criteria for high-grade pancreatic neuroendocrine tumors. High-grade neuroendocrine tumors are classified as small cell carcinomas and comprise less than 5% of pancreatic neuroendocrine tumors. These may produce ACTH and are associated with hypercalcemia. According to some authors, in general other pancreatic neuroendocrine tumors may be graded based on tumor size, mitotic index, Ki-67 index, angioinvasion, and the presence or absence of hormonal syndrome. **(p. 1090)**

A108. True

This can also be demonstrated by immunohistochemical staining of the tumor. **(p. 1090)**

A109. True

Therefore, cytokeratins, chromogranin, NSE, synaptophysin, neurofilaments, CD57 and other markers are usually positive. The tumors will also show immunoreactivity for their secretory product(s) (insulin, glucagon, somatostatin, pancreatic polypeptide, gastrin and vasoactive intestinal polypeptide). **(p. 1085)**

A110. False

Loss of heterozygosity at the *MEN I* gene locus at 11q13 has been found in about half of the sporadic endocrine neoplasms of foregut derivation, including pancreatic tumors, but not those of midgut or hindgut origin. 6q loss is associated with malignant insulinoma. **(p. 1085)**

A111. False

Only a small minority of patients with insulinoma have MEN I. **(p. 1085)**

A112. True

These are also characteristically small tumors and generally measure less than 1.5 cm. **(p. 1085)**

A113. False

Insulinomas characteristically show less expression of chromogranin than do other pancreatic neuroendocrine tumors. Also, their staining for insulin is less intense than that of normal β cells in the islets and only half of cases show reactivity for proinsulin. **(p. 1088)**

A114. False

Only up to 10% of insulinomas are malignant. **(p. 1088)**

A115. True

These tumors appear to secrete insulin-like growth factor II. **(p. 1088)**

A116. True

In contrast, non-syndromic glucagonomas are usually small, multiple, and nearly always benign. Interestingly, these non-syndromic small tumors show stronger immunoreactivity for glucagon than syndromic large tumors. **(p. 1088)**

A117. True

The symptoms are: normochromic normocytic anemia, abnormal glucose tolerance test, necrolitic migratory erythema, sore red tongue, angular stomatitis, severe weight loss, depression, DVT, and decreased immunity with overwhelming infections. **(p. 1088)**

A118. True

The tumors are most often present in the pancreas, followed by the duodenal wall and stomach. **(p. 1089)**

A119. False

These solitary tumors are often clinically malignant, whereas in contrast those arising in MEN I syndrome are usually located in the duodenum, multicentric, and less likely to be malignant. **(p. 1089)**

A120. True

However, Zollinger–Ellison syndrome, in addition to numerous peptic ulcers, is also frequently associated with diarrhea. **(p. 1089)**

A121. True

They are indistinguishable morphologically, histochemically and ultrastructurally. However, immunohistochemically these tumors show no expression of gastrin, but demonstrate immunoreactivity for vasoactive intestinal peptide (VIP), and often PP, calcitonin, and the α chain of hCG. **(p. 1089)**

A122. True

Somatostatin is an inhibitory hormone and therefore does not cause many symptoms. However, somatostatinoma syndrome is found in some patients and consists of diabetes, cholecystolithiasis, steatorrhea, indigestion, hypochlorhydria, and occasionally anemia. **(p. 1090)**

A123. False

Psammoma bodies are found in δ-cell tumors (somatostatinomas). **(p. 1090)**

A124. False

A secondary and minor component of PP cells is found in a high proportion of pancreatic neuroendocrine tumors. However, neoplasms composed predominately of PP-secreting cells are indeed rare. **(p. 1090)**

A125. False

Carcinoid tumors of the pancreas are rare and they arise from Kulchitsky's cells (serotonin-producing). **(p. 1090)**

A126. True

PNET has been described in the pancreas. **(p. 1091)**

A127. True

WHO proposed a classification in which 'well-differentiated endocrine tumors,' which are not clearly malignant, are further subdivided into 1) those that may have either benign behavior or uncertain behavior based on the presence of vascular invasion or proliferation rate; and 2) 'well-differentiated neuroendocrine carcinomas' (any with gross local invasion or metastases). The third group is that of small cell carcinoma. **(p. 1090)**

A128. True

Therefore, the main clinical manifestations are hyperparathyroidism, Zollinger–Ellison syndrome, and acromegaly or hypopituitarism. **(p. 1090)**

A129. True

Less common clinical manifestations include lipomas, multiple leiomyomas, nodular hyperplasia of the adrenal gland, and thyroid adenomas. **(p. 1091)**

A130. True

MEN II is caused by germline mutation of the *RET* proto-oncogene (which is also known as the *MEN II* gene). **(p. 1091)**

A131. False

MEN II has three distinct subtypes: MEN IIA, MEN IIB and familial medullary thyroid carcinoma-only (FMTC-only). **(p. 1091)**

A132. False

It is defined by the development of medullary thyroid carcinoma in at least four family members. **(p. 1091)**

A133. True

Also, MEN IIA patients do not have the phenotypic abnormalities of mucosal neuromas and marfanoid habitus found in MEN IIB patients. **(p. 1091)**

A134. True

Similarly, the pheochromocytomas of MEN IIA patients are nearly always benign. **(p. 1091)**

A135. True

However, primary lymphomas, including NK cell tumors, post-transplant lymphoproliferative disease and lymphoblastic lymphoma, have been described. **(p. 1091)**

A136. False

These tumors are very rare in the pancreas and may be equally rare or even more so than similar tumors in the salivary glands. Hemangioma, lymphangioma, solitary fibrous tumor, schwannoma and 'sugar' tumor have been described, among others. **(p. 1091)**

A137. False

It is possible that some anaplastic carcinomas were misdiagnosed as sarcomas, as some of these tumors do not show clear expression of cytokeratin or EMA in sarcomatous areas. **(p. 1091)**

A138. True

Often the tumor involves the pancreas by direct local spread rather than by distant metastases. **(p. 1091)**

A139. False

This image illustrates chronic pancreatitis with pseudoneoplastic proliferation of pancreatic endocrine cells, which should not be mistaken for invasive adenocarcinoma. The lack of significant cytologic atypia suggests the benign nature of the process. **(p. 1067)**

A140. False

Most of the time, perineural epithelial cells represent malignant tumor invading the perineural space. However, perineural extension of pancreatic endocrine cells has been described in chronic pancreatitis associated with extensive fibrosis. **(p. 1067)**

A141. True

If the biopsy shows only sarcoma-like areas one should still consider the diagnosis of sarcomatoid carcinoma as these tumors are far more frequent than true primary sarcomas of the pancreas. **(p. 1074)**

A142. False

This image illustrates a typical appearance of microcystic adenoma, which is not a mucinous lesion. **(p. 1075)**

A143. False

Marked cytologic atypia is not compatible with the diagnosis of mucinous cystic adenoma. This image illustrates papillary adenocarcinoma of the pancreas. **(p. 1079)**

A144. True

This image illustrates how, in a small biopsy, diagnosing acinar cell carcinoma may be a very difficult task. **(p. 1081)**

A145. True

However, it should not be forgotten that pancreatoblastoma, which is illustrated here, also frequently shows neuroendocrine differentiation. **(p. 1083)**

Ampullary region

A1. **False**

Ampullary carcinoma implies an origin from the intestinal-type mucosa of the ampullary region, often in a pre-existing villous adenoma of villoglandular polyp. It accounts for 5% of all GI malignancies. **(p. 1092)**

A2. **True**

This is frequently the case in advanced tumors. **(p. 1092)**

A3. **True**

However, some tumors have a mixed pattern, being both intra- and periampullary. **(p. 1092)**

A4. **True**

An association with adenomatous polyposis coli and neurofibromatosis has also been described. **(p. 1093)**

A5. **False**

Signet ring carcinoma is an uncommon histologic type in this region, but when present it is associated with poor prognosis. **(p. 1093)**

A6. **False**

These tumors often overexpress p53, but K-*ras* mutations and inactivation of the *DPC4* gene are uncommon. **(p. 1093)**

A7. **True**

Peak age is in the 70s, with men affected more often than women. **(p. 1092)**

A8. **False**

The 5-year survival rate after resection is 40–50%, and 80% if there are no nodal metastases; this is better than in pancreatic or bile duct carcinoma (with a 5-year survival rate of 10–20%). **(p. 1095)**

A9. **True**

Well-differentiated tumors have >95% glands, moderately differentiated have 50–95%, poorly differentiated have 5–49%, and undifferentiated tumors <5%. **(p. 1093)**

A10. **True**

However, the following criteria were found to be the most helpful: nuclear size variation of at least 4:1 between ductal epithelial cells, incomplete ductal lumina, and disorganized duct distribution. **(p. 1094)**

A11. **False**

MUC2+, CDX2+, DPC4+, MUC1–, MUC5AC–, CD17–, CK7–, and CK20– all distinguish this tumor from pancreatic ductal adenocarcinoma, which is MUC2–, CDX2–, DPC4– (50% cases), MUC1+, MUC5AC+, frequently CD17+, CK7+ and CK20+. **(p. 1093)**

A12. **True**

These lesions are best treated by local resection. **(p. 1095)**

A13. **False**

It is, in fact, more malignant than primary duodenal carcinoid. Somatostatin-producing tumors are common, have a glandular pattern (can be mucin positive), and are associated with psammoma bodies and neurofibromatosis; 50–70% of cases have nodal metastases. **(p. 1095)**

A14. **True**

However, this lesion should not be mistaken for well-differentiated papillary adenocarcinoma, the lesion with much greater cytologic atypia and, frequently, highly stratified lining. **(p. 1093)**

16 Adrenal gland and other paraganglia

Normal anatomy

Q1

The paraganglion system consists of the extra-adrenal paraganglia and the adrenal cortex.

Q2

The adrenal cortex secretes steroid hormones known as corticosteroids.

Q3

The adrenal cortex consists of three layers: glomerulosa, fasciculata and reticularis.

Q4

The zona glomerulosa secretes aldosterone, the zona fasciculata glucocorticoid, and the zona reticularis sex hormones.

Q5

'Spongiocytes' or 'clear cells' are characteristic of the zona reticularis.

Q6

The pheochromocyte is the predominant cell of the adrenal medulla.

Q7

The 'chief cells' of the paraganglion system are characterized by the presence of numerous cytoplasmic neurosecretory granules containing catecholamines.

Q8

Extra-adrenal paraganglia related to the orthosympathetic system are chromaffin and predominate in the retroperitoneum along the thoracolumbar para-aortic region.

Biopsy and cytology

Q1

Because of its low sensitivity (high false-negative rate), fine needle aspiration cytology is not recommended for the evaluation of tumor masses of the adrenal glands.

Lesions of adrenal cortex

Q1

Heterotopic (accessory) adrenal tissue can undergo marked hyperplasia and cause malignant hypertension.

Q2

Adrenal cortical heterotopia is most frequently located in the kidney.

Q3

The size and the number of 'micronodules' of the adrenal cortex is not associated with hypertension, diabetes and cardiovascular disease.

QUESTIONS

Q4

Congenital hyperplasia of the adrenal cortex is responsible for the large majority of cases of adrenogenital syndrome developing within the first year of life.

Q5

Adrenocortical congenital hyperplasia is an X-linked disorder and therefore occurs only in male children.

Q6

In congenital adrenocortical hyperplasia the basic defect is often an absence of the enzyme 21-hydroxylase, which results in an accumulation of 17OH-progesterone and its catabolite pregnanetriol and a deficiency of cortisol.

Q7

In all cases, the clinical picture of congenital adrenocortical hyperplasia is characterized by pure virilizing syndrome.

Q8

The pathologic change is the same in all types of congenital adrenocortical hyperplasia.

Q9

Acquired adrenocortical hyperplasia may be ACTH dependent or ACTH independent.

Q10

Carney's syndrome or complex consists of primary pigmented nodular adrenal cortical hyperplasia, Cushing's disease, spotty cutaneous pigmentation, cutaneous and cardiac myxoma, growth hormone-secreting pituitary adenomas, and psammomatous melanotic schwannomas.

Q11

Most adrenocortical tumors arise in children.

Q12

Very large tumors of the adrenal gland (palpable tumors) are malignant in practically every instance.

Q13

Grossly, adrenocortical adenomas are usually solitary encapsulated nodules, whereas nodular hyperplasia consists of numerous non-encapsulated nodules.

Q14

The most characteristic microscopic feature of adrenocortical adenoma is that mitoses are exceptionally rare or absent.

Q15

Hemorrhage is not a feature of adrenocortical adenoma.

Q16

Most 'black adrenocortical adenomas' are associated with primary aldosteronism.

Q17

Corticomedullary mixed tumor has features of adrenocortical and medullary differentiation.

Q18

Adrenocortical adenomas may be non-functional or functional and associated with diverse clinical syndromes.

Q19

Lipadenoma simply designates the presence of mature adipose tissue in the adrenocortical adenoma.

Q20

Sarcomatoid carcinoma and adenosquamous carcinomas have not been described as primary tumors, but they often metastasize to the adrenal gland.

Q21

Most adrenocortical tumors with oncocytic differentiation are malignant.

Q22

Myxoid features in an adrenocortical tumor strongly suggest malignancy.

Q23

Adrenocortical tumors are typically negative for EMA.

Q24

Adrenocortical tumors strongly express neural/neuroendocrine markers, including synaptophysin, neurofilaments, NSE and chromogranin.

Q25

Adrenocortical lesions under 100 g are generally cured by excision.

Q26

As in the colon, hyperplasia of the adrenal gland is associated with *ras* mutations.

QUESTIONS

Q27

In adrenocortical lesions, mitotic activity and venous invasion correlate best with recurrence or metastasis.

Q28

An adrenocortical tumor strongly positive for vimentin and only weakly positive or negative for low molecular weight cytokeratin (LMWCK) is likely to be a carcinoma.

Q29

The presence of aneuploidy strongly favors malignancy over a benign adrenocortical tumor.

Q30

Adrenocortical carcinoma can be distinguished from renal cell carcinoma immunohistochemically.

Q31

Histochemically, the identification of PAS-positive glycogen in tumor cells favors the diagnosis of renal cell carcinoma over adrenocortical carcinoma.

Q32

Chromogranin and low molecular weight cytokeratin (LMWCK) are most useful in distinguishing adrenocortical tumors from adrenomedullary tumors.

Q33

Metastases are present at the time of diagnosis in the great majority of adrenocortical carcinomas.

Q34

Regional lymph nodes are the most common site of metastatic involvement by adrenocortical carcinoma.

Q35

The prognosis of adrenocortical carcinoma is poor and the overall 5-year survival is only 60%.

Q36

Deficiency of the enzyme 11β-hydroxylase is a characteristic feature of adrenocortical carcinoma.

Q37

Conn's syndrome (primary aldosteronism) is usually caused by adrenocortical adenoma (70% of cases).

Q38

Conn's syndrome is characterized by hyperkalemia, hypertension and muscle weakness.

Q39

In Conn's syndrome the adenoma is typically unilateral, solitary (91%) and small.

Q40

Aldosterone-producing adenomas characteristically have a homogeneous golden-yellow cut surface.

Q41

Microscopically, aldosterone-producing adenomas most often have the appearance of zona glomerulosa.

Q42

In functional adrenocortical adenomas the surrounding adrenal cortex is usually atrophied, whereas in non-functional tumors the surrounding cortex is normal.

Q43

'Spironolactone bodies' are immunoreactive for aldosterone.

Q44

In contrast to Conn's syndrome, which is often caused by an adenoma, Cushing's syndrome is most frequently caused by adrenocortical hyperplasia.

Q45

Cushing's disease may be caused by either diffuse or nodular adrenocortical hyperplasia.

Q46

Cushing's syndrome may be part of Carney's syndrome.

Q47

Medullary carcinoma of the thyroid may cause Cushing's syndrome.

Q48

In contrast to secondary causes of Cushing's syndrome, primary adrenal lesions are characterized by more frequent hypokalemic alkalosis, very high urinary excretion of free cortisol, skin pigmentation, edema, and severe diabetes mellitus.

Q49

Excess androgens secreted by an adrenal lesion cause adult masculinity in male and female children, and in adult females.

Q50

Virilization of adrenal origin in adult females is usually the result of testosterone secretion by a tumor.

Q51

In adult females the probability that a virilizing adrenal cortical tumor is malignant is higher if the virilization is accompanied by Cushing's syndrome.

Q52

The most common cause of virilization in children is adrenocortical carcinoma.

Q53

Polycythemia can be caused by an adrenal cortical lesion (particularly carcinoma).

Q54

The finding of nuclear pleomorphism (left) in adrenocortical hyperplasia suggests focal malignant transformation.

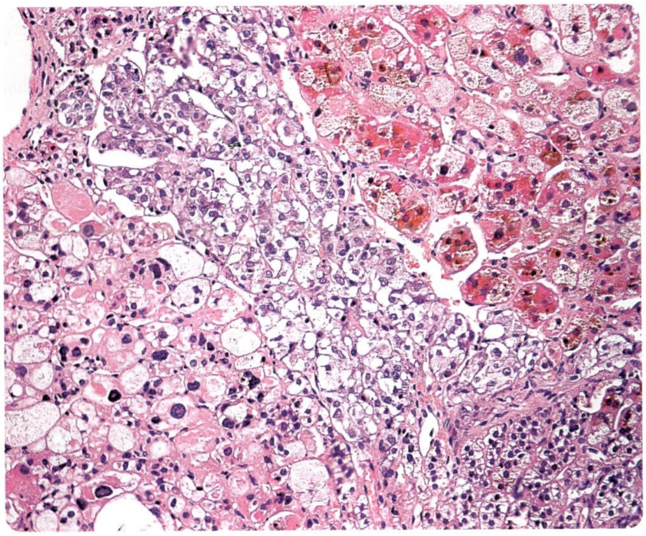

Fig. 16.1

Q55

The lesion of the adrenal cortex shown here is most likely malignant because it is large and shows areas of necrosis and hemorrhage.

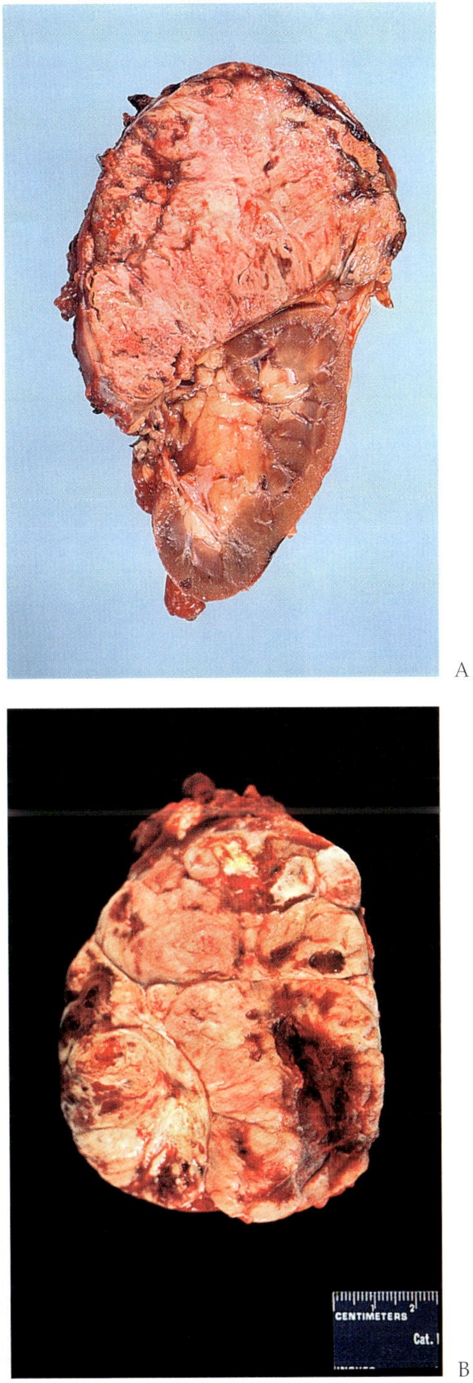

Fig. 16.2

Q56

Adrenal cortical adenoma as shown in this figure is histologically difficult to differentiate from adrenal cortical hyperplasia, or even from normal adrenal cortex.

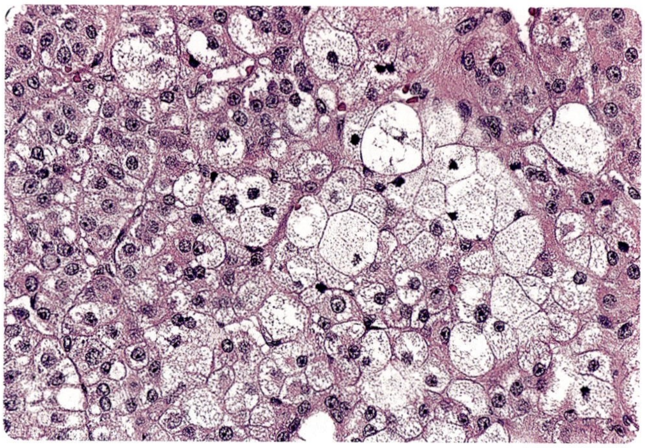

Fig. 16.3

Lesions of adrenal medulla

Q1

Generally speaking, all tumors and tumor-like conditions of the adrenal medulla arise from the embryonal neural line (sympathetic system).

Q2

Neuroblastoma, a tumor of the embryonal neural line, is very similar to another childhood tumor known as primitive neuroectodermal tumor (PNET) (also known as peripheral neuroblastoma).

Q3

Poorly differentiated tumors of embryonal neurons are more likely to arise in the adrenal medulla or close to the adrenal gland.

Q4

Neuroblastoma is an uncommon tumor of young children, with 80% of cases diagnosed by 4 years of age.

Q5

Neuroblastoma can be associated with neurofibromatosis.

Q6

Grossly, neuroblastomas are very similar to other malignant tumors of the adrenal gland; they are large, soft and gray, have areas of necrosis and hemorrhage, and may show cystic degeneration.

Q7

Neuroblastomas are frequently multifocal.

Q8

Homer Wright rosettes are commonly found in neuroblastoma and provide a diagnostic clue in most cases.

Q9

Homer Wright rosettes characteristically do not have central lumina but contain collections of neurites, which have a fibrillary appearance.

Q10

Generally speaking, neuroblastoma belongs to a group of 'small round blue cell tumors' and immunohistochemistry is very useful in the diagnostic work-up of this group of tumors.

Q11

Neuroblastoma causes an elevation in serum catecholamines.

Q12

High TRK-A expression in neuroblastoma correlates with favorable clinical stage, age <1 year, absence of 1p allelic loss, is more frequent in hyperdiploid or near-triploid tumors, and is inversely related to N-*myc* amplification.

Q13

In neuroblastoma, the most frequent site of distant metastases is the lung.

Q14

During the last two decades modern chemotherapy has significantly improved survival in neuroblastoma, and today the overall 3-year survival is about 60%.

Q15

Stage IV-S (S for *special*) have better survival than other stage IV patients despite radiologic evidence of bone metastases.

Q16

Microscopic grading of neuroblastoma is associated with the outcome.

Q17

The latest classification of neuroblastoma was issued in 1999 by the International Neuroblastoma Pathology Committee.

Q18

According to the International Neuroblastoma Pathology Committee classification, all 'neuroblastomas' are schwannian stroma poor and are further subtyped into undifferentiated (no ganglionic differentiation), poorly differentiated (<5% ganglion cells) and differentiating (>5% ganglion cells) neuroblastomas.

Q19

Cytogenetic analysis is not useful in neuroblastoma.

Q20

Ganglioneuroblastoma, like neuroblastoma, is most often located in the adrenal medulla.

Q21

Ganglioneuroblastoma has a heterogeneous appearance both microscopically and macroscopically.

Q22

There are two types of ganglioneuroblastoma: 'intermixed' and 'nodular.'

Q23

It is possible to use immunohistochemistry to determine the presence and the extent of differentiation in ganglioneuroblastoma.

Q24

Ganglioneuroblastomas have a better prognosis than neuroblastomas.

Q25

Ganglioneuromas are all benign tumors.

Q26

Ganglioneuromas are most frequently found in the posterior mediastinum and retroperitoneum.

Q27

Macroscopically, ganglioneuromas have the typical appearance of benign tumors: they are encapsulated and firm, with a homogeneous grayish-white cut surface.

Q28

Catecholamine synthesis is an almost constant feature of all ganglioneuromas, and leads to hypertension.

Q29

Primary malignant melanocytic tumors of the cervical, posterior mediastinal and lumbar sympathetic ganglia are malignant melanomas arising in the ganglia.

Q30

Hyperplasia of the adrenal medulla can be nodular or diffuse, unilateral or bilateral, and produces symptoms similar to pheochromocytoma.

Q31

Adrenal medullary hyperplasia is a precursor of both benign and malignant pheochromocytoma.

Q32

As in neuroblastoma, adrenal medullary hyperplasia has been reported associated with neurofibromatosis and Beckwith–Wiedemann syndrome.

Q33

Pheochromocytoma is a paraganglioma.

Q34

The term 'extra-adrenal pheochromocytoma' has been traditionally used for extra-adrenal paragangliomas connected to the parasympathetic system.

Q35

Pheochromocytoma, like neuroblastoma, is bilateral in 10% of cases and can be associated with neurofibromatosis.

Q36

In children, pheochromocytomas are more likely to be malignant.

Q37

Both pheochromocytomas and extra-adrenal paragangliomas secrete epinephrine.

Q38

Pheochromocytoma can be associated with renal artery stenosis, and this may affect the regulation of hypertension following excision of the pheochromocytoma.

Q39

The cardinal symptom of pheochromocytoma is hypertension, as a result of excessive catecholamine secretion.

Q40

Because hypertension is a very common disease, the clinical symptoms of pheochromocytoma are nonspecific and are not helpful in diagnosing this tumor.

Q41

Selective arteriography is the method of choice to detect pheochromocytoma because of the high vascularization of this tumor.

Q42

Pheochromocytomas are generally small tumors and are detected early because they are usually functional and produce a striking clinical presentation.

Q43

The microscopic appearance of pheochromocytoma is similar to that of neuroendocrine tumors.

Q44

Compared to their benign counterpart, malignant pheochromocytomas are usually larger, have more necrosis, and are composed of smaller cells.

Q45

An oncocytic variant of pheochromocytoma has been described.

Q46

Pheochromocytoma is a tumor of pheochromocytes and ganglion cells are not part of its make-up.

Q47

Pheochromocytoma can be associated with von Hippel–Lindau disease (the VHL gene is located on 3p; patients develop retinal and cerebellar hemangioblastomas, visceral cysts and renal cell carcinoma).

Q48

Paragangliomas do not express cytokeratin.

Q49

Detection of S-100 protein is important for the diagnosis of paraganglioma, including pheochromocytoma.

Q50

Pheochromocytoma can cause Cushing's syndrome.

Q51

No recurrent genetic changes have been detected in pheochromocytoma.

Q52

Malignant pheochromocytomas have a peculiar tendency to metastasize to the ribs and spine.

Q53

Tetraploid and aneuploid DNA content is associated with aggressive pheochromocytomas.

Q54

The presence of neoplastic rosettes, as shown here, helps in the histological diagnosis of neuroblastoma.

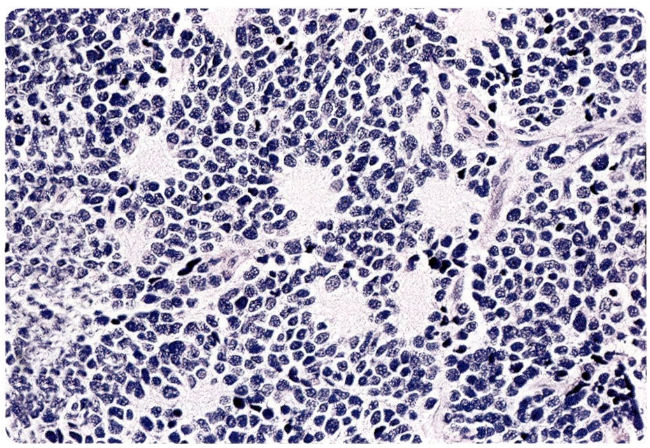

Fig. 16.4

Q55

This image shows ganglioneuroma, which, in contrast to neuroblastoma, is characterized by the presence of large ganglion cells rich in eosinophilic cytoplasm.

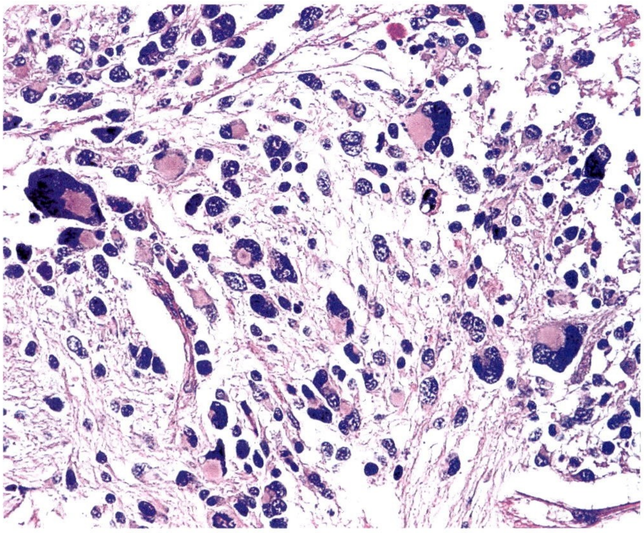

Fig. 16.5

Q56

A variegated cut surface with soft nodules and firm whitish bands is characteristic of a ganglioneuroblastoma.

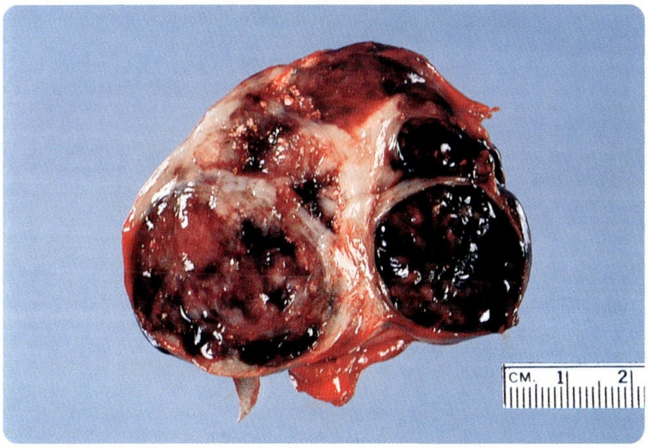

Fig. 16.6

Q57

Owing to the characteristic histological appearance ('Zellballen' structures), pheochromocytoma is usually diagnosed on the biopsy material.

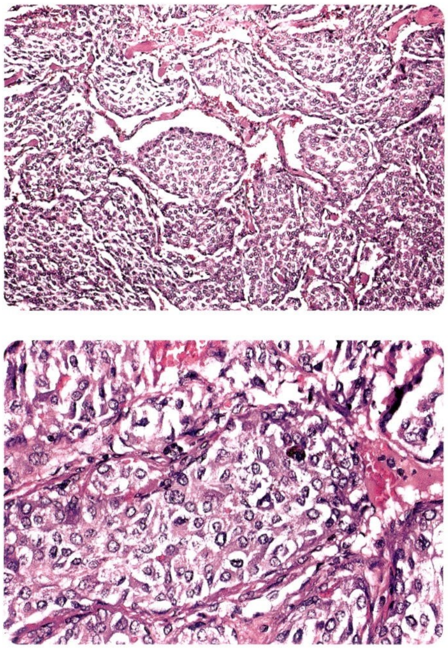

A

B

Fig. 16.7

Other adrenal lesions

Q1

Massive adrenal hemorrhage can present as a retroperitoneal mass and should be considered in the differential diagnosis of renal cell carcinoma.

Q2

Septicemia may cause massive adrenal hemorrhage.

QUESTIONS

Q3

It is clinically important to distinguish massive adrenal hemorrhage from hemorrhagic cysts of the adrenal gland.

Q4

Adrenal pseudocyst should be distinguished from bronchogenic cysts.

Q5

Adrenal cytomegaly refers to the cytopathic effects of cytomegalovirus (CMV).

Q6

Leydig cells can be found in the adrenal gland.

Q7

Tuberculosis is one of the classic causes of Addison's disease.

Q8

Myelolipoma of the adrenal glands is frequently bilateral and symptomatic.

Q9

Myelolipomas are clinically silent and are of little clinical significance.

Q10

Myelolipoma may be associated with Cushing's syndrome.

Q11

Mesenchymal tumors do not occur in the adrenal gland.

Q12

Tumors of the adrenal gland with melanin production are not melanomas, but rather adrenocortical or adrenomedullary tumors with pigment production.

Q13

This figure shows a black adenoma of the adrenal cortex.

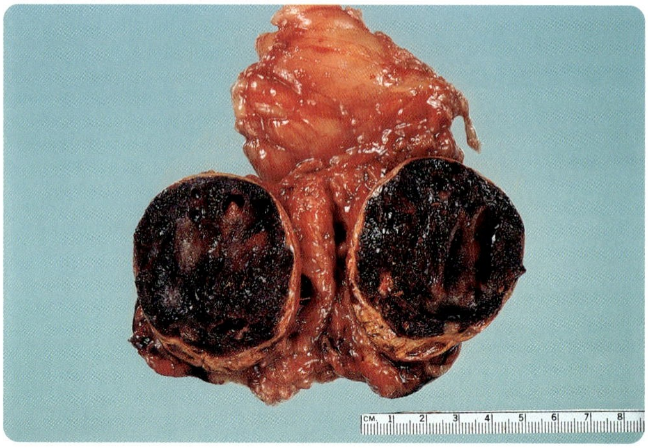

Fig. 16.8

Q14

Large tumor size, areas of hemorrhage and a variegated cut surface all favor the diagnosis of malignant adrenocortical tumor.

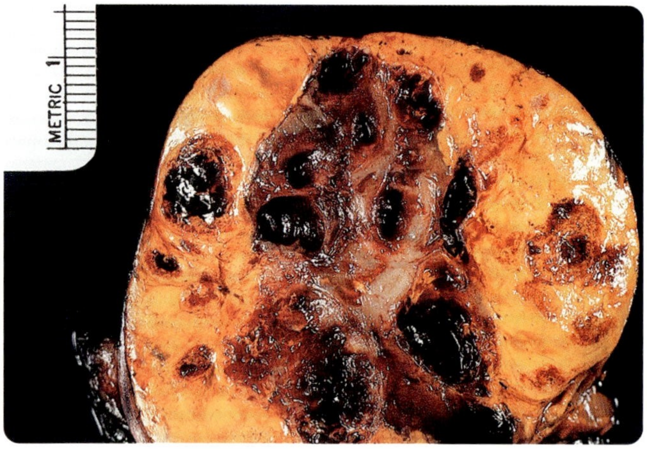

Fig. 16.9

Tumors and tumor-like lesions of other paraganglia

Q1

The term 'chemodectoma' can be properly applied only to carotid and aortic body paragangliomas.

Q2

Carotid body tumors and other paragangliomas of the head and neck region are 10 times more common in people living at high altitudes.

Q3

'Paragangliomatosis' is associated with von Hippel–Lindau disease.

Q4

The 'Carney triad' or 'Carney's syndrome' is a disease of young males.

Q5

The 'Carney triad' can be accompanied by adrenocortical tumors and is inherited in an autosomal dominant fashion.

Q6

Vascular invasion is a sign of malignancy in paraganglioma.

Q7

As in pheochromocytoma, about 10% of extra-adrenal paragangliomas are malignant.

Q8

Zuckerkandl's body paragangliomas are the most common extra-adrenal paragangliomas.

Q9

Carotid body hyperplasia has been described in association with cirrhosis of the liver.

Q10

'Glomus jugulare tumor' is a glomus tumor located in the adventitia of the jugular foramen.

Q11

Aortic body paragangliomas are probably more aggressive than other paragangliomas.

Q12

This histological appearance is diagnostic of lymphangioma, a rare tumor of the adrenal gland.

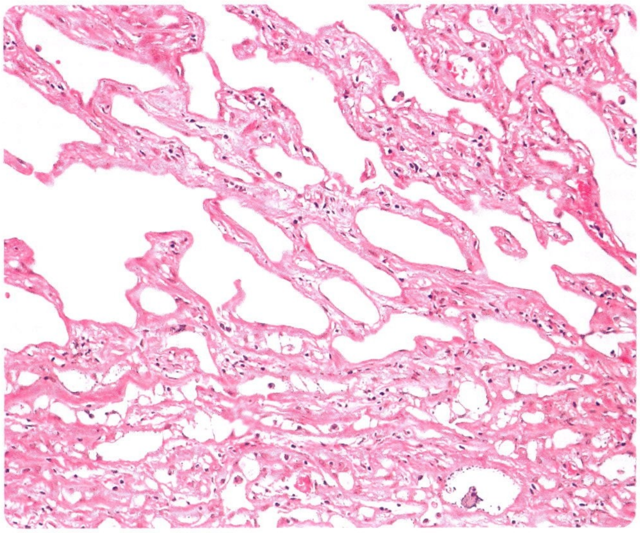

Fig. 16.10

Normal anatomy

A1. False

The paraganglion system consists of numerous collections of neuroepithelial cells ('chief cells') scattered throughout the body (the so-called extra-adrenal paraganglia) and the adrenal medulla, which is of neuroectodermal origin. This is in contrast to adrenal cortex, which is of mesodermal origin. **(p. 1117)**

A2. True

These hormones are classified into glucocorticoids, mineralocorticoids and adrenal androgen, and are all produced from cholesterol. **(p. 1115)**

A3. True

The zona glomerulosa is the most superficial, whereas the zone fasciculata forms a broad band with large cells arranged in two cell-wide cords. The zona reticularis, the innermost layer, consists of the cells that contain little or no lipid, in contrast to the other two zones. **(p. 1115)**

A4. False

Both zona fasciculata and zona reticularis secrete glucocorticoid and sex hormones, but glucocorticoid production dominates in the zona fasciculata. **(p. 1115)**

A5. False

These vacuolated clear cells with innumerable small lipid-containing vacuoles are found in the zona fasciculata, whereas 'compact' cells with little or no lipid are present in the zona reticularis. **(p. 1116)**

A6. True

This is a rather large chromaffin cell ('chromaffin' means that if the tissue is fixed in a solution containing chromium salts, these cells will turn brown owing to oxidation of catecholamines to melanin) that secretes norepinephrine and epinephrine. **(p. 1116)**

A7. True

These cells are arranged in well-defined nests ('Zellballen') encircled by a thin layer of S-100 protein-positive sustentacular cells. This cellular composition is recapitulated in paragangliomas, tumors of the paraganglia. **(p. 1117)**

A8. True

These retroperitoneal paraganglia probably represent lesser homologs of the adrenal medulla. The adrenal medulla is also related to the orthosympathetic system. **(p. 1117)**

Biopsy and cytology

A1. False

A sensitivity of 86% can be achieved using fine needle aspiration cytology. However, adrenal core biopsy is even better, with an overall sensitivity for malignancy reported at 94.6% and a specificity of 95.3%. **(p. 1117)**

Lesions of adrenal cortex

A1. False

Heterotopic adrenal tissue may undergo marked hyperplasia in patients with Nelson syndrome and other conditions associated with increased ACTH production, but heterotopic adrenal tissue almost never contains medulla, which secretes epinephrine. **(p. 1118)**

A2. False

Although it can be found in the kidney, the most common site is the retroperitoneal fat close to the adrenal gland. **(p. 1118)**

A3. True

These small nodules, which are located in the cortex or protrude through the capsule into the adjacent fat, do not have clinical significance. This is in contrast to hyperplasia, which can be associated with diverse clinical syndromes. **(p. 1118)**

A4. True

However, some cases may also first present clinically during adulthood. **(p. 1118)**

A5. False

Adrenocortical congenital hyperplasia is transmitted by an autosomal recessive gene and occurs with equal frequency in both males and females. **(p. 1118)**

A6. True

The absence of 21-hydroxylase accounts for 95% of cases. However, the inborn defect may occur in any of the five enzymatic steps required to synthesize cortisol from cholesterol. **(p. 1118)**

A7. False

Whereas in most cases the clinical picture is that of pure virilizing syndrome, the clinical presentation depends partly on which enzymatic step is defective, and certainly in some cases includes electrolyte disturbances and hypertension. **(p. 1118)**

A8. True

Congenital hyperplasia is always diffuse, in contrast to acquired hyperplasia, which may be diffuse or nodular. **(p. 1118)**

A9. True

ACTH-dependent acquired hyperplasia is diffuse and in most cases it is the pituitary that secretes ACTH, but ACTH may also be produced ectopically by lung tumors or other tumors. Nodular hyperplasia is characteristically ACTH-independent. **(p. 1118)**

A10. True

In addition, females may have multiple myxoid fibroadenomas of the breast and males may have large cell calcifying Sertoli and Leydig cell tumors of the testis. This is a rare cause of ACTH-independent Cushing's syndrome. **(p. 1119)**

A11. False

Most patients are adults, with a mean age of 50 years for carcinomas. **(p. 1119)**

A12. True

Most adenomas are small, rarely exceeding 5 cm in diameter or 50 g in weight, whereas carcinomas may reach >1000 g before being discovered. **(p. 1119)**

A13. True

Adrenocortical carcinomas are also usually solitary and may appear to be encapsulated, but are frequently characterized by areas of necrosis and hemorrhage, which are not found in adenomas. **(p. 1119)**

A14. True

Although the diagnostic value of finding bizarre nuclear forms is limited because atypical and bizarre nuclear forms can be occasionally found in adrenocortical adenoma, the presence of mitoses strongly suggests the diagnosis of carcinoma. **(p. 1119)**

A15. False

Small hemorrhagic foci are typical of adrenocortical adenomas containing foci of myelolipoma. **(p. 1120)**

A16. False

Most 'black adrenocortical adenomas' are non-functioning, but some may cause either primary aldosteronism or Cushing's syndrome. The black pigment is thought to represent either lipofuscin or neuromelanin. **(p. 1120)**

A17. True

Most of these tumors are benign. **(p. 1121)**

A18. True

Hyperfunctional zona glomerulosa results in increased mineralocorticoids and causes Conn's syndrome. Hyperfunctional zona fasciculata results in increased glucocorticoids and Cushing's syndrome, and hyperfunctional zona reticularis results in increased sex steroids and adrenogenital syndrome. **(p. 1124)**

A19. True

Such mature adipose tissue may also be found in adrenocortical hyperplasia. **(p. 1121)**

A20. False

Both of these high-grade tumors have been described as primary lesions of the adrenal gland, but are rare. **(p. 1121)**

A21. False

Most oncocytic tumors are benign and non-functional. **(p. 1121)**

A22. False

Both adenomas and carcinomas can show prominent myxoid features, but are otherwise typical of their respective types. **(p. 1121)**

A23. True

This is extremely useful in differentiating adrenocortical neoplasm from renal cell carcinoma, which practically always shows expression of EMA. In addition, CEA, B72.3, S-100 and Lewis blood group antigens are also typically negative in adrenocortical tumors. **(p. 1121)**

A24. False

Synaptophysin is typically weakly expressed, and although chromogranin is typically negative in adrenocortical tumors, it is readily positive in medullary adrenal pheochromocytoma. **(p. 1121)**

A25. False

Whereas most adrenocortical carcinomas weigh more than 10 g, lesions under 50 g are generally cured by excision. **(p. 1124)**

A26. False

Ras mutations have not been described in lesions of the adrenal cortex. **(p. 1122)**

A27. True

Specifically, a mitotic rate greater than 5 per 50 high-power fields (hpf), atypical mitoses, nuclear grade III or IV, necrosis, capsular invasion, vascular invasion (venous and sinusoidal invasion), a diffuse growth pattern, and the paucity or absence of clear cells are all suggestive of malignancy. These are the so-called 'Weiss criteria.' In addition, spindling of tumor cells also favors malignancy. **(p. 1119)**

A28. True

Most adrenocortical adenomas show strong expression of LMWCK and variable expression of vimentin. However, secondary tumors such as metastatic renal cell carcinoma and metastatic melanoma should also be considered, as both could be strongly vimentin positive and negative/focally weakly positive for LMWCK. **(p. 1121)**

A29. False

Aneuploidy has also been found in 20% of adrenocortical adenomas. Similarly, AgNOR counts, Ki-67 and DNA topoisomerase IIα, overexpression of p53, telomerase activity, and loss of heterozygosity cannot reliably distinguish between malignant and benign adrenocortical tumors. **(p. 1123)**

A30. True

Immunohistochemical positivity for low molecular weight cytokeratins, EMA, CD10, renal cell carcinoma marker (RCC Ma), and Lewis blood group isoantigen is found in renal cell carcinoma, whereas the expression of α-inhibin, MelanA/MART1, and synaptophysin favors adrenocortical carcinoma. **(p. 1123)**

A31. True

Histologically, the presence of glands that may contain red blood cells also strongly favors the diagnosis of renal cell carcinoma. **(p. 1123)**

A32. True

The adrenal cortex is typically negative for chromogranin and typically positive for LMWCK, but also for α-inhibin, MelanA/A103, bcl2, synaptophysin (weak), neurofilament and variable vimentin. The adrenal medulla is typically negative for vimentin and LMWCK, and is positive for chromogranin, synaptophysin, neurofilament, tyrosine hydroxylase, epinephrine and S-100 (only in sustentacular cells). **(p. 1123)**

A33. False

They are present in half of the cases. **(p. 1124)**

A34. False

The most common site is the liver (60%), followed by the lungs (40%) and the regional lymph nodes (40%). Peritoneal and pleural surfaces and bone are also commonly involved. **(p. 1124)**

A35. False

Half of the patients are dead within 2 years of presentation and the 5-year survival rate is only 20–35%. **(p. 1124)**

A36. True

It results in the production and release of steroid precursors such as dehydroepiandrosterone and 11-deoxycortisol. Deficiency of this enzyme is also the second most common cause of congenital adrenocortical hyperplasia. **(p. 1124)**

A37. True

Adrenocortical hyperplasia is responsible for most of the remaining cases; those cases caused by adrenocortical carcinomas are exceedingly rare. **(p. 1124)**

A38. False

Although hypertension and muscle weakness are typical, excessive aldosterone causes urinary loss of potassium and hypokalemia. **(p. 1124)**

A39. True

Because the lesions are unilateral and solitary, surgical excision is the primary treatment. **(p. 1124)**

A40. True

Most cortical adenomas have a homogenous yellow cut surface, but aldosterone-producing tumors characteristically have a somewhat darker, golden-yellow appearance. Exceptionally, they also can be 'black adenomas.' **(p. 1124)**

A41. False

Whereas normal zona glomerulosa produces aldosterone, most adenomas consist microscopically of cells that resemble zona fasciculata, or have hybrid features of both zona glomerulosa and zona fasciculata. **(p. 1124)**

A42. True

However, exceptions have been described. **(p. 1124)**

A43. True

These lamellar bodies occur in aldosterone-producing adenomas and in the zona glomerulosa of patients treated with spironolactone. Immunohistochemical positivity for aldosterone suggests that they bind this hormone. **(p. 1124)**

A44. True

And, just as in Conn's syndrome, adrenocortical carcinoma is the least common cause of Cushing's syndrome. **(p. 1125)**

A45. False

'Cushing's disease,' in contrast to Cushing's syndrome, designates only those patients with diffuse cortical hyperplasia secondary to pituitary hypersecretion of ACTH. Other cases of diffuse hyperplasia secondary to non-pituitary secretion of ACTH (small cell carcinoma of the lung, endocrine tumors of foregut origin and other tumors) are not diagnosed as 'Cushing's disease.' **(p. 1125)**

A46. True

This includes some cases of nodular adrenal hyperplasia independent of ACTH production. **(p. 1126)**

A5. False
Although the cytological appearance of some cells in the adrenal cortex bears resemblance to the cytopathic effect of CMV, these changes are associated with Beckwith–Wiedemann syndrome and are not infectious in nature. **(p. 1139)**

A6. True
Heterotopia of other tissues also occurs, and may include ovarian stroma, thyroid tissue and liver tissue. **(p. 1140)**

A7. True
The glands are enlarged, calcified, and replaced by granulomatous inflammation. **(p. 1140)**

A8. False
Myelolipomas are rarely bilateral and are usually clinically silent. **(p. 1140)**

A9. False
Although myelolipomas are usually clinically silent, they may be associated with other important clinical entities that need to be ruled out. These include adrenal cortical tumors, adrenal ganglioneuroma, and congenital adrenal hyperplasia. **(p. 1140)**

A10. True
Most cases of Cushing's syndrome in patients with myelolipoma are secondary to adrenal cortical tumors associated with the myelolipoma, but concurrent myelolipoma and Cushing's disease without adrenal cortical tumor has been described. **(p. 1140)**

A11. False
Rare cases of lipoma, angioma, schwannoma and various sarcomas have been described. **(p. 1141)**

A12. False
Although this is true for most pigmented tumors of the adrenal gland (for instance pheochromocytoma or black adenoma), malignant melanoma as a primary adrenal tumor is now accepted as an entity. Metastatic melanomas are far more common. **(p. 1142)**

A13. False
The adrenal gland is replaced by massive hemorrhage. There was no evidence of a tumor in any of the many sections taken. Massive adrenal hemorrhage may simulate a neoplasm clinically. **(p. 1139)**

A14. False
This is the typical gross appearance of myelolipoma, a truly benign lesion. **(p. 1140)**

Tumors and tumor-like lesions of other paraganglia

A1. True
These are the only two paragangliomas for which a chemoreceptor function has been demonstrated physiologically. **(p. 1142)**

A2. True
These are invariably benign and may represent a variant of hyperplasia secondary to hypoxia. **(p. 1142)**

A3. True
'Paragangliomatosis' refers to multifocal, bilateral paragangliomas. This includes pheochromocytoma. **(p. 1142)**

A4. False
First, the 'Carney triad' refers to extra-adrenal paraganglioma, gastric malignant stromal tumors and pulmonary chordoma, and is a disease of young females. It should not be confused with 'Carney's syndrome' (primary pigmented nodular adrenal cortical hyperplasia with Cushing's disease, spotty cutaneous pigmentation, cutaneous and cardiac myxomas, GH-secreting pituitary adenoma, psammomatous melanotic schwannoma, multiple myxoid fibroadenomas of the breast in females, and calcifying Sertoli cell tumors of the testis in males). **(p. 1142)**

A5. False
Although the Carney triad can be accompanied by adrenocortical tumors, it is rarely a familial disorder and should be distinguished from an autosomal disorder in which patients also develop paragangliomas and gastric stromal sarcomas. **(p. 1142)**

A6. False
As in pheochromocytoma, in extra-adrenal paragangliomas the only certain evidence of malignancy is metastatic disease. **(p. 1143)**

A7. True
However, some longer follow-up studies suggest that the percentage of malignant pheochromocytomas and extra-adrenal paragangliomas is probably higher. **(p. 1144)**

A8. False
Carotid body paraganglioma is the most common extra-adrenal paraganglioma. **(p. 1144)**

A9. True
Carotid body hyperplasia has also been described as a typical finding in people living at high altitudes. **(p. 1144)**

A10. False

'Glomus jugulare tumor' is not a glomus tumor, but rather a jugulotympanic paraganglioma, which most often presents as a mass in the middle ear or external auditory canal. In other instances it can cause enlargement of the jugular foramen. **(p. 1145)**

A11. True

Aggressive tumor growth has been described in about 45% of these tumors, with resultant impact on morbidity and death. **(p. 1145)**

A12. False

Despite being suggestive of lymphangioma, the presence of 'vascular spaces' without blood should bring into the differential diagnosis adenomatoid tumor, in which the spaces are lined by mesothelium, not endothelium. The diagnosis is confirmed by immunohistochemical analysis showing expression of calretinin and CK5/6, characteristic of mesothelial cells. **(p. 1141)**

Urinary tract 17

The renal biopsy and normal glomerulus

Q1

Ideally the kidney biopsy specimen should be divided into three parts: one for light microscopy, one for immunofluorescence microscopy and one for electron microscopy.

Q2

Semithin (1 μm thick) sections of the plastic-embedded tissue submitted for electron microscopy can be stained with toluidine blue and examined by light microscopy.

Q3

Immunofluorescence microscopy studies of kidney biopsies should be performed with antibodies to glomerular basement membrane antigens.

Q4

To be considered adequate the kidney biopsy performed for non-neoplastic diseases must contain at least 20 glomeruli.

Q5

The foot processes marked by arrows are located on the endothelial side of the basement membrane.

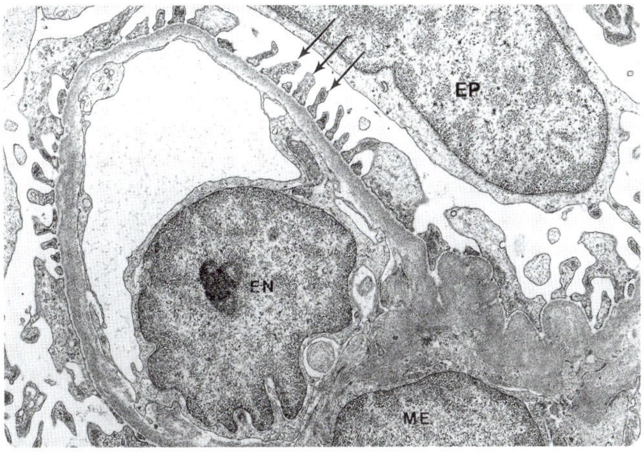

Fig. 17.1

Nephrotic syndrome

Q1

Nephrotic syndrome is almost always caused by immunologically mediated glomerulonephritis.

Q2

Membranous nephropathy is the most common cause of nephrotic syndrome in children.

Q3

Nephrotic syndrome caused by minimal change glomerulonephropathy responds favorably to treatment with corticosteroids.

Q4

The definitive diagnosis of minimal change glomerulonephropathy can be made only by electron microcopy.

Q5

Focal segmental glomerulosclerosis (FSG) may be primary (idiopathic) or secondary to other diseases.

Q6

In FSG the affected glomeruli as well as those that show no segmental lesions show a loss of epithelial foot processes.

Q7

Collapsing glomerulopathy is a variant of FSG, is diagnostic of HIV infection and has a favorable prognosis.

Q8

Membranous glomerulopathy is characterized by the position of immune complexes on the subepithelial side of the glomerular basement membrane.

Q9

In membranous glomerulopathy the mesangial areas typically contain proliferating mesangial cells and neutrophils.

Q10

Diabetic nephropathy and nephrotic syndrome are early signs of diabetes mellitus.

Q11

Nodular glomerulosclerosis (Kimmelstiel–Wilson lesion) is characterized by mesangial nodules composed of macrophages.

Q12

Primary amyloidosis is characterized by deposits of AA amyloid in the glomeruli.

Acute nephritis

Q1

Nephritis is clinically suspected when the urinary sediment appears 'active' and contains red blood cells, leukocytes, and red blood cell casts.

Q2

In acute poststreptococcal glomerulonephritis bacteria are typically found inside the glomeruli and can be cultured from the renal biopsy specimen.

Q3

In acute poststreptococcal glomerulonephritis the glomeruli are enlarged and hypercellular.

Q4

Idiopathic membranoproliferative glomerulonephritis type I is a chronic immune complex disease typically diagnosed in children and adolescents.

Q5

Membranoproliferative glomerulonephritis (MPGN) type I presents more often with nephritic syndrome, whereas membranoproliferative glomerulonephritis type II tends to present with nephrotic syndrome.

Q6

IgA nephropathy, the most common primary glomerulonephritis worldwide, is characterized by mesangial hypercellularity and mesangial deposits of IgA, IgG and C3.

Q7

Mesangial deposits of IgA can be found in chronic liver disease.

Q8

Crescentic glomerulonephritis is an extracapillary proliferative glomerulonephritis that presents clinically as rapidly progressive glomerulonephritis (RPGN).

Q9

Crescentic glomerulonephritis may be seen in some patients who have poststreptococcal glomerulonephritis, lupus nephritis or IgA nephropathy.

Q10

Crescentic glomerulonephritis is in most instances caused by an injury of glomerular basement membranes by the circulating antibodies to glomerular basement membrane (GBM) antigens.

Q11

Nephritis is a common complication of systemic lupus erythematosus, as evidenced by the fact that 40–80% of all patients with SLE have clinical or laboratory signs of renal involvement.

Q12

In SLE immune complexes are deposited only in the glomerular basement membranes, whereas other parts of the kidney are spared.

Q13

Diffuse proliferative glomerulonephritis (class IV lupus nephritis), found in 40–60% of patients, is characterized by a deposition of all immunoglobulins and complement in the mesangial areas and along the glomerular basement membranes of all (or almost all) glomeruli.

Vascular diseases

Q1

Takayasu's disease may involve the intrarenal arteries and arterioles.

Q2

Fibrinoid necrosis of the wall of large and medium-sized arteries is a typical feature of Henoch–Schönlein purpura.

Q3

The most common renal finding in mixed cryoglobulinemia is diffuse proliferative glomerulonephritis.

Q4

Diarrhea-related hemolytic uremic syndrome (D-HUS) is caused by *Salmonella* infection and is associated with crescentic glomerulonephritis and slowly evolving renal failure.

Q5

In the kidney systemic sclerosis affects predominantly the interlobar arteries, which show intimal thickening by loose, myxoid fibrous tissue.

Q6

Pre-eclampsia is typically caused by a deposition of antibodies to placental antigens in the subendothelial spaces of the glomerular capillaries.

Q7

Alport's syndrome is in most instances an X-linked nephropathy related to the mutation of one of the collagen type IV genes.

Q8

In male patients suspected of having Alport's syndrome the lack of an $\alpha 5$ chain of type IV collagen can be demonstrated by immunofluorescence microscopy of a skin biopsy, obviating the need for kidney biopsy.

Renal transplant rejection

Q1

Almost all cases of renal transplant failure are caused by immunologically mediated cellular transplant rejection.

Q2

In hyperacute renal transplant rejection there are thrombi in all the renal vessels, including the glomeruli.

Q3

Acute vascular rejection is characterized by changes that are most prominent in the glomeruli.

Q4

Acute interstitial allograft rejection is characterized by infiltration of the interstitium with basophils and mast cells.

Q5

Chronic rejection is the most common form of graft rejection after the initial 6–12-month period.

Q6

In chronic transplant rejection the blood vessels show obliterative fibrointimal proliferation.

Q7

Acute ciclosporin toxicity presents as nodular or diffuse hyalinosis of renal arterioles.

Q8

Tacrolimus (FK 506)-induced renal transplant changes can be distinguished from those induced by ciclosporin using renal biopsy.

Tubulointerstitial nephritis

Q1

Acute tubular necrosis is most often caused by ischemia due to hypoperfusion of the kidneys.

Q2

In acute pyelonephritis caused by ascending bacterial infection the inflammatory infiltrates are limited to the mucosa of the pyelon and the interstitium of the medullary part of the kidney.

Q3

Cortical and papillary scars overlying the dilated and blunted or deformed calices are typical features of chronic pyelonephritis.

Q4

In xanthogranulomatous pyelonephritis the renal parenchyma contains lobulated yellow masses replacing the normal parenchyma.

Q5

In malakoplakia the inflammatory infiltrate contains numerous plasma cells filled with Michaelis–Gutmann bodies formed of inspissated immunoglobulins.

Q6

Acute allergic tubulointerstitial nephritis is usually related to an adverse reaction to drugs.

Q7

Acute allergic tubulointerstitial nephritis is characterized by interstitial inflammatory infiltrates composed almost entirely of eosinophils.

Q8

Analgesic abuse nephropathy is complicated by bacterial renal infection in approximately 50% of cases.

Q9

Lead nephropathy is characterized by the appearance of intranuclear and cytoplasmic inclusions in tubular cells and can also be seen in the urinary sediment.

Q10

This ureteric lesion is best classified as a developmental disorder.

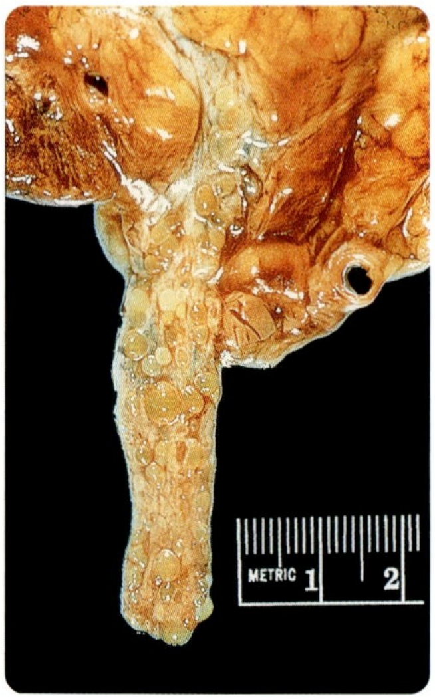

Fig. 17.2

Q11

Nephrolithiasis is more common in women than in men.

Q12

Bacterial infections with urea-splitting bacteria render the urine strongly acidic, thereby providing the conditions for the formation of uric acid stones.

Q13

Tubular casts formed in multiple myeloma are composed of light chains of monoclonal immunoglobulin found in this disease.

Q14

Hyaline arteriolosclerosis is diagnostic of severe malignant hypertension.

Q15

The most common cause of renal artery stenosis is atherosclerosis of the aorta.

Q16

Dysplastic lesions of the renal artery are bilateral in approximately 50% of cases, indicating that the lesions develop because of an underlying defect in vessel structure.

Q17

Renal artery injury caused by radiation is characterized by hyperplasia of smooth muscle cells causing narrowing of the lumen.

Q18

In chronically ischemic kidneys the juxtaglomerular (JG) apparati are enlarged and contain large granular JG cells, which are demonstrable by special stains.

Q19

Radiation nephropathy includes pathologic changes in the glomeruli, tubules and blood vessels.

Cystic diseases of the kidney

Q1

Multicystic renal dysplasia is the most common cause of abdominal masses in newborns.

Q2

In multicystic renal dysplasia the kidney is composed of cysts lined by columnar epithelium similar to the epithelium of collecting ducts.

Q3

Autosomal dominant polycystic kidney disease is common, accounting for approximately 10% of all cases of renal insufficiency requiring dialysis or transplantation.

Q4

In autosomal dominant polycystic kidney disease both kidneys are markedly enlarged and cystic.

Q5

In autosomal recessive polycystic kidney disease the liver is invariably affected.

Q6

In medullary sponge kidneys the cysts always arise from the collecting ducts in the medullary pyramids and the renal papillae, but they may be found only in some parts of one or both kidneys.

Q7

Nephronophthisis–medullary cystic kidney complex (NPH-MCKD) is a term that encompasses several genetic renal disorders with similar macroscopic and microscopic features.

Q8

Acquired renal cystic disease is found only in patients who have been on renal dialysis for more than 10 years.

Q9

In acquired renal cystic disease the cysts are usually solitary and limited to the renal cortex of one kidney.

Q10

Simple cysts are the most common cystic abnormality of the kidneys and their incidence increases with age.

Pediatric tumors and tumor-like conditions

Q1

Wilms' tumor is a tumor of infancy and early childhood; 50% of all tumors are diagnosed in children under the age of 3 years.

Q2

Some Wilms' tumors are bilateral and some are found in extrarenal locations.

Q3

The incidence of congenital urogenital anomalies is especially high in patients with Wilms' tumors diagnosed during the first year of life and those that have bilateral Wilms' tumors.

Q4

On cross-section Wilms' tumor often appears lobulated, but its color and consistency are highly variable.

Q5

Most Wilms' tumors are composed almost exclusively of small round-to-oval primitive cells resembling immature renal blastema.

Q6

Monophasic Wilms' tumor showing a blastematous growth pattern can be confused with neuroblastoma.

Q7

Predominantly epithelial Wilms' tumors may be confused with multicystic nephroma and renal cell carcinoma.

Q8

Wilms' tumors may occasionally resemble teratomas.

Q9

The presence of lung metastases in a young child with a retroperitoneal tumor strongly favors the diagnosis of Wilms' tumor over that of neuroblastoma.

Q10

Despite advances in chemotherapy only 50% of patients with Wilms' tumors survive 5 years, irrespective of the patient's age and the stage of the tumor at the time of diagnosis.

Q11

Increased relapse has been noticed in stage I tumors that show invasion of intrarenal vessels.

Q12

Anaplastic Wilms' tumors are more common in infants than in older children.

Q13

Mesoblastic nephroma is a tumor of older children and adolescents.

Q14

Most mesoblastic nephromas are located near the hilum of the kidney and on cross-section resemble uterine leiomyomas.

Q15

Mesoblastic nephromas are composed of mesenchymal cells resembling those of Wilms' tumor.

Q16

Cellular mitotically active tumors, called cellular or atypical mesoblastic nephromas, resemble infantile fibrosarcomas.

Q17

Multicystic nephroma usually presents with cysts replacing the entire kidney.

Q18

The cysts of multicystic nephroma are lined by clear cells, resembling renal cell carcinoma.

Q19

The stroma of multicystic nephroma may be indistinguishable from that in Wilms' tumors.

Q20

Nephroblastomatosis and nephrogenic rests are benign tumors composed of renal blastema and stroma.

Q21

Clear cell renal sarcoma tends to metastasize to the bones.

Q22

Clear cell renal sarcoma is in most instances composed of clear cells arranged into tubules.

Q23

Metastases of clear cell renal sarcoma tend to develop several years after removal of the primary tumor.

Q24

Rhabdoid tumors of the kidney are benign tumors that typically occur in adolescents and young adults.

Q25

The most remarkable feature of rhabdoid tumors of the kidney are the large cytoplasmic eosinophilic hyaline globules displacing the nuclei of the tumor cells laterally.

Adult tumors and tumor-like conditions

Q1

Renal cell carcinoma has a peak incidence around the age of 70 years and is more common in women than in men.

Q2

Renal cell carcinoma is a common malignancy in patients who have von Hippel–Lindau (VHL) disease.

Q3

Renal cell carcinoma may occasionally regress even without treatment.

Q4

Flank pain is the most common presenting complaint in patients with renal cell carcinoma.

Q5

On gross examination renal cell carcinoma typically appears golden yellow on cross-section.

Q6

Multicystic renal cell carcinoma is a low-grade tumor.

Q7

Renal cell carcinomas are typically composed of optically clear cells with sharply outlined boundaries, but may contain granular cells as well.

Q8

Most renal cell tumors are composed of cells forming tubules or solid nests, encased in scant stroma that contains sinusoid-like blood vessels.

Q9

Immunohistochemistry is of limited value in the differential diagnosis of renal carcinoma.

Q10

Most clear cell renal cell carcinomas show terminal deletion of the short arm of chromosome 3, a cytogenetic abnormality not seen in oncocytomas and most papillary tumors.

Q11

Clear cell renal cell carcinomas are more often bilateral and multicentric than papillary carcinomas.

Q12

Papillary carcinomas are often infiltrated with lymphocytes and plasma cells.

Q13

Papillary carcinomas have a worse prognosis than conventional clear cell renal cell carcinoma.

Q14

Collecting duct carcinomas are centered in the medulla, have a tubulopapillary architecture and evoke a strong desmoplastic reaction.

Q15

Renal medullary carcinoma is a highly aggressive renal cell tumor that occurs in persons who have sickle cell disease.

Q16

Chromophobe renal cell carcinomas are composed of polygonal cells that have a granular cytoplasm with focal clearing and sharply outlined cell membranes.

Q17

From the diagnostic point of view it is important to distinguish chromophobe carcinomas from oncocytomas, with which they share some common features.

Q18

Sarcomatoid renal cell carcinoma may resemble sarcomas of soft tissue and even contain cartilage or bone.

Q19

The most common sites of metastasis of renal cell carcinoma are the lungs and the bones.

Q20

Metastases of renal cell carcinoma occur irrespective of the size of the primary tumor.

Q21

Nuclear grading of renal tumors is of limited prognostic significance.

Q22

Metanephric adenomas are composed of cells that have abundant eosinophilic cytoplasm and are arranged into solid nests.

Q23

Renal oncocytomas are solid mahogany-brown tumors with a central fibrous scar.

Q24

Oncocytomas are composed of cells that have a scant bluish cytoplasm in standard hematoxylin- and eosin-stained slides.

Q25

Oncocytosis is a condition characterized by the presence of numerous oncocytic nodules in one or both kidneys.

Q26

Angiomyolipoma is a benign renal tumor composed of vessels, smooth muscle cells and fat cells, most often seen in patients who have tuberous sclerosis.

Q27

PECs (perivascular epithelioid cells) in angiomyolipomas react with the antibodies to melanocyte markers.

Q28

Angiomyolipomas composed of highly pleomorphic cells that show high mitotic activity and foci of necrosis should be considered potentially malignant.

Q29

Juxtaglomerular tumors typically present as small cortical nodules composed of blood vessels surrounded by spindle or polyhedral cells in a pattern reminiscent of hemangiopericytoma or glomus tumor.

Q30

Most juxtaglomerular tumors are functionally active and contain typical rhomboid crystalline granules.

Q31

The presumed cells of origin of medullary fibromas are medullary interstitial cells, known to produce prostaglandins and to regulate intrarenal blood pressure.

Q32

Renal sarcomas have the same histologic features as their equivalents in the soft tissues.

Q33

Renal lymphomas are often bilateral.

Q34

Transitional cell carcinoma of the renal pelvis is found often in patients who have other urothelial neoplasms.

Q35

Most transitional cell carcinoma of the renal pelvis are not invasive and are classified as grade I tumors.

Q36

Transitional carcinoma of the renal pelvis has an excellent prognosis.

Q37

Sarcomatoid carcinoma can be distinguished from sarcomas by finding foci of transitional carcinoma inside the tumor.

Q38

Urinoma results from the extravasation of urine into the perirenal fat tissue.

Bladder tumors

Q1

Inverted papilloma predisposes to the development of urothelial carcinoma.

Q2

Squamous papilloma is architecturally and cytologically similar to condyloma acuminatum.

Q3

Schistosoma haematobium is pathogenetically related to transitional cell (and squamous cell) carcinoma of the bladder.

Q4

HPV plays an important role in the pathogenesis of urothelial carcinoma.

Q5

When transitional cell carcinomas of the bladder occur in younger adults and children, they tend to be high grade and highly aggressive.

Q6

Detection of lamina propria invasion by transitional cell carcinoma is more important for the prognosis of tumors than the findings of invasion of the muscle payer (muscularis propria).

Q7

Prominent muscle fascicles always indicate muscularis propria in bladder biopsies.

Q8

Identification of tumor adjacent to fat cells indicates invasion into perivesical soft tissue.

Q9

The presence of focal glandular formation in transitional carcinoma is common and should not be regarded as adenocarcinoma.

Q10

Transitional cell carcinoma expresses both CK7 and CK20.

Q11

Genetic studies have shown similar changes between superficial papillary tumors and the invasive tumors that followed.

Q12

The pathology report of a bladder biopsy that contains a tumor should include the following information: grade, configuration, depth of penetration, presence of muscle, lymphatic and blood vessel invasion, and changes in adjacent mucosa if present.

Q13

The greatest value of exfoliative cytology of the urinary bladder is in the initial evaluation of most bladder tumors.

Q14

According to the 1998 WHO/ISUP classification, papillary neoplasms are classified as either low-grade or high-grade papillary carcinoma.

Q15

Invasive bladder carcinomas (especially high-grade tumors) are often associated with zones of atypical proliferation, carcinoma in situ, and early invasive carcinomas in areas remote from the main tumor mass.

Q16

Metastases of bladder cancer are most often found in the bones.

Q17

The term carcinoma in situ is used for all papillary transitional cell carcinomas that do not invade the stroma.

Q18

Total cystectomy is the treatment of choice for carcinoma in situ of the bladder.

Q19

Intravesical immunotherapy with bacillus Calmette–Guérin (BCG) is still a controversial therapy for superficial bladder carcinoma.

Q20

The microscopic grade of the tumor is the most important prognostic factor for transitional cell carcinomas of the urinary bladder.

Q21

Bladder adenocarcinomas are rare tumors, most of which develop from sequential changes in the surface transitional epithelium initiated by chronic inflammation.

Q22

Bladder adenocarcinoma is immunohistochemically indistinguishable from colorectal carcinoma.

Q23

Chronic schistosomiasis is most often associated with small cell carcinoma of the bladder.

Q24

The term squamous cell carcinoma should be reserved for those tumors that are squamous throughout.

Q25

Sarcomatoid carcinoma and carcinosarcoma are viewed as two different disease processes.

Q26

Transitional cell carcinoma is the most common malignant tumor of the bladder in children.

Q27

Most cases of metastatic tumor in the bladder are from breast carcinoma and malignant melanoma.

The renal biopsy and normal glomerulus

A1. True
One piece should be submitted fixed in formalin for light microcopy, one should be frozen for immunofluorescence microscopy, and the third should be fixed in glutaraldehyde for electron microscopy. **(p. 1164)**

A2. True
This tissue can be examined by light microscopy and can yield a great deal of information about the kidney that was biopsied. **(p. 1165)**

A3. False
Direct immunofluorescence microscopy is performed on tissue sections stained with fluorescein-tagged antibodies to immunoglobulins (IgG, IgA, IgM), complement (C3) and fibrin or fibrinogen. **(p. 1165)**

A4. False
Most renal diseases can be evaluated on much smaller specimens, even those containing approximately 10 glomeruli. Some diffuse lesions, such as membranous nephropathy, can be documented even if one single glomerulus is present in the biopsy. A biopsy that contains no glomeruli is considered to be inadequate. **(p. 1165)**

A5. False
The foot processes are part of the cytoplasm of the epithelial cell (EP) (podocytes) and are found on the epithelial side of the basement membrane. The cytoplasmic processes on the opposite side of the basement membrane belong to the endothelial cell, which lines the inside of the glomerular capillary (EN). **(p. 1167)**

Nephrotic syndrome

A1. False
Nephrotic syndrome can be caused by certain immunologic diseases, such as membranous nephropathy, but it can also be seen in metabolic diseases such as diabetes mellitus. **(p. 1169)**

A2. False
Approximately 80% of all cases of nephrotic syndrome in children are caused by minimal change glomerulopathy, a disease of unknown etiology. **(p. 1169)**

A3. True
Complete remission can be achieved in most instances within 8 weeks. However, after withdrawal of steroids about half of all patients have intermittent relapses, which are again treated with steroids. This period may be quite prolonged and may last up to 10 years. **(p. 1170)**

A4. True
On light microscopy the glomeruli appear normal, and immunofluorescence microscopy gives negative results. By electron microcopy one may see normal glomerular basement membrane, and the only abnormality is the extensive loss of epithelial cell foot processes. **(p. 1170)**

A5. True
The cause of idiopathic FSG is unknown. Secondary FSG can develop in the course of HIV infection, as a result of heroin addiction, morbid obesity, reflux obstructive uropathy or hypertension, to mention only the most common causes. **(p. 1172)**

A6. True
In this respect the glomerular changes resemble those seen in minimal change glomerulopathy. **(p. 1172)**

A7. False
Collapsing glomerulopathy is a variant of FSG that occurs in HIV patients, but also in drug addicts, and it may also be idiopathic. It has a poor prognosis and leads to rapid loss of renal function. **(p. 1173)**

A8. False
In membranous glomerulonephropathy the deposits of immune complexes are found on the subepithelial side of the basement membrane. **(p. 1175)**

A9. False
In membranous glomerulopathy the mesangial cells do not proliferate and there are no inflammatory cells in any part of the glomerulus. **(p. 1178)**

A10. False
Diabetic nephropathy develops in diabetics who have had the disease for at least 10 years. Such patients have proteinuria, but the nephrotic syndrome is found in 6–40% of them. Approximately 30% of diabetics die of chronic renal failure. **(p. 1178)**

A11. False
In diabetic nodular glomerulosclerosis the characteristic mesangial nodules are acellular and composed of hyalinized mesangial matrix. **(p. 1179)**

A12. False
Primary amyloidosis is a complication of multiple myeloma and is characterized by deposits of AL amyloid produced by plasma cells. It is called AL because it is derived from the light (L) chain of immunoglobulins. AA amyloid is deposited in secondary amyloidosis, which typically occurs as a complication of chronic inflammatory diseases. AA is derived from serum amyloid A precursor produced by the liver in response to various cytokines. **(p. 1181)**

Acute nephritis

A1. True
'Active' urinary sediment is a sign of glomerular inflammation and is typically seen in glomerulonephritis. **(p. 1188)**

A2. False
In acute poststreptococcal glomerulonephritis, an immunologically mediated inflammatory disease, the glomeruli contain immune complexes but no bacteria. The immune complexes may contain bacterial antigens, but in any case there are no living bacteria that could be cultivated from the renal biopsy specimen. **(p. 1189)**

A3. True
Mesangial cells, and to a lesser degree the endothelial cells, proliferate, causing glomerular hypercellularity and narrowing of the glomerular capillaries. Infiltrates of neutrophils and macrophages contribute further to glomerular enlargement and hypercellularity. **(p. 1189)**

A4. True
Approximately 90% of all patients are diagnosed in the 8–16-year age group. The disease is thought to be caused by chronic glomerular deposition of immune complexes. **(p. 1191)**

A5. False
It is actually MPGN type II that presents more often with nephritis, whereas MPGN type I tends to present with nephrotic syndrome. **(p. 1193)**

A6. True
IgA nephropathy , also known as Berger's disease, is the most common primary glomerulonephritis worldwide. It may present in several histologic forms, but in most instances it is characterized by proliferation of mesangial cells and deposits of IgA, accompanied by deposits of IgG and complement C3. **(p. 1195)**

A7. True
Deposits of IgA are found in chronic liver disease and several other conditions, such as celiac disease, Crohn's disease and HIV infection. **(p. 1195)**

A8. True
These three terms are actually used interchangeably for a group of glomerular inflammatory diseases characterized by proliferation of cells inside the urinary space between the capillary loops of the glomerulus and the Bowman capsule. The hypercellularity of these glomerular 'crescents' is increased by the exudation of macrophages, which are intermixed with proliferating epithelial cells of the glomerulus. **(p. 1197)**

A9. True
Crescentic glomerulonephritis may occur in severe cases of essentially all immunologically mediated glomerulonephritis, including among others poststreptococcal glomerulonephritis, lupus nephritis and IgA nephropathy. **(p. 1199)**

A10. False
Anti-GBM antibodies account only for 10–20% of all crescentic glomerulonephritides. In most cases crescentic glomerulonephritis is classified as pauci-immune and is associated with antineutrophil cytoplasmic antibodies (ANCA). **(p. 1199)**

A11. True
Nephritis is common in patients with SLE and it is likely that that the clinical assessment of these patients actually underestimates the actual frequency of histologic changes in the glomeruli. Glomerular changes may namely present even when the urinalysis is essentially normal. **(p. 1200)**

A12. False
Immune complexes are deposited primarily in the glomeruli, but they may be found along the tubular basement membrane and in the wall of the renal vessels as well. The pathologic findings are variable and may occur in all four renal compartments: glomeruli, tubules, interstitium and blood vessels. **(p. 1200)**

A13. True
Deposition of Ig, IgA, IgM and complement (often referred to as a 'full-house' pattern) is considered to be characteristic. Class IV lupus nephritis is diagnosed in approximately half of all biopsies of SLE patients. **(p. 1202)**

Vascular diseases

A1. False

Large vessel vasculitis such as Takayasu's disease involves the aorta and may cause narrowing of the main renal arteries, but it does not involve the intrarenal arteries. Intrarenal arteries are involved in medium-sized vessel vasculitis, such as polyarteritis nodosa or Kawasaki's disease. Small vessel vasculitides, such as microscopic polyangiitis, or Wegener's granulomatosis, often cause glomerulonephritis. **(p. 1205)**

A2. False

Henoch–Schönlein purpura involves small blood vessels and in the kidney it causes glomerulonephritis. It does not affect the large or medium-sized muscular arteries. **(p. 1208)**

A3. True

Diffuse proliferative glomerulonephritis, the most common renal finding in mixed cryoglobulinemia, often has a membranoproliferative pattern. Focal and segmental glomerulonephritis may also occur, but is less common. **(p. 1208)**

A4. False

D-HUS, the most common form of HUS in the US, is related to infection with verotoxin-producing *Escherichia coli* infection, following eating undercooked meat or unpasteurized apple juice. It is characterized by fibrinoid necrosis or thrombi in the small arteries and arterioles. Glomeruli show ischemic changes, mesangiolysis or an ultrastructurally visible subendothelial electron-lucent zone. Inflammatory changes in the glomeruli are not prominent and there is no crescentic glomerulonephritis. **(p. 1210)**

A5. True

These fibrotic changes in the interlobar arteries may be accompanied by deposits of fibrin and glomerular ischemia. **(p. 1212)**

A6. False

Pre-eclampsia is characterized by swelling of endothelial cells ('endotheliosis') in the glomeruli, and occasional deposits of fibrin, but there are no deposits of immunoglobulins. After delivery these changes usually disappear and the prognosis for complete recovery is generally very good. Renal biopsy is rarely performed to document glomerular changes in pre-eclampsia. **(p. 1212–1213)**

A7. True

In over 80% of cases Alport's syndrome is linked to the mutation of COL4A5 located on the long arm of the X chromosome encoding the α5 chain of type IV collagen. This mutation leads to structural changes in the glomerular basement membrane. **(p. 1214)**

A8. True

The α5 chain of type IV collagen is normally found in the epidermal basement membrane of the skin. In patients with Alport's syndrome this collagen chain is missing and the defect can be demonstrated by immunofluorescence microscopy of the skin biopsy. **(p. 1215)**

Renal transplant rejection

A1. False

The transplanted kidney may fail for many reasons, including immunologically mediated rejection, nephrotoxicity of immunosuppressive drugs, acute tubular necrosis, obstruction of the vasculature or urinary outflow tract, or recurrent or de novo glomerular disease. **(p. 1219)**

A2. True

These thrombi develop as a result of endothelial injury by preformed antibodies circulating in the recipient. **(p. 1220)**

A3. False

In acute vascular rejection, also called acute humoral rejection, the most severe changes are seen in the small arteries, arterioles and veins. The vessels wall is infiltrated with mononuclear cells, which cause both endothelial and medial changes. Inside the vessel one may find thrombi or foci of endothelial proliferation. **(p. 1220)**

A4. False

Acute interstitial allograft rejection, also called cellular rejection, is characterized by severe interstitial edema and infiltrates composed of lymphocytes, plasma cells and macrophages. Eosinophils and granulocytes may be present but are not prominent. If present, one should consider pyelonephritis. Basophils are not prominent at all. **(p. 1221)**

A5. True

It is, however, not a distinct entity but rather the end stage of repeated episodes of acute vascular or interstitial rejections. **(p. 1222)**

A6. True

Microscopically these changes involving the interlobular and arcuate arteries are similar to those seen in nephrosclerosis. They cause ischemic changes in the glomeruli and the tubules and a loss of functioning nephrons. **(p. 1222)**

A7. False

Nodular or diffuse hyalinosis of renal arterioles is a feature of chronic ciclosporin toxicity. In acute toxicity there is isometric vacuolization of proximal tubules. Furthermore, there is often degeneration of individual smooth muscle cells in the arterioles and narrowing of the arteriolar lumen. **(p. 1224)**

A8. False

Tacrolimus (FK 506)-induced changes in renal transplants are identical to those induced by ciclosporin. **(p. 1224)**

Tubulointerstitial nephritis

A1. True

Acute tubular necrosis can be subdivided into two groups: ischemic and toxic. Ischemic tubular necrosis is more common and is usually caused by hypotension that occurs in the course of surgery, after trauma, after loss of fluid in burned persons, in septic shock and many other conditions. **(p. 1225)**

A2. False

Ascending bacterial infection does not respect anatomic borders and can affect the entire kidney, including the cortical tissue. The inflammatory exudate may be found in the interstitial spaces, but also inside the tubules and even inside the Bowman capsule of the glomeruli. **(p. 1226)**

A3. True

Chronic pyelonephritis is characterized by fibrous scarring that deform the kidney, calices and renal pelvis. **(p. 1226)**

A4. True

Xanthogranulomatous pyelonephritis is a chronic renal infection characterized by infiltrates of foamy histiocytes forming large aggregates that can be seen on cross-sections of the kidney. The histiocytes contain lipids, which account for the yellow color of these masses. **(p. 1227)**

A5. False

In malakoplakia Michaelis–Gutmann bodies are found in the cytoplasm of macrophages. These bodies are PAS positive and contain calcium salts. By electron microscopy these bodies have a targetoid appearance. **(p. 1227)**

A6. True

Acute allergic tubulointerstitial nephritis may occur as an adverse reaction to a number of drugs, most often β-lactam antibiotics, NSAIDS and diuretics. **(p. 1228)**

A7. False

The interstitial infiltrates in acute allergic tubulointerstitial nephritis consist of lymphocytes, plasma cells, macrophages and eosinophils. **(p. 1228)**

A8. True

Renal infection is found in approximately 50% of patients who have analgesic abuse nephropathy. Both conditions predispose to renal papillary necrosis, which is found in some cases. **(p. 1229)**

A9. True

These inclusions consist of a lead protein complex that stains red in Giemsa-stained tubular cells in the urinary sediment. The inclusions also have a typical fibrillar ultrastructural appearance. **(p. 1229)**

A10. False

This figure shows the typical features of ureteritis cystica, an inflammatory condition characterized by cystic dilatation of epithelial buds of urothelium that have grown downwards into the stroma of the wall of the ureter. Ureteritis cystica is not related to renal developmental disorders, such as the autosomal dominant polycystic kidney disease. **(p. 1230)**

A11. False

Men are affected approximately four times more often than women. **(p. 1230)**

A12. False

Bacterial infections with urea-splitting bacteria render the urine alkaline, predisposing to the formation of struvite stones composed of magnesium ammonium phosphate. Uric acid stones form in non-infected urine containing increased amounts of urates that is only slightly acidic **(p. 1231)**

A13. True

Immunoglobulin light chains are filtered in the glomeruli and reabsorbed in the tubules. Excess of immunoglobulin light chains filtered through the glomeruli in multiple myeloma exceeds the capacity of the tubules to reabsorb the light chains and they form intratubular casts. These casts occlude the tubules and cause renal failure. **(p. 1232)**

A14. False

Hyaline arteriolosclerosis develops in the kidneys of aging persons and is accelerated and more prominent in those who have benign hypertension or diabetes. In malignant hypertension the arterioles show myointimal hypertrophy and hyperplasia, or fibrinoid necrosis. **(p. 1232)**

A15. True

Atheromatous plaques of the aorta located at the orifice of the renal arteries are the most common cause of renal artery stenosis. Atherosclerosis does not extend into the renal arteries. **(p. 1234)**

A16. True

The reasons for the renal artery dysplasia are not known. The fact that both renal arteries are involved in approximately half of all cases suggests that the lesions develop in structurally defective arteries. **(p. 1234)**

A17. False

Radiation-induced injury of renal arteries is characterized by a loss of smooth muscle cells and an intense fibrosis of all layers of the blood vessel. **(p. 1235)**

A18. True

Ischemia stimulates juxtaglomerular cells, which appear enlarged and contain granules visible in specially stained slides or by electron microscopy. **(p. 1236)**

A19. True

The changes vary, but in principle all components of the kidney are affected. The glomerular changes include scarring, which may be global or segmental, and fibrinoid necrosis or thickening of glomerular capillary walls. Mesangiolysis and occasional crescents can also be seen. Arterioles and small arteries show fibrinoid necrosis, or narrowing due to foamy cells. Tubules may show desquamation of the tubular cells or atrophy and hyalinization. **(p. 1236)**

Cystic diseases of the kidney

A1. True

Multicystic renal dysplasia, a developmental disorder that is most often unilateral, is the most common abdominal mass in newborns. **(p. 1237)**

A2. False

Histologic features of multicystic renal dysplasia include immature glomeruli and tubules intermixed with immature mesenchymal tissue focally differentiating into cartilage or fibromuscular tissue. **(p. 1237)**

A3. True

Autosomal dominant polycystic kidney disease is also known as the adult form of renal polycystic disease, because it becomes clinically manifest in adulthood. It is an important cause of renal insufficiency, accounting for approximately 10% of all those requiring dialysis or transplantation. **(p. 1237)**

A4. True

The disease involves both kidneys, which enlarge to approximately the same size. The cystic kidneys may be huge and weigh 3–5 kg each. **(p. 1237)**

A5. True

Essentially, all patients with this disease have liver changes. In the neonatal period the renal symptoms predominate, but in later life the patient may present with liver problems. Histologically the liver shows signs of hepatic fibrosis and biliary dysgenesis or ectasia. **(p. 1238)**

A6. True

Medullary sponge kidney may affect both kidneys, only one kidney, or only parts of one or both kidneys. The cysts always arise from the dilatation of medullary and papillary collecting ducts. **(p. 1239)**

A7. True

NPH-MCKD is a name give to a group of diseases that have the same morphologic features but differ from one another genetically and clinically. The term nephronophthisis is used for renal diseases of early onset. It includes three autosomal recessive disorders called juvenile (MPH1), infantile (MPH2), and adolescent (MPH3). The term medullary cystic kidney disease is a disease of adult age and includes MCKD1 and MCKD2, with a median age of onset of end-stage renal disease of 62 and 32 years, respectively. **(p. 1239)**

A8. False

Acquired renal cystic disease is found in over 80% of all patients who have been on renal dialysis for more than 10 years, but also in 40% who have had dialysis for only 3 years and up to 20% of chronic renal patients who never had any dialysis at all. **(p. 1240)**

A9. False

In acquired renal cystic disease the kidneys contain numerous small cysts, found in cortex and the medulla. Both kidneys are involved. **(p. 1240)**

A10. True

The occurrence of simple renal cysts increases with age from 0.1% in children to 20% in those older than 50 years. They are less than 5 cm in diameter and are usually asymptomatic. They can be solitary or multiple, and are usually unilocular and located in the cortex. **(p. 1240)**

Pediatric tumors and tumor-like conditions

A1. True

The histogenesis of Wilms' tumor recapitulates the embryogenesis of the kidney, and thus it is no surprise that the tumor occurs mostly at an early age. Approximately 50% are diagnosed in children younger than 3 years, and 90% are found in those less than 6 years of age. **(p. 1240)**

A2. True

Approximately 5–10% of all Wilms' tumors are bilateral. Rarely, Wilms' tumors may arise in extrarenal sites, such as the retroperitoneum, sacrococcygeal region, mediastinum, testis and uterus. **(p. 1240)**

A3. True

These facts cannot be fully explained, but are probably all linked to the *WT1* tumor suppressor gene, which plays a role in the histogenesis of Wilms' tumors. The *WT1* gene encodes a zinc finger transcription factor that is expressed at a high rate in the developing urogenital tract, and its mutation probably causes some of the developmental anomalies. **(pp. 1240 and 1243)**

A4. True

Many Wilms' tumors appear lobulated on cross-section, but the gross features of these tumors are highly variable. Some are gray-tan, some are brown and some are yellow. Some tumors are rubbery and firm, and some are soft. Areas of necrosis and hemorrhage may be prominent, and some tumors are even cystic. **(p. 1241)**

A5. False

Most tumors are triphasic, i.e. they have three major components: undifferentiated blastema, mesenchyma (stromal) and epithelial tissue. Some are biphasic and some are monophasic. **(p. 1241)**

A6. True

Blastematous Wilms' tumor may be composed of small blue cells only and thus can be confused with neuroblastoma, an adrenal or retroperitoneal tumor that also occurs in infants and young children. **(p. 1241)**

A7. True

The differential diagnosis for predominantly epithelial Wilms' tumors, especially in older patients, should include multicystic nephroma and renal cell carcinoma. It is well known that Wilms' tumor can occasionally occur in adults as well. Furthermore, foci of renal cell carcinoma have been described in otherwise typical Wilms' tumors. **(p. 1242)**

A8. True

Wilms' tumors may contain various epithelial and mesenchymal and even neuroepithelial structures. These tumors, called teratoid Wilms' tumors, cannot always be reliably distinguished from teratomas. **(p. 1243)**

A9. True

Wilms' tumor most often metastasizes to the lungs, and only 15% of metastases are found in local lymph nodes. In contrast, neuroblastomas are prone to metastasize to the bones. Bones are involved in only 1% of all Wilms' tumors. **(p. 1243)**

A10. False

Most patients with Wilms' tumors respond favorably to chemotherapy, and 80–90% of infants and children are cured. The stage is the most important prognostic determinant. Infants and children under the age of 2 years have a better prognosis **(p. 1244)**

A11. True

Four histologic findings have been associated with increased relapse of stage I Wilms' tumors. In addition to invasion of intrarenal vessels, the other predictors of relapse are the presence of an inflammatory pseudocapsule, invasion of the renal sinus, and extensive infiltration of the renal capsule. **(p. 1244)**

A12. False

Anaplasia is rare in Wilms' tumors of infancy and children younger than 2 years of age. This is probably the reason for the better prognosis of tumors in that age group than in older children. The signs of anaplasia are threefold: a marked enlargement of nuclei (at least three times over normal) in all three components of the tumor; hyperchromasia of nuclei; and multipolar mitoses. Overexpression of the *p53* gene correlates with the anaplasia of the tumor. **(p. 1244–1245)**

A13. False

Mesoblastic nephromas are diagnosed in infants and children younger than 6 months of age. Vary rarely they can occur in older children, and even in adults. **(p. 1245)**

A14. True

The tumors are perihilar, solid, firm, and have a whorled configuration on cross-section, resembling uterine leiomyomas. **(p. 1245)**

A15. False

Mesoblastic nephromas are composed of fibroblasts, myofibroblasts and smooth muscle cells, occasionally entrapping glomeruli and renal tubules. **(p. 1245)**

A16. True

These tumors tend to invade the surrounding tissues and show areas of necrosis and hemorrhage. They contain a chromosomal translocation that is also found in infantile fibrosarcomas. However, as the classic mesoblastic nephroma contains the same translocation, cytogenetic data do not justify the distinction between cellular and classic mesoblastic nephroma. **(p. 1245–s1246)**

A17. False

Most multicast nephromas are sharply delineated from the uninvolved renal parenchyma, although in some instances the entire kidney may be replaced by tumor, as shown in Figure 17.3. **(p. 1246–1247)**

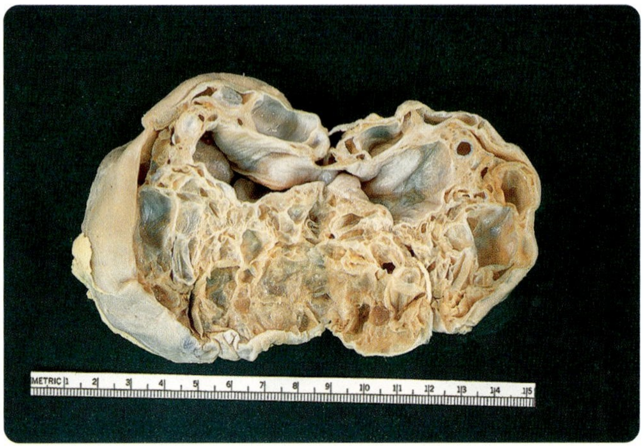

Fig. 17.3

A18. False

The cysts of mesoblastic nephroma are lined by tubular epithelium ranging in height from cylindrical to extremely flat, as in lymphangiomas. Most often the cells have a hobnail quality. **(p. 1247)**

A19. True

The stroma between the cysts is usually fibroblastic and nondescript, but may contain smooth muscle cells, skeletal muscle, cartilage, and even blastematous elements similar to Wilms' tumor. It has been suggested that multicystic nephroma represents the end of a spectrum of differentiation of Wilms' tumor, i.e. that it represents a fully differentiated Wilms' tumor. **(p. 1246)**

A20. False

Nephroblastomatosis and nephrogenic rests are composed of renal blastema and stroma. They result from developmental disorders and are not considered to be neoplastic. They are found in 1% of all neonatal kidneys. Nephroblastomatosis is found in 30% of kidneys with Wilms' tumor, and in these cases both the tumor and the embryonic rest show the same mutations of the *WT1* gene. **(p. 1248)**

A21. True

The tumor is also known as bone metastasizing renal tumor. Previously considered a variant of Wilms' tumor it is now recognized as a specific entity, with a propensity to metastasize to bones in particular. As noted earlier, Wilms' tumor metastasizes to the bones extremely rarely. **(p. 1249)**

A22. False

Despite its name, clear cells predominate only in 20% of tumors. Most tumors are composed of small cells with round normochromic nuclei, and have a light-staining eosinophilic cytoplasm. The cells line arborizing fibrovascular cores and alveoli or form nests, palisades, cords and trabeculae. The distinct alveolar and arborizing vascular stroma is considered to be a more important diagnostic finding than the finding of clear cells. **(p. 1249)**

A23. True

Distant metastases may be found 5 or more years after removal of the primary tumor. In this respect the tumor also differs from Wilms' tumor, which metastasizes early and does not show this long delay in the appearance of metastases. **(p. 1249)**

A24. False

Rhabdoid tumors, previously considered variants of Wilms' tumor, are tumors of infancy and early childhood; most are diagnosed before the age of 18 months. **(p. 1250)**

A25. True

The tumor cells are called rhabdoid because of the prominent eosinophilic globules reminiscent of cytoplasmic aggregates of myofilaments in rhabdosarcoma cells. Immunohistochemically, the cytoplasmic globules react with the antibodies to vimentin and usually keratin, and show no muscle-specific differentiation. **(p. 1250)**

Adult tumors and tumor-like conditions

A1. False

Renal cell carcinoma has a peak incidence in the 55–60-year age group and is twice as common in men as in women. **(p. 1251)**

A2. True

Approximately 50% of patients with VHL disease will develop renal cell carcinomas. VHL disease is related to mutations or deletions of the VHL gene on chromosome 3. This tumor-suppressor gene plays a role in the pathogenesis of renal cell carcinoma, even in patients who do not have VHL disease. **(p. 1251)**

Bladder tumors

A1. False

There is no evidence that inverted papilloma predisposes to the development of carcinoma, but the occasional coexistence of the two lesions suggests a pathogenetic relationship. **(p. 1326)**

A2. False

Squamous papilloma is architecturally similar to condyloma acuminatum but lacks cytopathic epithelial changes and is negative for HPV DNA, suggesting a lack of relationship between the two lesions; most occur in elderly women and follow a benign clinical course, with occasional local recurrences. **(p. 1326)**

A3. True

Schistosoma haematobium is also thought to be pathogenetically related to transitional cell (and squamous cell) carcinoma of the bladder, as the greatest concentration of such carcinomas occurs in areas of the world infested by this parasite. **(p. 1327)**

A4. False

The role of HPV remains controversial, but most of the available evidence suggests that it does not play a significant role in the genesis of this tumor. **(p. 1327–1328)**

A5. False

Most cases of transitional cell carcinoma of the bladder present in patients over the age of 50, but they can also occur in younger adults and children. The latter tend to be low-grade indolent neoplasms, but occasional highly aggressive examples have been recorded in this age group. **(p. 1328)**

A6. False

Stromal invasion by transitional cell carcinoma proceeds in two stages: invasion of the lamina propria and invasion of the muscle layer. Detection of the former is a difficult and somewhat subjective exercise. Conversely, detection of muscle invasion is of great consequence because of its relevance for the therapy and prognosis of bladder tumors. **(p. 1328)**

A7. False

Care should be exercised not to misinterpret the inconsistent but sometimes prominent fascicles of muscularis mucosae (particularly common in women) as belonging to the muscularis propria. **(p. 1328)**

A8. False

It is also important not to misinterpret the mature adipose tissue commonly present in the lamina propria or muscularis propria as perivesical soft tissue, in order to avoid a tumor adjacent to fat in a biopsy specimen being badly overstaged. **(p. 1329)**

A9. True

Foci of glandular metaplasia are common, usually in the form of intracytoplasmic mucin-containing vacuoles. Exceptionally, a microcystic pattern develops as the result of enlargement of the mucin-filled cavities, which can reach a diameter of 1 mm or more. Ward found that 25–30% of transitional cell carcinomas had evidence of focal mucin production, and that a similar number (but not necessarily the same cases) showed some glandular formation. These tumors, sometimes incorrectly designated 'mixed carcinomas,' behave as conventional transitional cell carcinomas of equivalent grades. A clear distinction should be made between them and the pure adenocarcinomas of the bladder. **(p. 1329)**

A10. True

There is consistent expression of CK20, in stark contrast with the morphologically similar transitional cell carcinomas of the ovary. This CK20 positivity is particularly common and strong in the high-grade tumors. The coordinate expression of CK7 and CK20 is a particularly reproducible feature of transitional cell carcinoma and is usually maintained in the metastatic foci. **(p. 1329)**

A11. True

Genetic analyses have shown concordant changes between superficial papillary tumors and the invasive tumors that followed, supporting the time-honored belief regarding the progression of one tumor into the other. **(p. 1330)**

A12. True

All these pathologic findings should be included to provide clinicians with complete information about bladder tumors. **(p. 1330)**

A13. False

Exfoliative cytology is important for the initial diagnosis of bladder tumors but is of little practical value in the evaluation of most bladder tumors, which can be readily performed by urologists. The greatest value of urinary bladder cytology is in the follow-up evaluation of patients who have received surgery or radiotherapy for bladder carcinoma. In some cases the recurrence may not become clinically apparent until more than a year after the malignant cells have been detected in the urine. **(p. 1330–1331)**

A14. False

The WHO/ISUP classification recognizes four papillary bladder tumors, as follows: papilloma (with the variant inverted papilloma); papillary neoplasm of low malignant potential; low-grade papillary carcinoma; and high-grade papillary carcinoma. **(p. 1331)**

A15. True

Invasive bladder carcinomas are often associated with neoplastic changes at a distance from the main tumor mass. Molecular studies analyzing the *p53* tumor-suppressor gene and the pattern of X-chromosome inactivation suggest that in most instances these apparently multifocal urothelial tumors are derived from a single progenitor cell. **(p. 1332)**

A16. False

Metastases are most often found in pelvic lymph nodes. Such metastases are found with approximately 25% of invasive tumors. The most common sites of distant metastasis are the lungs, liver, bone and central nervous system. **(p. 1333)**

A17. False

By convention, the term carcinoma in situ (Tis) of the bladder is reserved for high-grade lesions showing pronounced cytologic atypia but lacking a papillary configuration. One should realize that papillary transitional cell carcinomas that do not invade the stroma are also carcinomas in situ (Ta), but they are not designated as such to avoid lumping together two conditions with markedly different morphologic features, natural history, and probably molecular pathways. **(p. 1334)**

A18. True

The recommended treatment for carcinoma in situ is total cystectomy, except for small and apparently localized lesions; for these, intravesical chemotherapy may induce temporary and sometimes complete remission; however, in 40–70% of cases new tumors will develop, usually within 6–12 months. **(p. 1335)**

A19. False

Immunotherapy with BCG is now a widely accepted form of therapy for superficial bladder carcinomas, whether papillary or in situ. This therapy results in superficial mucosal erosion, submucosal granulomatous inflammation and reactive epithelial atypia. **(p. 1335)**

A20. False

Stage is by far the most important prognostic determinant, as the pioneer studies of Jewett and others have demonstrated. **(p. 1335)**

A21. True

Bladder adenocarcinomas constitute approximately 2% of the malignant tumors of this organ. Most develop from sequential changes in the surface transitional epithelium initiated by chronic inflammation – from Brunn's islands to cystitis glandularis and cystica, and finally to adenocarcinoma, which is usually mucin secreting. **(p. 1337)**

A22. False

Immunohistochemically, primary bladder adenocarcinoma differs from colorectal carcinoma by the fact that the β-catenin, if present, is primarily membranous (and some cytoplasmic) rather than nuclear. It is also more commonly positive for keratin 7 (6.5% vs 0%) and less commonly for keratin 20 (53% vs 94%). **(p. 1337)**

A23. False

Chronic schistosomiasis is most often associated with squamous cell carcinoma of the bladder, as reported from Egypt, Sudan and several other countries. **(p. 1340)**

A24. True

Because focal squamous cell changes are common in high-grade transitional cell tumors, the term squamous cell carcinoma should be reserved for those tumors that are squamous throughout. **(p. 1340)**

A25. False

Sarcomatoid carcinoma (spindle cell, metaplastic) carcinoma is a high-grade neoplasm of the bladder in which a malignant epithelial component, clearly identifiable as such (of transitional, glandular, squamous, or undifferentiated type), coexists with areas having a sarcoma-like appearance. The latter may have a nonspecific spindle cell or pleomorphic look (sometimes admixed with osteoclast-like giant cells) or may exhibit specific features of mesenchymal differentiation, such as rhabdomyosarcoma, chondrosarcoma, osteosarcoma, liposarcoma or malignant fibrous histiocytoma. When such specific features are present the tumor may be designated as carcinosarcoma, but we view this as a variation of the same basic process. Whether areas of specific mesenchymal differentiation occur or not, transitions may be seen between the two major components, suggesting that the sarcoma-like areas are also epithelial in nature. Further evidence of the epithelial nature of these proliferations is provided by the immunoreactivity for keratin often detected in the sarcoma-like component. **(p. 1340)**

A26. False

Embryonal rhabdomyosarcoma (particularly the botryoid subtype) is the most common malignant tumor of the bladder in children. **(p. 1341)**

A27. True

Breast carcinoma and malignant melanoma are the most common tumors found in patients with metastases in the bladder. Metastases from other sites have also been reported, including primary tumors of the lung, kidney, stomach, pancreas and ovary. **(p. 1343)**

Male reproductive system 18

PROSTATE

Normal anatomy

Q1

The prostate gland may be divided into peripheral and central zones.

Q2

The capsule of the prostate consists of a fibromuscular layer and is not well developed.

Q3

PSA (prostate-specific antigen) is produced by prostatic glands and is a useful marker for both screening diagnostic procedures and diagnostic immunophenotyping in the diagnosis of prostate carcinoma.

Q4

PAP (prostatic acid phosphatase) is used clinically in the same way as PSA.

Q5

Prostatic secretion is a neutral mucosubstance.

Q6

Prostate acini and ducts are lined by basal cells (which do not have contact with the lumina of the glands) and secretory cells.

Q7

Basal cells are precursors of secretory cells of the prostate.

Q8

Basal cells form a thin and continuous layer that separates the secretory epithelium from the basement membrane.

Q9

Basal cells and secretory cells of the prostate express PSA.

Q10

Basal cells express high molecular weight cytokeratins, which may be detected by antibodies to CK5/6 and 34βE12.

Q11

Expression of high molecular weight cytokeratin in the glands of the prostate rules out prostate carcinoma.

Q12

Neuroendocrine cells of the prostate express PSA.

Q13

The large ducts of the prostate are lined by transitional epithelium, which is identical to the epithelium found in the urinary bladder.

Q14

Prostatic stroma is notable for its large content of smooth muscle.

Q15

Myoepithelial cells of the prostate express both S-100 protein and PSA.

Non-neoplastic disorders

Q1

Ectopic prostate tissue can frequently be found in the seminal vesicles and also in the retrovesical space.

Q2

The central zone accounts for only 25% of the overall prostate volume, but is the most frequent site of benign nodular hyperplasia of the prostate.

Q3

50% of 50-year old men have nodular hyperplasia of the prostate.

Q4

Castration is a predisposing factor for nodular hyperplasia.

Q5

There are no immunohistochemical differences between normal prostate and prostate tissue in nodular hyperplasia.

Q6

p27 protein expression levels are low in both more aggressive adenocarcinomas of the prostate and benign prostatic hypertrophy (BPH), suggesting a molecular link between these two common disorders of the prostate.

Q7

As benign prostatic hypertrophy progresses, it gradually involves all anatomical compartments/ zones of the prostate.

Q8

The earliest change in benign prostatic hypertrophy is the appearance of small, rather vascular stromal nodules around the urethra.

Q9

In BPH, glandular hyperplasia is typically preceded by stromal hyperplasia.

Q10

A mild chronic perivascular inflammatory infiltrate is common in BPH, indicating the role of chronic inflammation in the induction of the disease.

Q11

In BPH there is no correlation between the relative predominance of stromal or glandular tissues and the degree of urinary obstruction.

Q12

Transurethral resection (TUR) is a common treatment modality for BPH, which reduces the volume of the prostatic tissue, relives urinary obstruction and decreases the risk of adenocarcinoma of the prostate.

Q13

Infarct of the prostate usually occurs in large prostates involved by BPH, and is usually focal, sparing most of the organ.

Q14

In the milder form of prostatic infarct, the infarcted tissues show glandular necrosis with sparing of the prostate stroma.

Q15

Ducts surrounding the infarcted prostate tissue typically show squamous metaplasia.

Q16

Most prostatic infarcts are clinically silent because of their small size.

Q17

Inflammation of the prostate gland is clinically divided into acute and chronic prostatitis.

Q18

Acute bacterial prostatitis is usually associated with predisposing conditions such as bladder outlet obstruction secondary to benign prostatic hypertrophy or an immunosuppressed state.

Q19

Prostate biopsy is contraindicated in acute prostatitis.

Q20

In acute prostatitis there is diffuse infiltration by neutrophils.

Q21

Eosinophilic prostatitis occurs in the setting of hypereosinophilic syndrome.

Q22

'Granulomatous prostatitis' is caused by either fungi or mycobacteria.

Q23

A prostate biopsy demonstrating well-formed granulomas is most likely involved by tuberculous prostatitis.

Q24

The prostate may be involved by various specific infections, including blastomycosis, coccidioidomycosis, actinomycosis, cryptococcosis, histoplasmosis, aspergillosis and candidiasis.

Q25

An abscess of the prostate is usually caused by a sexually transmitted infection.

Q26

Prostate calculi, like stones in the gallbladder, are radio-opaque and easily detectable on plain X-rays.

Q27

Prostatic calculi are most commonly seen in patients with nodular hyperplasia.

Q28

Nodular hyperplasia of the prostate is illustrated in this figure.

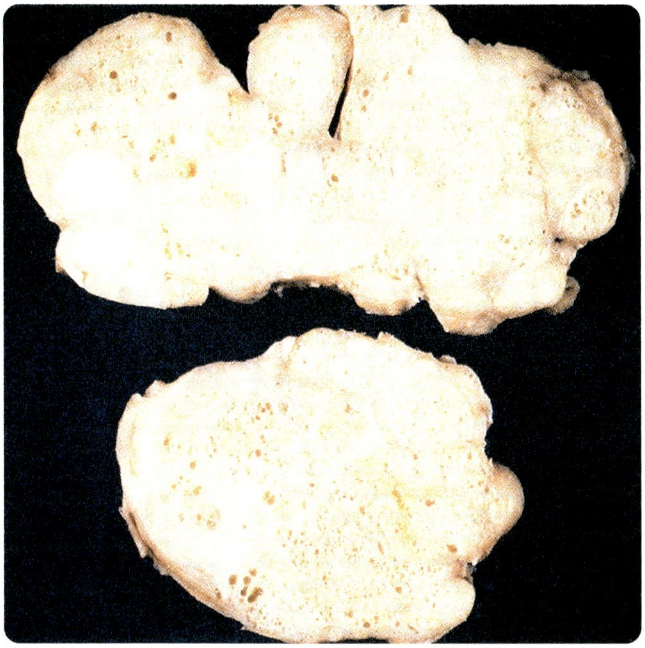

Fig. 18.1

Q29

This figure depicts squamous cell carcinoma, a rare lesion.

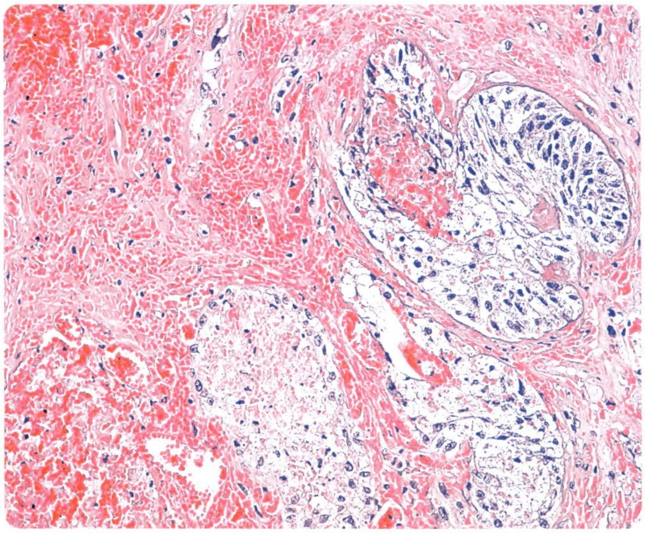

Fig. 18.2

Q30

Mycobacteria are frequently demonstrated in the giant cells of granulomatous prostatitis.

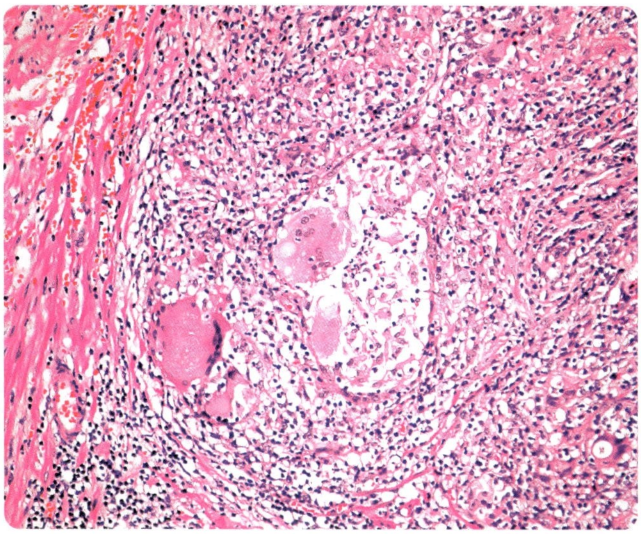

Fig. 18.3

QUESTIONS

Tumor-like conditions of prostate and prostatic urethra

Q1
Postoperative spindle cell nodule is sometimes referred to as inflammatory pseudotumor.

Q2
Postoperative spindle cell nodule, like inflammatory pseudotumor of the prostate, is smooth muscle actin and vimentin positive.

Q3
It is not possible to distinguish histologically between postoperative spindle cell nodule and inflammatory pseudotumor of the prostate.

Q4
Postoperative spindle cell nodule may resemble Kaposi's sarcoma and other sarcomas.

Q5
The differential diagnosis of benign stromal lesions of the prostate includes inflammatory pseudotumor, postoperative spindle cell nodule, benign stromal nodule with and without cellular atypia in BPH, and leiomyoma with atypia.

Q6
Inflammatory pseudotumor of the prostate can show three main histologic patterns: nodular fasciitis-like, fibrous histiocytoma-like, and desmoid or scar tissue type.

Q7
Urethral polyps are polypoid masses of prostate tissue arising in the verumontanum.

Q8
Urethral polyps are an example of prostatic ectopy.

Q9
Melanosis of the prostate is also known as blue nevus of the prostate.

Q10
Extramedullary hematopoiesis can be found in the prostate.

Q11
Demonstration of cytokeratin expression in spindle cell lesions of the prostate supports the diagnosis of sarcomatoid carcinoma.

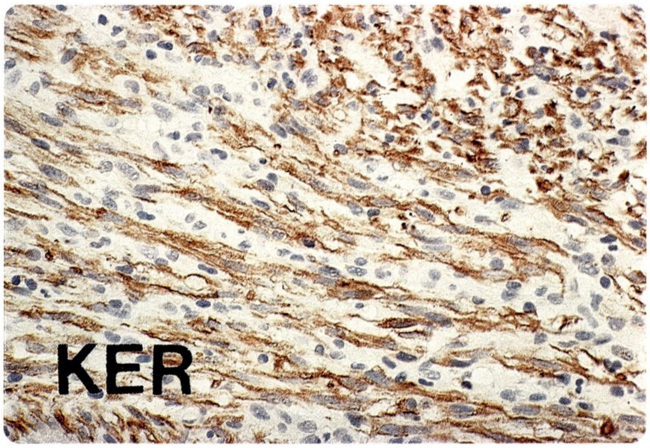

Fig. 18.4

Carcinoma

Q1
Carcinoma of the prostate is the most common internal malignancy among men in the United States, but is not responsible for large numbers of deaths owing to its very slow progression and relatively benign clinical behavior.

Q2
Prostate carcinoma is testosterone related.

Q3
Prostate carcinoma is more common in men who smoke and in men with numerous venereal diseases.

Q4
Prostate carcinoma has been associated with age, race, and the presence of nodular hyperplasia of the prostate.

Q5
Transrectal ultrasonography per se is a sensitive method of detecting prostate carcinoma.

Q6
PSA, a glycoprotein secreted by the luminal epithelium of prostate glands, can be detected in the serum by biochemical testing. PSA levels = 4 ng/mL are strongly suggestive of prostate carcinoma.

Q7

PSA levels <4 ng/mL are common in nodular hyperplasia and a biopsy of the prostate is not indicated in these cases.

Q8

Adenocarcinoma of the prostate can be divided into two major categories based on the site of origin: carcinoma originating in the small ducts and acini, and carcinoma originating in the large ducts.

Q9

Most adenocarcinomas of the small ducts and acini cause obstruction of the prostatic urethra because they arise in the transitional zone.

Q10

Macroscopically, adenocarcinoma of the prostate can be seen as a gray or yellowish, poorly delineated, firm area.

Q11

Microscopically, adenocarcinoma of the prostate may be divided into those that create regular glandular units (each neoplastic cell is in contact with the stroma on one side and the glandular lumen on the other, and laterally it is in contact with other epithelial cells) and those that create irregular glandular units (loss of contact with either the stroma or the glandular lumen, or both).

Q12

Cytological features are irrelevant in the grading of prostate carcinoma.

Q13

Cytological features are irrelevant to the diagnosis of prostate carcinoma.

Q14

Intraluminal crystalloids are diagnostic of prostate carcinoma.

Q15

Intraluminal mucin, demonstrated by Alcian blue at pH 2.5, is diagnostic of prostate carcinoma.

Q16

The absence of basal cells (morphologically and immunohistochemically) is diagnostic of prostate carcinoma.

Q17

Multiple tumor foci are not unusual in prostate cancer and are due to intraglandular tumor spread ('intraglandular metastases').

Q18

Perineural invasion found in a needle biopsy specimen is a good predictor of capsular invasion by the tumor.

Q19

In prostate adenocarcinoma the stroma surrounding neoplastic glands may show a combination of hypercellularity and deposition of a basophilic ground substance ('mucinous fibroplasia' or 'collagenous micronodules').

Q20

The presence of corpora amylacea rules out the diagnosis of adenocarcinoma of the prostate.

Q21

Atypical small acinar proliferation (ASAP) represents a morphologic entity that can be further classified as benign or malignant using immunostaining for high molecular weight cytokeratins.

Q22

Signet-ring cell carcinoma is a special subtype of prostate adenocarcinoma.

Q23

Primary transitional cell (urothelial) carcinoma of the prostate cannot usually be differentiated morphologically or immunohistochemically from urothelial carcinoma of the urinary bladder or urethra spreading into the prostate.

Q24

Mixed adenocarcinoma–transitional cell carcinoma of the prostate has been described.

Q25

CK7 and CD20 could be helpful in differentiating prostatic adenocarcinoma from urothelial carcinoma.

Q26

In contrast to PSA, expression of PSMA (prostate-specific membrane-bound glycoprotein) increases with progression from benign epithelium to high-grade PIN to adenocarcinoma.

Q27

Expression of CD57 (Leu7) in prostate adenocarcinoma indicates neuroendocrine differentiation.

Q28

In atypical acinar proliferation, expression of high molecular weight cytokeratin (as detected by 34βE12 or CK5/6 antibodies) rules out malignancy.

Q29

Prostatic carcinomas demonstrate expression of steroid receptors.

Q30

P504S is a marker that detects α-methylacyl-CoA racemase, which is expressed exclusively in adenocarcinoma of the prostate and therefore has great diagnostic value.

Q31

No specific molecular abnormalities have been found in prostate carcinoma.

Q32

Prostate carcinomas with neuroendocrine differentiation have a worse prognosis than those without.

Q33

Small cell carcinoma of the prostate is biologically similar to that of the lung.

Q34

Mucinous adenocarcinoma is defined as an adenocarcinoma of the prostate with abundant extracellular mucin in >50% of the tumor.

Q35

Signet-ring cell carcinoma of the prostate is diagnosed when more than 50% of the tumor is composed of signet-ring cells.

Q36

Adenosquamous carcinoma has been described after radiation therapy for prostate carcinoma.

Q37

Adenoid basal cell tumor is also known as adenoid cystic-like tumor.

Q38

Basaloid carcinoma is a low-grade carcinoma of the prostate.

Q39

Sarcomatoid carcinoma of the prostate may contain areas of cartilage and bone formation.

Q40

Prostatic intraepithelial neoplasia (PIN) is divided into three grades and two categories.

Q41

As in Gleason's grading of adenocarcinoma of the prostate, architectural features are the most important feature in grading prostatic intraepithelial neoplasia (PIN).

Q42

High-grade PIN can be differentiated from invasive carcinoma by the presence of basal cells.

Q43

Repeat prostatic biopsy is indicated in PIN grade 2.

Q44

The demonstration of acidic mucin is diagnostically helpful in differentiating atypical adenomatous hyperplasia from adenocarcinoma of the prostate, which can have a similar histologic appearance.

Q45

The presence of carcinoma in the TUR specimen may indicate spread from the peripheral zone.

Q46

Lobular atrophy is a lesion of the peripheral zone that is difficult to distinguish from adenocarcinoma.

Q47

High-grade adenocarcinomas of the prostate do not have benign mimics.

Q48

Radiation therapy of prostate adenocarcinoma may cause cytological atypia of the benign stroma and glands, which may be difficult to differentiate from residual adenocarcinoma.

Q49

Basal cell hyperplasia is limited to the transition zone.

Q50

Transitional cell hyperplasia is composed of stratified epithelium.

Q51

Cribriform hyperplasia or 'clear cell cribriform hyperplasia' can present a diagnostic problem in needle biopsy.

Q52

The basal cells of the prostate do not express the S-100 protein.

Q53

Nephrogenic adenoma is a lesion of the prostatic urethra.

Q54

Nephrogenic adenoma can mimic prostate adenocarcinoma.

Q55

No histologic features are helpful in distinguishing nephrogenic adenoma from adenocarcinoma of the prostate.

Q56

Post-atrophic hyperplasia refers to a crowded focus of small, atrophic glands that may have prominent nucleoli and mimic adenocarcinoma.

Q57

The incidence of invasion of the prostate capsule by adenocarcinoma correlates very positively with total tumor size and the percentage of high-grade tumor (Gleason grades 4 and 5).

Q58

The most common sites of prostate adenocarcinoma metastases are the lung and the liver.

Q59

Metastatic prostate carcinoma may mimic primary lung carcinoma.

Q60

Primary breast carcinoma can develop in prostatic carcinoma patients treated with estrogen.

Q61

The occult prostate carcinoma is that which is unsuspected clinically and found incidentally at autopsy or in prostatectomy biopsies performed for nodular hyperplasia or other benign disorders.

Q62

Gleason's score refers to the sum of the predominant histologic grade ('primary pattern') and the second most predominant histologic grade ('secondary pattern').

Q63

The therapeutic options for prostate carcinoma include radiation therapy, prostatectomy and hormonal manipulation.

Q64

Positive surgical margins in a prostatectomy specimen correlate with tumor progression in prostate carcinoma.

Q65

Stage for stage, black males have a higher mortality from prostatic carcinoma than white males.

Q66

In general, younger patients have more aggressive prostate carcinomas.

Q67

Prostate carcinomas diagnosed on TURP have higher rates of dissemination than those diagnosed by needle biopsy.

Q68

The preoperative PSA level is a proven prognostic factor in prostate carcinoma.

Q69

The histologic type of prostate carcinoma and DNA ploidy status of the tumor appear to be independent predictors of outcome.

Q70

The presence of perineural invasion is associated with a worse outcome in prostate carcinoma.

Q71

Alveolar rhabdomyosarcoma is the most common malignant tumor of the prostate in infancy and childhood.

Q72

Most patients with embryonal rhabdomyosarcoma die of their disease.

Q73

The histological appearance of embryonal rhabdomyosarcoma is nonspecific and hence the diagnosis is fully dependent on immunohistochemical studies.

Q74

Benign neoplasms of the adult prostate are more common than malignant tumors.

Q75

The most common primary lymphoma of the prostate is small lymphocytic lymphoma.

Q76

Prostate adenocarcinoma may be appreciated macroscopically as firm, solid areas that are yellowish in color, as shown here.

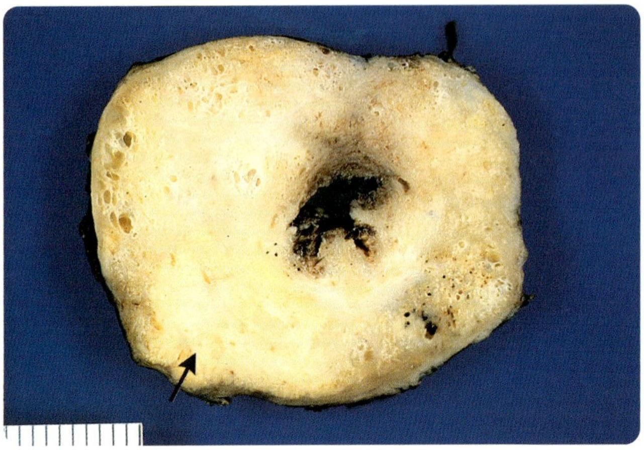

Fig. 18.5

Q77

Intraglandular crystalloid is illustrated. This finding is diagnostic of prostate adenocarcinoma and is usually present in high-grade tumors.

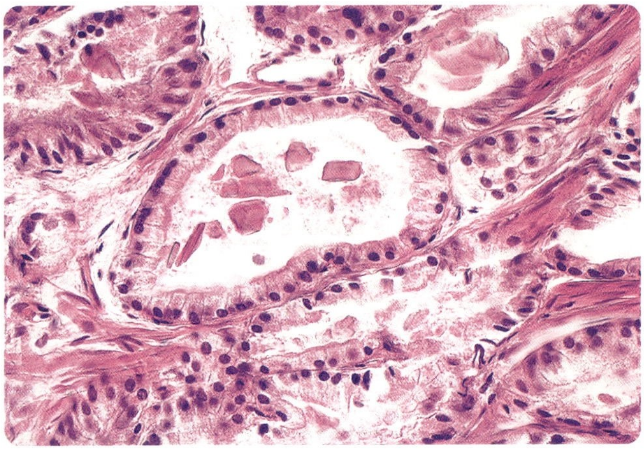

Fig. 18.6

Q78

Large prostate ducts involved by pagetoid spread of adenocarcinoma are shown.

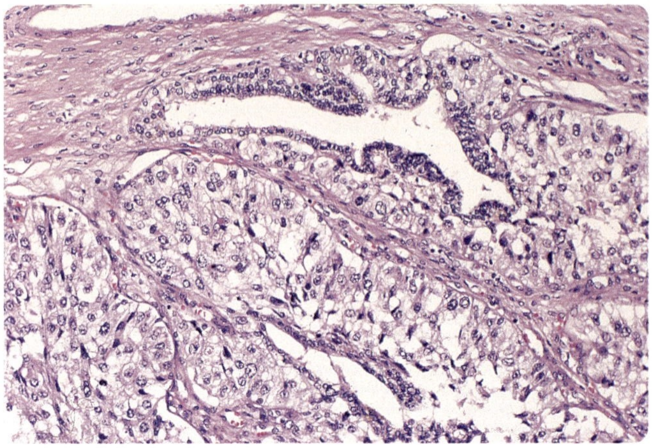

Fig. 18.7

Seminal vesicles and Cowper's glands

Q1

The cytoplasm of the epithelial cells in the seminal vesicles characteristically contains large amounts of lipofuscin pigment, by which this organ can always be distinguished from prostate tissue.

Q2

'Monstrous' cells are a common feature of the seminal vesicle epithelium and should not be confused with malignancy.

Q3

Amyloidosis of the seminal vesicle has been linked to hormonal treatment of prostate carcinoma.

Q4

Hyaline globules, which can be found in the muscular stroma of the seminal vesicles, have been linked to radiation treatment of prostate carcinoma.

Q5

Primary carcinomas of the seminal vesicles are PSA negative and show expression of CK7 and CA-125.

Q6

In contrast to nephrogenic adenoma, normal Cowper's glands in the prostate are easy to identify histologically.

TESTIS

Normal anatomy

Q1

The growth and development of the testis can be divided into three phases: static, growth, and development.

Q2

The age of the individual cannot be determined by histologic study of the testis.

Q3

The testis has a capsule that consists of three layers.

Q4

The mediastinum of the testis contains blood and lymph vessels and the mediastinal portion of the rete testis.

Q5

Each convoluted seminiferous tubule is surrounded by loose connective tissue to form a lobule of the testis.

Q6

Type B spermatogonia are stem cells.

Q7

Maturation arrest is diagnosed when not all stages of differentiation are found in the seminiferous tubule.

Q8

The degree of spermatogenesis in a testicular biopsy can be estimated by establishing the germ cell:Sertoli cell ratio and by counting spermatids per tubule cross-section.

Q9

Charcot–Bottcher crystalloids are found in Leydig cells.

Q10

Sertoli cells do not express cytokeratin and desmin, and therefore their tumors are typically negative for cytokeratin and desmin.

Q11

Cryptorchidism refers to a testis that is undescended at birth.

Q12

In adults, undescended testes are located outside the scrotum but are histologically normal.

Q13

A cryptorchid testis is twice as likely to develop a malignant neoplasm as a normally placed testis.

Q14

Testicular regression syndrome can develop post vasectomy.

Q15

Testicular biopsy is useful in the evaluation of the patient with infertility.

Q16

Open surgical biopsy provides much more information than punch biopsy of the testis in the evaluation of infertility.

Q17

Spermatocytic arrest is by far the most common finding in biopsy specimens from infertile men with azoospermia.

Q18

Generalized fibrosis of the testis is an exceptionally rare finding in testicular biopsies from infertile men with azoospermia.

QUESTIONS

Q19
Multinucleated giant stromal cells of a reactive nature have been observed in cases of testicular atrophy after radiation therapy.

Q20
Testes in Klinefelter's syndrome (XXY karyotype) characteristically show Leydig cell hyperplasia.

Q21
Hypogonadotrophic eunuchoidism is the most common diagnosis in biopsies done because of a lack of sperm count resulting from endocrine abnormalities.

Q22
In oligospermia the biopsy regularly shows 'sloughing and disorganization.'

Q23
Fine needle aspiration (FNA) biopsy is a minimally invasive test and may replace biopsy of the testis.

Q24
Infarcts of the testis usually result from torsion of the spermatic cord.

Q25
Granulomatous orchitis is often caused by mycobacterial infection.

Q26
Malakoplakia is secondary to bacterial infection of the testis.

Q27
Michaelis–Gutmann bodies are associated with juvenile xanthogranuloma.

Q28
Ectopic spleen can be found in the testis.

Q29
In cystic dysplasia, numerous irregular cystic spaces are found in the mediastinum testis.

Q30
Epidermoid cyst of the testis is most commonly found in patients over 50 years of age.

Q31
Epidermoid cyst of the testis may represent monodermal teratoma.

Q32
The microscopic features of epidermoid cyst are shown, but epidermoid cyst of the testis can be diagnosed by gross examination.

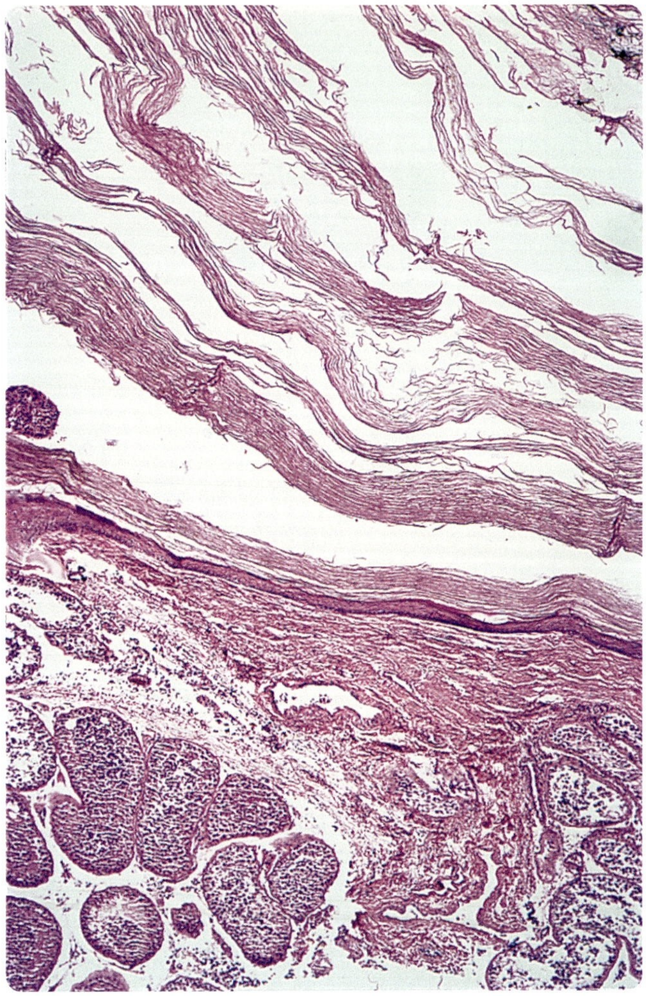

Fig. 18.8

Tumors

Q1
Germ cell tumors are the most common tumors of the testis.

Q2
Germ cell tumors are generally divided into seminoma and non-seminomatous germ cell tumors, both of which arise from the same precursor.

Q3

Non-seminomatous germ cell tumors are more aggressive than seminomas.

Q4

Spermatocytic seminoma is a relatively benign disease of old men and is frequently bilateral.

Q5

Grossly, classic seminoma frequently shows areas of cystic change, necrosis and hemorrhage.

Q6

Classic seminoma consists of large but uniform mononuclear cells with very prominent nucleoli.

Q7

A granulomatous reaction with Langhans'-type multinucleated giant cells and epithelioid cells may be present in classic seminoma.

Q8

PLAP immunoreactivity distinguishes classic seminoma from a poorly differentiated carcinoma.

Q9

Cytokeratin positivity rules out seminoma.

Q10

Seminoma is strongly positive for vimentin.

Q11

Spermatocytic seminoma, like classic seminoma, typically consists of tumor cells intermixed with small lymphocytes and is PLAP positive.

Q12

The histological finding of tubule formation in classic seminoma indicates the presence of a non-seminomatous component to the germ cell tumor, or the admixture of a sex cord–stromal tumor.

Q13

Classic seminomas show no specific molecular abnormalities.

Q14

Abundant glycogen is a typical finding in classic seminoma.

Q15

The presence of elevated serum hCG or AFP has no clinical significance in an otherwise histologically typical classic seminoma.

Q16

At presentation, about half of classic seminomas involve the entire testis, including the tunica albuginea.

Q17

When giant cells (hCG positive) are found in an otherwise classic seminoma, the tumor should be classified as classic seminoma and choriocarcinoma.

Q18

The anaplastic variant of spermatocytic seminoma is biologically similar to spermatocytic seminoma with a sarcomatous component.

Q19

Many of the features of anaplastic spermatocytic seminoma cause diagnostic difficulty, and in particular it may be difficult to distinguish this lesion from embryonal carcinoma with a solid growth pattern.

Q20

Grossly, embryonal carcinoma is gray or white and shows areas of hemorrhage and necrosis.

Q21

There are various histological patterns of growth of embryonal carcinoma.

Q22

The pure form of embryonal carcinoma is the most common.

Q23

Embryonal carcinoma, even when it grows in patterns resembling adenocarcinoma, can be distinguished from adenocarcinoma by immunophenotyping.

Q24

Teratomas of the testis are rare non-seminomatous germ cell tumors and are most common in very young children.

Q25

Teratomas of the testis are associated with several syndromes.

Q26

Dermoid cyst is the most common type of testicular teratoma.

Q27

Epidermoid cyst and dermoid cyst of the testis are synonyms.

Q28

Polyembryoma is a subtype of teratoma.

Q29

Teratocarcinoma refers to a teratoma with focal malignant transformation.

Q30

Choriocarcinoma is usually fatal if pure. Fortunately, this is very rarely the case.

Q31

The diagnosis of a choriocarcinoma requires the presence of a biphasic tumor that consists of both cytotrophoblast and syncytiotrophoblast.

Q32

Among germ cell tumors, cytokeratin 7 appears to be specific for choriocarcinoma.

Q33

Cytotrophoblasts have clear cytoplasm and bland nuclear features, whereas syncytiotrophoblasts are multinucleated cells with eosinophilic cytoplasm.

Q34

Yolk sac tumor, just like pure teratoma, is a tumor of small children (usually <2 years of age).

Q35

Schiller–Duval bodies are diagnostic of yolk sac tumor.

Q36

Hyaline intracytoplasmic and extracytoplasmic inclusions are consistently seen in yolk sac tumors.

Q37

Immunohistochemical demonstration of cytoplasmic expression of AFP is useful in the diagnosis of yolk sac tumor.

Q38

Intratubular germ cell neoplasia is a germ cell neoplasm in situ and is frequently found in the testes of elderly men without any other pathologic findings.

Q39

The microscopic appearance of intratubular germ cell neoplasia depends on the type of associated invasive germ cell tumor.

Q40

Intratubular germ cell neoplasia is infrequently found with teratomas and other germ cell tumors in very young children.

Q41

Germ cell tumors in the mediastinum are not associated with intratubular germ cell neoplasia of the testis.

Q42

When atypical germ cells are present at the base of the seminiferous tubules only, this type of intratubular germ cell neoplasia is designated as 'unclassified.'

Q43

Intratubular germ cell neoplasia shows immunoreactivity for PLAP and CD117.

Q44

Chromosomal aberrations are rare in germ cell tumors.

Q45

Fas gene mutations are common in yolk sac tumors.

Q46

Chromosome 12 abnormalities designate progression of germ cell neoplasms because they are not present in intratubular germ cell neoplasia, and are seen only in invasive germ cell tumors.

Q47

In germ cell tumors it is very common for metastases to have a different histological appearance from the primary tumor.

Q48

The microscopic appearance of lung metastases after treatment is associated with prognosis.

Q49

Chemotherapy is widely used for the treatment of germ cell tumors.

Q50

The prognosis of germ cell tumors is excellent.

Q51

Serum levels of hCG, AFP and LDH are usually detected in patients with germ cell tumors, but these levels do not correlate with the clinical prognosis.

Q52

Regardless of histological type, both extension of the tumor through the tunica vaginalis and into the spermatic cord, and vascular invasion adversely influence prognosis.

Q53

Sex cord–stromal cell tumors are derived from somatic cells, including Sertoli/granulose cells of sex cord origin and Leydig/theca–lutein cells of mesenchymal origin.

Q54

PLAP is the most useful marker to distinguish between germ cell tumors and sex cord–stromal cell tumors.

Q55

All sex cord–stromal cell tumors show expression of α-inhibin.

Q56

Micronodules of Leydig cells are frequently seen in certain conditions associated with severe decrease of spermatogenesis or germinal aplasia, such as the so-called Sertoli cell-only syndrome (Del Castillo syndrome), cryptorchidism and Klinefelter syndrome.

Q57

Leydig cell tumors are frequently accompanied by Leydig cell hyperplasia.

Q58

About half of Leydig cell tumors are malignant.

Q59

Malignant Leydig cell tumors usually occur in children.

Q60

Leydig cell tumors usually produce testosterone and may cause gynecomastia.

Q61

The diagnosis of malignant Leydig cell tumor cannot be made histologically. As in adrenal tumors, only the presence of metastatic disease indicates malignant biology.

Q62

Malignant Leydig cell tumors are hormonally active.

Q63

Adrenal rests in the testis are hormonally active, secrete androgens, and may resemble Leydig cell tumors or hyperplasia.

Q64

Leydig cell tumors may occur in Carney complex.

Q65

Sertoli cell tumors are frequently found in association with two distinct multiple neoplasm syndromes, Carney complex and Peutz–Jeghers syndrome.

Q66

Sertoli cell tumors in Peutz–Jeghers syndrome can be difficult to distinguish from those found in Carney complex on the basis of histology.

Q67

Sclerosing Sertoli cell tumors are small and show no endocrine activity.

Q68

Sertoli cell tumors are classified as large cell calcifying, sex-cord tumors with annular tubules, sclerosing, and Sertoli cell tumors, not otherwise specified (NOS).

Q69

Sertoli cell adenomas are associated with testicular feminization.

Q70

As in granulosa cell tumors, the neoplastic cells of Sertoli cell tumors express α-inhibin, CD99, and antimüllerian hormone.

Q71

Sertoli cell hyperplasia occurs in cryptorchid testes.

Q72

10% of Sertoli cell tumors are malignant.

Q73

Large cell calcifying Sertoli cell tumor is S-100 positive.

Q74

In Sertoli–Leydig cell tumors Leydig cells are prominent and a pronounced stromal component distinguishes it from pure Sertoli cell tumors.

Q75

Juvenile granulosa cell tumor of the testis occurs in first few months after birth.

QUESTIONS

Q76

Adult-type granulosa cell tumor of the testis is a very rare disease.

Q77

Sex cord–stromal tumors and germ cell tumors are always EMA negative, which is useful in the differential diagnosis from (adeno)carcinoma.

Q78

Gonadoblastoma is a mixed germ cell–sex cord–stromal tumor.

Q79

Malignant lymphoma is the most common testicular tumor in elderly persons.

Q80

Diffuse large B-cell lymphoma is by far the most common type of malignant lymphoma of the testis.

Q81

Leukemic involvement of the testis is most common in acute myeloid leukemia.

Q82

Primary carcinoid tumors of the testis are associated with carcinoid syndrome because they produce serotonin.

Q83

The presence of sarcomatoid morphology in a testicular tumor should first prompt consideration of a Sertoli cell tumor or spermatocytic seminoma.

Q84

Lung and prostate are the two most common primary tumors to give rise to testicular metastases.

Q85

The gross appearance of embryonal carcinoma is shown.

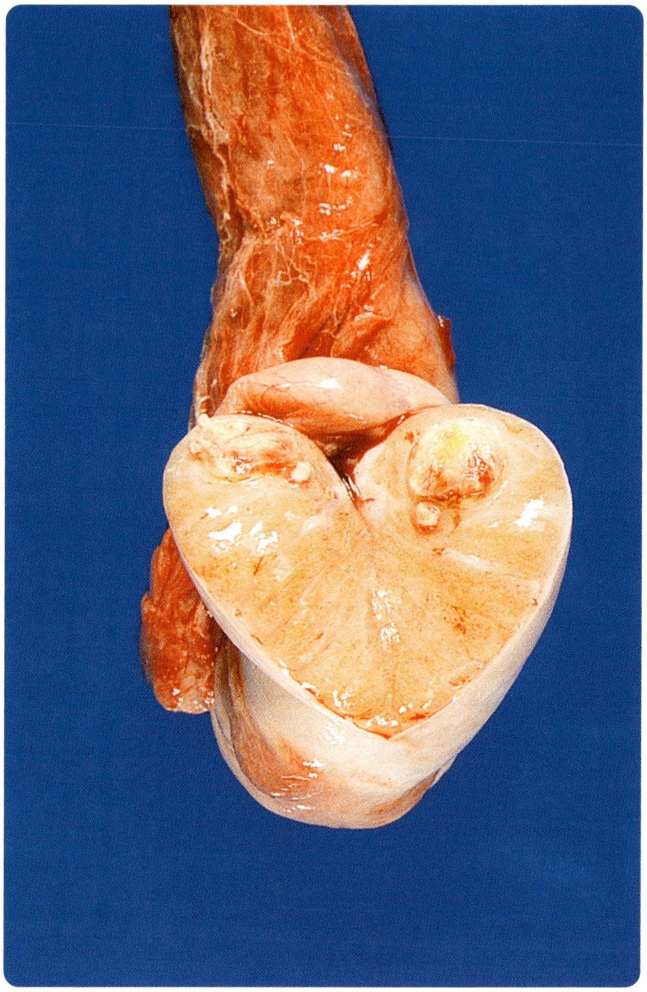

Fig. 18.9

Q86

Classic seminoma is shown. Tumor cells are seen admixed with smaller lymphocytes.

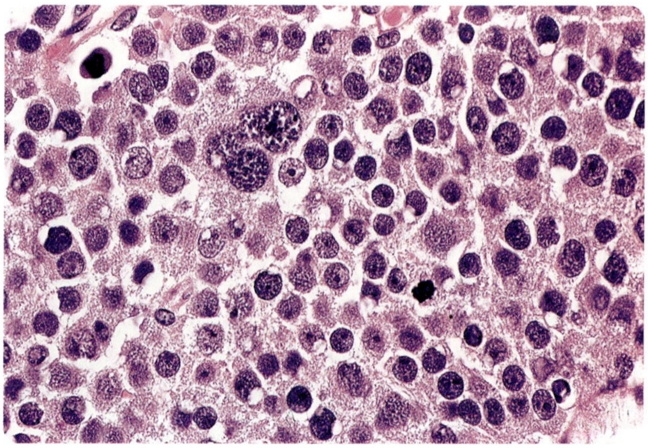

Fig. 18.10

Q87

A Schiller–Duval body in a yolk sac tumor of the testis is illustrated.

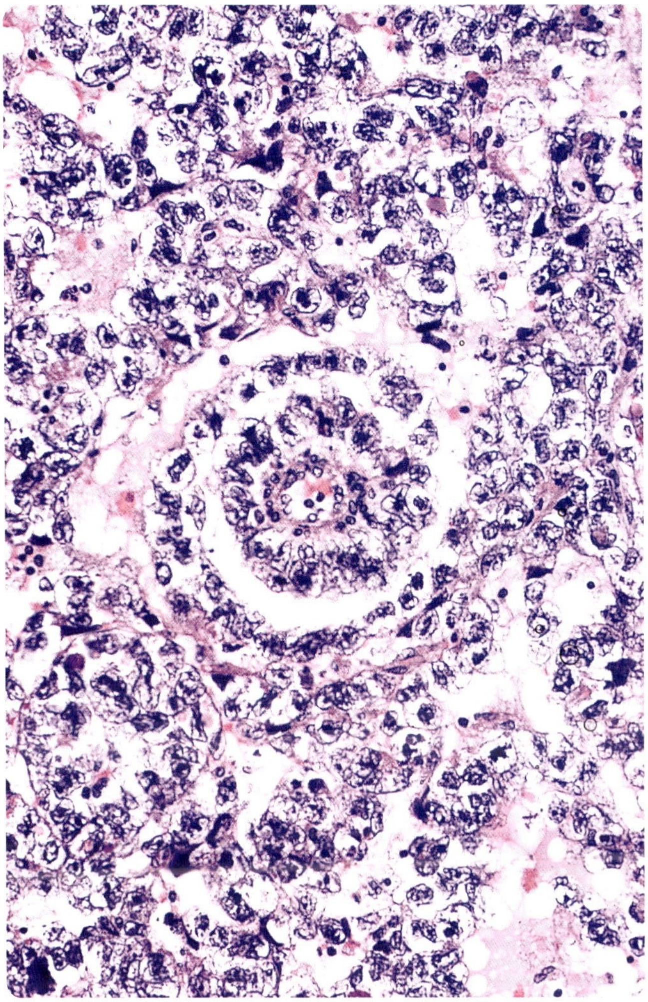

Fig. 18.11

Q88

Melanoma of the testis is shown.

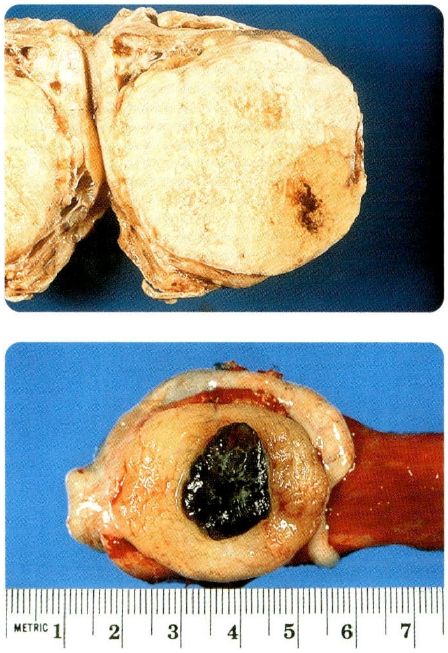

A

B

Fig. 18.12

TESTICULAR ADNEXA

Non-neoplastic lesions

Q1

The rete testis has three components: septal, mediastinal and extratesticular.

Q2

The rete testis empties into the ductuli afferentes.

Q3

The epididymis connects the ductuli efferentes with the vas deferens.

Q4

The epithelium of the epididymis shows four types of cell: tall columnar cells with cilia, narrow darker-staining columnar cells, basal cells and clear cells.

Q5

The vas deferens connects the epididymis to the prostatic urethra.

Q6

The appendix testis is attached to the tunica vaginalis at the lower pole of the testis.

Q7

The appendix epididymis is a remnant of the caudal portion of the müllerian duct.

Q8

The vas aberrans and paradidymis are remnants of the mesonephric tubules.

Q9

Rete testis dysgenesis is sometimes present in cryptorchid testes.

Q10

Cystic dilatation of the rete testis is present as a secondary change due to obstruction of the epididymis by varicocele.

Q11

Adenomatous hyperplasia of the rete testis is usually an incidental finding in testes removed for prostate carcinoma.

Q12

Adenomatous hyperplasia of the rete testis may show hyaline globules, simulating the appearance of yolk sac tumor.

Q13

Adenocarcinoma of the rete testis can originate in a cystadenoma of the rete testis.

Q14

Chlamydial epididymitis tends to be destructive and abscess forming.

Q15

Tuberculosis of the epididymis may occur as a result of hematogenous spread or spread from the prostate. The latter usually spares the tail of the epididymis and the vas deferens.

Q16

Spermatic granuloma is clinically silent.

Q17

Granulomatous ischemic lesions involve the tail of the epididymis.

Q18

The typical gross appearance of adenomatoid tumor of the epididymis is illustrated.

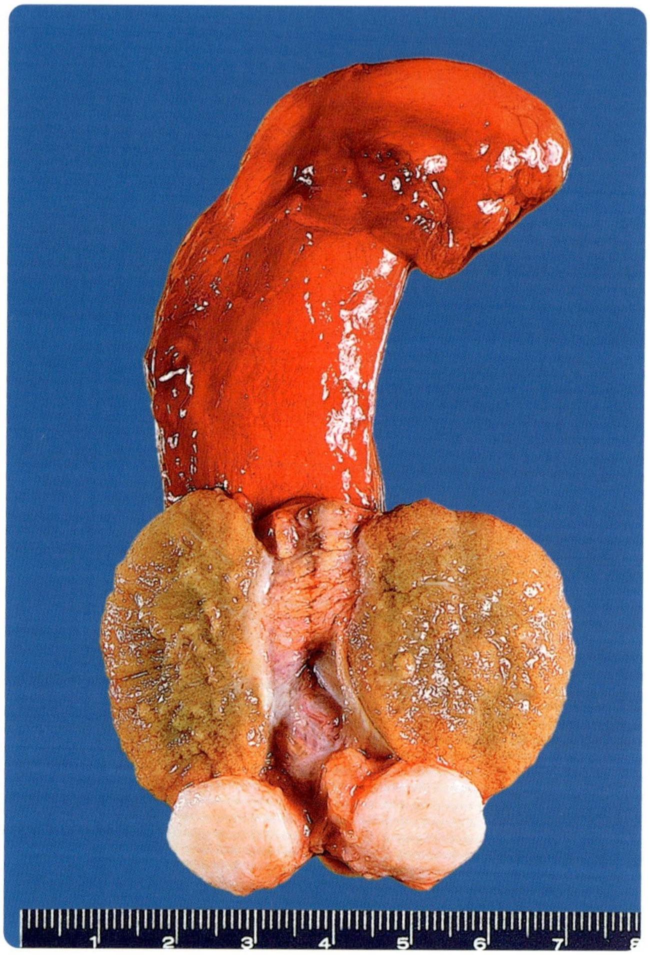

Fig. 18.13

Tumors

Q1

Adenomatoid tumor is the most common tumor of the epididymis.

Q2

Adenomatoid tumor of the epididymis is a large, but well circumscribed and encapsulated, benign tumor.

Q3

Adenomatoid tumor frequently shows vacuolization of the cytoplasm and may simulate vascular tumors.

Q4

Mesothelioma has been described in the same region(s) as adenomatoid tumor.

Q5

Papillary cystadenoma of the epididymis occurs in Carney complex.

Q6

Papillary cystadenoma of the epididymis can be either cystic or solid.

Q7

Torsion of the spermatic cord may cause testicular infarct.

Q8

Vasitis nodosa is a condition related to polyarteritis nodosa of the vas deferens.

Q9

Inguinal herniorrhaphy may be associated with proliferative funiculitis.

Q10

Lipoma is the most common tumor of the spermatic cord.

Q11

Well-differentiated liposarcoma is the most frequent malignant tumor of the spermatic cord in children.

Q12

Leiomyosarcoma of the paratesticular region and desmoplastic small round cell tumor of the same locale occur in patients in the same age group.

PENIS AND SCROTUM

Penis

Normal anatomy

Q1

The penis consists of the corpus, glans and prepuce.

Q2

'*Dartos*' is an elastic sheet that separates the penis into dorsal and ventral portions.

Q3

The male urethra is divided into two parts, prostatic and penile.

Q4

The *fossa navicularis* is the part of the prostatic urethra immediately distal to the verumontanum.

Q5

The urethra is lined by transitional epithelium.

Q6

Cowper's glands are present along the full length of the corpus spongiosum.

Non-neoplastic lesions

Q1

Median raphe cyst of the glans is a mucoid, cystic dilatation of the small accessory urethral canal present in the central aspect of the glans.

Q2

Mucoid cyst of the prepuce or glans penis is lined by stratified columnar epithelium.

Q3

Mucinous metaplasia is usually seen in the elderly and is associated with severe chronic inflammation.

Q4

Inflammation of Littré's glands may clinically simulate a penile tumor.

Q5

The inflammatory infiltrate of primary syphilis is characterized by a granulomatous reaction to spirochetes.

Q6

Granulomatous inflammation due to tuberculosis may present clinically as penile nodules.

Q7

The simultaneous appearance of genital and oral ulcers should prompt consideration of Behçet's disease.

Q8

Peyronie's disease is a form of localized fibromatosis.

Q9

Almost all polypoid lesions of the male urethra are examples of condyloma acuminatum.

Q10

Almost all HPV-related lesions of the penis are polypoid.

Q11

HPV-related lesions of the penis are characteristically associated with typical viral cytopathic effects in the form of koilocytosis.

Q12

Pearly penile plaques are associated with HPV infection.

Tumors

Q1

Bowen's disease and erythroplasia of Queyrat are both squamous cell carcinoma in situ.

Q2

Squamous cell carcinoma in situ of the penis is treated by penectomy.

Q3

Bowen's disease and bowenoid papulosis are the same disease.

Q4

Circumcision done shortly after birth protects against squamous cell carcinoma of the penis.

Q5

Most squamous cell carcinomas of the penis arise in the glans.

Q6

Generally, endophytic squamous cell carcinoma of the penis is better differentiated than exophytic squamous cell carcinoma.

Q7

Squamous cell carcinoma of the penis is divided into usual type, warty (condylomatous), verrucous, and papillary NOS.

Q8

By definition, verrucous carcinoma is – at least focally – a grade I tumor.

Q9

Basaloid carcinoma of the penis is clinically similar to basal cell carcinoma.

Q10

Vascular invasion is the most important predictor of outcome in squamous cell carcinoma of the penis.

Q11

Microscopic type, but not microscopic grade, is a prognostic factor in squamous cell carcinoma of the penis.

Q12

Paget's disease may be difficult to differentiate from malignant melanoma or Bowen's disease.

Q13

Leiomyoma is common in the male urethra.

Q14

Transitional cell carcinoma is the most frequent malignancy of the male urethra.

Q15

The prognosis and treatment of urethral carcinoma depend greatly on the histological type of the malignancy.

Q16

Malignant melanoma of the urethra is typically polypoid.

Q17

Hirsutoid papillomas are HPV-related changes on the corona of the glans.

Q18

Bowen's disease is illustrated.

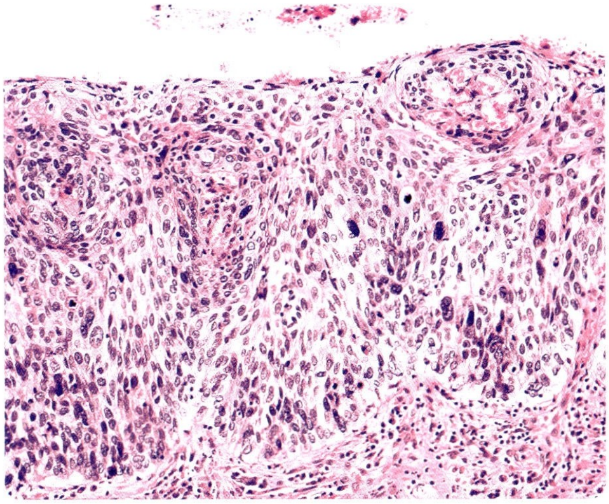

Fig. 18.14

Q19

Verrucous carcinoma of the penis is illustrated.

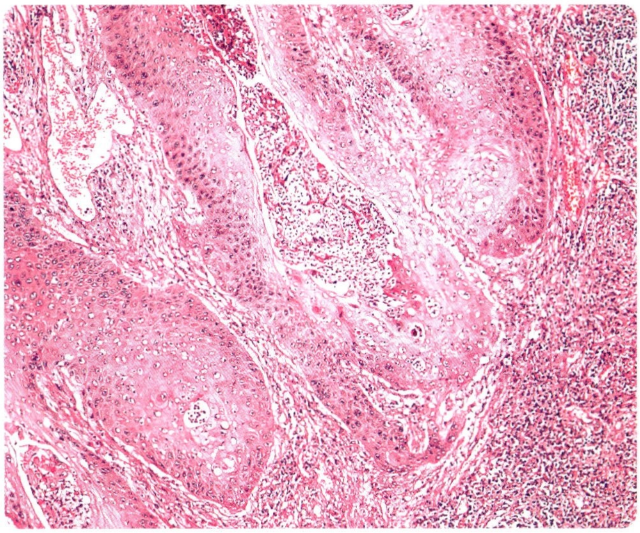

Fig. 18.15

Scrotum

Non-neoplastic lesions

Q1

Hydroceles are differentiated from spermatoceles by the type of cyst lining.

Q2

Idiopathic calcinosis of the scrotum is associated with hypercalcemia.

Q3

Fibrous pseudotumor is a form of fibromatosis of the scrotum.

Q4

Some cases of fibrous pseudotumor are examples of solitary fibrous tumor.

Q5

Sclerosing granuloma of the scrotum is an example of fat necrosis of unknown etiology.

Q6

Crohn's disease can manifest in the scrotum.

Q7

In patients with hematological malignancy, chemotherapy can cause Fournier's gangrene of the scrotum.

Tumors

Q1

Most scrotal tumors are benign cutaneous tumors.

Q2

Aggressive angiomyxoma is a well-circumscribed tumor with a high rate of metastases.

Q3

Squamous cell carcinoma of the scrotum is rare.

Q4

Malignant mesothelioma is the most common malignant tumor of the tunica dartos.

Q5

Angiomyofibroblastoma is positive for PR, ER, CD34, desmin and actin.

QUESTIONS

Q6

Fat necrosis of the scrotum is illustrated.

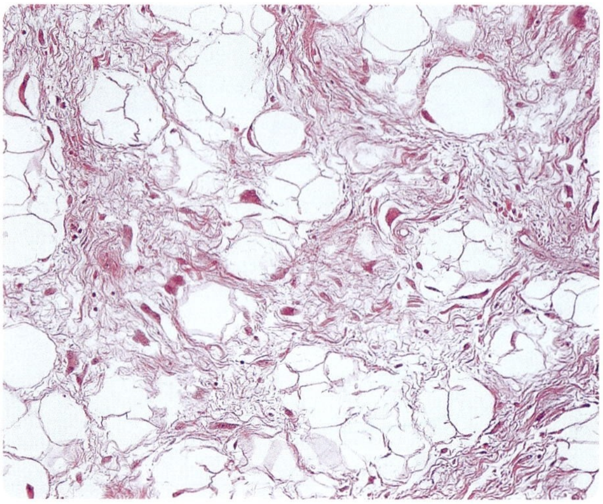

Fig. 18.16

PROSTATE

Normal anatomy

A1. False
The prostate consists of the peripheral zone, transitional zone, periurethral zone and central zone. **(p. 1361)**

A2. True
The 'prostatic capsule' consists of a fibromuscular layer most prominent along the base and posterior portion of the lateral borders, and is an inseparable component of the prostatic stroma. **(p. 1361)**

A3. True
Biochemical tests are used for prostate carcinoma screening in the general population, and also for follow-up of patients with a known diagnosis of prostate carcinoma. This marker is widely used to confirm the prostatic origin of metastatic carcinoma of unknown primary origin. **(p. 1362)**

A4. False
PAP is widely used for diagnostic work-up of tumors of unknown primary origin, but is less specific than PSA and is not used as a biochemical marker of prostate carcinoma. **(p. 1362)**

A5. True
This is important as carcinomas usually produce acid mucins, which are occasionally secreted into the lumina of the carcinomatous glands and will stain blue with Alcian blue histochemical stain. This may be of diagnostic help. **(p. 1362)**

A6. True
In addition, scattered neuroendocrine cells are also present. **(p. 1362)**

A7. False
It is believed that both are terminally differentiated cells originating from the same precursor, i.e. the stem cells located in the basal cell epithelial compartment. **(p. 1362)**

A8. True
However, the basal layer may become discontinuous in some benign diseases of the prostate. **(p. 1362)**

A9. False
Only secretory cells of the prostate express PSA. Also, basal cells do not express PAP. **(p. 1362)**

A10. True
In addition, the basal cells – but not secretory cells – show nuclear expression of p63. **(p. 1362)**

A11. False
The cells of prostate carcinoma may be positive for high molecular weight cytokeratins, including CK5/6 and 34βE12, and it is the presence of basal cells that can be identified in the prostate acini and small ducts which rules out the diagnosis of malignancy. **(p. 1362)**

A12. True
Interestingly, they do not express androgen receptor. **(p. 1362)**

A13. False
The difference is that the large ducts lined by transitional epithelium do not have umbrella cells on the surface, but rather are lined by a single layer of columnar cells that are immunoreactive for both PSA and PAP. These may give rise to primary transitional carcinoma of the prostate. **(p. 1362)**

A14. True
It also is hormonally regulated and regularly expresses androgen receptors. Although estrogen receptors (both α and β) and progesterone receptors can also be found, these are generally expressed to a much lesser degree. **(p. 1362)**

A15. False
Normal prostate does not contain any myoepithelial cells. However, S-100-positive cells that resemble myoepithelial cells may be found in the rare condition known as 'sclerosing adenosis of the prostate.' **(p. 1362)**

Non-neoplastic disorders

A1. False
Ectopic prostate tissue can be found in the seminal vesicles, retrovesical space, urinary bladder, epididymis, testis and other organs, but it is a very rare phenomenon. **(p. 1362)**

A2. False
Nodular hyperplasia (or benign prostatic hypertrophy) is a disease of the periurethral and transitional zones of the prostate. **(p. 1363)**

A3. True
This number increases to 75% by the eighth decade. **(p. 1362)**

A4. False
Nodular hyperplasia is an androgen-dependent process, and even though it is one of the most common diseases of men no predisposing factors have been identified. **(p. 1362)**

A5. False
p27 protein (a cell cycle inhibitor) is not expressed in nodular hyperplasia but is regularly detected in the normal prostate. **(p. 1363)**

A6. False
In BPH both protein levels and mRNA levels of this gene are low, whereas in prostate carcinoma only protein levels are low. Epidemiological and genetic studies show no association between these two disorders. **(p. 1374)**

A7. False

The periurethral and transitional zones enlarge and push aside the peripheral zone, which is involved by BPH only in a very small number of cases. **(p. 1363)**

A8. True

The content of smooth muscle in these nodules varies depending on their 'maturation.' Very early lesions are very vascular and have scant smooth muscle, whereas more mature nodules are larger, richer in smooth muscle and less vascular. **(p. 1363)**

A9. True

It appears that stromal hyperplasia induces glandular hyperplasia. Several studies have showed possible roles for IGF2, FGF7, PGR and other molecules that function in growth regulation and differentiation. The upregulated signaling molecules in BPH all appeared to be expressed in the prostatic stroma more than in the epithelium. **(p. 1363)**

A10. False

The role of the mild chronic perivascular inflammatory infiltrate, which is commonly found in prostates with BPH, is not known. The diagnosis of chronic prostatitis is not warranted merely by the presence of this infiltrate. **(p. 1363)**

A11. False

It was found that symptomatic patients have significantly higher ratios of stromal-to-epithelial hyperplasia. However, the total weight/size of the gland shows no direct correlation with the degree of obstruction. **(p. 1364)**

A12. False

The risk of prostate adenocarcinoma is not reduced by TUR, which only removes newly formed tissues in the periurethral and transitional zones and not in the peripheral zone, where 80% of carcinomas arise. **(p. 1364)**

A13. True

In about 20% of prostates with BPH microscopic examination reveals the presence of infarcted tissue. **(p. 1364)**

A14. False

By definition, the prostate stroma should also be necrotic. As with infarcts, 'glandular necrosis only' may also be found in BPH, but it is not caused by ischemic necrosis. **(p. 1364)**

A15. True

Squamous metaplasia at the periphery of the infarct should not be confused with squamous cell carcinoma. **(p. 1364)**

A16. True

However, in some cases pre-existing urinary obstruction may become more severe owing to the development of edema around the urethra, whereas in others the infarct may cause gross hematuria. **(p. 1364)**

A17. False

There are four clinical entities of prostatitis: acute bacterial, chronic bacterial, non-bacterial (or abacterial) and prostatodynia. **(p. 1365)**

A18. True

Gram-positive bacteria are the most common pathogens in cultures from the prostatic fluid. Some cases follow urethral catheterization or gonococcal urethritis. **(p. 1365)**

A19. True

The acutely inflamed prostate is swollen and enlarged, warm, firm, and very tender. Both vigorous massage and biopsy may cause bacteremia and sepsis and should therefore be avoided. **(p. 1365)**

A20. False

Neutrophils are usually confined to the glands. The prostatic stroma is usually infiltrated by lymphocytes, macrophages and plasma cells. The number of eosinophils is usually very low to absent. **(p. 1365)**

A21. False

'Eosinophilic prostatitis' is a term used for four conditions: 'iatrogenic granuloma,' which occurs after TURP or other surgical procedures and has no systemic symptoms; 'allergic granuloma of the prostate,' usually with a history of asthma or allergy and associated with peripheral eosinophilia, elevated PSA levels, and occasionally vasculitis; secondary to infestation by metazoa; and 'granulomatous prostatitis.' **(p. 1366)**

A22. False

'Granulomatous prostatitis' is an immune-mediated inflammatory reaction to prostate secretions released into the prostate tissue by rupture of obstructed ducts. Therefore, it is most commonly seen in nodular hyperplasia. **(p. 1366)**

A23. False

In the prostate involved by tuberculosis there is very little tendency to form classic granulomas. Rather, the findings of large areas of caseous necrosis and frequent cavitation are typical for the prostate involved by tuberculosis. However, well-formed granulomas may be found in patients treated with intravesical bacillus Calmette–Guérin (BCG) for bladder carcinoma. **(p. 1365)**

A24. True

These infections are more common in patients with AIDS or other immunodeficiences. Dimorphic fungi usually reach the prostate by hematogenous dissemination. **(p. 1366)**

A25. False

Currently, abscesses of the prostate, which can be detected on digitorectal examination as fluctuation of the prostatic tissue, are most commonly caused by *Escherichia coli* secondary to urinary tract obstruction. Historically, it was often due to gonorrhea. **(p. 1365)**

A26. False

Although it is true that prostate stones are radio-opaque and easily seen on plain X-rays, only 15–20% of gallstones are visible on plain radiographs. **(p. 1367)**

A27. True
There is no evidence that patients with renal/bladder stones or gallbladder stones have a higher incidence of prostate stones. **(p. 1367)**

A28. True
Macroscopically nodular hyperplasia is characteristically nodular, microcystic and focally solid. **(p. 1363)**

A29. False
Squamous cell carcinoma is a rare lesion in the prostate. Shown in this image is squamous metaplasia at the edge of an infarct, which is a common finding. **(p. 1365)**

A30. False
Granulomatous prostatitis is not caused by mycobacterial infection. **(p. 1366)**

Tumor-like conditions of prostate and prostatic urethra

A1. False
Inflammatory pseudotumor (also known as pseudosarcomatous fibromyxoid tumor of the prostate) is not temporally related to surgical manipulation of prostate tissue, but may share some histological and immunohistochemical characteristics with postoperative spindle cell nodule, as both appear to be of myofibroblastic origin. **(p. 1367)**

A2. True
However, postoperative spindle cell nodule is also strongly positive for cytokeratin in up to 20% of cases, which is not the case with inflammatory pseudotumor. ALK-1 may be expressed in inflammatory pseudotumors. **(p. 1367)**

A3. False
Postoperative spindle cell nodule – unlike inflammatory pseudotumor – generally shows higher mitotic counts (up to 25/10 hpf and up to 50% of cells Ki-67+) and significant cytological atypia. Also, inflammatory pseudotumor is usually a much larger lesion than postoperative spindle cell nodule. However, the history of a recent operative procedure is the most important discriminator. **(p. 1367)**

A4. True
Postoperative spindle cell nodule, more often than inflammatory pseudotumor, may resemble malignant sarcomas. Most often, postoperative spindle cell nodule resembles leiomyosarcoma, but Kaposi's sarcoma should be excluded in cases of postoperative spindle cell nodule with prominent extravasation. **(p. 1367)**

A5. True
In stromal nodules with or without atypia in BPH, as well as in leiomyoma with atypia, androgen receptor is positive. Conversely, it is negative in inflammatory pseudotumor and postoperative spindle cell nodules. S-100 and NSE are positive in stromal nodules of BPH without atypia, and pan-cytokeratin is positive in some postoperative spindle cell nodules. Desmin and actin are variable in all of the above and are not helpful. ALK-1 expression would strongly favor inflammatory pseudotumor. **(p. 1367)**

A6. True
These are the patterns that may be seen in inflammatory pseudotumor in any organ in the body. Although the most common pattern is nodular fasciitis-like, most often a mixture of patterns is found. **(p. 1367)**

A7. True
The columnar epithelium of urethral polyps is strongly PSA and PAP positive. This is a relatively common cause of hematuria in young males. **(p. 1367)**

A8. False
Urethral polyps once were thought to represent ectopic prostate tissue, but it is currently believed that they are hyperplastic–metaplastic in nature. True prostatic ectopic tissue is found in the urachal remnants, bladder trigone, root of the penis and pericolic fat. **(p. 1367)**

A9. True
Histologically, this lesion looks like blue nevus of the skin. **(p. 1368)**

A10. True
This is a rare condition in patients with agnogenic myeloid metaplasia. However, the prostate may also be involved by granulocytic sarcoma, chronic lymphocytic leukemia and other hematological diseases. **(p. 1368)**

A11. False
Cytokeratin is typically also expressed in postoperative spindle cell nodules. **(p. 1367)**

Carcinoma

A1. False

Despite screening, carcinoma of the prostate is responsible for 10% of all deaths in men, and it is second only to lung carcinoma as the leading cause of cancer-related death. **(p. 1368)**

A2. True

Eunuchs castrated before puberty never develop prostate carcinoma. Patients with high estrogen levels resulting from liver cirrhosis infrequently develop prostate carcinoma. **(p. 1368)**

A3. False

No association has been found with smoking, venereal diseases, diet, occupational exposure or sexual habits. **(p. 1368)**

A4. False

It is well known that prostate carcinoma is a disease of aging men and is more common in the black population. However, whereas prostate carcinoma is relatively common in nodular hyperplasia there is no evidence that patients with nodular hyperplasia have a higher risk of developing prostate carcinoma. They are found together because they are both common disorders of the prostate in aging men. **(p. 1368)**

A5. False

Transrectal ultrasonography detects about 70% of prostate carcinomas as hypoechoic lesions. However, 30% of lesions are isoechoic and are missed by this method. **(p. 1369)**

A6. True

However, other lesions, such as prostatitis, infarct of the prostate or recent trauma (surgical or not), may also cause transitory elevations of PSA, which should resolve with treatment. Importantly, >50% of men with PSA values >10 ng/mL have disease beyond the prostate. **(p. 1369)**

A7. False

Although different clinical centers may have different protocols for the management of patients with increased PSA levels, it is worth noting that 20% of patients with histologically proven prostate carcinoma have PSA levels <4 ng/mL. **(p. 1369)**

A8. True

However, adenocarcinoma originating in the large ducts accounts for <1% of carcinomas of the prostate. It has been previously known as 'endometrioid carcinoma of the prostate' because of its histological similarities to endometrial carcinoma. **(p. 1369)**

A9. False

Most of these adenocarcinomas arise in the peripheral zone, and for some reason have difficulty crossing the boundary between the peripheral and transitional zones, thereby selectively 'avoiding' the transitional zone. Only very large tumors, most of which are already metastatic, cross into the transitional zone. **(p. 1369)**

A10. True

However, it is very important to understand that in many cases it is not possible to identify the tumor grossly. Therefore, a large number of sections are needed in prostatectomy specimens so as not to underestimate the tumor's volume and stage, which are the most important prognostic factors in this carcinoma. **(p. 1369)**

A11. True

This statement summarizes all the other features that are used to discriminate between Gleason grades 1–3 (low-grade tumor) and grades 4–5 (high-grade tumor). Furthermore, regular glandular units may be large (usually grade 2) or small (usually grade 3), whereas irregular glandular units demonstrate a large number of variants (cribriform, glomeruloid, papillary etc.). **(p. 1370)**

A12. True

Under the Gleason's grading system, which currently holds international recommendation, cytological features are not important. WHO grading, which takes into account the nuclear features of the neoplastic cells, is no longer in use. **(p. 1371)**

A13. False

Cytological features are often crucial for the correct diagnosis of prostate carcinoma, especially in small biopsies, small tumor foci and in unusual histological types (e.g. adenocarcinoma with atrophic features, pseudohyperplastic prostatic adenocarcinoma etc.). **(p. 1370)**

A14. False

Intraluminal crystalloids are highly suggestive of prostate adenocarcinoma. These are usually found in Gleason grade 2 carcinoma (low-grade tumors) and are almost never found in metastatic prostate carcinoma. However, they have also been described in benign lesions. **(p. 1371)**

A15. False

The presence of intraluminal mucin, which can be demonstrated by Alcian blue at pH 2.5, is highly suggestive of malignancy and is usually present in Gleason grade 4 carcinoma (high-grade tumors). However, it has rarely been found in benign prostate tissue. **(p. 1371)**

A16. False

The absence of basal cells favors the diagnosis of adenocarcinoma. However, true absence of basal cells has been described focally in atypical adenomatous hyperplasia. Scattered circumferential loss of basal cell staining in morphologically benign glands (average, two to three glands) is not unusual and can be seen in 15–30% of cases, depending on the antibody used for their detection. **(p. 1373)**

A17. False

Multiple tumor foci are frequent, but are currently believed to represent true multicentricity rather than intraglandular spread. This is supported by their genetic heterogeneity, and also by the fact that they are more common in early prostate carcinoma, rather than in tumors with large volume. **(p. 1371)**

A18. True

However, perineural glandular tissue per se is not indicative of malignancy as the presence of benign glands in perineural spaces has also been described. **(p. 1371)**

A19. True

Interestingly, most often there is no obvious stromal response to invasive adenocarcinoma in the prostate tissue. **(p. 1371)**

A20. False

It used to be dogma that the finding of corpora amylacea was not compatible with the diagnosis of adenocarcinoma. Unfortunately, this is not the case. **(p. 1371)**

A21. False

Up to 5% of prostate needle biopsies may have small foci suspicious for, but not diagnostic of, adenocarcinoma which cannot be resolved by using immunohistochemistry. This finding warrants a second biopsy. **(p. 1371)**

A22. True

However, this is basically adenocarcinoma of small ducts and acini, Gleason grade 4. **(p. 1376)**

A23. True

However, in most cases it is possible clinically to determine the origin of the tumor. Also, primary urothelial carcinoma of the prostate does not demonstrate 'umbrella cells.' Primary urinary bladder transitional carcinomas may show immunoreactivity for PAP and PSA as the tumor spreads into the prostate. The latter is likely induced by the prostatic stroma through the mechanism of mesenchymal-epithelial interaction. **(p. 1372)**

A24. True

This rare lesion has been described under the name 'prostatic adenocarcinoma with urothelial (transitional cell) carcinoma features.' Most patients present with high-stage disease. **(p. 1372)**

A25. True

However, the findings are useful only for those tumors that show either both markers positive (urothelial carcinoma) or both markers negative (prostate carcinoma). PSA and PAP are also useful in this setting (see Question 22). **(p. 1373)**

A26. False

Adenocarcinoma of the prostate secretes about 10 times more PSA than benign prostate tissue. However, the most undifferentiated (highest grade) prostate adenocarcinomas and metastatic prostate adenocarcinomas may lose expression of PSA, which is usually not the case with PSMA. However, immunohistochemical detection of PSMA has not become routine practice in most laboratories. **(p. 1373)**

A27. False

Benign prostate epithelium shows expression of CD57, and this is also the case for most prostatic adenocarcinomas. As such, it does not indicate neuroendocrine differentiation. **(p. 1373)**

A28. False

Expression of high molecular weight cytokeratin may be seen in prostate carcinoma cells. It is the absence of basal cells, which regularly show strong expression of high molecular weight cytokeratin (and also nuclear expression of p63), that strongly suggests the malignant nature of the lesion. **(p. 1374)**

A29. True

Almost all cases show expression of androgen receptors and many the expression of estrogen receptor-β. Progesterone receptor also may be expressed, but estrogen receptor-α is seen only exceptionally. **(p. 1373)**

A30. False

This racemase is expressed in many malignant tumors. Although it was previously believed that P504S never stained benign prostate tissue, newer studies have indicated that α-methylacyl-CoA racemase can be expressed by benign prostate glands. Therefore, the diagnostic value of this marker is limited; however, it is still considered useful if strict guidelines for the interpretation of the immunostaining results are followed. **(p. 1373)**

A31. True

Despite a very large number of studies, only nonspecific abnormalities (e.g. *TP53* gene mutation, *Rb* tumor suppressor gene mutation, *Her-2/neu* amplification and altered telomerase activity) have been described. **(p. 1374)**

A32. True

Neuroendocrine differentiation has been described in 10–33% of otherwise typical adenocarcinomas of the prostate. **(p. 1374)**

A33. True

Small cell carcinoma of the prostate may be found together with an ordinary adenocarcinoma of the prostate. As in the lung, these tumors may produce Cushing's syndrome and inappropriate ADH secretion. **(p. 1375)**

A34. False

In colorectal adenocarcinoma a cut-off point of 50% is used for the diagnosis of mucinous adenocarcinoma. In prostate, however, the cut-off point is 25%. **(p. 1375)**

A35. False

Whereas in colorectal carcinoma the criterion is >50% cells with signet-ring features, in the prostate no such specific level has been defined. For this diagnosis in the prostate, the tumor must demonstrate a 'great majority of cells' with signet-ring morphology. **(p. 1376)**

A36. True

Some cases have been described de novo. This is similar to the very rare squamous cell carcinoma of the prostate, which has been described after hormonal therapy. **(p. 1376)**

A37. True

This lesion is histologically similar to the tumor of the salivary glands. Interestingly, this tumor in the prostate has never given rise to metastatic lesions. **(p. 1376)**

A38. False

This is a highly aggressive, rare malignancy of the prostate with histological features similar to those of the so-called 'cloacogenic carcinoma' of the anal canal. Elevated bcl-2 and high Ki-67 distinguish it immunohistochemically from adenoid basal cell tumor. **(p. 1376)**

A39. True

Whether a specific mesenchymal component is present or not, this tumor is probably epithelial in derivation. **(p. 1376)**

A40. True

It is divided into grades 1–3, and into low-grade category (including grades 1 and 2) and high-grade category (including grade 3 only). **(p. 1377)**

A41. False

In contrast to Gleason's grading, high-grade PIN (grade 3) is defined cytologically by the presence of macronucleoli, regardless of the architecture. **(p. 1377)**

A42. True

It is most difficult to differentiate between high-grade PIN with cribriform architecture and invasive adenocarcinoma Gleason grade 4. Fortunately, basal cells should be found in PIN, albeit potentially decreased in number and partly disconnected from each other. **(p. 1377)**

A43. False

In the first place, as a low-grade neoplasm, PIN grade 2 should not be reported in the prostate biopsy. Only high-grade PIN has been associated with an increased incidence of adenocarcinoma in follow-up biopsy (30% if PIN grade 3 was found in only one core; up to 75% if PIN grade 3 was found in more than three cores). **(p. 1378)**

A44. False

Acidic mucin can be found in atypical adenomatous hyperplasia and does not support the diagnosis of carcinoma. In addition, this lesion may also demonstrate small glands without basal cells. Consequently, in a small biopsy atypical adenomatous hyperplasia can closely mimic carcinoma; the lack of macronucleoli, however, should prevent misdiagnosis. **(p. 1378)**

A45. True

However, this applies only to high-grade tumors (Gleason grades 4 and 5) in TUR. Gleason grade 1–2 tumors (and most likely even grade 3 tumors) probably represent primaries within the transition zone and often have 'clear cell' features with optically clear cytoplasm. **(p. 1378)**

A46. False

It is usually very easy to distinguish lobular atrophy from adenocarcinoma. However, in more challenging cases the demonstration of basal cells by immunohistochemistry is very useful, as basal cells are not present in 'atrophic adenocarcinoma of the prostate.' **(p. 1379)**

A47. False

Sometimes it is difficult to distinguish cholesterol-laden macrophages from a small focus of Gleason grade 4 adenocarcinoma. Also, treacherous artifact closely mimicking signet-ring cells may be seen in the stromal cells and stromal lymphocytes of TUR specimens. **(p. 1379)**

A48. True

These changes may last many months after cessation of the radiation therapy. **(p. 1379)**

A49. False

It is usually seen in the transition zone, but may also be present in the peripheral zone. **(p. 1379)**

A50. True

The cells characteristically have a perpendicular orientation to the lumina. **(p. 1380)**

A51. False

Cribriform hyperplasia belongs to a group of atypical cribriform lesions, but is not found on needle biopsy because it is usually seen in the transition zone. The cells show no cytologic atypia (no macronucleoli), have clear cytoplasm, and possess an obvious basal cell layer. Normal central zone glands are very similar and show no cytologic atypia; they can be distinguished by their tall, pseudostratified nuclei and eosinophilic cytoplasm. **(p. 1380)**

A52. True

However, in the prostate lesion known as 'sclerosing adenosis,' basal cells show myoepithelial metaplasia and expression of S-100 protein. Sclerosing adenosis is more common in the transition zone and therefore is rarely present in the needle biopsy. **(p. 1380)**

A53. True

However, this lesion is not really an adenoma. Therefore, it is better to use the terms adenomatoid metaplasia or (so-called) nephrogenic metaplasia. It represents an uncommon alteration of the urothelium associated with prior trauma and/or chronic infection. **(p. 1380)**

A54. True

The problem is that about 40% of cases may be negative for high molecular weight cytokeratins and focally show PSA and PAP staining. The cells rarely may have prominent nucleoli. Additional worrying features include the presence of tubules, cords, signet ring-like tubules, muscle involvement, and blue-tinged mucinous secretions. **(p. 1380)**

A55. False

Features useful in the diagnosis of nephrogenic adenoma include the following: distinctive nephrogenic patterns, such as papillary and 'vascular;' adjacent urothelium; thyroidization; peritubular sheaths; associated inflammation; and positivity for cytokeratin 7 and, in some cases, 34βE12. **(p. 1380)**

A56. True

This is an important lesion, because like adenocarcinoma it is most often seen in the peripheral zone of the apex/mid-prostate. Its association with elastosis (a basophilic tinge to the stroma) and the presence of basal cells demonstrable by immunohistochemistry are useful diagnostically. **(p. 1379)**

A57. True

This is also true for seminal vesicle involvement and the presence of distant metastases. **(p. 1381)**

A58. False

The most common metastases are those to the lymph nodes and bone. Bone metastases are typically osteoblastic, not osteolytic. **(p. 1381)**

A59. True

Lung metastases are not as rare as was previously thought. Massive pleural effusion may be the initial symptom. **(p. 1382)**

A60. True

However, prostate carcinoma metastasizing to the breast needs to be ruled out by immunohistochemistry (PSA, PAP). **(p. 1382)**

A61. False

Latent carcinoma is unsuspected clinically and found incidentally at autopsy or in prostatectomy specimens performed for nodular hyperplasia or other benign disorders. The occult prostate carcinoma is that which presents with metastatic disease, but the primary tumor remains clinically undetected. **(p. 1382)**

A62. True

When the tumor has the same grade throughout, its score is obtained by doubling the grade. **(p. 1383)**

A63. True

Chemotherapy has shown no benefits in prostate carcinoma. However, 'watchful waiting' is an option in patients with low-volume, low-grade (Gleason sum up to 4) incidental tumors found in TURP specimens. **(p. 1384)**

A64. True

The status of the surgical margins is dependent on both the tumor volume and the surgical technique. **(p. 1386)**

A65. False

When stratified by stage and grade, there is no difference in mortality between the races. **(p. 1386)**

A66. False

In general, there is no difference in the biology of prostate carcinoma in different age groups. However, a very small group of very young patients (men under 35 years) has been identified with poorly differentiated and biologically very aggressive disease. **(p. 1386)**

A67. False

Low-grade clear cell adenocarcinomas of the transition zone do not have high rates of dissemination. The above statement refers only to high-grade large-volume carcinomas of the peripheral zone that involve the transitional zone only once they are quite advanced. **(p. 1386)**

A68. True

Other proven factors include the stage of prostate carcinoma, Gleason's score, status of the surgical margins, and volume of the tumor (particularly high-grade volume). **(p. 1386)**

A69. True

However, more evidence is needed and these studies must be validated before they enter clinical practice. **(p. 1387)**

A70. False

In prostate carcinoma the prognostic value of perineural invasion remains controversial. **(p. 1387)**

A71. False

The most common malignant tumor of the prostate in infancy and childhood is embryonal rhabdomyosarcoma. **(p. 1388)**

A72. False
80% of patients are cured by multidrug chemotherapy combined with limited surgery and radiation. However, most stage 4 patients still die of their disease. **(p. 1388)**

A73. False
This type of tumor typically has high perivascular cellularity, which alternates with myxoid/edematous areas and necrosis. The tumor cells are small and rounded, or spindly, or may show bizarre forms. The cytoplasm is abundant and eosinophilic, and variable cross-striations are usually found. Immunohistochemical analysis is needed for the confirmation of this diagnosis. **(p. 1388)**

A74. False
Benign neoplasms of the adult prostate are practically non-existent. **(p. 1388)**

A75. False
Small lymphocytic lymphoma/chronic lymphocytic leukemia is the most common secondary lymphoma of the prostate, as it involves the prostate in about 20% of cases. The most common primary lymphoma is diffuse large B-cell lymphoma, and it is a very rare disease. **(p. 1389)**

A76. True
However, it is impossible to determine the tumor borders accurately without microscopic examination. **(p. 1369)**

A77. False
Intraglandular crystalloids are usually associated with low-grade adenocarcinoma of the prostate. However, they can also be found in benign lesions of the prostate. **(p. 1371)**

A78. False
The figure shows primary transitional cell carcinoma of the prostate involving large suburethral prostatic ducts. **(p. 1372)**

Seminal vesicles and Cowper's glands

A1. False
Occasionally prostate epithelium may contain large amounts of lipofuscin pigment. However, this finding favors a seminal vesicle origin for the cells. **(p. 1389)**

A2. True
These cells, as in the rest of seminal vesicle epithelium, contain lipofuscin pigment, which is a clue to their correct interpretation. **(p. 1390)**

A3. True
Otherwise, the presence of amyloid in seminal vesicles does not indicate the presence of systemic amyloidosis. **(p. 1390)**

A4. False
These hyaline globules have no known clinical significance or association. **(p. 1459)**

A5. True
These are very rare lesions. Histologically, they most often have a papillary growth pattern. **(p. 1390)**

A6. True
They have the appearance of mucinous minor salivary glands embedded in skeletal muscle and do not mimic prostate carcinoma. However, very rarely adenocarcinoma of the Cowper's gland has been described. This is a mucin-producing PSA-negative tumor. **(p. 1390)**

TESTIS

Normal anatomy

A1. True
The static phase occurs between birth and age 4, the growth phase between ages 4 and 10 years, and the development phase between age 10 and puberty. **(p. 1412)**

A2. False
In general, the age of the individual cannot be determined by histological study of the testis after the age of 12 years. **(p. 1412)**

A3. True
Most superficially there is the tunica vaginalis (serosal covering, loose connective tissue layered by mesothelium), followed by the tunica albuginea (thick fibrous connective tissue) and the tunica vasculosa (loose connective tissue with vessels). **(p. 1412)**

A4. True
The rete testis is comprised of a labyrinthine system of cavities in the mediastinum that are in continuation from straight tubules, the *tubuli recti*. **(p. 1412)**

A5. False

Up to four seminiferous tubules form a lobule of the testis. The usual testicular biopsy is composed of three to five lobules. **(p. 1412)**

A6. False

Type A spermatogonia are stem cells which, with each division, produce type A and type B spermatogonia. Type B spermatogonia undergo mitosis to produce primary spermatocytes. **(p. 1412)**

A7. False

Spermatogenesis proceeds in an orderly, overlapping helical pattern along the length of the tubule; as a consequence, not all stages of germ cell differentiation are seen in any one cross-sectional view of a seminiferous tubule. **(p. 1412)**

A8. True

The germ cell:Sertoli cell ratio is relatively constant at about 13:1, and an average of 12 Sertoli cells per tubular cross-section is considered normal. Also, spermatid count per tubule cross-section correlates well with the sperm count in the seminal fluid. **(p. 1413)**

A9. False

Charcot–Bottcher crystalloids, which are formed from the intermediate filament vimentin, are found in Sertoli cells. Reinke crystalloids, which show immunohistochemical reactivity for inhibin and Melan-A, are found in Leydig cells. **(p. 1413)**

A10. False

Whereas in the adult testis Sertoli cells show no immunoreactivity for cytokeratin or desmin, both of these intermediate filaments are expressed in the fetal testis and may reappear in pathologic conditions. **(p. 1413)**

A11. False

About 10% of boys are born with a testis that has not descended into the scrotum. Only 10% of these infants will still have an undescended testis after age 1, which is then diagnosed as cryptorchidism. Cryptorchidism is unilateral in about 80% of cases. **(p. 1413)**

A12. False

Undescended testes are small, brown, undeveloped and show hyperplasia of the Sertoli cells. Germ cells are frequently atypical at the base of the tubule, which is referred to as intratubular germ cell neoplasia. **(p. 1414)**

A13. False

A cryptorchid testis is 30–50 times more likely to develop a malignant neoplasm. Even if cryptorchid testes are surgically placed into the scrotum after 6 years of age, the risk of malignancy is still higher than in a control population. This is why cryptorchid testes need to be removed surgically if they were not placed into scrotum before mid-adolescence. **(p. 1414)**

A14. False

In testicular regression syndrome the patient has only a rudimentary epididymis and spermatic cord with vas deferens; testicular tissue is replaced by a fibrovascular nodule, possibly owing to testicular infarct. Post vasectomy, changes are mild and consist of reduced spermatids and Sertoli cells, thickening of the tubular wall and variable interstitial fibrosis, but most of the testicular tissue is well preserved. **(p. 1414)**

A15. True

It is particularly useful in individuals with azoospermia and normal endocrine findings. **(p. 1414)**

A16. True

Punch biopsy is not nearly as satisfactory as an open surgical biopsy. However, punch biopsy is clinically preferred. **(p. 1414)**

A17. False

Spermatocytic arrest, germ cell aplasia (Sertoli cell-only syndrome) and normal spermatogenesis have the same incidence (about 25–30%). **(p. 1415)**

A18. False

It is found in up to 20% of cases. **(p. 1415)**

A19. False

These multinucleated giant stromal cells are typically found after estrogen therapy. **(p. 1415)**

A20. True

There is also tubular fibrosis and prominent basement membrane thickening. Klinefelter's syndrome is associated with an increased incidence of breast carcinoma, possibly Leydig cell tumors, and mediastinal germ cell tumors. **(p. 1415)**

A21. True

This diagnosis accounts for 60% of cases, followed by Klinefelter's syndrome (30%) and testicular aplasia (10%). The biopsy shows small infantile tubules with few/no Leydig cells, scattered spermatogonia and Sertoli cells. **(p. 1415)**

A22. False

There are many different biopsy findings in oligospermia. 'Sloughing and disorganization,' in which spermatogenesis has a disorderly appearance and the tubular lumina are filled with desquamated immature cells, is a nonspecific finding. It may even be artifactual, and result from mechanical damage to the specimen. **(p. 1415)**

A23. True

FNA has been proposed as an alternative to testicular biopsy. **(p. 1415)**

A24. True

Other causes of testicular infarction include venous thrombosis secondary to pyogenic epididymo-orchitis, and vasculitis associated with various causes (e.g. Crohn's disease). **(p. 1415)**

A25. False

Although some patients may develop granulomatous orchitis secondary to TB, syphilis, sarcoidosis, leprosy and brucellosis, most patients with granulomatous orchitis have a history of recent trauma. It appears that there is a granulomatous response to the products of disintegrated sperm. **(p. 1416)**

A26. True

Coliform organisms are frequently found, and electron microscopy shows bacteria in the phagolysosomes of the macrophages. Malakoplakia is frequently associated with abscess formation and venous thrombosis, and is therefore very symptomatic. **(p. 1416)**

A27. False

Michaelis–Gutmann bodies are intracellular and extracellular round structures containing iron and calcium, and are found in malakoplakia. In juvenile xanthogranuloma, clustered comma-shaped bodies are occasionally observed on electron microscopy but are not specific for this very rare disease of the testis. **(p. 1416)**

A28. True

Splenogonadal fusion syndrome (which also occurs in females) is a congenital malformation occurring at the stage when the splenic and gonadal Anlagen are topographically close. **(p. 1416)**

A29. True

In this congenital defect, the cystic spaces are lined by a single layer of cuboidal epithelium. **(p. 1416)**

A30. False

This is a benign tumor of patients between 10 and 39 years of age. **(p. 1416)**

A31. True

Therefore, epidermoid cyst of the testis is not an epidermal inclusion cyst. It is necessary to sample thoroughly for adnexal structures, because lesions without adnexal structures require only a conservative surgical approach, as metastases never occur under these circumstances. **(p. 1416)**

A32. False

The absence of skin adnexal structures needs to be documented histologically. **(p. 1417)**

Tumors

A1. True

Germ cell tumors comprise about 90% of all testis tumors. Other tumor categories include sex cord–stromal tumors, mixed germ cell–sex cord–stromal tumors, primary tumors nonspecific to the testis, and metastatic tumors. **(p. 1417)**

A2. True

Both types of germ cell tumor arise from germinal (seminiferous) epithelium of the mature or maturing testis. **(p. 1417)**

A3. True

60% of patients with non-seminomatous germ cell tumors present with stage 2 or 3 disease and their tumors metastasize earlier than seminomas, using the hematogenous route. However, with modern chemotherapy, even in the face of metastases, the cure rate is between 49% and 95%. **(p. 1417)**

A4. False

The mean age of spermatocytic seminoma patients is only 55 years, but this is still older than that of 'classic seminoma,' which has a mean age of 40 years. Spermatocytic seminoma is bilateral in only 10% of cases and appears to be benign in almost all cases. Interestingly, it occurs only in the descended testis (never in the mediastinum!). **(p. 1424)**

A5. False

The cut surface of classic seminoma is very uniform: a homogeneous, solid, light-yellow tumor. Thorough sampling is necessary to rule out non-seminomatous components if there are any alterations in color or consistency. **(p. 1420)**

A6. True

Groups of these cells are typically surrounded by a lymphocytic infiltrate, which may represent host reaction to the tumor. **(p. 1420)**

A7. True

Occasionally it is so extensive as to obscure the neoplastic nature of the process. **(p. 1420)**

A8. False

PLAP is characteristically present in seminoma, but many other tumors, typically including adenocarcinomas, may show expression of PLAP. **(p. 1421)**

A9. False

Most testicular seminomas are cytokeratin negative, but focal positivity may be present and is far more common in mediastinal seminomas. Therefore, to distinguish between carcinoma and seminoma it is better to use EMA, which has never been described in seminoma or germ cell tumors in general. **(p. 1421)**

A10. False

Seminoma typically shows a variable expression of vimentin, often found only in the form of 'dot-like' positivity. **(p. 1421)**

A11. False

In contrast to classic seminoma, spermatocytic seminoma has no lymphoid cells and is not PLAP positive. **(p. 1425)**

A12. False

Rarely, classic seminoma may show tubule formation ('tubular seminoma'), but it can only be differentiated from non-seminomatous components by immunohistochemistry (yolk sac tumor and embryonal carcinoma are vimentin negative, yolk sac tumor is AFP positive, and embryonal carcinoma is CD30 and cytokeratin positive; Sertoli cell tumors are PLAP negative). **(p. 1420)**

A13. True

K-*ras* mutations and *TP53* mutations are common. **(p. 1422)**

A14. True

It can be demonstrated by PAS histochemical staining. **(p. 1421)**

A15. False

Although the presence of elevated serum hCG does not change the classification and has no clinical significance, elevated AFP indicates a non-seminomatous germ cell component (or liver disease), even if this is not seen histologically. **(p. 1424)**

A16. False

Although it is true that about half of patients show the entire testis replaced by seminoma, the tumor is very well demarcated and involves the tunica albuginea in only 10%. **(p. 1434)**

A17. False

If cytotrophoblasts are not present the best diagnosis is 'seminoma with trophoblastic giant cells,' this diagnosis accounting for 10–20% of seminomas. Giant cells are often related to blood vessels, and the hCG serum level is not very high (<1000 u/L). It is uncertain whether these tumors have a tendency to more aggressive behavior or not. **(p. 1424)**

A18. False

Despite the anaplastic appearance (cells with large vesicular nuclei and macronucleoli, multinucleated tumor giant cells, a high mitotic index, abnormal mitotic figures, blood vessel invasion, invasion of tunica albuginea, and necrosis), the clinical course of the anaplastic variant is not different from that of an usual spermatocytic seminoma, whereas those tumors with a sarcomatous component (undifferentiated spindle cells, or cells with rhabdomyosarcomatous differentiation) have a very aggressive clinical course. **(p. 1426)**

A19. True

However, immunohistochemical analysis is helpful. The lack of diffuse immunoreactivity for PLAP and cytokeratin strongly supports the diagnosis of the much more benign anaplastic spermatocytic seminoma. **(p. 1426)**

A20. True

However, no gross features are helpful in diagnosis. **(p. 1426)**

A21. True

Most often the pattern is solid or has differentiation toward embryonal structures. Overall, it looks more like 'carcinoma' than the other germ cell tumors. **(p. 1426)**

A22. False

Pure tumors represent only 2% of germ cell tumors; 85% of non-seminomatous tumors have a component of embryonal carcinoma. **(p. 1426)**

A23. True

Embryonal carcinomas show no mucin production, have CD30 expression and are EMA negative. Expression of cytokeratin and PLAP are not useful in this differential diagnosis. **(p. 1426)**

A24. True

These tumors are benign in children but assumed to be malignant in adults. **(p. 1427)**

A25. True

Teratomas of the testis are associated with Down and Klinefelter syndromes, spina bifida, xeroderma pigmentosa and hemihypertrophy. **(p. 1426)**

A26. False

This type of teratoma is commonly seen in the ovary and is extremely rare in the testis. **(p. 1427)**

A27. False

Epidermoid cyst designates a lesion without adnexal structures. **(p. 1416)**

A28. False

Polyembryoma is an immature germ cell tumor with multiple embryoid bodies, and resembles embryonic yolk sac. It is classified as a mixed germ cell tumor rather than as a separate entity, as it does not appear in a pure form but rather in association with mature and immature teratoid structures and primitive embryonic tissue, as seen in embryonal carcinoma. **(p. 1428)**

A29. False

Teratocarcinoma is an obsolete term which referred to a tumor that is a mixture of teratoma and embryonal carcinoma. Today, this tumor should be diagnosed as a mixed non-seminomatous germ cell tumor, followed by a list of the proportions of the relative components. **(p. 1428)**

A30. True

Only up to 1% of germ cell tumors are pure choriocarcinoma. **(p. 1428)**

A31. True

Isolated cells of syncytiotrophoblast or groups of syncytiotrophoblast cells can be seen in other germ cell tumors and do not suffice for the diagnosis of choriocarcinoma. **(p. 1428)**

A32. True

Other germ cell tumors do not show expression of cytokeratin 7. **(p. 1428)**

A33. True

Cytotrophoblasts are also characterized by polygonal/round cell morphology and distinct cell borders. Correct histological recognition of cytotrophoblasts is diagnostically important. **(p. 1429)**

A34. True

Yolk sac tumor may be considered a unilateral teratoma mimicking embryonal yolk sac tissue. **(p. 1430)**

A35. True

This distinctive feature represents an attempt by the yolk sac tumor to recapitulate yolk sacs. However, these are present in only 50% of tumors. **(p. 1430)**

A36. True

(p. 1430)

A37. True

However, pediatric tumors can be AFP negative. GATA-4 and cytokeratin are also expressed in yolk sac tumors. **(p. 1431)**

A38. False

This is an in situ germ cell neoplasm, but it is usually seen together with invasive germ cell malignancy. **(p. 1431)**

A39. False

Intratubular germ cell neoplasia has the same appearance regardless of the morphology of the invasive component. **(p. 1431)**

A40. True

This refers particularly to mature teratoma and pure yolk sac tumor of childhood. **(p. 1431)**

A41. False

Intratubular germ cell neoplasia has been observed in association with primary germ cell tumors of the mediastinum. **(p. 1431)**

A42. True

This is in contrast to 'intratubular seminoma' (in which the atypical cells pack the tubules and totally replace the normal Sertoli and germ cells), and the very rare 'intratubular embryonal carcinoma.' Intratubular germ cell neoplasia with extratubular extension is referred to as 'microinvasive intratubular germ cell neoplasia.' **(p. 1431)**

A43. True

These two markers are the most useful for making the correct diagnosis of intratubular germ cell neoplasia in a small biopsy. **(p. 1431)**

A44. False

Mature teratoma of the prepubertal testis is the only germ cell neoplasm lacking gross chromosomal aberrations. **(p. 1432)**

A45. False

Fas gene mutations are common in embryonal carcinoma. **(p. 1434)**

A46. False

Chromosome 12 abnormalities, specifically isochromosome of the short arm [i(12p)] and deletions of the long arm [del(12q)], are associated with both in situ and invasive germ cell tumors. **(p. 1433)**

A47. True

However, metastatic classic seminoma usually resembles classic seminoma. **(p. 1434)**

A48. True

Patients with histologically more mature metastases have a better prognosis than those whose metastases appear immature or possess sarcomatous elements. **(p. 1435)**

A49. False

Chemotherapy is used only for patients presenting with advanced disease or who have a relapse after radiation therapy. **(p. 1435)**

A50. True

90% of patients with newly diagnosed disease are cured. **(p. 1435)**

A51. False

Serum levels of hCG, AFP and LDH have been found to be independent prognostic factors for germ cell tumors. This is also true of the presence of non-pulmonary visceral metastases. **(p. 1435)**

A52. True

Therefore, pathologists need to carefully search for these features. **(p. 1435)**

A53. True

Many of these tumors have these components admixed. **(p. 1436)**

A54. False

α-Inhibin is the most useful marker to distinguish between germ cell tumors and sex cord–stromal cell tumors. **(p. 1437)**

A55. False

Fibromas, myxomas and sclerosing stromal tumors are negative for α-inhibin. **(p. 1437)**

A56. True
The distinction between Leydig cell hyperplasia and Leydig cell tumors is based on size (tumors are >0.5 cm) and multifocality (tumors are not multifocal). **(p. 1437)**

A57. False
Leydig cell tumors are not accompanied by Leydig cell hyperplasia. **(p. 1437)**

A58. False
Only about 10% of the tumors give rise to metastases. **(p. 1437)**

A59. False
Malignant Leydig cell tumors occur exclusively in adults. **(p. 1437)**

A60. True
In about 10% of children and 30% of adults with Leydig cell tumors, gynecomastia is secondary to estrogen excess as a result of aromatase activity in some of the tumors, or due to peripheral aromatization of testosterone. **(p. 1436)**

A61. False
The presence of cytologic atypia, necrosis, angiolymphatic invasion, increased mitotic activity, atypical mitotic figures, infiltrative margins and extension beyond the testicular parenchyma is associated with metastatic behavior in Leydig cell tumors and should be reported by the pathologist. **(p. 1436)**

A62. False
Malignant Leydig cell tumors are hormonally active only in exceptional cases. **(p. 1437)**

A63. True
This lesion is always bilateral (in contrast to unilateral Leydig cell tumors) and the patient can be effectively treated by appropriate glucocorticoid substitution, which leads to gradual regression of the 'tumor' in 75% of cases. **(p. 1437)**

A64. True
Leydig cell tumors in Carney complex can have endocrine manifestations. **(p. 1440)**

A65. True
The syndromic Sertoli cell tumors are usually bilateral and benign. **(p. 1438)**

A66. True
However, Peutz–Jeghers tumors of the testis may have features of ovarian sex-cord tumors with annular tubules, and can be associated with gynecomastia. **(p. 1438)**

A67. True
This variant of Sertoli cell tumor is seen in younger patients and is rarely malignant. **(p. 1440)**

A68. True
Sertoli cell tumors (NOS) arise in descended testes and can cause gynecomastia. **(p. 1438)**

A69. True
They consist of elongated tubules lined by Sertoli-like cells. **(p. 1438)**

A70. True
In contrast to germ cell tumors, they show no expression of PLAP or CD117 (c-*kit*). **(p. 1439)**

A71. True
Half of cryptorchid testes show Sertoli cell hyperplasia. **(p. 1437)**

A72. True
This is exactly the same percentage as in Leydig cell tumors. **(p. 1439)**

A73. True
S-100 is not expressed in Leydig cell tumors. **(p. 1440)**

A74. False
Leydig cells are often difficult to recognize in these tumors. **(p. 1440)**

A75. True
Prominent differentiation into follicles distinguishes this lesion from Sertoli cell tumors (NOS) that show tubular differentiation. **(p. 1440)**

A76. True
In contrast to the juvenile granulosa cell tumor, which is non-functional, the adult form is functional and 20% of patients show gynecomastia; 10% of adult cases are malignant, but none of the juvenile forms is malignant. **(p. 1440)**

A77. True
Alternatively, cytokeratin is widely expressed and not useful in this differential diagnosis. **(p. 1440)**

A78. True
This tumor occurs mainly in association with gonadal dysgenesis or male pseudohermaphroditism. **(p. 1441)**

A79. True
However, it can occur at any age. **(p. 1441)**

A80. True
However, rare variants of T-cell lymphoma and NK-cell malignancies have been described. **(p. 1442)**

A81. False
Acute lymphoblastic leukemia more commonly involves the testes, and is microscopically identified in about 20% of patients. Testicular involvement may also occur as the first sign of relapse. **(p. 1442)**

A82. False
These tumors produce serotonin, but the patients do not develop carcinoid syndrome. **(p. 1443)**

A83. True
True primary sarcomas of the testes are very rare in both children and adults. **(p. 1443)**

A84. True

Kidney, stomach and melanoma may also metastasize to the testes. In children, metastatic neuroblastoma may be found in the testes. **(p. 1443)**

A85. False

This is the typical gross appearance of seminoma (uniform, yellow, no hemorrhage or cysts). Embryonal carcinoma is usually white or gray and frequently shows cystic degeneration and hemorrhage. **(p. 1421)**

A86. False

This is spermatocytic seminoma showing an admixture of medium-sized cells, giant cells and small lymphocyte-like cells. These are the three typical cell types of spermatocytic seminoma. **(p. 1425)**

A87. True

These organoid formations are present in only 50% of cases. **(p. 1430)**

A88. False

This is the gross appearance of a Leydig cell tumor. These tumors may be dark brown. However, metastatic melanomas to the testes have been described. **(p. 1436)**

TESTICULAR ADNEXA

Non-neoplastic lesions

A1. True

The extratesticular component is also known as 'bullae retis.' **(p. 1457)**

A2. False

The rete testis empties into the *ductuli efferentes*. **(p. 1457)**

A3. True

It consists of three parts: head, body and tail. **(p. 1457)**

A4. True

The tall columnar cells with cilia are the principal lining cells of the epididymis. **(p. 1457)**

A5. True

The vas is lined by pseudostratified epithelium with ciliated columnar cells and basal cells. **(p. 1457)**

A6. False

The appendix testis is attached to tunica vaginalis at the upper pole of the testis. It is also known as the hydatid of Morgagni and represents a remnant of the cranial portion of the müllerian duct. **(p. 1457)**

A7. False

This is remnant of the cranial portion of the mesonephric duct. **(p. 1457)**

A8. True

The vas aberrans is also known as the organ of Haller; the paradidymis has been termed the organ of Giraldes. **(p. 1457)**

A9. False

Rete testis dysgenesis is the rule in cryptorchid testes. **(p. 1457)**

A10. True

The cystic dilatation of the rete testis should not be confused with cystic dysplasia of the testis, which is a congenital condition. **(p. 1457)**

A11. True

However, it can present as a grossly evident solid or cystic mass in the testicular hilum. **(p. 1457)**

A12. True

Positivity for EMA and negativity for AFP and PLAP in adenomatous hyperplasia helps distinguish these two lesions. **(p. 1457)**

A13. False

These are two unrelated disorders of the rete testis. Adenocarcinoma of the rete testis is a very rare disease that needs to be distinguished from the slightly more common mesothelioma of the tunica vaginalis. **(p. 1457)**

A14. False

Chlamydial epididymitis tends to be proliferative, whereas bacterial epididymitis tends to be destructive and abscess forming. **(p. 1458)**

A15. False

Hematogenous spread preferentially involves the head of the epididymis and spares the tail and vas deferens, whereas spread through the prostate, which is more common, preferentially involves the tail of the epididymis and the vas deferens. **(p. 1458)**

A16. False

It presents clinically as a nodule measuring up to 3 cm. **(p. 1458)**

A17. False

Granulomatous ischemic lesions involve the head of the epididymis and are accompanied by partial necrosis of the ductal wall. As the name suggests, they are not infectious but probably rather ischemic in pathogenesis. **(p. 1458)**

A18. True

These tumors appear well circumscribed, but are not encapsulated. **(p. 1459)**

Tumors

A1. True
It is most often seen in middle-aged men. **(p. 1459)**

A2. False
Adenomatoid tumor of the epididymis is usually a small and unencapsulated tumor, which may extend into the adjacent testis. However, this tumor is benign. **(p. 1459)**

A3. True
Immunohistochemical analysis will reveal the mesothelial nature of these cells, whereas vascular tumors will show vascular markers. **(p. 1459)**

A4. True
These two lesions show the immunophenotype of mesothelial cells (CK7+, HBME-1+, and calretinin+). Therefore, morphologic findings are vital to distinguish the two. **(p. 1460)**

A5. False
It occurs in von Hippel–Lindau disease and it may be bilateral. **(p. 1460)**

A6. True
Histologically it may resemble renal cell carcinoma owing to its high vascularity and abundant clear cytoplasm. **(p. 1460)**

A7. True
This occurs either in the first year of life or close to puberty. Clinically, the differential diagnosis includes torsion of the testicular appendage (most often the appendix testis). **(p. 1461)**

A8. False
Although systemic vasculitides may involve the vessels of the vas deferens, vasitis nodosa refers to spermatic granuloma of the vas deferens. It may occur after vasectomy or herniorrhaphy. **(p. 1462)**

A9. True
Proliferative funiculitis is a pseudosarcomatous myofibroblastic proliferation of the spermatic cord. It shows the microscopic features of nodular fasciitis and runs a benign course. **(p. 1462)**

A10. True
It is surrounded by the tunica vaginalis and derives its blood supply from the vessels of the cord. **(p. 1462)**

A11. False
Well-differentiated liposarcoma is the most frequent malignant tumor of the spermatic cord in adults, with a mean age of 63 years. In children, the most common malignant tumor of spermatic cord is embryonal rhabdomyosarcoma. **(p. 1462)**

A12. False
The mean age of patients with leiomyosarcoma in the paratesticular region is 62 years, whereas the mean age for desmoplastic small round cell tumor in this region is 28 years. **(p. 1462)**

PENIS AND SCROTUM

Penis

Normal anatomy

A1. True
Furthermore, the corpus consists of two corpora cavernosa and one corpus spongiosus. **(p. 1466)**

A2. False
'*Dartos*' is a discontinuous smooth muscle layer covering the corpora and midpart of the foreskin. It is Buck's fascia, a fibroelastic and vascular membrane that separates the penis into dorsal and ventral portions. **(p. 1466)**

A3. False
The male urethra is divided into three parts: prostatic, membranous and penile. The membranous part extends from the lower pole of the prostate to the bulb of the corpus spongiosum. **(p. 1466)**

A4. False
The fossa navicularis is the most distal part of penile urethra, and is somewhat wider than the more proximal parts. **(p. 1466)**

A5. False
Only the prostatic portion of the urethra is lined by transitional epithelium. The distal portion – corresponding to the fossa navicularis – is lined by stratified squamous epithelium, and the rest of the canal is lined by stratified or pesudostratified columnar ciliated epithelium. **(p. 1466)**

A6. False
Cowper's glands are present at the level of the membranous urethra only, but Littré's glands are present along the full length of the corpus spongiosum. **(p. 1466)**

Non-neoplastic lesions

A1. True
It is usually found in young men. **(p. 1466)**

A2. True
It is often associated with intraepithelial mucous glands. **(p. 1466)**

A3. True
It is usually associated with Zoon's balanitis, also called balanitis circumscripta, which is characterized by epidermal atrophy and a dense inflammatory infiltrate rich in plasma cells. **(p. 1466)**

A4. True
Along the same line of thinking, Zoon's balanitis may resemble Bowen's disease, Wegener's granulomatosis can present as localized disease and mimic carcinoma, and amyloidosis may present as a localized mass and thus simulate penile tumor. **(p. 1467)**

A5. False
Although spirochetes may be detected by the Warthin–Starry silver stain in primary syphilis, the inflammation is characterized by a dense lymphocytic and plasma cell infiltrate as well as very typical endarteritis obliterans. Granulomas are not formed in primary syphilis. **(p. 1467)**

A6. True
Granulomas due to other causes may have an identical clinical appearance. **(p. 1467)**

A7. True
In addition, Behçet's disease may cause either anterior uveitis (inflammation in the front of the eye) or posterior uveitis (inflammation in the back of the eye), and sometimes both. Most symptoms are the result of the underlying vasculitis. **(p. 1467)**

A8. True
It is localized to the penis and causes plastic induration, pain, and curvature toward the side of the lesion on penile erection. **(p. 1467)**

A9. False
Only about one-third of polypoid lesions of the male urethra are examples of condyloma acuminatum. **(p. 1468)**

A10. False
'High-risk' HPV types (16, 18, 31, 33, 35) are mainly associated with macular lesions (about 60%); one-quarter are papular and <10% are acuminate. **(p. 1468)**

A11. False
Many HPV-associated lesions of the penis do not show these characteristic histological/cytological changes, which are much more frequently seen in the cervix uteri. **(p. 1468)**

A12. False
The histologic changes resemble the papular type of condyloma, but no HPV is demonstrable in these lesions. **(p. 1469)**

Tumors

A1. True
HPV DNA has been consistently found in these lesions. Both arise in the same location (glans or prepuce), but differ in that Bowen's disease is grossly scaly whereas erythroplasia of Queyrat is smooth, shiny and velvety. **(p. 1469)**

A2. False
Only clearly invasive tumors are treated by penectomy. **(p. 1469)**

A3. False
Bowen's disease is a squamous cell carcinoma in situ, whereas Bowenoid papulosis demonstrates various degrees of dysplasia but still shows maturation. The lesions of bowenoid papulosis are multiple, have a more prominent viral cytopathic effect, and tend to involve the upper portions of sweat glands while sparing the upper portions of pilosebaceous units. The opposite is true of Bowen's disease. **(p. 1469)**

A4. True
Squamous cell carcinoma of the penis is more common in patients with a long phimotic foreskin. Association with HPV infection is well documented. **(p. 1470)**

A5. True
The next most frequent site of origin is the prepuce, followed by the coronal sulcus. **(p. 1470)**

A6. False
Exophytic tumors are better differentiated. **(p. 1470)**

A7. True
However, the last three categories are characterized by a similar exophytic pattern of growth. **(p. 1470)**

A8. False
By definition, verrucous carcinoma is a grade I tumor throughout. If only part of the tumor has verrucous morphology, the term 'hybrid tumor' can be applied. **(p. 1472)**

A9. False
Basaloid carcinoma is a very aggressive type of squamous cell carcinoma which, together with sarcomatoid carcinoma, has a high rate of nodal metastases and poor survival. Basal cell carcinoma has never been reported to metastasize in this location. **(p. 1472)**

A10. False

Vascular invasion is an indicator of poor prognosis, but clinical stage is the most important predictor. For example, if metastases are present in two or more lymph nodes, the chances of survival are very small. **(p. 1473)**

A11. False

These two parameters are closely related, and both microscopic grade and microscopic type show very good correlation with prognosis. **(p. 1473)**

A12. True

Immunohistochemical evaluation for CEA and low molecular weight cytokeratins (which are positive in the atypical cells in Paget's disease), high molecular weight cytokeratins (which are positive in Bowen's disease) and Melan-A (and/or HMB-45, which are positive in melanoma), should provide a definitive diagnosis. **(p. 1473)**

A13. False

Leiomyoma is more common in the female urethra. **(p. 1473)**

A14. False

Squamous cell carcinoma accounts for 75% of malignancies. **(p. 1473)**

A15. False

In the male urethra, prognosis and treatment depend more heavily on location and stage of disease than on histological type. Anterior and distal lesions have a better outcome than proximal and posterior lesions. **(p. 1474)**

A16. True

The prognosis is exceedingly poor. **(p. 1474)**

A17. False

Hirsutoid papillomas are fibroepithelial polyps on the corona of the glans and are not HPV related. **(p. 1474)**

A18. True

This is the typical appearance of full-thickness dysplasia or squamous cell carcinoma in situ. **(p. 1469)**

A19. False

This is a moderately differentiated squamous cell carcinoma of the penis. Verrucous carcinoma is always a well-differentiated tumor. **(p. 1471)**

Scrotum

Non-neoplastic lesions

A1. True

Although it has been said that the presence of sperm defines the spermatocele, the sperm may be washed out during tissue processing. However, the lining of the hydrocele is mesothelial, whereas that of the spermatocele is epithelial. This difference can be demonstrated by immunohistochemistry if necessary. **(p. 1475)**

A2. False

It appears that this condition may represent calcification of multiple keratinous cysts. **(p. 1475)**

A3. False

Fibrous pseudotumor is a peritesticular fibrosis of unknown etiology, which results in diffuse or nodular thickening and may grossly simulate the appearance of a tumor. **(p. 1475)**

A4. True

However, most cases are probably the result of a smoldering nonspecific inflammation ('nodular periorchitis'). **(p. 1475)**

A5. True

In this condition, fat necrosis is associated with extensive areas of fibrosis and hyalinization. Fat necrosis of the scrotum may also be the result of exposure to cold. **(p. 1476)**

A6. True

It presents as an erythematous non-tender swelling. **(p. 1476)**

A7. True

This is a necrotizing subcutaneous infection of the perineum and external genitalia. Some cases are idiopathic and some are related to urethral strictures. **(p. 1476)**

Tumors

A1. True

These tumors are similar to skin tumors in other locations. **(p. 1477)**

A2. False

As in the female genital tract, this is a poorly circumscribed soft tissue tumor with a tendency for local recurrence, but it does not metastasize. **(p. 1477)**

A3. True

However, it is notably associated with certain occupations (including chimney sweeps, paraffin workers, tar workers and cotton mill workers). **(p. 1477)**

A4. False

Malignant mesothelioma is the most common malignant tumor of the tunica vaginalis. The tunica dartos does not contain any mesothelium. **(p. 1477)**

A5. True

This is a superficial tumor (in contrast to aggressive angiomyxoma) and has features of vulvovaginal angiomyofibroblastoma and spindle cell lipoma. It involves the scrotum or inguinal region in men with a median age of about 60 years. **(p. 1477)**

A6. False

This is a well-differentiated liposarcoma involving the scrotum. Atypical cells, not foamy macrophages, are present between the more normal-appearing adipocytes. **(p. 1478)**

Female reproductive system 19

VULVA

Normal anatomy

Q1

Adnexal structures, such as apocrine and sebaceous glands, are usually not identified in the labia minora.

Q2

Bartholin's gland is the major vestibular gland.

Q3

Skene's or periurethral glands are analogous to the male vas deferens.

Q4

Most of the vulvar lymphatics drain to the deep pelvic nodes.

Congenital abnormalities

Q1

Ectopic mammary tissue can occur in the vulvar region, along the primitive milk line.

Inflammatory diseases

Q1

Granuloma inguinale is a chronic infection caused by *Chlamydia*.

Chronic vulvar dystrophies

Q1

Lichen sclerosus (et atrophicus) of the vulva may occur in any age group, including children.

Q2

Lichen sclerosus represents a precancerous lesion in more than 90% of cases.

Q3

Squamous hyperplasia (keratosis) of the vulva is characterized microscopically by acanthosis, hyperkeratosis and the absence of atypia.

Human papillomavirus and vulvar pathology

Q1

Vulvar condyloma is a venereal disease caused by HPV, usually type 16.

Q2

Flat vulvar condyloma is a subtype that is less common than papillary condyloma acuminatum.

Q3

Koilocytosis of the vulvar epithelium is not as florid in vulvar condyloma as it tends to be in condyloma of the cervix.

Q4

A typical condyloma shows microscopic features of basal atypia, lack of epithelial maturation and numerous atypical mitoses.

Squamous intraepithelial lesions

Q1

Vulvar Bowen's disease shows only mild basal dysplasia, thus corresponding to a CIN-I type cervical lesion.

Q2

VIN-III, high-grade vulvar dysplasia shows a high propensity to progress to invasive carcinoma.

Invasive squamous cell carcinoma

Q1

Vulvar carcinoma occurring in older women is typically related to HPV infection.

Q2

Invasive squamous cell carcinoma located in the clitoris tends to be more anaplastic, and is known to metastasize directly into the deep pelvic nodes.

Q3

Regional lymph node metastases occur in 20% of cases with vulvar squamous cell carcinoma.

Q4

Treatment of an early vulvar squamous cell carcinoma, using wide local excision with at least 1 cm tumor-free surgical margin, results in a high rate of local control.

Q5

The most significant prognostic parameter in cases with vulvar squamous carcinoma is lymph node status.

Q6

The term microinvasive vulvar squamous cell carcinoma has been applied to tumors in which the depth of penetration is less than 5 mm.

Q7

Vulvar verrucous carcinoma has a typical exophytic appearance, is well differentiated and can mimic condyloma acuminatum.

Q8

Verrucous carcinomas show cytologic atypia and infiltrative margins.

Paget's disease

Q1

Paget's disease is a benign tumor of the vulva that originates from deep dermal adnexal structures.

Q2

Vulvar Paget's disease expresses keratin, EMA, CEA, B72.3 and GCDF-15.

Other epithelial tumors

Q1

Hidroadenoma papilliferum of the vulva is a benign tumor that probably arises from ectopic breast tissue.

Q2

Basal cell carcinoma of the vulva presents as nodular masses in the labia majora.

Melanocytic tumors

Q1

Malignant melanoma is the most common malignant tumor of the vulva.

Aggressive angiomyxoma and related lesions

Q1

Aggressive angiomyxoma is a polypoid soft tissue neoplasm that arises in the perineum.

Q2

Vulvar angiomyofibroblastoma is a benign tumor characterized by alternating hyper- and hypocellular areas with admixed small blood vessels.

Q3

Cellular angiofibroma has infiltrating margins and is composed mostly of fat and large pleomorphic cells.

Other tumors and tumor-like conditions

Q1

Fibroepithelial polyp is a superficially located lesion composed of a loose myxoid stroma covered by normal squamous epithelium.

Q2

Metastases to the vulva usually originate from the breast.

Lesions of Bartholin's glands and related structures

Q1

Cysts and abscesses of Bartholin's glands are the result of chronic bacterial inflammation, especially associated with gonorrhea.

Q2

Carcinomas of the Bartholin's glands are usually of basaloid type.

Lesions of the female urethra

Q1

Urethral caruncle has the appearance of a small raspberry protruding from the meatus; it bleeds easily and may become infected.

Q2

Urethral carcinoma occurs in younger patients and is associated with chronic inflammation.

QUESTIONS

VAGINA

Normal anatomy

Q1

The vagina derives from the paired müllerian ducts and is composed of three main layers: mucosa, muscularis and adventitia.

Q2

The vaginal epithelium is responsive to steroid hormones.

Q3

The wolffian duct in the vagina is represented by Gartner's duct.

Q4

The complex vaginal lymphatics drain mostly into the inguinal nodes.

Adenosis and related lesions

Q1

Grossly, adenosis appears as yellow granular spots or patches.

Q2

Adenosis represents partial or complete conversion of the vaginal mucosa from squamous to any kind of müllerian-type glandular epithelium.

Q3

Foci of adenosis are often accompanied by squamous metaplasia and chronic inflammation.

Q4

A firm relation between vaginal adenosis and in-utero exposure to diethylstilbestrol (DES) has not been established.

Q5

Transverse ridges of the vagina and cervix are another structural anomaly related to exogenous steroid administration.

Q6

Other known DES-related lesions are immature squamous metaplasia, atypical metaplasia and VAIN I.

Other non-neoplastic lesions

Q1

Indolent vaginal infections with *Candida* and *Trichomonas* spp. are relatively rare during pregnancy.

Q2

Vaginal xanthogranulomatous reaction and malakoplakia may occur as a result of minor mechanical injury and can present as ulcers.

Q3

Following vaginal hysterectomy the tubal fimbria can be entrapped in the healing vaginal apex and must not be confused with a neoplastic process.

Q4

Vaginal endometriosis typically follows scars from multiple laparoscopic procedures.

Benign epithelial tumors

Q1

Squamous papillomas are probably of viral/HPV etiology.

Squamous intraepithelial lesions

Q1

Vaginal intraepithelial lesions usually arise from metaplastic epithelium.

Invasive squamous cell carcinoma

Q1

Primary vaginal carcinoma is much less common than carcinoma of the vulva and cervix.

Q2

Most primary vaginal squamous cell carcinomas are grossly ulcerative or nodular.

Q3

The most common sites of origin of the vaginal carcinoma are the lower and posterior vaginal walls.

Clear cell (adeno)carcinoma

Q1

Clear cell carcinoma occurs in the anterior or lateral wall of the upper vagina or in the cervix of children, adolescents and young adults.

Q2

In two-thirds of patients with clear cell carcinoma there is a history of prenatal exposure to progesterone.

Q3

There is a very common association of clear cell carcinoma with vaginal adenosis, cervical ectropion, and occasional transverse vaginal or cervical ridges.

Q4

The major microscopic differential diagnoses of clear cell carcinoma are microglandular hyperplasia and Arias–Stella reaction.

Q5

Microscopically, clear cell carcinoma is composed of tubules with solid and papillary formations, with hobnail-shaped cells containing mostly glycogen and mucin.

Q6

The immunohistochemical profile of clear cell carcinoma shows consistent positivity for CK20 and CD30, and negativity for CK7.

Other carcinoma types

Q1

Verrucous carcinoma is an extremely well differentiated variant of squamous cell carcinoma that is known to invade locally but is almost never associated with distant metastases.

Q2

Spindle cell or sarcomatoid vaginal carcinoma is the subtype often found in tumors of the lower digestive tract.

Q3

Endometrioid adenocarcinoma of the vagina is thought to arise on the basis of vaginal transverse ridges.

Q4

Small cell neuroendocrine carcinoma can occur in the vagina, either in a pure form or associated with squamous/glandular elements.

Q5

Immunohistochemical evidence of neuroendocrine differentiation is typically not observed in vaginal small cell carcinoma.

Q6

Malignant mixed tumor of the vagina is characterized by a biphasic pattern of malignant glands admixed with spindle cells.

Mesenchymal tumors and tumor-like conditions

Q1

Vaginal fibroepithelial polyps (FP) are seen only in the third decade.

Q2

FP are not true neoplasms but rather hormone-induced localized hyperplasia of the loose subepithelial vaginal connective tissue.

Q3

FP can show a microscopic picture of markedly edematous stroma or sometimes hypercellular tissue with scattered highly atypical stellate shape stromal cells mimicking other malignant tumors, such as botryoid rhabdomyosarcoma.

Q4

Postoperative spindle cell nodule is a pseudosarcomatous vaginal lesion that occurs few weeks after hysterectomy.

Q5

The microscopic appearance of postoperative spindle cell nodule has a strong resemblance to Kaposi's sarcoma or leiomyosarcoma.

Botryoid rhabdomyosarcoma

Q1

Botryoid rhabdomyosarcoma (BR) is a rare ulcerative vaginal tumor that usually arises from the posterior vaginal wall.

Q2

Approximately 90% of cases of BR occur in patients over 60 years of age.

Q3

Microscopically, botryoid rhabdomyosarcoma contains myxoid stroma with small round or spindle cells exhibiting eosinophilic cytoplasm, with a racquet- or strap-shaped form and sometimes cross-striations.

Q4

The subepithelial dense zone of malignant rhabdomyoblasts, the so-called 'cambium layer,' represents an important diagnostic feature.

Q5

Foci of neoplastic cartilage in botryoid rhabdomyosarcoma are associated with a worse prognosis.

Melanocytic tumors

Q1

Malignant melanoma presents as a soft polypoid mass, blue or black, in the lower third of the vagina.

Q2

Vaginal melanomas are mostly ulcerated, with the microscopic appearance of an undifferentiated and anaplastic, largely amelanotic, neoplasm.

Q3

Melanoma typically originates from an intraepithelial component of lentiginous appearance ('junctional activity')

Metastatic tumors

Q1

Metastatic carcinoma to the vagina arises most commonly in the uterine cervix and endometrium.

UTERUS–CERVIX

Normal anatomy

Q1

Most of the exocervix is covered by non-keratinizing squamous epithelium that is composed of three layers: basal cell, midzone and superficial.

Q2

The morphological appearance of the various layers of cervical squamous mucosa is independent of age.

Q3

Glandular and basal cells of the cervical mucosa are immunoreactive for estrogen receptors.

Remnants and ectopias

Q1

Mesonephric rests are remnants of wolffian ducts, composed of tubules lined by a single row of cuboidal cells that typically contain an inspissated, deeply eosinophilic secretion in the lumen, and are seen in more than half of women.

Squamous and other metaplasias

Q1

The most common type of cervical metaplasia is squamous metaplasia.

Q2

Most commonly, squamous metaplasia involves all three layers of the squamous epithelium.

Q3

Complex patterns of squamous metaplasia may result in an overdiagnosis of squamous cell carcinoma or dysplasia.

Q4

Transitional cell metaplasia is seen in older women, involves the entire thickness of the exocervix, and is often associated with atrophy.

Q5

Tubal metaplasia represents aberrant differentiation following injury.

QUESTIONS

Inflammatory lesions

Q1

Herpes simplex infection is a relatively common infection marked by the presence of diagnostic multinucleated cells with intranuclear inclusions.

Q2

Chlamydia trachomatis is endemic in Africa and Central America.

Non-neoplastic glandular lesions

Q1

Endocervical polyps are true neoplasms that can reach several centimeters in diameter.

Q2

Tunnel clusters are the results of localized proliferation of endocervical glands (clefts), with side channels growing out from them.

Q3

Microglandular hyperplasia can be confused with carcinoma owing to its solid growth and mitotic activity.

Q4

Features distinguishing Arias–Stella reaction from carcinoma are the lack of desmoplastic stromal reaction, lack of a mass-forming lesion, and no infiltrative pattern.

Q5

Lobular endocervical glandular hyperplasia is a premalignant precursor for endocervical adenocarcinoma.

Non-neoplastic stromal lesions (including endometriosis and related processes)

Q1

Decidual reaction usually presents as yellow spots on the cervix.

Q2

Areas of decidual reaction are keratin positive, whereas placental site nodules are keratin negative.

Q3

Endometriosis spots within the cervix are always composed of stroma and glands.

HPV and the lower genital tract

Q1

HPV comprises a family of DNA viruses of which more than 60 types have been characterized, the most common being 6 and 12.

Q2

The 'gold standard' for identification of HPV is immunohistochemical staining.

Q3

The morphologic hallmark of HPV infection is koilocytosis, also known as koilocytic atypia.

Q4

There is evidence of overdiagnosis of HPV infection on the basis of the microscopic presence of perinuclear clearing.

Q5

The presence of koilocytosis is indicative of low-grade dysplasia.

Q6

HPVs are currently divided into three major categories, depending on their level of association with CIN and invasive squamous cell carcinoma.

Q7

Condyloma acuminatum is a grossly polypoid lesion characterized by papillomatosis, achantosis, koilocytosis and a variable degree of stromal inflammation.

Q8

Squamous papilloma, in at least some instances, represents condyloma in which recognizable changes of HPV infection have subsided.

Tumors

Q1

Almost all invasive cervical carcinomas are preceded by a stage in which the abnormal cells are confined to the epithelium (intraepithelial stage).

Q2

Most severe forms of dysplasia will inevitably lead to invasive carcinoma.

Q3

Dysplastic foci can be so small that occasionally they can be removed by biopsy.

Q4

The microscopic criteria for cervical intraepithelial neoplasia are different for pregnant women and non-pregnant women.

Q5

The term CIN III encompasses both severe dysplasia and carcinoma in situ.

Q6

The Bethesda classification introduced a new term, squamous intraepithelial neoplasia (SIL), with subdivision into low- and high-grade lesions.

Q7

All patients with low-grade CIN require therapy.

Q8

Invasive squamous carcinoma in which the depth of invasion is less than 5 mm is considered microinvasive.

Q9

The overall risk for lymph node metastasis in microinvasive carcinoma is 1%.

Q10

The single most important risk factor for invasive squamous cell carcinoma is number of sexual partners.

Q11

The bulky carcinomas that grow out of the cervix are more likely to invade surrounding structures.

Q12

Microscopically there are three major categories of cervical squamous cell carcinoma.

Q13

Some squamous cell carcinomas can be associated with peripheral eosinophilia.

Q14

The *p53* gene is often mutated in cervical squamous cell carcinomas.

Q15

Cervical carcinoma characteristically spreads by direct extension to the adjacent organs, and subsequently by lymphatic spread.

Q16

Cervical carcinomas are usually resistant to radiotherapy.

Q17

The most important prognostic determinant for invasive squamous cell carcinoma is clinical stage.

Q18

The presence of endometrial extension of squamous cell carcinoma reduces survival by 10–20%.

Q19

Verrucous carcinoma is a highly differentiated variant of squamous cell carcinoma with a polypoid pattern of growth, an extremely well differentiated cytologic appearance, and a capacity for local invasion but not metastatic spread.

Q20

There is no evidence of HPV infection in spindle cell carcinoma.

Q21

Primary cervical adenocarcinoma comprises only 1% of all carcinomas of the cervix.

Q22

Adenocarcinoma of the cervix is cytokeratin, EMA, CEA and p16 positive.

Q23

HPV infection (particularly HPV 16 and 18) is found in most endocervical adenocarcinomas.

Q24

The overall prognosis for cervical adenocarcinoma is worse than that of squamous cell carcinoma.

Q25

The differential diagnosis between endometrial adenocarcinoma and cervical adenocarcinoma is not a diagnostic problem.

Q26

The most important diagnostic features of adenocarcinoma in situ are cytologic atypia, increased mitotic activity and the presence of apoptotic bodies.

Q27

The generally strong positivity for p16 supports a strong association of in situ cervical adenocarcinoma with HPV infection.

Q28

Conization is an adequate treatment for cervical adenocarcinoma, and the status of the surgical margins is a good indicator of the adequacy of excision.

Q29

Adenoma malignum is a type of cervical adenocarcinoma so well differentiated structurally and cytologically that it could be diagnosed as malignant only because of the presence of distorted glands with irregular outlines deeply positioned in the cervix, and the fact that a portion of the infiltrating tumor is associated with a stromal response.

Q30

Adenoma malignum is usually positive for CEA, HPV and p53.

Q31

Adenosquamous (mixed) carcinomas have a worse prognosis than pure squamous cell carcinoma when compared stage by stage.

Q32

Glassy cell carcinoma has been described as a distinct type of well-differentiated squamous cell carcinoma.

Q33

Adenoid cystic and adenoid basal cell carcinomas are both associated with a poor prognosis. **(p. 1544)**

Q34

Clear cell carcinoma is the most common form of cervical carcinoma in young females.

Q35

Neuroendocrine carcinomas show a strong association with HPV infection as well as a common association with adjacent CIN.

Q36

The large majority of neuroendocrine cervical neoplasms are morphologically and clinically aggressive.

Q37

The Pap smear was first described by George Papanicolau at Cornell University.

Q38

The currently used Bethesda classification groups HPV-associated changes, mild dysplasia and CIN I in one group under term low-grade intraepithelial lesions (LGSIL).

Other tumors and tumor-like conditions

Q1

Botryoid rhabdomyosarcoma of the cervix presents in children and adolescents as a myxoid polypoid mass covered by attenuated epithelium.

Q2

Malignant lymphoma of the cervix is usually T-cell in type.

Q3

Metastatic carcinoma to the cervix is rare; however, the most common sites are the ovary, large bowel, stomach, breast and kidneys.

ENDOMETRIUM

Normal anatomy

Q1

The endometrial mucosa is divided into a deeply seated basal layer and a superficial functional layer, which is further subdivided into compactum and spongiosum.

Q2

For subnuclear vacuolization to be regarded as evidence of ovulation, it should be present in at least 50% of the functional glands present in the section.

Q3

The basal layer of the endometrium and the mucosa of the lower uterine segment are two areas most sensitive to progesterone effect.

Q4

Arias–Stella reaction is an exaggerated expression of gestational hyperplasia and is most commonly seen in postabortion curettings.

Q5

A decidual reaction is seen exclusively in women of childbearing age.

Curettage and biopsy

Q1

Fractional curettage is essential in determining the endocervical extension of endometrial carcinoma.

Q2

Asherman's syndrome is a common complication of the dilatation and curettage procedure.

Effects of hormone administration

Q1

Endometrial hyperplasia is present in 15–30% of postmenopausal women receiving estrogen therapy alone.

Q2

Small atrophic glands and decidualized stroma are the features seen in continuous combined contraceptive programs.

Q3

The sequential contraceptive program is still considered the most effective and is widely used.

Q4

Tamoxifen can have both an estrogenic and an antiestrogenic effect on endometrium.

Q5

The most characteristic feature of tamoxifen-associated endometrial lesions is endometrial hyperplasia.

Endometritis

Q1

The presence of neutrophils in the endometrium is a diagnostic sign of acute endometritis.

Q2

Identification of plasma cells is the most important criterion for the diagnosis of chronic endometritis.

Q3

The presence of neutrophils in the endometrial surface is a good predictor of pelvic inflammatory disease (PID).

Q4

An intrauterine device inserted for the purpose of contraception does not change the appearance of the endometrium on biopsy.

Q5

Mechanical cervical occlusion can lead to pyometra and hematometra.

Q6

Tuberculous granulomatous endometritis usually spreads to the myometrium.

Endometrial metaplasia

Q1

Endometrial metaplasias are benign lesions not associated with an increased risk for adenocarcinoma.

Q2

Ciliated (tubal) metaplasia may be seen in an otherwise normal endometrium but occurs more commonly in the setting of endometrial hyperplasia.

Q3

Intestinal metaplasia is a common form of endometrial metaplasia associated with endometriosis.

Adenomyosis and endometriosis

Q1

Adenomyosis and endometriosis are closely related disorders that usually occur together.

Q2

Many pathogenetic theories have been proposed over the years, but the most probable mechanism of endometriosis is mechanical implantation of the endometrium.

Q3

Adenomyosis can affect leiomyomatous lesions.

Q4

By convention, the diagnosis of adenomyosis should be reserved for those cases in which endometrial glands and stroma are seen in the myometrium at a distance of at least one low-power field from the endometrial–myometrial junction.

Q5

Endometriosis occurs in 1–7% of women in the USA.

Q6

Spontaneous cutaneous endometriosis is limited to the umbilical and inguinal areas.

Q7

Perineural invasion can be seen only with invasive carcinomas.

Q8

Endocervicosis represents endometriosis of the cervix.

Q9

Endometriosis is subject to any of the metaplastic, hyperplastic or neoplastic changes that may supervene in the orthotopic endometrium.

Dysfunctional uterine bleeding and hyperplasia

Q1

Bleeding associated with an organic cause in postmenopausal women is called dysfunctional uterine bleeding.

Q2

Inadequate proliferative-phase bleeding occurs in the absence of ovulation and is the most common type of dysfunctional uterine bleeding (DUB)

Q3

An anovulatory cycle can be recognized in its earliest stage by finding a proliferative endometrium at the time of the cycle when the secretory pattern would be expected.

Q4

Most commonly, prolonged unremitting estrogen stimulation results in endometrial hyperplasia.

Q5

Despite the shortcomings of the current classification for endometrial hyperplasia by Kurman and Norris, it is still the most used.

Q6

A cystic endometrial gland is always a sign of simple hyperplasia.

Q7

Endometrial hyperplasia is most commonly seen in postmenopausal women.

Q8

The presence of true intraglandular cellular bridges containing stromal support is highly indicative of well-differentiated endometrioid carcinoma.

Q9

The term atypical secretory hyperplasia has been applied to a pattern of architectural abnormalities and cellular atypia within a secretory endometrium, with the atypical glands resembling those seen in the 16th to 17th days of a normal cycle.

Q10

Most cases of endometrial carcinoma of the endometrioid type are preceded by a stage of hyperplasia, but overall relatively few patients with hyperplasia will subsequently develop a carcinoma.

Q11

The more severe the hyperplasia, the more likely it is to be followed by carcinoma.

Tumors

Q1

Endometrial polyps are true neoplasms representing a tumoral form of endometrial hyperplasia.

Q2

Endometrial polyps occur with an increase incidence after tamoxifen exposure.

Q3

Atypical polypoid adenomyomas are associated with Klinefelter syndrome.

Q4

Carcinoma of the endometrium is the most common gynecologic malignancy in developed countries.

Q5

It is currently believed that endometrial carcinoma can be divided into two major categories, one as a result of estrogenic excess and another that occurs de novo independent of estrogenic effect.

Q6

Grossly, carcinoma of the endometrium is always polypoid, in the form of broad-based polypoid masses.

Q7

Microscopically, 80% of endometrial malignant epithelial tumors are conventional adenocarcinomas.

Q8

A collection of foamy histiocytes in an endometrial curettage specimen is highly indicative of tumor necrosis and the presence of endometrioid adenocarcinoma.

Q9

Spread of endometrial carcinoma into the cervix occurs in over 50% of cases, usually by direct extension.

Q10

Adenoacanthoma is an older name for adenosquamous (mixed) carcinoma.

Q11

Secretory carcinoma is characterized by neoplastic glands having subnuclear vacuolization resembling that of a normal 17-day secretory endometrium and accompanied by a late secretory pattern in the adjacent endometrium.

Q12

Mucinous adenocarcinoma is a tumor subtype characterized by abundant mucin secretion.

Q13

Psammoma bodies are always indicative of a papillary–serous adenocarcinoma.

Q14

Clear cell carcinoma of the endometrium shares similar morphological features and an association with intrauterine diethylstilbestrol exposure with clear cell tumors of other sites, such as the vagina and cervix.

Q15

Small cell carcinomas of the endometrium are morphologically and etiologically different from their counterparts in other body sites.

Q16

Giant cell carcinoma shows strong positivity for hCG in the large giant cells.

Q17

The routine Pap smear is as effective in detecting endometrial adenocarcinoma as in detecting cervical carcinoma.

Q18

Coexpression of vimentin and keratin is common in endometrioid carcinoma.

Q19

All endometrial adenocarcinomas are ER/PR positive.

Q20

HER2/neu is present in approximately 20% of endometrial adenocarcinomas.

Q21

The four major abnormalities that have been detected in endometrioid carcinomas are microsatellite instability in the PTEN, K-*ras*, β-catenin and *p53* genes.

Q22

The most common sites of extrauterine spread of endometrioid carcinoma are the pelvic and para-aortic lymph nodes and ovaries.

Q23

The most common sites of recurrence of endometrial carcinoma are the vaginal vault and pelvis.

Q24

Approximately 28% of endometrial carcinomas are accompanied by a simultaneous ovarian carcinoma.

Q25

The usual treatment for endometrial carcinoma is total abdominal hysterectomy with bilateral salpingo-oophorectomy followed by radiation therapy.

Q26

Adenocarcinomas associated with hyperplasia have worse prognosis than ones not associated with hyperplasia.

Q27

Papillary serous adenocarcinoma and clear-type adenocarcinoma are the most aggressive subtypes of endometrial carcinoma.

Q28

The recently described markers that promise to be of importance in the identification and differential diagnosis of endometrial stroma tumors and smooth muscle tumors are CD10 and h-caldesmon.

Q29

Endometrial stromal tumors have been divided according to their microscopic appearance into endometrial stromal nodule and stromal sarcoma.

Q30

A proposal has been made to subdivide endometrial stromal sarcomas into low-grade and high-grade types according to their mitotic activity.

Q31

The most valuable prognostic factor for endometrial stromal sarcoma is mitotic rate.

Q32

The term 'uterine tumors resembling ovarian sex-cord tumors' refers to endometrial stromal tumors with epithelium-like formations.

Q33

Plexiform tumors, or tumorlets, are separate stromal tumors of neuroendocrine origin similar to their lung counterparts.

Q34

Tumors with the appearance of endometrial stromal tumors can be seen exclusively within the uterus.

Q35

Poorly differentiated endometrial stromal sarcoma shows a marked degree of nuclear pleomorphism and atypicality and lacks the vascular pattern and other distinctive features of endometrial stromal sarcoma.

Q36

Mixed malignant müllerian tumors (MMMT) are usually polypoid tumors in postmenopausal women presenting with bleeding and uterine enlargement.

Q37

The appearance of the epithelial component is the basis for the division of MMMTs into homologous and heterologous varieties.

Q38

It is the epithelial portion of MMMTs that shows the greatest capability for invasion and metastasis.

Q39

Because of their sarcomatous component, especially in heterologous varieties, the differentiation of MMMTs from teratomas can be difficult.

Q40

Tumors having only homologous stromal elements have been found to have a slightly better prognosis than those with heterologous elements.

Q41

A history of pelvic radiation is commonly observed in patients with MMMT.

Q42

MMMT can arise in extrauterine locations.

Q43

Müllerian adenosarcoma is considered a high-grade variant of MMMT.

Q44

Müllerian sarcomas resemble phylloides tumors of the breast microscopically.

Q45

Cases of müllerian adenosarcoma have been reported in association with tamoxifen therapy.

Q46

Criteria found to be useful in distinguishing müllerian adenosarcomas from müllerian adenofibromas include two or more standard stromal mitoses per hpf.

Q47

Clinically apparent leiomyomas are more common in nulliparous than parous and postmenopausal women than in premenopausal women.

Q48

Myoma nascens is a polypoid myoma that fills the endometrial cavity and emerges from the cervical canal.

Q49

Malignant transformation of leiomyomas is common and therefore surgical removal of larger leiomyomas is always necessary.

QUESTIONS

Q50

An alternative to surgical treatment of leiomyoma is arterial embolization and leuprolide medical therapy.

Q51

Stellate zones of recent hemorrhage within leiomyomas are rare.

Q52

Cellular leiomyomas have increased cellularity, no coagulative necrosis, atypia or an excessive number of mitotic figures.

Q53

Epithelioid (clear cell) leiomyoma is positive for CD117.

Q54

Cotyledonoid dissecting leiomyoma is an exophytic bulky tumor that extends from the uterine wall into the broad ligament and pelvic cavity, with vascular invasion and unpredictable clinical behavior.

Q55

Parasitic leiomyoma is smooth muscle proliferation formed as a result of schistosomal parasitization of the uterus.

Q56

Intravenous leiomyomatosis is an extremely rare condition characterized by the growth of mature smooth muscle inside the lumina of the uterine and pelvic wall vessels.

Q57

Benign metastasizing leiomyoma is another term for parasitic leiomyoma.

Q58

It has been proved that separate 'metastasizing' foci of the benign leiomyoma are separate independent nodules.

Q59

The majority of leiomyosarcomas are solitary lesions.

Q60

Microscopically, typical leiomyosarcomas are hypercellular, with nuclear atypia and pleomorphism, mitotically active and with areas of necrosis.

Q61

There is constant positivity for smooth muscle actin, h-caldesmon vimentin and low molecular weight keratin (CAM 5.2) in leiomyosarcomas.

Q62

Most valuable prognostic factors for the clinical behavior of leiomyosarcomas are tumor stage, microscopic grade, and number of mitosis.

Q63

The presence or absence and type of necrosis within smooth muscle tumors are of prognostic significance.

Q64

In the coagulative type of necrosis there is an abrupt transition between necrotic and viable cells.

Q65

Adequate sampling is essential for the correct interpretation of smooth muscle tumors.

Q66

'High-power field' is usually a combination of 20× eyepiece and 40× objective.

Q67

Tumors with marked and diffuse atypia, even with a lack of mitotic activity and coagulative necrosis, should be regarded as malignant.

Q68

Tumors with increased mitotic activity but lacking atypia and coagulative necrosis should be regarded as mitotically active.

Q69

Tumors with diffuse moderate to severe atypia and more than 10 mitoses per hpf should not be regarded as malignant without the presence of coagulative necrosis.

Q70

Myxoid leiomyosarcoma is an exception to the rule in which malignancy is to be diagnosed even without the presence of coagulative necrosis, increased mitotic activity and severe atypia.

Q71

Extramedullary hematopoiesis can occur in the endometrium associated with hematological or systemic diseases.

Q72

Adenomatoid tumors of the uterus can simulate lymphangiomas.

Q73

The most frequent metastatic carcinomas to the uterus from extrapelvic sites are breast, gastrointestinal tract, kidney and skin.

FALLOPIAN TUBE

Normal anatomy

Q1

The fallopian tube is divided into three segments: intramural, isthmus and ampulla.

Q2

The broad ligament is the peritoneal fold that supports the uterus on either side.

Q3

The round ligament is the peritoneal fold attached to the superior lateral border of the uterus that passes over the external iliac vessels and the inguinal ligament.

Inflammation

Q1

Rupture of a tubo-ovarian abscess requires prompt surgical intervention.

Q2

Pelvic inflammatory disease (PID) is the generic term used for inflammatory processes in which the ovary is the epicenter of inflammation.

Q3

Tuberculosis of the fallopian tube develops by the hematogenous route.

Torsion

Q1

Torsion of the fallopian tube is usually secondary to inflammation or tumor, but occasionally it develops in a previously normal organ.

Tubal pregnancy

Q1

Owing to the increased use of antibiotics and the prevention of PID, the incidence of tubal pregnancy has markedly decreased in recent times.

Q2

Tubal implantation usually occurs in the infundibular region of the tube.

Q3

The necrotic trophoblastic tissue may be retained within fallopian tube for a long time and appear as hyalinized ghost outlines of chorionic villi.

Other non-neoplastic processes

Q1

Paratubal cysts are commonly seen as small round cysts attached by a pedicle to the fimbriated end of a tube.

Q2

Decidual reaction of the tubal mucosa is a common finding.

Q3

Salpingitis isthmica nodosa is unilateral well-delimited nodular enlargement of the isthmic portion of the tube.

Q4

Metaplastic papillary tumor is encountered in tubes removed in the immediate postpartum period.

Proliferative epithelial lesions

Q1

The diagnosis of atypical tubal epithelial hyperplasia requires the presence of moderate or severe atypia without atypical mitosis.

Carcinoma

Q1

A growing number of cases of fallopian tube carcinoma have been reported in carriers of *BRCA1* and *BRCA2* mutations.

Q2

In the diagnosis of fallopian tube carcinoma, cervicovaginal smear is not a good diagnostic method.

Q3

The most common type of fallopian tube carcinoma is clear cell carcinoma.

Q4

The prognosis of tubal carcinoma depends largely on the stage.

Other tumors

Q1

Adenomatoid tumor is a benign lesion that can show a marked degree of smooth muscle hypertrophy.

Q2

Tubal teratomas are common.

Tumors and tumor-like conditions of the broad and round ligaments

Q1

Wolffian adnexal tumor is a distinct lesion seen within the leaves of the broad ligament.

Q2

The round ligament is only rarely the site of a primary tumor.

OVARY

Normal anatomy

Q1

The ovary is covered by a single layer of modified mesothelium known as surface, celomic or germinal epithelium.

Q2

The ovarian stroma is divided into a cortical and a basilar region.

Q3

The maturing ovarian follicle is composed of granulosa cells.

Q4

At the ovarian hilus there are clusters of cells analogous to testicular Leydig cells, known as ovarian hilus cells.

Gonadal dysgenesis

Q1

Features of Turner syndrome with a 45,XY karyotype are represented by large ovaries having a thickened stroma.

Q2

Testicular feminization represents a rare form of female pseudohermaphroditism.

Cysts, stromal hyperplasia and other non-neoplastic lesions

Q1

Follicular cysts form by distension of developing or atretic follicles and are usually smaller than 10 cm.

Q2

Large solitary luteinized follicular cyst is a rare lesion presenting in younger age groups.

Q3

Polycystic (sclerocystic) ovaries are characterized by multiple follicular cysts covered by a thick fibrous capsule.

Q4

Stromal hyperplasia is characterized by a diffuse or nodular proliferation of plump ovarian cortical stromal cells.

Q5

Ectopic decidual reaction can occur in the ovary during the normal menstrual cycle.

Q6

So-called luteomas of pregnancy are hemorrhagic nodules typically encountered during the first trimester.

Q7

Developmental ovarian cysts derive from wolffian and müllerian remnants, and are common in the region of the ovarian hilus.

Inflammation

Q1

Granulomatous infections such as tuberculosis occur in the ovary.

Q2

Autoimmune oophoritis is a poorly understood disorder characterized microscopically by giant cell reaction.

Q3

Endometriosis presents grossly as small, slightly raised blueberry-like spots on the ovarian surface.

Q4

The endometrial lining in endometriosis may be the site of reactive atypia ('atypical endometriosis') that stains negative for p53.

Ovarian biopsy

Q1

Ovarian biopsy obtained by laparotomy or surgical culdoscopy was carried out in the past for the evaluation of selected patients with amenorrhea and sterility resulting from anovulation.

Tumors

Q1

Surface epithelial tumors represent a rare group of ovarian neoplasms.

Q2

The ovarian surface epithelium, when involved in metaplastic or neoplastic conditions, often undergoes müllerian differentiation.

Q3

Serous tumors make up about one-quarter of all ovarian tumors, and approximately 30–50% are bilateral.

Q4

Serous cystadenoma contains cysts and papillae lined by multiple layers of atypical cells with high mitotic activity.

Q5

Ovarian surface tumors showing some or all of the features associated with carcinoma but lacking definite stromal invasion are called borderline tumors.

Q6

The decision whether an ovarian serous neoplasm is malignant or borderline in nature should be made purely on the basis of the morphologic features of the primary tumor, regardless of whether or not peritoneal lesions, lymph node metastases, or even lung deposits exist.

Q7

The microinvasive foci appear as individual cells or clusters of cells with large nuclei and scant clear cytoplasm.

Q8

Micropapillary serous carcinoma represents a category of serous neoplasms placed between borderline tumors and cystadenocarcinomas.

Q9

Prognostically, the presence and type (invasive versus non-invasive) of peritoneal implants are more important than whether the primary tumor is conventional or micropapillary carcinoma subtype.

Q10

In a specific type of malignant serous neoplasm called cystadenofibroma the fibroblastic stromal component is prominent, appearing grossly as solid, white, nodular and cystic.

Q11

Serous psammocarcinoma is a rare variant of serous carcinoma characterized by a massive presence of psammoma bodies and high-grade cytologic atypia; the behavior of these tumors closely resembles that of serous carcinoma.

Q12

Immunohistochemically, the typical keratin profile of serous tumors is CK7–/CK20+.

Q13

Important negative markers for serous tumors are CK20 and cytoplasmic CEA (in contrast to primary and metastatic mucinous tumors).

Q14

Mucinous neoplasms are less common than serous and are bilateral in only 10–20% of cases.

Q15

Ovarian mucinous tumors tend to be smaller than the serous types.

Q16

Microscopically, ovarian mucinous tumors (particularly those of borderline nature) have been divided into two major types, endocervical and serous.

Q17

The malignant type of mucinous tumor is characterized by cell atypia, increased layering of cells, complex glands, and areas of stromal invasion.

Q18

The existence and clinical significance of borderline mucinous tumors are more difficult to define than for their serous counterparts.

Q19

Some authors have proposed the following rules for the distinction between borderline and malignant mucinous tumors: if there is an unquestionable invasion, the tumor is classified as a carcinoma; if invasion is uncertain, the tumor is classified as borderline when the atypical epithelium is less than four cells thick, and as carcinoma when more than four atypical layers are present.

Q20

Immunohistochemically, the tumor cells of ovarian mucinous tumors express vimentin, SMA and inhibin.

Q21

Mucinous cystadenocarcinomas tend to metastasize to distant areas and do not invade locally.

Q22

Endometrioid carcinoma presents grossly as a cystic/solid hemorrhagic mass.

Q23

Microscopically, the appearance of endometrioid carcinoma resembles that of the ordinary type of endometrial carcinoma.

Q24

Immunohistochemically, endometrioid carcinomas express CEA, whereas EMA and vimentin are usually negative.

Q25

At the molecular level the difference between uterine and ovarian carcinomas is a mutation leading to β-catenin deregulation, found in nearly half of ovarian endometrioid carcinomas.

Q26

In some endometrioid carcinomas the neoplastic cells often form signet ring cells, suggesting a common tumor subtype.

Q27

As a group, endometrioid carcinoma has a prognosis twice as good as that of serous or mucinous carcinomas.

Q28

Clear cell (mesonephroid) adenocarcinoma is a distinctive ovarian tumor with a grossly spongy, often cystic, appearance.

Q29

Benign and borderline ovarian clear cell tumors are very rare.

Q30

Benign Brenner tumors, composed microscopically of solid and cystic nests of epithelial cells resembling transitional epithelium, are often accompanied by signs of hyperestrinism, such as uterine bleeding from endometrial hyperplasia.

Q31

Borderline or low malignant potential Brenner tumor shows low-grade cytologic atypia.

Q32

Cytologically malignant neoplasms associated with stromal invasion are referred to as malignant Brenner tumors.

Q33

Malignant mixed müllerian tumor (MMMT) of the ovary differs grossly and microscopically in every respect from its less common uterine counterpart.

Q34

Almost all ovarian MMMTs are seen in postmenopausal patients.

Q35

The most important differential diagnosis of ovarian MMMT with heterologous elements is immature teratoma.

Q36

Ovarian carcinoma accounts for the greatest number of deaths from malignancies of the female genital tract.

Q37

The majority of sporadic ovarian cancers are due to mutations in the *BRCA1* or the *BRCA2* genes.

Q38

Telomerase activity is found in virtually all carcinomas and borderline tumors.

Q39

Oncogenes reported to be amplified in ovarian carcinomas are HER2/*neu*, cyclin D, cyclin A, *p21* and *MDM2*.

Q40

DNA ploidy analyses have shown that benign and borderline tumors are usually aneuploid.

Q41

The most common site of involvement of ovarian serous carcinoma are the ureters, leading to a clinical presentation of hydronephrosis.

Q42

So-called 'Sister Joseph's nodule' represents an early manifestation of the disease, with widespread pelvic metastases.

Q43

The spread of borderline serous tumors is mainly in the form of invasive or non-invasive peritoneal implants.

Q44

Most peritoneal proliferative epithelial lesions have features of benign inclusion cysts.

Q45

Most germ cell tumors are seen in children and young adults, with approximately 95% of such tumors being benign cystic teratomas.

Q46

Some ovarian dysgerminomas arise in trisomies 13 and 18.

Q47

Dysgerminomas are more common on the right side and are often large and encapsulated, with a smooth, often convoluted, surface.

Q48

Immunohistochemically, dysgerminoma tumor cells are reactive for CEA and CD34.

Q49

Like testicular seminoma, ovarian dysgerminoma may exhibit signs of early differentiation towards other types of germ cell elements: scattered hCG-positive syncytiotrophoblastic cells, carcinomatous differentiation towards anaplastic dysgerminoma, or abortive yolk sac elements with serum elevation of α-fetoprotein.

Q50

Yolk sac tumor (endodermal ovarian sinus tumor) is a neoplasm generally seen in young children.

Q51

Microscopically, the appearance of yolk sac tumors is very variable.

Q52

Ovarian yolk sac tumors also stain with CK20 and EMA.

Q53

Embryonal carcinoma presents clinically with often (but not always) elevated serum α-fetoprotein, whereas chorionic gonadotropin levels are invariably high.

Q54

On gross examination embryonal carcinomas show extensive areas of necrosis and hemorrhage.

Q55

Microscopically, embryonal carcinoma has a similar appearance to testicular seminoma.

Q56

Most choriocarcinomas involving the ovary represent metastases from uterine tumors.

Q57

Immature (malignant) teratoma is defined as malignant ovarian tumor composed of a mixture of embryonal and adult tissues derived from all three germ layers.

Q58

The most significant prognostic factors in immature teratomas are size and stage of the tumor.

Q59

Grade I immature ovarian teratomas are composed of abundant mature tissues, intermixed with loose mesenchymal tissue with occasional mitoses, immature cartilage and tooth Anlagen.

Q60

Mature solid teratomas are clinically always malignant.

Q61

Mature cystic teratomas make up almost 20% of all ovarian tumors.

Q62

In mature teratomas the teeth tend to be located in a well-defined nipple-like structure, known as Rokitansky's protuberance.

Q63

Mature cystic teratomas may coexist with serous cystadenoma and adenofibroma.

Q64

Mature cystic teratomas can rupture into the abdominal cavity, with keratin and sebum provoking a prominent foreign body reaction.

Q65

Peritoneal implants composed exclusively of mature glial tissue, a condition known as gliomatosis peritonei, are associated only with immature teratomas.

Q66

The most common malignant change in cystic teratoma is squamous cell carcinoma, followed by carcinoid tumor and adenocarcinoma.

Q67

Epidermoid cyst of the ovary, a rare tumor entity, probably arises from ovarian epithelial cell nests.

Q68

Struma ovarii is the expression of the dominant growth of thyroid tissue in a teratoma.

Q69

Carcinoid tumor can be seen in the ovary only as a metastasis of a primary tumor, often located in the gastrointestinal tract.

Q70

Grossly, pure primary carcinoid tumors have a mean diameter of 10 cm, with a predominantly solid, yellow and homogeneous cut surface.

Q71

Strumal carcinoid is an ovarian neoplasm combining the features of carcinoid tumor and struma ovarii.

Q72

Granulosa cell tumor is an ovarian neoplasm showing differentiation toward follicular granulosa cells.

Q73

Adult granulosa cell tumors are usually cystic and occur during childhood.

Q74

The microscopic appearance of granulosa cell tumors is extremely variable, including the following patterns: microfollicular (with Call–Exner bodies), macrofollicular, trabecular, insular, solid and diffuse (sarcomatoid).

Q75

An important microscopic diagnostic feature of granulosa cell tumors is the presence of nuclear folds or grooves, resulting in a 'coffee-bean' appearance.

Q76

Positive immunohistochemical markers of granulosa cell tumors include chromogranin, EMA and CEA.

Q77

Cytogenetically, the cells of the adult granulosa cell tumor show consistent trisomy for chromosome 12.

Q78

Juvenile granulosa cell tumors show morphologic features similar to those of an adult subtype.

QUESTIONS

Q79

The differential diagnosis of granulosa cell tumor (particularly of the adult variety) includes poorly differentiated carcinoma of surface epithelial origin, carcinoid tumor, and tumors of endometrial stromal type.

Q80

The prognosis of granulosa cell tumors is largely dependent on the patient's age.

Q81

As a group, juvenile granulosa cell tumors behave more aggressively than their adult counterparts.

Q82

Thecoma presents before the menopause, is usually bilateral and has a cystic appearance.

Q83

Microscopically, thecomas are composed of fascicles of spindle cells with pale cytoplasm embedded within stroma showing significant collagen deposition and focal hyaline formation.

Q84

Masson trichrome and iron stains are used to highlight theca cells in dense stroma.

Q85

Fibromas are common benign tumors with a firm, solid, white cut surface, microscopically composed of closely packed spindle stromal cells arranged in a storiform pattern.

Q86

Ovarian fibroma (especially if large) can be associated with ascites, sometimes in combination with right-sided pleural effusion (Meigs' syndrome).

Q87

Sclerosing stromal tumor occurs in older age groups and has significant malignant potential.

Q88

Massive edema of the ovary is probably not a neoplasm but is important because of its gross similarities to fibroma.

Q89

The endometrium of patients with granulosa cell tumors or thecomas exhibits changes consistent with progestin effects.

Q90

Small cell carcinoma as a primary ovarian neoplasm has two well described types: gastric and hypocalcemic.

Q91

Hypercalcemic-type small cell carcinoma, which is more common, is a high-grade ovarian malignancy that may be confused with granulosa cell tumor (especially the juvenile subtype).

Q92

The tumor cells in small cell ovarian carcinoma may express keratin, EMA, vimentin and chromogranin, but not inhibin and S-100.

Q93

Sertoli–Leydig cell tumors are very common ovarian neoplasms.

Q94

Well- to intermediately differentiated Sertoli–Leydig cell tumors are composed mostly of tubules and cords.

Q95

Among many (at least six patterns) microscopic types of Sertoli–Leydig cell tumor, poorly differentiated types are composed of mostly Leydig cells.

Q96

Sertoli–Leydig cell tumor with heterologous elements is composed of tissues such as mucinous epithelium of gastrointestinal type, liver, skeletal muscle or cartilage.

Q97

Immunohistochemically, the areas of Sertoli cell differentiation stain for keratin but not for EMA, PLAP, CEA, CA19-9, CA-125 or S-100, whereas the gonadal stromal component is strongly positive for inhibin.

Q98

Almost half of the cases of Sertoli–Leydig cell tumor are accompanied by signs of estrogen excess.

Q99

Lipid cell ovarian tumors are manifested by an abundant eosinophilic or vacuolated cytoplasm that is often positive for fat stains.

Q100

Lipid cell tumors are usually bilateral and are composed of dark nodules.

Q101

Lipid cell tumor can occur at any age, and is typically associated with defeminization, amenorrhea and Cushing's syndrome.

Q102

Gynandroblastoma is the term used for sex cord–stromal tumors composed of primitive teratomatous elements.

Q103

Sex cord tumor with annular tubules is a distinctive ovarian tumor composed of a mixture of cells suggestive of granulosa cell tumor with a pattern of growth reminiscent of Sertoli cells.

Q104

Wolffian adnexal tumor was originally described as occurring in the broad ligament, retroperitoneum and ovary.

Q105

Gonadoblastoma is a tumor composed of a combination of germ cells and epithelial cells.

Q106

The risk of neoplasia in dysgenetic gonads is very low.

Q107

Nearly all ovarian lymphomas are of Hodgkin's type.

Q108

Secondary ovarian involvement by generalized lymphoma or leukemia is well recognized.

Q109

Primary sarcomas of the ovary are very common neoplasms.

Q110

Fibrosarcomas are distinguished from fibromas mainly on the basis of their cellularity.

Q111

The ovary is a common site of involvement for metastases.

Q112

Adenocarcinomas of the large bowel are particularly important because of their high frequency and their ability to simulate primary ovarian carcinomas, mainly of the mucinous and endometrioid types.

Q113

Features favoring ovarian metastasis from the large bowel are bilaterality, surface involvement by tumor cells, hilar involvement, single cell invasion, signet ring cells, and a cribriform glandular growth pattern with 'dirty' necrosis.

Q114

Metastatic large bowel carcinoma is characteristically CK7+/CK20–, CEA–, CA-125+, MUC2–.

Q115

The eponym Krukenberg tumor is used to designate an ovarian neoplasm, usually unilateral and characterized grossly by a large cystic ovarian mass.

Q116

The tubular variant of Krukenberg tumor, with its prominent tubular pattern and occasional virilization, may lead to a mistaken diagnosis of Sertoli–Leydig cell tumor.

Q117

Most examples of Krukenberg tumor occur before the age of 40.

Q118

The diagnosis of Krukenberg tumor is usually based on H&E recognition pattern.

Q119

Metastatic malignant melanomas in the ovaries are usually easy to recognize.

PREGNANCY, TROPHOBLASTIC DISEASE AND PLACENTA

Normal anatomy

Q1

The bulk of the umbilical cord is made up of highly mucoid connective tissue known as Wharton's jelly, in which two veins and a single artery are embedded.

Q2

The chorion associated with the membranes is referred to as chorion laeve.

Q3

Both syncytiotrophoblasts and cytotrophoblasts are positive for keratin stains.

Q4

The villous vessels contain only nucleated red blood cells at about 8 weeks and after 12 weeks they are virtually absent.

Q5

Decidual cells are reactive for vimentin, desmin and α_1-antitrypsin and are non-reactive with keratin.

Abortion

Q1

A monoamnionic placenta is indicative of monozygotic twins.

Q2

Immunohistochemical staining for hCG, hPL, SP1 and keratin can be useful in determining the presence of a product of conception when no definitive morphologic evidence is present on routine histological sections.

Q3

The Arias–Stella reaction is a physiologic response to viable trophoblastic tissue.

Q4

Hydropic changes are characterized by enlarged villi without trophoblastic proliferation and cistern formation.

Gestational trophoblastic disease

Q1

The nuclei of the trophoblastic cells in complete mole are composed exclusively of paternal DNA, whereas all cytoplasmic DNA is maternal.

Q2

The risk of complete mole can be reduced by increased consumption of carotene.

Q3

Clinically the uterus involved by a complete mole is usually smaller than expected for the stage of pregnancy.

Q4

By flow cytometry 75% of complete moles are diploid.

Q5

The presence of villi or atypical trophoblasts following the evacuation of molar pregnancy indicates the presence of an invasive mole.

Q6

Partial mole is more common than complete mole.

Q7

The volume of the placental tissue in partial mole is not as abundant as in complete mole, and grossly vesicular villi are mixed with normal-appearing villi.

Q8

Immunostaining for p57 is useful in distinguishing partial mole from complete mole.

Q9

Flow cytometry of placentas showing a triploid karyotype is a definitive proof of partial molar pregnancy.

Q10

The term invasive mole refers to a hydatidiform mole that is mostly of the partial type in which villi penetrate deeply into the myometrium and/or its vessels.

Q11

Invasive mole has all of the biologic features of a malignant neoplasm except that it is self-limited.

Q12

10–15% of complete moles are followed by choriocarcinoma.

Q13

There is a striking relationship between the incidence and prognosis of choriocarcinoma and the ABO groups of both the woman and her husband.

Q14

The presence of villi within classic choriocarcinoma is a good prognostic sign.

Q15

Microscopic grading of choriocarcinoma is of little value.

Q16

Choriocarcinoma cells are positive for hCG and keratin.

Q17

The survival rate is close to 100% in cases of choriocarcinoma restricted to the uterus and approximately 83% for patients with metastatic disease.

Q18

About 75% of cases of placental site trophoblastic tumor (PSTT) follow a normal pregnancy.

Q19

Grossly, PSTT presents mostly as a well-localized mass.

Q20

The morphological and immunohistochemical features of cells in PSTT correspond to those of intermediate trophoblasts.

Q21

The mortality of PSTT is 10–20% if not treated properly.

Q22

Epithelioid trophoblastic tumor shows extensive geographic necrosis and hemorrhage grossly.

Q23

Epithelioid trophoblastic tumor shows strong positivity for both hCG and hPL.

Q24

Exaggerated placental site reaction is a result of excessive but otherwise normal infiltration of the implantation site by intermediate trophoblasts.

Q25

Placental site nodules are yellow plaques and well-circumscribed nodules occurring exclusively in the endometrium.

Non-neoplastic lesions of term placenta

Q1

Placenta increta may result in spontaneous uterine rupture and fatal hemoperitoneum.

Q2

Amnion nodosum presents as small plaques on the amniotic surface, formed by squamous cells and fibrin.

Q3

The absence of an umbilical artery is associated with different congenital anomalies.

Q4

The acute inflammatory infiltrate situated mostly within peripheral membranes and chorionic plate is mostly contributed by maternal circulation.

Q5

The most common cause of placental infection is hematogenous spread of bacterial infection.

Q6

Acute funisitis is a sign of fetal inflammatory response.

Q7

Grossly, fresh placental infarct is whitish with a firm consistency.

Q8

An increased number of syncytial knots in the placenta can be seen in diabetic women.

Q9

Placental iron deposits are always a pathologic finding and are usually a sign of chronic placental bleeding.

Tumors and tumor-like conditions of term placenta

Q1

Hemangiomas of the placenta may be associated with hydramnios, hemorrhage, premature delivery, premature placental separation and placenta previa.

Q2

Metastatic tumors of maternal origin can lodge in the placenta in the form of distinct nodules.

VULVA

Normal anatomy

A1. True
The adnexal structures are usually not present in labia minora, but occasional sweat gland and sebaceous glands can be encountered. **(p. 1483)**

A2. True
Bartholin's gland is a major vestibular gland made up of acini with mucus-secreting columnar cells and transitional epithelium-lined ducts. **(p. 1483)**

A3. False
Skene's glands are analogous to the prostate gland. **(p. 1483)**

A4. False
Most of the vulvar lymphatics drain to the superficial inguinal nodes, but those in the clitoris empty directly into the deep chain. **(p. 1483)**

Congenital abnormalities

A1. True
The primitive milk line extends in embryo from the axilla to the groin. **(p. 1483)**

Inflammatory diseases

A1. False
Granuloma inguinale is a chronic infection caused by *Calymmatobacterium granulomatis*, a Gram-negative encapsulated bacillus. **(p. 1484)**

Chronic vulvar dystrophies

A1. True
Lichen sclerosus does occur in any age group, with a high percentage of spontaneous involution during puberty. **(p. 1485)**

A2. False
The consensus is that only a minimal risk exists for cancerous transformation of lichen sclerosus. **(p. 1485)**

A3. True
The absence of atypia in specimens with hyperplasia and a mild dermal chronic infiltrate represent a typical microscopic finding. **(p. 1485)**

Human papillomavirus and vulvar pathology

A1. False
Vulvar condyloma is usually caused by type 6 HPV. **(p. 1486)**

A2. False
Flat condyloma is more common than condyloma acuminatum. **(p. 1486)**

A3. True
(p. 1487)

A4. False
Condyloma shows minimal atypia, orderly maturation and mitoses that can be numerous but not atypical. **(p. 1487)**

Squamous intraepithelial lesions

A1. False
Bowen's disease corresponds to CIN-III cervical dysplasia involving the entire epithelial thickness. **(p. 1487)**

A2. False
Only a small percentage (10%) of cases progress to invasive carcinoma. **(p. 1488)**

Invasive squamous cell carcinoma

A1. False
There are two types of vulvar carcinoma: the most common, occurring in older women, is keratinizing tumor not related to HPV. The other type, in younger women, is frequently HPV related. **(p. 1488)**

A2. True
These carcinomas are known to metastasize directly into the deep pelvic nodes. **(p. 1489)**

A3. True
Tumors of the labia spread first to the inguinal lymph nodes, whereas those located in the clitoris may metastasize directly into the deep nodes. **(p. 1489)**

A4. True
The overall 5-year survival rate in patients treated for vulvar squamous cell carcinoma has been in the range 50–75%. **(p. 1490)**

A5. True
Lymph node status is more significant prognostic parameter than depth of invasion. **(p. 1490)**

A6. True
Even for microinvasive carcinoma the recommended treatment is surgery combined with inguinal lymphadenectomy. Perhaps the only invasive vulvar squamous cell carcinomas for which conservative surgery is indicated are those that are both well differentiated and very superficial (3 mm or less). **(p. 1490)**

A7. True
These tumors can be very large, with practically non-existent metastases. **(p. 1490)**

A8. False
These tumors invade stroma in a well-circumscribed 'pushing' fashion, and show no evidence of cytologic atypia. **(p. 1491)**

Paget's disease

A1. False
Pagets' disease is a malignant tumor that originates from the multipotential cells located along the epidermal basal layer. **(p. 1491)**

A2. True
Other useful stains in this neoplasm that are important in differentiating from melanoma are S-100, which is positive in one-third of Paget's disease cases, and negative HMB-45 stain. **(p. 1492)**

Other epithelial tumors

A1. True
This tumor shows remarkable morphologic similarity to intraductal papilloma of the breast and nipple duct adenoma. **(p. 1493)**

A2. True
These masses can grow very large and are known to ulcerate. Their behavior and microscopic appearance are the same as those of basal cell carcinoma elsewhere in the skin. **(p. 1494)**

Melanocytic tumors

A1. False

Melanoma is the second most common vulvar malignant tumor, following squamous cell carcinoma. Mostly, these lesions are already advanced at the time of diagnosis. **(p. 1495)**

Aggressive angiomyxoma and related lesions

A1. True

Microscopically, these tumors show hypocellular stroma devoid of mitotic activity, with hyalinized vessels. **(p. 1495)**

A2. True

These cells are immunoreactive for vimentin, desmin and hormone receptors, but usually not for actin and keratin. **(p. 1496)**

A3. False

Angiofibromas have well-circumscribed margins and are composed of uniform, bland spindle mesenchymal cells accompanied by numerous thick-walled vessels and inconspicuous islands of mature fat. **(p. 1496)**

Other tumors and tumor-like conditions

A1. True

Microscopically the tumor is sometimes composed of bizarre stellate multinucleated cells. **(p. 1496)**

A2. False

Most vulvar metastases originate from the cervix (50%), endometrium, kidney or gastrointestinal tract. **(p. 1497)**

Lesions of Bartholin's glands and related structures

A1. True

The lining of the cyst, which is usually transitional or squamous in type, can be obscured by the inflammatory infiltrate. **(p. 1498)**

A2. False

These carcinomas may take the form of squamous cell carcinoma (the most common), adenocarcinoma, transitional cell carcinoma, small cell or adenoid cystic carcinoma. **(p. 1498)**

Lesions of the female urethra

A1. True

This is not a true neoplasm, rather a reactive polypoid lesion with chronic inflammation and hyperplastic epithelium. **(p. 1498)**

A2. False

Urethral carcinoma occurs in elderly patients and presents with dysuria and bleeding. Microscopically, most carcinomas are of the squamous cell type, followed by transitional, columnar and clear cell adenocarcinoma. **(p. 1499)**

VAGINA

Normal anatomy

A1. True
The squamous epithelium, which is responsive to steroid hormones, can be divided, as in the exocervix, into three main zones: basal, intermediate and superficial. **(p. 1508)**

A2. True
This epithelium is responsive to steroid hormones, its appearance depending on the age of the patient and the time of the menstrual cycle. **(p. 1508)**

A3. True
Gartner's duct runs deeply along the lateral vaginal walls. **(p. 1508)**

A4. False
The major vaginal lymphatics drain into pelvic, rectal, aortic, iliac and femoral nodes. **(p. 1508)**

Adenosis and related lesions

A1. False
Adenosis grossly appears as red spots. **(p. 1508)**

A2. True
Originally adenosis of the vagina was described as the conversion of squamous to endocervical-type glandular epithelium. This concept was later expanded to embrace the presence of any müllerian-type glandular epithelium. Grossly, adenosis appears as red granular spots or patches that do not stain with Lugol's solution. **(p. 1508)**

A3. True
Sometimes the squamous metaplasia is so extensive that the only evidence of a pre-existing adenosis is found in the form of rare pools of intracellular droplets of mucin. **(p. 1509)**

A4. False
A clear relation between adenosis and in-utero exposure to DES has been established. **(p. 1509)**

A5. False
Transverse ridges are also related to DES administration. **(p. 1509)**

A6. True
These DES-related lesions usually revert to normal following biopsy or therapy. **(p. 1509)**

Other non-neoplastic lesions

A1. False
These infections are very common during pregnancy. **(p. 1509)**

A2. False
The above-mentioned lesions may occur as a result of an unusual bacterial infection and lead to pseudotumorous formation or stricture. **(p. 1509)**

A3. True
The tubal prolapse with granulation tissue typically occurs within 6 months post hysterectomy. **(p. 1510)**

A4. False
Vaginal endometriosis is seen in connection with episiotomy scars. **(p. 1510)**

Benign epithelial tumors

A1. True
Papillomas may be seen in the adult vagina, but less commonly than in the cervix. **(p. 1510)**

Squamous intraepithelial lesions

A1. False
Intraepithelial vaginal dysplasia arises from native epithelium. **(p. 1511)**

Invasive squamous cell carcinoma

A1. True
It is largely a disease of the elderly, and often represents an extension of cervical carcinoma. **(p. 1511)**

A2. True
The upper third and the anterior or lateral vaginal walls are the most common sites of primary squamous cell carcinoma. **(p. 1511)**

A3. False
The most common sites of origin of vaginal carcinoma are the upper third, anterior or lateral vaginal walls. **(p. 1511)**

Clear cell (adeno)carcinoma

A1. True
The average age at the time of diagnosis is 17 years. **(p. 1512)**

A2. False
Exposure to DES shows a correlation with clear cell carcinoma. **(p. 1512)**

A3. True
These features strongly suggest the existence of a DES-related disturbance. **(p. 1512)**

A4. True
Microglandular hyperplasia and Arias–Stella reaction both contain clear cytoplasm and occur in a background of pregnancy or progestational agents. **(p. 1512)**

A5. True
Hobnail-shaped cells in clear cell carcinoma can be detected by cytologic examination, but can be missed in patients with vaginal smears. **(p. 1512)**

A6. False
Tumor cells show positivity for CK7, CD15, CAM-5.2, and negativity for CK20 and CK30. **(p. 1512)**

Other carcinoma types

A1. True
The tumor invades locally and can reach the rectum and coccyx. **(p. 1513)**

A2. False
Sarcomatoid carcinoma with similar microscopic features is found in the upper aerodigestive tract. **(p. 1513)**

A3. False
These tumors arise from the foci of vaginal endometriosis. **(p. 1513)**

A4. True
These tumors can also occur in a background of atypical adenosis. **(p. 1513)**

A5. False
Positive neuroendocrine immunohistochemical markers are usually observed in vaginal small cell carcinomas. **(p. 1513)**

A6. True
Some of these tumors have been located in the upper lateral vaginal area, suggesting the possibility that they may arise from Gartner's ducts or related mesonephric rests. **(p. 1514)**

Mesenchymal tumors and tumor-like conditions

A1. False
FP is seen in adult women during pregnancy or in neonates. **(p. 1514)**

A2. True
Fibroepithelial polyps can also represent the end stage of granulation tissue. **(p. 1514)**

A3. True
The slow pace of growth and the fact that a cambium layer, epithelial invasion and cross-striations are absent are among the distinguishing features of this benign tumor. **(p. 1514)**

A4. True
Grossly, it presents as a small friable reddish mass in the vaginal vault. **(p. 1515)**

A5. True
Clues to the recognition of postoperative spindle cell nodule are a distinct fascicular pattern, the absence of pleomorphism, typical mitoses, and – most importantly – a history of recent surgery. **(p. 1515)**

Botryoid rhabdomyosarcoma

A1. False
BR is a polypoid tumor and arises from the anterior vaginal wall. **(p. 1515)**

A2. False
Most cases (90%) occur in girls under 5 years of age. **(p. 1515)**

A3. True
Cross-striations may or may not be present. **(p. 1515)**

A4. True
This important diagnostic feature is typically seen beneath non-neoplastic epithelium. **(p. 1516)**

A5. False
Foci of neoplastic cartilage within BR are associated with a better prognosis. **(p. 1516)**

Melanocytic tumors

A1. True
Melanomas typically occur as primary vaginal tumors in elderly patients. **(p. 1517)**

A2. True
Vaginal melanomas tend to show greater anaplasia and pleomorphism than their cutaneous counterparts. **(p. 1517)**

A3. True
An intraepithelial component of melanoma can be destroyed by the tumor ulceration. **(p. 1517)**

Metastatic tumors

A1. True
Some cases represent direct extension, and others are distant metastases. **(p. 1517)**

UTERUS–CERVIX

Normal anatomy

A1. True

The midzone is also called the stratum spongiosum. Another layer of cells situated just above the basal layer (suprabasal layer) can be demonstrated by silver staining and is considered by some authors to be the 'stem cell' of the cervical squamous mucosa. **(p. 1523)**

A2. False

In postmenopausal women the cervix shows atrophic changes morphologically similar to cervical intraepithelial neoplasia (CIN I). **(p. 1523)**

A3. True

The glandular mucosa of the endocervix is formed by a layer of columnar mucus-secreting cells with histochemical reactivity for mucin, depending on the time of the menstrual cycle. **(p. 1523)**

Remnants and ectopias

A1. False

Mesonephric rest are seen in about a third of women. **(p. 1524)**

Squamous and other metaplasias

A1. True

Squamous metaplasia describes the focal or extensive replacement of mucus-secreting glandular epithelium by stratified squamous epithelium. **(p. 1524)**

A2. False

Most commonly, squamous metaplasia involves only the superficial layer of the squamous epithelium and is recognized by the presence of squamous epithelium overlying the endocervical glands. **(p. 1525)**

A3. True

Although most cervical carcinomas arise in areas of cervix that at some time in the past had been involved by squamous metaplasia; the latter process has no premalignant connotation. **(p. 1525)**

A4. True

This condition has been somewhat controversial, as some authors regard it as nothing but an atrophic form of CIN. However, follow-up data have not supported this alternative interpretation. **(p. 1525)**

A5. True

It is commonly seen after conization. **(p. 1526)**

Inflammatory lesions

A1. False

Only rarely are diagnostic multinucleated cells with intranuclear inclusions encountered. **(p. 1526)**

A2. False

Chlamydia trachomatis is now recognized as the most common venereal infection in the western world. **(p. 1526)**

Non-neoplastic glandular lesions

A1. False
Endocervical polyps are the result of chronic inflammatory changes and are not considered true neoplasms. **(p. 1527)**

A2. True
Tunnel clusters, originally described by Fluhmann, have been divided into type A (non-cystic) and type B (cystic) and are the result of localized proliferation of endocervical glands (clefts), with side channels growing out from them. **(p. 1527)**

A3. True
Microglandular hyperplasia can be confused with carcinoma because of its solid growth and mitotic activity. However no significant atypia is present. **(p. 1528)**

A4. True
Owing to significant morphological atypia Arias–Stella reaction can be confused with carcinoma. However, lack of a mass-forming lesion, stromal reaction and infiltrative pattern is the main morphological distinction. **(p. 1528)**

A5. False
Lobular endocervical glandular hyperplasia is a benign, distinctly lobular proliferation of small to medium-sized glands around a larger central gland with no premalignant potential. **(p. 1529)**

Non-neoplastic stromal lesions (including endometriosis and related processes)

A1. True
Decidual spots usually occur in pregnancy and present as friable yellow spots that bleed easily. **(p. 1529)**

A2. False
Placental site nodules are composed of intermediate trophoblasts showing cytoplasmic vacuolization and have been characteristically positive for keratin. Decidual spots are negative for keratin staining. **(p. 1529)**

A3. False
On occasion the process is composed almost exclusively of endometrial stroma and is referred to as 'stromal endometriosis.' **(p. 1530)**

HPV and the lower genital tract

A1. False
HPV comprises a family of DNA viruses, of which more than 60 types have been characterized, the most common being 6 and 11. **(p. 1530)**

A2. False
The test currently regarded as the gold standard for the detection of HPV is Southern blot hybridization. **(p. 1530)**

A3. True
Koilocytes were first described by Finnish workers Esco Purola and Eeva Savia, and then the term koilocytic atypia was introduced by Leopold Koss and Grace Durfee. The word itself stems from the Greek *koilos*, which means 'hollow.' **(p. 1530)**

A4. True
Perinuclear clearings can be seen in postmenopausal squamous atypia and are not associated with HPV infection. **(p. 1530)**

A5. False
The features in a cervical biopsy exhibiting the signs of HPV infection that indicate the additional presence of CIN are atypia along the basal layers, a disorderly pattern of maturation, and abnormal mitotic figures. Koilocytic atypia alone is not enough for a diagnosis of CIN. **(p. 1531)**

A6. True
The three major groups are the 'high-risk' types, primarily 16 and 18, but also 31, 33, 35, 39, 45, 51, 52, 56, 58, 59, 68, 73 and 82. HPV types 16, 53 and 66 have been classified as 'probably high risk,' and types 6, 11, 40, 42, 43, 44, 54, 61, 70, 72, 81 and CP6108 are included in the 'low-risk' category. **(p. 1531)**

A7. True
A mild degree of atypia can also be seen, but need not be mentioned; if more severe atypia is present it should be evaluated and graded by same criteria as flat squamous intraepithelial lesions. **(p. 1531)**

A8. True

The true nature of the lesion is not clear; however, it has to be differentiated from the papillary form of CIN, verrucous carcinoma and well-differentiated squamous cell carcinoma. **(p. 1532)**

Tumors

A1. True

The intraepithelial stage shows a monomorphic population of dysplastic cells affecting the full epithelial thickness. **(p. 1532)**

A2. False

This assumption is unproven. In fact, the milder forms are particularly unstable. **(p. 1532)**

A3. True

Dysplastic foci often end abruptly and their extent is highly variable, but they can be focal and small and therefore removed completely by biopsy. However, in rare instances dysplasia can extend into the vagina as far as the endometrial cavity, and even to the fallopian tubes. **(p. 1532)**

A4. False

The morphological criteria for the diagnosis of CIN should be the same regardless of the circumstances. **(p. 1533)**

A5. True

The difference between severe dysplasia and carcinoma in situ is based on rather subtle and subjective criteria that vary according to the individual pathologist and institution. The term CIN was proposed in hope of eliminating some of those problems. **(p. 1534)**

A6. True

The low-grade lesions correspond to CIN I (as well as some HPV-induced lesion that do not qualify as CIN), whereas the high-grade lesions correspond to CIN II and CIN III. **(p. 1534)**

A7. False

Whether all patients with low-grade CIN require therapy remains contentious. **(p. 1534)**

A8. True

Such carcinomas have been also designated as 'superficially invasive,' or carcinomas with 'early stromal invasion.' **(p. 1535)**

A9. True

Benson and Norris have found that the overall risk for lymph node metastasis in microinvasive carcinoma is 1%. However, Hasumi et al. further subdivided microinvasion into those that invade up to 3 mm and those that invade from 3.1 to 5 mm. Their research showed an increased percentage of lymph node metastases in the latter group (13.9% vs 0.9%) This evidence encouraged the cut-off point for microinvasion to be 3 mm. **(p. 1535)**

A10. False

The single most important factor is age at first intercourse. **(p. 1535)**

A11. False

In fact, bulky carcinomas that grow out of the cervix are less likely to invade the surrounding structures. **(p. 1535)**

A12. True

There are three morphological subtypes of squamous cell carcinoma: large cell non-keratinizing, keratinizing, and small cell variant. Small cell variant needs to be differentiated from small cell neuroendocrine carcinoma. Admixtures and intermediate forms of these three subtypes usually exist in the same tumor. **(p. 1536)**

A13. True

On occasion cervical squamous cell carcinoma is associated with intense infiltration by eosinophils with or without accompanying peripheral eosinophilia. The production of eosinotactic or eosinopoietic substances by the tumor is suggested as a pathogenetic mechanism. **(p. 1536)**

A14. False

Squamous cell carcinoma often expresses p63, which is a homolog of p53 that is preferentially expressed in basal and immature cervical squamous epithelium. **(p. 1537)**

A15. True

The pattern of involvement is usually sequential, represented by paracervical, hypogastric, obturator and external iliac groups, and the second by the sacral, common iliac, aortic and inguinal groups. The incidence of nodal involvement is related directly to the stage of the disease. **(p. 1537)**

A16. False

Invasive carcinoma of the cervix can be treated by surgery, irradiation, or a combination of both. They are mostly radiosensitive; however, lack of a prompt response to radiation therapy is a predictor of likely recurrence and an indicator that adjuvant therapy should be considered. **(p. 1537)**

A17. True

Besides the clinical stage, which is the most significant risk factor, microscopic grade and type of carcinoma, tumor-associated eosinophilia, HPV status and cell proliferation index are other risk factors, but are considered to be of controversial significance. **(p. 1539)**

A18. True

Cervical carcinoma spreads characteristically by direct extension to the vagina, endometrium or myometrium, parametrium, lower urinary tract and uterosacral ligaments. **(p. 1539)**

A19. True

Verrucous carcinoma must be differentiated from condyloma acuminatum and ordinary squamous cell carcinoma with papillary growth. **(p. 1539)**

A20. False

Spindle cell carcinoma is a variant of squamous cell carcinoma with sarcomatoid-like stroma. Often there is evidence of HPV infection. **(p. 1539)**

A21. False

Primary cervical adenocarcinoma comprises 10–15% of all carcinomas. The percentage has been higher in Jewish women and has been increasing in the general population. **(p. 1540)**

A22. True

In addition, overexpression of p53 is common and a quarter of cases are positive for ER and PR. **(p. 1540)**

A23. True

The few negative tumors tend to be non-mucinous and occur in older women. **(p. 1541)**

A24. False

The overall prognosis in cervical adenocarcinoma depends on the clinical stage, the amount of tumor, microscopic grade and nodal status, and is usually better than the prognosis for squamous cell carcinoma. **(p. 1541)**

A25. False

Morphologically both tumors are very similar; however, the presence of in situ adenocarcinoma in the cervical glands, diffuse mucin with CEA positivity, negativity for vimentin, estrogen and progesterone receptors, and the presence of HPV by in situ hybridization favors endocervical adenocarcinoma. **(p. 1541)**

A26. True

In addition, most lesions are positive for CEA, less than half for keratin, and the lesions usually show increased MIB-1 proliferative index. **(p. 1541)**

A27. True

HPV plays an important role in the pathogenesis of cervical squamous and adenocarcinoma in situ. **(p. 1542)**

A28. False

In most cases conization is an adequate treatment for cervical adenocarcinoma; however, negative surgical margins do not always indicate that no tumor is left behind. **(p. 1542)**

A29. True

In addition, half of the cases have small foci with a less differentiated appearance. Vascular and perineural invasion can be seen. **(p. 1542)**

A30. False

Adenoma malignum is positive for CEA, which is a useful feature in differentiating it from benign lesions such as microglandular hyperplasia or tubal metaplasia. However, adenoma malignum usually lacks evidence of high-risk HPV and p53 mutations. **(p. 1543)**

A31. False

Even though some series have shown the worst overall prognosis of adenosquamous carcinomas, when compared stage by stage there does not seem to be a prognostic difference between squamous and adenosquamous carcinomas. **(p. 1543)**

A32. False

Glassy cell carcinoma is considered as a distinct type of poorly differentiated adenosquamous carcinoma. **(p. 1543)**

A33. False

The two entities share some similar morphological features, but adenoid cystic carcinoma is associated with particularly poor prognosis whereas adenoid basal carcinoma is a low-grade lesion with an excellent prognosis. **(p. 1545)**

A34. True

However, it has a second peak at age 70. It shows a relationship with intrauterine diethylstilbestrol (DES) exposure in younger patients and occurs in the absence of exposure to this hormone in older women. **(p. 1545)**

A35. False

Even though the association with HPV is strong in cases of neuroendocrine carcinomas, CIN changes in the adjacent mucosa are extremely rare. **(p. 1546)**

A36. True

A definite relationship exists with the degree of microscopic differentiation, with clinical outcome being particularly grim for small cell carcinomas. **(p. 1546)**

A37. False

The Pap smear was first described by Romanian pathologist Aureli Papes and then popularized by Papanicolau. **(p. 1546)**

A38. True

The rationale for such grouping is based on many morphological similarities between the lesions, which make their separation difficult. **(p. 1548)**

Other tumors and tumor-like conditions

A1. True

The appearance is similar to that of its vaginal counterpart; however, cervical tumors are associated with a better prognosis. **(p. 1549)**

A2. False

Most cervical lymphoma present with vaginal bleeding without obvious ulceration, and most are diffuse large B-cell lymphomas. **(p. 1550)**

A3. True

Metastatic carcinomas can originate from genital or extragenital organs, and some of them can simulate primary cervical carcinoma. **(p. 1551)**

ENDOMETRIUM

Normal anatomy

A1. True

The basal layer is equivalent to the reserve cell layer and is responsible for the regeneration of the endometrium following menstruation. It is made up of weakly proliferative endometrium and spindled stroma. The functional layer undergoes a series of sequential changes in the course of the ovulatory cycle. **(p. 1569)**

A2. True

Subnuclear vacuolization appears on the 16th day of ovulation, and in order for this feature to be diagnostic of ovulation 50% of cells should contain subnuclear vacuoles. **(p. 1570)**

A3. False

On the contrary, only the functional layer is prone to hormonal influence, whereas the basal layer and the lower uterine segment mucosa are not subject to the influence of progesterone. **(p. 1570)**

A4. True

These changes are almost always focal and may occur in the cervix, endocervical polyps, adenomyosis and endometriosis. **(p. 1571)**

A5. False

Exceptionally, decidual reaction is seen in postmenopausal endometrium even in the absence of an exogenous or endogenous source of progesterone excess. **(p. 1571)**

Curettage and biopsy

A1. False

Fractional curettage is a method of separate sampling from the endometrium and endocervix, and even though the method is helpful, small isolated tumor fragments can be found in endocervical samples without actual infiltration. In such cases the presence of cancer in material submitted is reported without a definitive statement about invasion. **(p. 1572)**

A2. False

Ashernman's syndrome is the development of adhesions resulting in amenorrhea and other menstrual abnormalities. It is an exceptional complication of endometrial curettage, but is seen most often after postpartum or postabortion curettages, and is thought to be the result of a subclinical uterine infection. **(p. 1572)**

Effects of hormone administration

A1. True

Furthermore, several studies have linked the exogenous administration of estrogen to the subsequent appearance of endometrial adenocarcinoma. The addition of progestin to the medication protects the endometrium and reduces the incidence of hyperplasia and carcinoma. **(p. 1572)**

A2. True

Not only endometrium, but also endometriotic foci have a similar change, which must be borne in mind whenever pelvic lesions are evaluated for pathology. **(p. 1572)**

A3. False

The sequential program was discontinued in the United States and Canada in 1976 because of several reports suggesting that it promoted the development of endometrial adenocarcinoma. **(p. 1573)**

A4. True

It has antiestrogenic effects on the endometrium when competing with ovarian estrogen secretion, but also a paradoxical estrogenic effect in the absence of ovarian estrogen secretion. **(p. 1573)**

Endometritis

A1. False

Neutrophils are normally present in the endometrium on days 26, 27 and 28 of the menstrual cycle. **(p. 1573)**

A2. True

Plasma cells are indicators of chronic inflammation in endometrial biopsy. Lymphoid follicles with or without germinal centers can be seen in normal endometrium. **(p. 1573)**

A3. True

The presence of neutrophils in the endometrial surfaces is a good predictor of PID, especially if combined with plasma cells in the endometrial stroma. **(p. 1574)**

A4. False

In an old series, only 29% of symptomatic patients and 40% of asymptomatic patients had a normal endometrial appearance on biopsy. The most common change is focal or extensive endometritis, which can be accompanied by necrosis and squamous metaplasia. One of the agents involved in the inflammatory process is *Actinomyces*. **(p. 1574)**

A5. True

Pyometra refers to the accumulation of pus in the endometrial cavity, and hematometra represents the accumulation of blood within the endometrial cavity. Both are usually a consequence of cervical occlusion. **(p. 1574)**

A6. False

Tuberculous granulomas tend to concentrate in the superficial functional layer, whereas in sarcoidosis granulomas are spread within the myometrium. **(p. 1575)**

Endometrial metaplasia

A1. False

Like endometrial hyperplasia, metaplasias are associated with endometrial carcinoma and are more common in populations already at high risk for the development of this tumor. The presence of p53 overexpression in a significant number of metaplasias has been documented. This was an unexpected finding, usually associated with malignant tumors. **(p. 1575)**

A2. True

Scattered ciliated cells are normally present in the endometrium. **(p. 1575)**

A3. False

Intestinal metaplasia is an exceptionally rare form that resembles intestinal mucosa. It is not associated with endometriosis. **(p. 1576)**

Adenomyosis and endometriosis

A1. False

Even though these lesions are regarded as closely related they often occur independently of each other. Adenomyosis is usually composed of non-functional endometrium, whereas the endometriosis is composed of functional endometrium. **(p. 1576)**

A2. False

The most common and important mechanism is metaplastic change of the secondary müllerian system. **(p. 1576)**

A3. True

In elderly women the uterus may appear atrophic despite extensive adenomyosis. **(p. 1577)**

A4. True

Microscopically, the diagnosis of adenomyosis depends on the threshold used by the individual pathologist. Because of the normally irregular interphase between endometrium and myometrium such interpretations can be very diverse. **(p. 1578)**

A5. True

Endometriosis can be located in the cervix, vagina, vulva, rectovaginal septum, ovary, fallopian tube, uterine ligaments and other sites. **(p. 1578)**

A6. True

In other areas it practically always arises in surgical scars. **(p. 1578)**

A7. False

Some morphological features of endometriosis can be confusing to interpret, and one of these is perineural invasion. Other morphological variants are micronodular stromal form, stromal elastosis and prominent myxoid change. **(p. 1579)**

A8. False

Endocervicosis is a subtype of endometriosis in which glands undergo prominent mucinous metaplasia, a change that can result in a mistaken diagnosis of well-differentiated mucinous adenocarcinoma. The combination of endometriosis and endocervicosis is sometimes referred as müllerianosis. **(p. 1579)**

A9. True

Benign, borderline and malignant tumors can develop within endometriosis, with endometrioid and clear cell carcinoma being the most common types. **(p. 1579)**

Dysfunctional uterine bleeding and hyperplasia

A1. False

Bleeding *not* associated with an organic cause in women of childbearing age belongs to the large category of dysfunctional uterine bleeding. **(p. 1580)**

A2. False

Cases of DUB can be divided into those associated with ovulation and those in which ovulation has not occurred. Inadequate proliferative-phase bleeding belongs to the ovulatory group and is recognized by a disparity between the endometrial pattern observed and that expected for the time of the cycle. **(p. 1580)**

A3. True

Absence of tortuous secretory glands is a significant microscopic finding in this entity. **(p. 1580)**

A4. True

All gradations of this phenomenon occur, ranging from abnormal exuberant proliferative endometrium (so-called disordered proliferative endometrium) to an atypical one that approaches the appearance of adenocarcinoma. **(p. 1580)**

A5. True

Kurman and Norris divided endometrial hyperplasia into simple and complex on the basis of architecture, and further subdivided the groups into typical and atypical on the basis of cytological atypia. A particular concern was the reproducibility of the classification, especially in the category of simple atypical hyperplasia. However, it was felt that no other classification was ready to replace the current one. **(p. 1581)**

A6. False

Cystic glands can be seen in cystic endometrial atrophy, a condition known as retrogressive hyperplasia usually seen in postmenopausal women. **(p. 1581)**

A7. False

Endometrial hyperplasia is most commonly seen in perimenopausal women, but it can occur in younger patients, even adolescents. **(p. 1581)**

A8. False

The distinction between complex hyperplasia and a well-differentiated carcinoma can be very difficult. The presence of true intraglandular cellular bridges *devoid* of stromal support is indicative of carcinoma. Other morphological features favoring carcinoma are marked pleomorphism with loss of polarity, a complex ramification of disorderly arranged glands, extensive papillary formations, a confluent glandular pattern with solid or cribriform appearance, and a desmoplastic stromal response. **(p. 1582)**

A9. True

The natural history of this condition is not yet well known, and it would seem that a conservative therapeutic approach is justified. **(p. 1582)**

A10. True

All patients with endometrioid carcinoma who had adequate previous biopsies had an abnormal endometrioid pattern before the development of carcinoma. However, the mere presence of hyperplasia is not an indication for hysterectomy. **(p. 1583)**

A11. True

This is particularly true with regard to cytologic atypia. When this is coupled with architectural atypia the risk is even higher. **(p. 1583)**

Tumors

A1. False

Most endometrial polyps are not true neoplasms and only represent circumscribed foci of hyperplasia. **(p. 1583)**

A2. True

Such polyps are usually fibrotic, multiple, and may exhibit stromal decidualization and mucinous metaplasia. At the molecular level they show a higher frequency of K-*ras* mutation. **(p. 1584)**

A3. False

Some are associated with Turner syndrome. They tend to occur in younger women and present with vaginal bleeding. Glands occurring between the endometrial stroma and smooth muscle bundles exhibit varying degree of hyperplasia, atypia and squamous morules, which can be misdiagnosed as adenocarcinoma with myometrial invasion. **(p. 1584)**

A4. True

The highest incidence is in the USA and Canada, with a recent decline in both incidence and mortality. **(p. 1585)**

A5. True

Those at high risk of estrogenic excess-related endometrial carcinoma include obese, hypertensive, diabetic and infertile patients. **(p. 1585)**

A6. False

Endometrial carcinoma can also present grossly as diffuse infiltration within the myometrium. Usually extensive myometrial invasion is accompanied by clinically detectable uterine enlargement; however, sometimes deep myometrial extension is accompanied by a normal-sized uterus. **(p. 1586)**

A7. True

They are usually divided into well differentiated (grade I), moderately differentiated (grade II) and poorly differentiated (grade III). **(p. 1586)**

A8. False

The stroma of an endometrioid adenocarcinoma may contain collections of foamy cells, which are probably the result of tumor necrosis and a good marker for the presence of carcinoma. However, such cells can also be seen in hyperplasia and in the absence of proliferative epithelial changes. **(p. 1586)**

A9. False

Extension to the cervix occurs in over 10%, mostly by direct extension, but allegedly also by implantation following dilatation and curettage.

A10. False

Adenoacanthomas contain areas of benign squamous elements derived from a benign metaplastic process, whereas adenosquamous carcinomas contain malignant-appearing elements. Morphologic studies have suggested that adenoacanthoma and adenosquamous carcinoma represent a spectrum of squamous metaplasia in a single tumor, rather than two independent entities. However, for the time being they are considered different neoplasms. **(p. 1588)**

A11. True

This tumor is not believed to be a specific type of endometrial carcinoma but rather the expression of a pattern that may be present diffusely or focally in a well-differentiated endometrioid carcinoma, usually as a result of progesterone stimulation. **(p. 1588)**

A12. True

It is distinguished from mucinous metaplasia by virtue of its architectural and cytologic atypia, although on occasion it can be deceptively bland in appearance. **(p. 1589)**

A13. False

Occasionally psammoma bodies can be seen in endometrioid carcinoma. Key features of papillary serous adenocarcinoma are the consistently high-grade nature of its cytologic features, complex papillary growth, numerous mitoses and extensive necrosis. **(p. 1589)**

A14. False

Even though clear cell tumors of the various sites share morphological features, clear cell tumors of the vagina and cervix are the only ones associated with intrauterine diethylstilbestrol exposure. **(p. 1590)**

A15. False

Small cell carcinomas of the endometrium are morphologically, immunohistochemically and ultrastructurally identical to their counterparts in other body sites. Their behavior is very aggressive, as seen in lung, cervix and in other sites. **(p. 1590)**

A16. False

Endometrioid carcinoma with trophoblastic differentiation shows positivity for hCG, whereas giant cell carcinoma is hCG negative. **(p. 1591)**

A17. False

The positive rate in detecting endometrial carcinoma by PAP smear is only 50%. Several cytologic methods have been employed to increase this rate, such as endometrial aspiration, tampon smear, endometrial lavage, endometrial brushing and suction curettage. However, the widespread applicability of any of these methods to mass screening remains problematic. **(p. 1592)**

A18. True

Some tumor cells have also been found to contain GFAP. **(p. 1592)**

A19. False

Endometrioid adenocarcinomas show the highest degree of positivity, followed by papillary serous adenocarcinoma and clear cell carcinoma. High-grade adenosquamous carcinomas are consistently negative. **(p. 1592)**

A20. True

Expression of CD114 (c-*kit*) has been also found in about half of adenocarcinomas, but is present in over 90% of normal proliferative endometria. **(p. 1592)**

A21. False

Microsatellite instability in the PTEN, K-*ras* and β-catenin is seen in endometrioid carcinomas, but *p53* mutation is seen in papillary serous adenocarcinoma. **(p. 1592)**

A22. True

Nodal metastases occur in approximately 5–25% of stage I tumors and are more likely to occur in invasive, high-grade tumors. **(p. 1593)**

A23. True

Distant metastases of endometrial carcinomas are more common in the lung, liver, bone, skin and central nervous system. **(p. 1593)**

A24. False

Only 8% of endometrial carcinomas are accompanied by a simultaneous ovarian carcinoma. When they are of similar microscopic types it becomes difficult to decide whether there are two independent tumors or whether one of the sites represents a metastasis. Features favoring a metastatic nature for the ovarian tumor are smaller size, bilateral involvement, multinodular growth pattern, the presence of associated surface implants, and prominent lymphatic vascular invasion within ovarian stroma. **(p. 1593)**

A25. False

The usual treatment of endometrial carcinoma is total abdominal hysterectomy with bilateral salpingo-oophorectomy. Radiation therapy is no longer favored routinely, except for patients with poor prognostic factors that put them at high risk of recurrence. **(p. 1593)**

A26. False

It is exactly the reverse. Endometrial papillary serous carcinomas are not associated with hyperplasia and have a much worse prognosis than endometrioid carcinomas usually associated with endometrial hyperplasia. **(p. 1594)**

A27. True

Among the various morphologic variants the papillary serous adenocarcinoma and the clear-type adenocarcinoma are the most aggressive subtypes of endometrial carcinoma, the former having a definite tendency for upper abdominal spread. **(p. 1594)**

A28. True

In endometrial stromal tumors CD10 is consistently positive, but h-caldesmon is negative. The reverse pattern is seen in smooth muscle tumors. **(p. 1595)**

A29. False

The division is primarily based on growth pattern and type of margins. Endometrial stromal tumor has smooth margins, whereas stromal sarcoma has infiltrating margins. A third category has been proposed for tumors with irregular but not infiltrative margins, designating them endometrial stromal tumors with limited infiltration. **(p. 1595)**

A30. True

Low-grade tumors would be those with fewer than 10 mitoses/hpf, and high grade those with more than 10 mitoses/hpf. **(p. 1596)**

A31. False

Size of tumor, extrauterine extension and mitotic activity are important prognostic factors; however, mitotic rate does not seem to be as important as was previously believed. **(p. 1596)**

A32. True
Their immunohistochemical and ultrastructural profile varies considerably; however, some cases have shown positivity with CD99 and A13. They mostly behave in a benign fashion. **(p. 1597)**

A33. False
Plexiform tumors are small – less than 1 cm – nodules showing smooth muscle differentiation. Tumorlets of the lung are usually multiple small neuroendocrine nodules. **(p. 1597)**

A34. False
They can be found in the ovary, cervix, pelvis and retroperitoneum. Some of these are presumably associated with endometriosis. **(p. 1598)**

A35. True
It is an altogether different neoplasm that behaves in a very aggressive manner and which may actually have a closer relationship to malignant mixed müllerian tumor, the sarcoma-like component of which it greatly resembles. **(p. 1598)**

A36. True
They usual location is the uterine body, particularly the posterior wall in the region of the fundus. **(p. 1599)**

A37. False
It is the appearance of the sarcomatoid component that divides these tumors into homologous (resembling endometrial stroma, leiomyosarcoma or fibrosarcoma) and heterologous (skeletal muscle, cartilage, bone and fat) varieties. **(p. 1599)**

A38. True
This suggests that perhaps these tumors should be regarded as carcinomas rather than sarcomas. **(p. 1599)**

A39. False
MMMTs are easily distinguished from teratomas by their occurrence in an older age group and by the absence of skin appendages, glia, thyroid and other tissues. **(p. 1600)**

A40. True
However, the difference between the two is small and in some studies absent, and far outweighed by the stage of disease. **(p. 1600)**

A41. True
Norris and Taylor made the disturbing observation that 30% of patients with heterologous MMMTs and 13% of those with homologous tumors had a history of previous irradiation to the pelvic area, with the median interval of 16.4 years. **(p. 1600)**

A42. True
The most common sites are the ovaries and pelvic structures. **(p. 1601)**

A43. False
It is considered a low-grade variant of MMMT. **(p. 1602)**

A44. True
The stroma usually resembles endometrial stroma and the epithelial component appears bland. **(p. 1602)**

A45. True
Also of interest is a report of a cluster of müllerian adenosarcomas in the Washington DC metropolitan area. **(p. 1602)**

A46. True
Also included are marked cellularity and atypia. **(p. 1603)**

A47. False
It is the opposite. Clinically apparent leiomyomas are more common in multiparous than nulliparous women and in premenopausal than postmenopausal women. **(p. 1603)**

A48. True
Under these circumstances the surface of the myoma is ulcerated and infected, the gross appearance thus simulating that of a malignant neoplasm. **(p. 1603)**

A49. False
Malignant transformation is such a rare event that it can be disregarded. Most asymptomatic leiomyomas need not be excised. **(p. 1604)**

A50. True
Administration of gonadotropin-releasing hormone analogs may result in a reduction in size. Embolization leads to massive necrosis accompanied by a foreign body-type reaction to the injected material and calcifications. **(p. 1604)**

A51. False
Hemorrhage can be seen in apoplectic leiomyoma and red degeneration, especially in pregnant patients or with the use of contraceptive drugs. **(p. 1604)**

A52. True
Their natural history is similar to that of ordinary leiomyomas. At the cytogenetic level they have been accompanied by loss of almost the entire short arm of chromosome 1. **(p. 1605)**

A53. False
Epithelioid leiomyoma is partially or totally composed of rounded or polygonal cells, and it has a similar appearance to its most common counterpart in the gastrointestinal tract. However, it does not show positivity for c-*kit* (CD117) **(p. 1606)**

A54. False
Despite its dissecting gross nature it does not show vascular invasion and it is benign in nature. **(p. 1607)**

A55. False
Parasitic leiomyoma is the term given to a uterine leiomyoma that has become separate from the uterus and has acquired vascular connections with the omentum. **(p. 1607)**

A56. True
The clinical and gross features are similar to those of endometrial stromal sarcoma, but grossly apparent involvement of veins is more prominent. **(p. 1607)**

A57. False
Benign metastasizing leiomyoma is the name given to a leiomyoma with benign morphological features which is accompanied by nodules in the lung, regional lymph nodes and other sites. **(p. 1608)**

A58. False
This theory has been postulated; however, nodules have been found to be clonally related, thus speaking in favor of metastases from the uterine tumor. **(p. 1608)**

A59. True
In a large series it has been shown that 67% of all leiomyosarcomas are solitary lesions. **(p. 1609)**

A60. True
However, not all leiomyosarcomas will exhibit all of these features simultaneously. **(p. 1609)**

A61. False
Positivity for keratins is common but not constant, especially in epithelioid variants, a feature that may lead to a mistaken interpretation of carcinoma. **(p. 1609)**

A62. False
Although tumor stage is an important prognostic factor, no constant correlation has been found between survival and histological grade of the tumor. There is some evidence that DNA ploidy may be of some prognostic significance. **(p. 1610)**

A63. True
Generally two types of necrosis can be seen in smooth muscle tumors. Hyaline type or 'infarction' necrosis is usually seen in benign tumors and coagulative necrosis is commonly present in malignant smooth muscle tumors. **(p. 1610)**

A64. True
As opposed to the hyaline type, where there is a zonal pattern reminiscent of an evolving infarct with a center of 'bland' necrosis, a periphery of granulation tissue and a layer of hyalinized collagen in between. On low power coagulative necrosis appears as a cuff of preserved cells around large vessels surrounded by large expanses of necrotic tumor. **(p. 1610)**

A65. True
Recommended is a total of at least 10 sections, or one section per centimeter of diameter, whichever is the greater. **(p. 1611)**

A66. False
'High-power field' is usually a combination of 10× eyepiece and 40× objective. **(p. 1611)**

A67. False
Such tumors should be regarded as atypical or bizarre, or at most borderline if the change is extensive. Without mitotic activity and coagulative necrosis a diagnosis of malignancy is not warranted. **(p. 1612)**

A68. True
Mitotically active tumors with no coagulative necrosis represent benign neoplasms. **(p. 1612)**

A69. False
Severe atypia and mitotic activity warrant a diagnosis of malignant smooth muscle tumor. **(p. 1612)**

A70. True
This subtype of leiomyosarcoma represents an exception from the rule applied to the conventional type of leiomyosarcoma. **(p. 1612)**

A71. False
Extramedullary hematopoiesis can occur in the endometrium even without an association with hematological or systemic diseases. **(p. 1613)**

A72. True
Adenomatoid tumors with cystic patterns can be morphologically similar to lymphangiomas. However, the lining of adenomatoid tumors is mesothelial in origin. **(p. 1613)**

A73. True
The myometrium is more often involved than the endometrium. **(p. 1613)**

FALLOPIAN TUBE

Normal anatomy

A1. False

The fallopian tube is divided into four segments: intramural (inside the uterus), isthmus (2–3 cm, thick walled), ampulla (a thin-walled expanded area) and infundibulum (a trumpet-shaped ending that opens into the peritoneal cavity through the ostium and is fringed by the fimbriae). **(p. 1636)**

A2. True

This structure and the adjacent areas contain a variety of tubular structures related to the müllerian and wolffian systems. **(p. 1636)**

A3. False

The round ligament is a fibrous cord, not a peritoneal fold. **(p. 1636)**

Inflammation

A1. True

The rupture of such abscesses may lead to localized or generalized peritonitis and requires prompt intervention. **(p. 1637)**

A2. False

Pelvic inflammatory disease (PID) is the generic term used for inflammatory processes in which the fallopian tube is the epicenter of inflammation. **(p. 1637)**

A3. True

Most patients with fallopian tube tuberculosis are young, and infertility is common. **(p. 1637)**

Torsion

A1. True

It has been suggested that if torsion occurs in a previously normal ovary, it is due to the fact that the infundibulopelvic ligament extends along the edge of the ovarian ligament so that the tube and ovary hang on a very narrow stalk. **(p. 1639)**

Tubal pregnancy

A1. False

The actual incidence of tubal pregnancy has increased. It is often the consequence of chronic salpingitis, which leads to inflammatory destruction of the lining folds and retention of the ovum. **(p. 1639)**

A2. False

Tubal implantation usually occurs in the ampulloisthmic or midtubal portion. **(p. 1639)**

A3. True

On occasion the appearance of these retained tissues corresponds to that of so-called placental site nodule, as described in the uterine corpus. **(p. 1640)**

Other non-neoplastic processes

A1. True
Paratubal cysts are traditionally known as hydatids of Morgagni, their wall is paper-thin and their content clear. Most are lined by tubal columnar epithelium. **(p. 1640)**

A2. True
Decidual reaction of the tubal mucosa is common, especially in specimens of tubal ligation obtained at the time of cesarean section. **(p. 1640)**

A3. True
Microscopically, cystically dilated gland-like formations are seen surrounded by hypertrophic muscle. It has been postulated that the lesion is inflammatory in nature; however, some authors propose a pathogenesis analogous to that of uterine adenomyosis. **(p. 1641)**

A4. True
This is a distinctive lesion characterized by mucinous and eosinophilic metaplasia of the mucosa, resulting in a sharply outlined papillary configuration. Its behavior is benign. **(p. 1641)**

Proliferative epithelial lesions

A1. True
Mild degrees of proliferative and atypical changes of the tubal epithelium are extremely common and are seen in up to 83% of all tubes examined. However, more florid changes with moderate or severe atypia are usually seen associated with other lesions, such as salpingitis, carriers of *BRCA1* mutations, exogenous and endogenous estrogen stimulation, and serous borderline tumors of the ovary. **(p. 1642)**

Carcinoma

A1. True
These findings are leading some authors to recommend not only prophylactic hysterectomy/oophorectomy, but also bilateral salpingectomy. **(p. 1642)**

A2. True
Cervicovaginal cytology will be positive in only a minority of patients; however, endometrial scraping will reveal malignant cells. **(p. 1642)**

A3. False
The most common type of fallopian tube carcinoma is papillary serous carcinoma. **(p. 1643)**

A4. True
The staging system currently used is adapted from the FIGO staging system for ovarian carcinoma. **(p. 1643)**

Other tumors

A1. True
This feature can actually obscure the true mesothelial nature of the tumor. **(p. 1643)**

A2. False
Only 50 cases of tubal teratoma have been described. **(p. 1644)**

Tumors and tumor-like conditions of the broad and round ligaments

A1. True

The tumor is thought to be of wolffian derivation and is composed of epithelial cells growing in diffuse, trabecular or tubular patterns. It has a generally good clinical prognosis. **(p. 1644)**

A2. True

Cases of leiomyoma, fibroma and benign mesenchymoma have been reported. **(p. 1645)**

OVARY

Normal anatomy

A1. True

This epithelium is immunoreactive for keratin, EMA, Ber-EP4, CA-125, vimentin, estrogen and progesterone receptors and FSH. **(p. 1649)**

A2. False

Ovarian stroma contains cortical and medullary regions, two indistinct components. **(p. 1649)**

A3. True

Granulosa cells form small rosette-like formations known as Call–Exner bodies, which are immunoreactive for vimentin, keratin and desmoplakin. **(p. 1650)**

A4. True

The ovarian hilus cells may contain Reinke's crystalloids, lipids and lipochrome pigment. **(p. 1650)**

Gonadal dysgenesis

A1. False

Turner syndrome (45,XO) is associated with bilateral gonads represented by a streak of fibrous tissue that vaguely resembles ovarian stroma. **(p. 1650)**

A2. False

This familial syndrome is the most common type of male pseudohermaphroditism in individuals with a normal male chromosome constitution and an end-organ defect (androgen insensitivity). **(p. 1652)**

Cysts, stromal hyperplasia and other non-neoplastic lesions

A1. True

The cyst wall is lined by theca with or without an inner granulosa layer. **(p. 1653)**

A2. False

These large cysts, with a median diameter of 25 cm, present during pregnancy and the puerperium. **(p. 1653)**

A3. True

Various clinical syndromes may develop in patients with polycystic ovaries, including Stein–Leventhal syndrome accompanied by endometrial hyperplasia and frank virilism. **(p. 1654)**

A4. True

These cells can be involved in patchy or diffuse luteinization. **(p. 1654)**

A5. False

Ovarian decidual reaction is typically seen during pregnancy. **(p. 1655)**

A6. False

They have been encountered during cesarean section in multiparous women. **(p. 1655)**

A7. True

According to some authors it is possible to distinguish these two types of remnant within cystic tissues, based on microscopic grounds. **(p. 1656)**

ANSWERS

Inflammation

A1. True
Other infectious agents responsible for granulomatous oophoritis are *Actinomyces*, *Schistosoma* and *Enterobius vermicularis*. **(p. 1656)**

A2. False
Autoimmune oophoritis shows microscopic evidence of lymphocytic and plasma cell infiltration in relation to developing follicles. **(p. 1657)**

A3. True
Microscopically, endometriotic foci are composed of endometrial glands, endometrial stroma, and fresh and old (hemosiderin-containing) hemorrhagic areas. **(p. 1657)**

A4. True
Interestingly, p53 is absent in the epithelial cells of benign uncomplicated endometriotic cysts, but present in about half of the carcinomas arising from them as well as in the adjacent non-neoplastic epithelium. **(p. 1658)**

Ovarian biopsy

A1. True
Nowadays, ovarian biopsies are rarely if ever performed in women with premature ovarian failure and a normal karyotype. **(p. 1659)**

Tumors

A1. False
Numerically these tumors are the most important group of ovarian neoplasms, thought to derive from the celomic or germinal epithelium. **(p. 1659)**

A2. True
As a result of this differentiation, the ovarian surface epithelium may produce any of the adult structures formed by müllerian ducts, including tubal, endometrial and endocervical mucosa. **(p. 1659)**

A3. True
30–50% of bilateral tumors support the theory of a clonal origin for these neoplasms. **(p. 1659)**

A4. False
Serous cystadenoma is a benign tumor composed of cysts and papillae lined by a single layer of cells, without atypia. **(p. 1660)**

A5. True
These tumors make up approximately 15% of all serous tumors. **(p. 1660)**

A6. True
The additional proposal has been made that tumors should still be placed into the borderline category even if they show foci of stromal microinvasion. **(p. 1661)**

A7. False
The microinvasive foci show clusters of cells with abundant eosinophilic cytoplasm; these tumors have a prognosis similar to that of non-invasive serous borderline tumors. **(p. 1661)**

A8. True
This neoplasm represents a controversial entity characterized microscopically by a filigree pattern of highly complex micropapillae arising from large papillary structures. **(p. 1661)**

A9. True
The significance of this prognostic sign is important because of general agreement that micropapillary serous tumors are associated with a higher rate of recurrence. **(p. 1662)**

A10. False
Adenofibromas and cystadenofibromas are benign lesions. **(p. 1662)**

A11. False
Serous psammocarcinoma shows low-grade cytologic atypia and a clinical behavior similar to that of borderline tumors. **(p. 1662)**

A12. False
It is CK7+ and CK20–. **(p. 1663)**

A13. True
Colonic carcinoma represents a typical metastatic tumor staining positive for CK20. **(p. 1664)**

A14. True
These bilateral tumors also seem to be clonal in nature. **(p. 1664)**

A15. False
Grossly, they tend to be larger, often multiloculated, with viscous material present in the lumen. **(p. 1664)**

A16. False
The two major subtypes of mucinous tumor are intestinal and endocervical or müllerian. **(p. 1665)**

A17. True
As stromal invasion may be present in only a small area of the tumor, thorough sampling for microscopic examination is essential. **(p. 1665)**

A18. True
In mucinous borderline tumors stromal invasion is difficult to evaluate in cases with a complex interaction of stroma and glands. **(p. 1666)**

A19. True
Some independent studies have confirmed the prognostic utility of this arbitrary and biologically questionable criterion, but others have not. **(p. 1666)**

A20. False
The tumor cells of ovarian mucinous neoplasms express CEA, keratin (CK7), EMA and MUC5AC. **(p. 1667)**

A21. False
These tumors are known to implant on and locally invade bowel, abdominal wall and bladder, sometimes creating extensive deposits of intra-abdominal mucin (pseudomyxoma peritonei). **(p. 1667)**

A22. True
The content of this cystic area tends to be hemorrhagic rather than serous or mucinous. **(p. 1667)**

A23. True
Most endometrioid carcinomas are well differentiated with or without papillary formations, with half of the tumors expressing foci of squamous metaplasia. **(p. 1667)**

A24. False
These tumor cells are positive for EMA and vimentin, but CEA is usually negative or weak. **(p. 1668)**

A25. True
This difference suggests a different genetic pathway for their formation. **(p. 1668)**

A26. False
Several morphological variants of endometrioid carcinoma present with cords and tubular structures, mimicking a Sertoli–Leydig cell tumor. Others contain squamous metaplasia and yolk sac elements, adding another group of differential diagnoses. Signet ring carcinoma is not a defined subtype of endometrial carcinoma. **(p. 1668)**

A27. True
This seems to be mainly a function of the fact that many of these tumors are stage I and well differentiated. **(p. 1669)**

A28. True
These tumors are composed of tubular or papillary to solid structures, lined by large cells protruding into the lumina, resulting in a 'hobnail' configuration, and a clear cytoplasm. **(p. 1669)**

A29. True
Borderline clear cell tumors show a moderate to marked degree of epithelial atypia and proliferation in the absence of recognizable stromal invasion. **(p. 1670)**

A30. True
These tumors vary in size and are typically unilateral, white and firm. **(p. 1671)**

A31. False
Borderline Brenner tumors are composed of highly proliferating sheaths of cells associated with a greater degree of atypia (equivalent to a grade III transitional cell carcinoma). In comparison, proliferating Brenner tumor shows only low-grade cytologic atypia (grades I–II). **(p. 1672)**

A32. True
These tumors are usually associated with a typical, benign, metaplastic, proliferating, or borderline component. **(p. 1672)**

A33. False
Ovarian MMMT resembles its more common uterine counterpart both grossly and microscopically. **(p. 1673)**

A34. True
Postmenopausal patients with MMMT often present with a history of low parity. **(p. 1674)**

A35. True
Some heterologous elements of MMMT can resemble neuroectodermal differentiation, typically seen in immature teratoma. **(p. 1674)**

A36. True
It is the fifth leading cause of cancer deaths in women. **(p. 1674)**

A37. False
BRCA1 and *BRCA2* mutations are associated with familial not sporadic forms of ovarian cancer. Another familial syndrome associated with an increased risk of ovarian carcinoma is Lynch type II syndrome. **(p. 1675)**

A38. True
Telomerase activity is not found in benign cystadenomas. **(p. 1676)**

A39. True
In addition, EGFR and the M-CSF receptors are expressed along with the respective ligands in some cases. **(p. 1676)**

A40. False
Aneuplody is associated with the majority of invasive carcinomas, whereas benign tumors are usually diploid. **(p. 1676)**

A41. False
The most common sites of involvement are the contralateral ovary, peritoneal cavity, para-aortic and pelvic lymph nodes, and liver. **(p. 1676)**

A42. False
'Sister Joseph's nodule' represents an early umbilical metastasis. **(p. 1676)**

A43. True
Implants can also involve lymph nodes of the neck, lung and pleura. **(p. 1676)**

A44. False
Peritoneal proliferative epithelial lesions can theoretically represent spread from an ovarian tumor, or can have an autochthonous origin from the lower abdominal mesothelium. **(p. 1676)**

A45. True
The younger the patient, the more likely the germ cell tumor will be malignant. **(p. 1681)**

A46. False
Approximately 5% of dysgerminomas arise in abnormal gonads as a result of gonadoblastoma or testicular feminization syndrome. **(p. 1681)**

A47. True
Microscopically, these tumors resemble testicular seminomas, with large pleomorphic tumor cells within well-defined nests separated by fibrous strands infiltrated by lymphocytes. **(p. 1681)**

A48. False
These tumors are reactive for PLAP, CD117, often for keratin, and sometimes for GFAP and desmin. **(p. 1682)**

A49. True
As with equivalent testicular examples, it is not clear whether any of these changes alters the prognosis of dysgerminoma. **(p. 1682)**

A50. False
These are neoplasms of children and young adults (median age 19 years) that have also been described in the elderly. **(p. 1683)**

A51. True
Most of the tumors show reticular and microcystic areas formed by a loose meshwork lined by flat-to-cuboidal cells, rounded pseudopapillary processes with central vessels, and Schiller–Duval bodies. **(p. 1683)**

A52. False
Yolk sac tumors stain for pankeratin, but not for CK7, CK20 or WT-1. **(p. 1684)**

A53. True
Chorionic gonadotropin levels are sometimes so high that a positive pregnancy test results. **(p. 1685)**

A54. True
The external surface of these tumors is smooth and glistening. **(p. 1685)**

A55. False
Microscopically, these tumors are composed of solid sheets and nests of large primitive cells, occasionally forming papillae and abortive glandular elements with scattered syncytiotrophoblast-like tumor cells. **(p. 1685)**

A56. True
Primary ovarian choriocarcinomas are exceedingly rare. **(p. 1685)**

A57. True
The main immature component is usually primitive neuroepithelium, but mesodermal elements are also common. **(p. 1686)**

A58. False
The microscopic grade of the primary tumor is the best prognostic factor. **(p. 1686)**

A59. True
The grading system (I–III) often correlates with various types of karyotypic abnormalities. **(p. 1686)**

A60. False
These solid tumors with small cystic areas are composed entirely of adult tissues and should be extensively sampled to rule out grade I immature teratoma, and have an excellent prognosis. **(p. 1687)**

A61. True
These tumors are grossly multiloculated, with a greasy cystic content, largely composed of keratin, sebum and hairs. **(p. 1687)**

A62. True
This structure should be sampled for microscopic examination because it will exhibit the greatest variety of tissue structures. **(p. 1687)**

A63. False
Mature teratomas typically coexist with serous cystadenoma, Brenner tumor and fibrothecoma. **(p. 1688)**

A64. True
Prominent foreign body reaction can look like metastatic cancer to the surgeon. **(p. 1688)**

A65. False
Mature as well as immature cystic and solid teratomas may be accompanied by gliomatosis peritonei. **(p. 1689)**

A66. True
Other, more rare malignant transformations are malignant melanoma, Paget's disease, sarcomas and glioblastoma multiforme. **(p. 1689)**

A67. True
It is distinguished from mature cystic teratoma on thorough sampling by the absence of skin adnexal and other tissues. **(p. 1689)**

A68. True
Grossly the mass, which is often cystic, looks like thyroid tissue and can show pathological changes of thyroiditis, carcinoma and even lymphoma. **(p. 1690)**

A69. False
Carcinoid tumors can be seen in association with metastatic tumor, as a component of adult cystic teratoma, or as a pure primary ovarian neoplasm. **(p. 1690)**

A70. True
The large majority of primary carcinoids are unilateral and have better prognosis than metastatic tumors. The paraneoplastic syndrome is more common in large tumors. **(p. 1690)**

A71. True
This lesion has also been observed in association with multiple endocrine neoplasia (MEN) type IIA. **(p. 1691)**

A72. True
Whether these tumors arise from granulosa cells in pre-existing follicles or from specialized ovarian stroma is debatable. **(p. 1692)**

A73. False
Adult granulosa cell tumor is usually diagnosed during the childbearing years, is solid on gross examination, and is associated with hyperestrinism. **(p. 1692)**

A74. True
This variable microscopic appearance is seen even within the same neoplasm. **(p. 1693)**

A75. True
Occasionally, bizarre nuclei and multinucleated giant cells ('floret type') are seen. **(p. 1693)**

A76. False
Granulosa cell tumor shows positive immunohistochemical staining with inhibin, vimentin, desmoplakin, CD99 and A103. **(p. 1693)**

A77. True
Other less common karyotypic aberrations of this tumor are trisomy 14 and monosomy 22. **(p. 1694)**

A78. False
The tumor is composed of macrofollicular cystic-like spaces, lager tumor cells with a paucity of nuclear grooves, and often high mitotic activity. **(p. 1694)**

A79. True
Strong immunoreactivity for inhibin in tumor cells strongly suggests a granulosa cell tumor. **(p. 1694)**

A80. False
The prognosis is largely dependent on clinical stage. Other significant prognostic signs are size, tumor rupture, and the presence of nuclear atypia. **(p. 1695)**

A81. True
In nearly 80% of cases these tumors are diagnosed during the first two decades of life. **(p. 1695)**

A82. False
Thecomas occur after the menopause, are usually unilateral, and have a well-defined capsule with a firm solid cut surface showing a predominance of yellow areas alternating with whitish foci. **(p. 1695)**

A83. True
The degree of tumor cellularity varies considerably, and some tumors in young women are heavily calcified. **(p. 1695)**

A84. False
With Oil-Red-O stain the cells of thecomas show abundant intracytoplasmic neutral fat, and silver stains usually demonstrate reticulin fibers surrounding individual cells. **(p. 1695)**

A85. True
Fibromas can exhibit a great deal of cellularity and even increased mitotic activity. These are called cellular fibromas if the mitotic activity does not exceed 3/10 hpf. **(p. 1697)**

A86. True
The mechanism for the pleural effusion is said to be related to intrathoracic negative pressure and transdiaphragmatic passage of fluid through peritoneal lymphatics. **(p. 1697)**

A87. False
These are benign, less cellular ovarian tumors than fibromas/thecomas and occur in younger age groups. **(p. 1697)**

A88. True
Most patients present with pain, an abdominal mass, and even Meigs' syndrome. **(p. 1697)**

A89. False
In about a quarter of cases with these tumors the endometrium exhibits various degrees of hyperplasia. **(p. 1698)**

A90. False
There are two types of primary ovarian small cell carcinoma: hypercalcemic and pulmonary. **(p. 1698)**

A91. True
The tumor is large and solid with areas of necrosis and hemorrhage, and is associated with hypercalcemia in two-thirds of cases. **(p. 1699)**

A92. True

The keratin and EMA positivity, the negativity for inhibin, and the finding of K-*ras* mutations suggest an epithelial origin. Most surprisingly, this tumor has been found to have a diploid DNA pattern. **(p. 1699)**

A93. False

These are very rare neoplasms seen in young patients (average age 25 years) and comprise less than 0.1% of all ovarian tumors. **(p. 1700)**

A94. True

The presence of cords and tubules is a characteristic sign of early tumor recognition. **(p. 1700)**

A95. False

Poorly differentiated tumors are composed of masses of spindle-shaped cells arranged in a sarcomatoid pattern. **(p. 1701)**

A96. True

Sertoli–Leydig cell tumor with heterologous elements is also known as teratoid androblastoma. **(p. 1701)**

A97. True

Knowledge of this profile is useful in the differential diagnosis between Sertoli–Leydig cell tumors with heterologous elements and carcinosarcoma. **(p. 1701)**

A98. False

More than half of cases are associated with androgen excess, and clinical signs of masculinization. **(p. 1702)**

A99. True

These steroid-producing tumors are composed of steroid-producing cells, such as thecal, stromal, hilar and adrenocortical. **(p. 1702)**

A100. False

These tumors are usually unilateral, grossly deep brown nodules reminiscent of a renal oncocytoma, separated by fibrous trabeculae. **(p. 1702)**

A101. True

Only few cases are associated with estrogenic or progestogenic manifestations such as endometrioid carcinoma. **(p. 1703)**

A102. False

This term describes tumors composed of mixture of granulosa–theca cells and Sertoli–Leydig cell elements. **(p. 1703)**

A103. True

Its morphologic hallmark is the presence of annular tubules containing eosinophilic intraluminal bodies. This tumor is often associated with Peutz–Jeghers syndrome. **(p. 1703)**

A104. True

Grossly, this tumor is cystic or solid and microscopically it shows epithelial cells forming elongated glandular structures within stroma composed of spindle to oval cells. **(p. 1704)**

A105. False

This tumor is composed of germ cells combined with sex cord–stromal cells. It almost always occurs in sexually abnormal individuals. **(p. 1704)**

A106. False

One-quarter of dysgenetic gonads will develop a neoplastic process, from dysgerminoma to Sertoli cell tumors. **(p. 1704)**

A107. False

Most ovarian lymphomas are B-cell lymphomas of non-Hodgkin's type. In children, undifferentiated (small non-cleaved) types predominate; in adults most are large cell, diffuse or follicular in type. **(p. 1705)**

A108. True

Primary ovarian lymphomas and leukemias are much more rare. **(p. 1705)**

A109. False

These are extremely rare and need to be rather distinguished from undifferentiated carcinomas, malignant mixed müllerian tumors, Krukenberg tumors with strong stromal reaction, and sarcomatoid forms of sex cord–stromal tumors. **(p. 1705)**

A110. False

Fibrosarcomas are distinguished from cellular fibromas on the basis of their mitotic activity (four or more per 10 hpf in fibrosarcomas). **(p. 1705)**

A111. True

Over half of metastatic tumors are bilateral. The most common sources are stomach, large bowel, appendix, breast, uterus and skin. **(p. 1706)**

A112. True

Immunohistochemical stains are an important tool in differentiating primary from metastatic ovarian tumors. **(p. 1706)**

A113. True

Primary ovarian tumors show an expansile pushing pattern of invasion, a complex papillary architecture and a smooth external surface. **(p. 1707)**

A114. False

Colonic carcinoma shows reactivity for CK20+, CEA+ and MUC2+. In contrast, primary ovarian mucinous carcinomas are nearly always CK7+, CA-125+ and MUC5AC+. **(p. 1707)**

A115. False

Krukenberg tumor is almost always bilateral and metastatic in origin, characterized by solid multinodular enlargement of the ovaries and microscopically by diffuse infiltration of signet ring cells and marked stromal proliferation. **(p. 1707)**

A116. True

The diagnosis of Krukenberg tumor requires the histochemical identification of intracytoplasmic mucin and the immunohistochemical detection of epithelial markers. **(p. 1708)**

A117. False

These tumors occur after the age of 40, usually arising from the stomach, large bowel, appendix and breast. **(p. 1708)**

A118. False

Diagnosing Krukenberg tumor often requires the histochemical identification of intracytoplasmic mucin and the immunohistochemical detection of epithelial markers. **(p. 1708)**

A119. True

Recognition of malignant melanomas is based upon their pigmentation, nodular growth pattern and cytologic features. **(p. 1709)**

PREGNANCY, TROPHOBLASTIC DISEASE AND PLACENTA

Normal anatomy

A1. False

The umbilical cord contains two arteries and one vein. **(p. 1737)**

A2. True

The chorion associated with the membranes is referred to as chorion laeve and that located in the placenta proper is called chorion frondosum. **(p. 1737)**

A3. True

In addition, syncytiotrophoblasts are also strongly reactive for hCG, PLAP, hPL (variable stain) and inhibin, whereas cytotrophoblasts are non-reactive with those stains. **(p. 1737)**

A4. True

The presence of nucleated red blood cells after week 12 is a sign of fetal distress. **(p. 1737)**

A5. False

On occasion decidual cells are positive for keratin, PLAP and β-hCG. **(p. 1738)**

Abortion

A1. False

A monochorionic placenta is indicative of monozygotic twins and a dichorionic placenta of dizygotic twinning. **(p. 1738)**

A2. True

This may be of great clinical significance in the differential diagnosis of intrauterine and ectopic pregnancy. **(p. 1739)** However, it should be mentioned that under exceptional circumstances one could find a few villi in the uterine curettage specimen of a patient with ectopic pregnancy. **(p. 1740)**

A3. True

It characteristically develops during pregnancy, but it may also follow the use of progestational agents and other exogenous hormones. **(p. 1740)**

A4. True

Gross villous swelling is not appreciated in hydropic change. Proliferation is present: usually it is polar, has an orderly arrangement and lacks significant nuclear atypia. **(p. 1740)**

Gestational trophoblastic disease

A1. True
Complete mole is caused by abnormal gametogenesis and fertilization. The process is fertilization of an 'empty' ovum either by two haploid sperms or by one haploid sperm that duplicates. **(p. 1741)**

A2. True
Patients with complete mole tend to be older than 30 years and more likely to have a diet deficient in vitamin A. This could explain the striking geographic variations in the incidence of molar pregnancy, with significantly higher rates noted in Mexico, India and Taiwan. **(p. 1741)**

A3. False
The uterus is usually larger than expected; grossly the specimen is abundant, weighing more than 200 g, with enlarged vesicles measuring from 1 to 30 mm. **(p. 1741)**

A4. False
By flow cytometry 50% of complete moles are diploid, 43% are tetraploid, 3.6% are polyploid and 1.7% are triploid. **(p. 1741)**

A5. False
The presence of villi or atypical trophoblasts following the evacuation of a molar pregnancy indicates the presence of persistent trophoblastic disease. The decision whether to give chemotherapy or not still depends largely on the hCG level. **(p. 1742)**

A6. False
15–35% of all molar pregnancies are partial mole. **(p. 1742)**

A7. True
Gross examination represents an important initial tool in the recognition of molar pregnancy. **(p. 1742)**

A8. True
It has been shown that p57, a cell cycle inhibitor and tumor suppressor encoded by a strongly paternally imprinted gene, is positive in cytotrophoblasts of normal pregnancy, spontaneous abortion and partial moles, but is absent or markedly decreased in complete mole. **(p. 1742–1743)**

A9. False
Although most partial moles are triploid, not all placentas of triploid conceptuses show partial molar transformation; in fact, some (perhaps the majority) have a normal morphologic appearance. **(p. 1743)**

A10. False
The invasive mole is mostly of the complete type and occasionally of the partial type. **(p. 1743)**

A11. True
Invasive mole invades the stroma, produces tumor emboli, and metastasizes distantly. It differs from choriocarcinoma by the presence of chorionic villi. **(p. 1744)**

A12. False
Only 1–2% of complete moles are followed by choriocarcinoma. The tumor is more common in the areas of the world where mole is more prevalent. **(p. 1744)**

A13. True
The highest risk is for women of group A and a man of the same group, with a relative risk of 10.4 : 1. Women and men with the same blood group had the highest incidence of spontaneous regression of trophoblasts after the evacuation of a hydatidiform mole. **(p. 1744)**

A14. False
Villi are characteristically absent, and their presence is said to rule out the diagnosis of choriocarcinoma no matter how atypical the trophoblastic cells may be. **(p. 1745)**

A15. True
Few attempts at correlating various patterns have been made; however, of these, the most convincing finding of a slightly improved prognosis is observed in tumors with an intense inflammatory infiltrate at the interface between tumor and stroma. **(p. 1745)**

A16. True
They also may be positive for hPL, SP1 and CEA. **(p. 1745)**

A17. True
When treated by surgery the cure rate is significantly lower; however, with the use of chemotherapy (methotrexate, actinomycin D and chlorambucil) the rates are significantly improved. **(p. 1746)**

A18. True
Only 5% of patients had molar pregnancy before the PSTT. **(p. 1746)**

A19. False
Grossly it can present as a well-localized or ill-defined mass. **(p. 1746)**

A20. True
Immunoreactivity is consistent with intermediate trophoblastic cells showing strong positivity for hPL and focal staining for hCG. **(p. 1747)**

A21. True
Some cases have resulted in widespread metastases. **(p. 1747)**

A22. True
The gross appearance closely simulates carcinoma. It was originally described as a peculiar change in the metastatic foci of treated choriocarcinoma, but is now known to occur de novo. **(p. 1747)**

A23. False

Both of those markers are negative in epithelioid trophoblastic tumor. It shows diffuse reactivity with keratin, E-cadherin, EMA, and α-inhibin. **(p. 1747)**

A24. True

(p. 1748)

A25. False

They can also occur in the cervix and fallopian tubes. **(p. 1748)**

Non-neoplastic lesions of term placenta

A1. False

It is placenta percreta that can cause uterine rupture, as its villous infiltration extends throughout the thickness of myometrium. In placenta increta villi invade the myometrium superficially. **(p. 1749)**

A2. True

Ultrastructural and other studies suggest that amnion nodosum originates from the deposition of desquamated fetal squamous cells in the presence of oligohydramnios. **(p. 1749)**

A3. True

The abnormalities may involve the cardiac, renal or other systems, and it is seen in approximately 30% of cases with one umbilical artery. **(p. 1749)**

A4. True

Inflammation concentrated along the umbilical cord and fetal surface vessels is usually contributed by the fetal circulation. **(p. 1750)**

A5. False

The most common route is ascending from the maternal vaginal tract. Bacterial infection is the most common cause of placental infection; however, other infections, such as herpes virus or *Candida* can also cause ascending chorioamnionitis. **(p. 1750)**

A6. True

The association with fetal infection is stronger in preterm than in term placentas. **(p. 1751)**

A7. False

Old placental infarct is whitish with a firm consistency, whereas fresh infarct is dark red and firmer. **(p. 1751)**

A8. True

An increased number of syncytial knots is a sign of chronic ischemic change and can be seen in diabetics. **(p. 1752)**

A9. False

Placental iron deposits in the form of granular structures along the trophoblastic basement membrane are normal; their presence in 7.5% or more of the villi is abnormal and can be associated with fetal growth anomalies. **(p. 1752)**

Tumors and tumor-like conditions of term placenta

A1. True

Small hemangiomas are usually asymptomatic; however, larger ones (>5 cm) can be associated with hydramnios, hemorrhage, premature delivery, premature placental separation and placenta previa. The left-to-right shunting may lead to transient congestive heart failure in the infant. **(p. 1753)**

A2. True

Most often this phenomenon is seen in malignant melanomas, lymphomas and leukemias. **(p. 1753)**

Breast 20

Normal anatomy

Q1

The breast is a glandular organ composed of two major parts, the terminal duct–lobular unit (TDLU) and the large duct system.

Q2

The TDLU is composed of the lobule and terminal ductule and represents the secretory portion of the gland.

Q3

The entire ductal–lobular epithelial system of the breast is covered by a specialized single cell-type epithelial lining.

Q4

Myoepithelial cells react with HMB-45 and CEA.

Q5

The nipple has a very characteristic microscopic appearance, with large collecting ducts opening onto the surface and numerous sebaceous glands.

Q6

Pregnancy-related lactational changes in the mammary lobule with marked cytoplasmic vacuolization, large nuclei and dilated lumina is a condition that can simulate other breast conditions of greater significance.

Q7

Another clinically inconsequential alteration is a clear cell change of the ductal or lobular epithelium that is often associated with lupus.

Ectopia, inflammatory and related lesions

Q1

Ectopic breast tissue has been reported often within the umbilical region.

Q2

Mammary duct ectasia has also been referred to as comedomastitis, varicocele tumor, periductal mastitis and granulomatous mastitis.

Q3

Fat necrosis is often associated with hormonal replacement therapy.

Q4

Lymphocytic mastitis is an unusual breast lesion consisting microscopically of dense perilobular and perivascular lymphocytic infiltrates associated with lobular atrophy and sclerosis.

Q5

Tuberculosis of the breast may be secondary to either bloodstream dissemination or extension from an adjacent tuberculous process.

Q6

Breast infarct is typically associated with trauma.

Benign proliferative breast disease

Q1

Fibroadenoma is a sharply demarcated benign breast tumor typically occurring in patients between the ages of 20 and 35.

Q2

Malignant changes in fibroadenomas are found in more than 50% of cases.

QUESTIONS

Q3

Tubular adenoma presents in young adults as a solitary, well circumscribed, firm mass that is tan-yellow.

Q4

Intraductal papilloma arises within large or small ducts of the breast and occurs at an average age of 48 years.

Q5

Microscopically, papillomas are simple structures with florid necrosis and papillary fronds containing one cell type only.

Q6

Microscopic morphologic variations sometimes encountered in intraductal papillomas include infarcts, squamous and apocrine metaplasia, sebaceous metaplasia, and the presence of atypical ductal hyperplasia and ductal carcinoma in situ.

Q7

Nipple adenoma, also known as florid papillomatosis of the nipple ducts, is a variant of tubular adenoma.

Q8

Clinically, nipple adenoma patients can present with an eroded nipple, and the disease can be confused with Paget's disease.

Q9

The term adenosis can be applied to any hyperplastic process that primarily involves the glandular component of the breast.

Q10

Sclerosing adenosis is a benign form of adenosis that occurs in patients older than 60 years.

Q11

Microscopically, the most important diagnostic feature of sclerosing adenosis is its architecture as seen at very low magnification, with nodules retaining a round or oval lobular configuration.

Q12

Micronodular adenosis is a common form of adenosis with large dilated tubules.

Q13

Microglandular adenosis is an indolent condition that should be treated conservatively.

Q14

Fibrocystic disease of the breast is an extremely important lesion because of its high frequency and the ability to simulate the appearance of carcinoma.

Q15

Epithelial hyperplasia is the least important component of fibrocystic disease.

Q16

Florid ductal hyperplasia shows no evidence of necrosis, with the oval shape of the nuclei and the parallel arrangement resulting in 'streaming,' and prominent peripheral clefts within the glandular lumina.

Q17

Collagenous spherulosis represents a curious lesion that may be also seen in salivary gland tumors.

Q18

Sclerosing ductal lesions are seen in association with infarcts.

Q19

Microscopically, sclerosing ductal lesions (often called radial scar) show a densely fibrotic center with small ductular formations that are disorganized but still composed of two cell types.

Q20

Atypical ductal hyperplasia (ADH) is a lesion with cytologic (monomorphic cells with round nuclei) and architectural (micropapillae, tufts, bridges, fronds, solid and cribriform patterns) features indistinguishable from low-grade DCIS, but intimately admixed with usual ductal hyperplasia and/or showing only partial involvement of the TDLU.

Carcinoma

Q1

Breast carcinoma is the second most common malignant tumor among women in the USA.

Q2

The incidence of breast carcinoma among women is also very high in most Asian and African countries.

Q3

Risk factors for the development of breast carcinoma have been established, including country of birth, family history, reproductive history, fibrocystic disease and epithelial hyperplasia, exogenous estrogens, contraceptive use and radiation.

Q4

Two genes responsible for approximately two-thirds of familial breast carcinomas are *BRCA2* and *BRCA3*.

Q5

Analysis of the breast carcinomas developing in carriers of *BRCA1* mutations has shown a higher percentage of tumors with medullary features (high grade, mitotically active, pushing margins, negative estrogen receptors, syncytial growth pattern).

Q6

Approximately 50% of breast carcinomas are located in the lower outer quadrant.

Q7

Multicentricity of breast carcinoma is more common in lobular than in ductal carcinoma.

Q8

Mammography can detect breast tumors if not smaller than 5 mm.

Q9

The incidence of calcifications in breast carcinoma is approximately 80%, and is almost absent in benign breast disease.

Q10

Two methods have been used to obtain cytologic material from the breast: aspiration of nipple secretions and fine needle aspiration.

Q11

Whereas nipple secretion aspiration cytology has limited value and is used mostly for screening purposes, fine needle aspiration is a highly reliable method with an average sensitivity of 87% and specificity close to 100%.

Q12

Fine needle aspiration is very useful in differentiating between in situ and invasive ductal carcinoma.

Q13

Needle core biopsy for the non-operative diagnosis of breast carcinoma has been generally favored over FNA.

Q14

Well known pitfalls of the needle core procedure include missing infiltrating lobular carcinoma.

Q15

The two key determinations to make in the morphologic study of breast carcinoma are whether the tumor is in situ or invasive, and whether it is ductal or lobular in type.

Q16

Several morphologic variants of ductal carcinoma in situ (DCIS) exist, mostly originating in large ducts.

Q17

Comedocarcinoma presents grossly as a cluster of thick-walled ducts plugged by necrotic tumor reminiscent of that seen in comedones.

Q18

The term extensive intraductal carcinoma (EIC) has been proposed for tumors in which the intraductal component comprises 75% or more of the area encompassed by the infiltrating tumor and is also present in the surrounding breast tissue.

Q19

[In situ] papillary carcinoma makes up only a small percentage of breast carcinomas and occurs in an older age group.

Q20

Microscopically, features favoring papillary carcinoma are spindle epithelial cells, the presence of two cell types and squamous metaplasia.

Q21

The presence within papillary carcinoma of large pale eosinophilic cells (known as clear or globoid cells), which can be mistaken for myoepithelial cells, represents an important diagnostic trap.

Q22

It seems likely that most papillary carcinomas arise within areas of atypical ductal hyperplasia.

Q23

The micropapillary variety of DCIS is more likely than others to involve multiple quadrants of the breast.

Q24

The cystic hypersecretory form is a variation of DCIS characterized by an adjacent invasive process.

Q25

Lobular cancerization is a term that refers to the presence, in a structure identifiable as a lobule, of carcinoma with the features of DCIS.

Q26

The rare morphologic variation of DCIS also known as endocrine DCIS (E-DCIS) is often accompanied by adjacent fat necrosis.

Q27

Immunohistochemically, two important features of DCIS (in relation to the differential diagnosis from LCIS) are the presence of E-cadherin and scantiness or the absence of high molecular weight keratin.

Q28

The assumed implication of a diagnosis of DCIS is that, if left untreated, the lesion will not progress to invasive carcinoma.

Q29

Lobular carcinoma in situ (LCIS) has no distinguishing features on gross examination and is usually found incidentally.

Q30

Microscopically, LCIS shows lobules distended and completely filled by relatively uniform, round, small to medium-sized cells with normochromatic nuclei.

Q31

Terminal ducts adjacent to LCIS often exhibit proliferation of cells similar to those in LCIS, a change referred to as Paget's disease.

Q32

LCIS can be also found in fibroadenomas and in foci of sclerosing adenosis or collagenous spherulosis.

Q33

The only conventional special stains of some significance for the evaluation of LCIS are those for mucin, which shows positivity in scattered tumor cells in about three-quarters of cases.

Q34

Approximately 80% of patients with LCIS will develop invasive lobular carcinoma.

Q35

The gross size, shape and consistency of breast carcinoma are highly dependent on the relative amounts of tumor cells and stroma.

Q36

The presence of malignant gland formations is necessary to establish the diagnosis of ductal carcinoma.

Q37

The most common type of tumor invasion seen in ductal carcinoma is perineural invasion.

Q38

Breast carcinomas can be positive for S-100.

Q39

The majority of infiltrating ductal carcinomas contain intraluminal or intracellular mucin.

Q40

Microscopically, tubular carcinoma simulates a benign condition because of the well-differentiated nature of the glands, the absence of necrosis or mitoses, and scanty pleomorphism.

Q41

Cribriform carcinoma shows a high incidence of multricentricity, a history of bilateral breast carcinoma and a family history of breast carcinoma.

Q42

The mucin content of mucinous ductal carcinomas is almost exclusively intracellular.

Q43

Pure mucinous carcinomas are associated with a very low incidence of nodal metastases.

Q44

Medullary carcinoma can be grossly and clinically mistaken for a fibroadenoma.

Q45

A constant microscopic component of medullary carcinoma is a prominent lymphoplasmacytic infiltrate at the periphery of the tumor.

Q46

Medullary carcinomas are almost always ER positive.

Q47

The prognosis of medullary carcinoma is slightly worse than that for invasive ductal carcinoma NOS.

Q48

Apocrine change is always associated with benign lesions.

Q49

Juvenile secretory carcinoma occurs exclusively in children and adolescents.

Q50

Carcinomas with neuroendocrine features are often associated with an intraductal component and mucin secretion.

Q51

Mucinous carcinoma, small cell neuroendocrine carcinoma and NOS infiltrating ductal carcinoma can express neuroendocrine features.

Q52

Metaplastic carcinoma is a generic term for breast carcinoma of ductal type in which the predominant component has an appearance other than epithelial and glandular and more in keeping with another cell type, such as squamous cell carcinoma, sarcomatoid carcinoma, chondrosarcoma, osteosarcoma, carcinoma with osteoclast-like giant cells, etc.

Q53

Molecular studies support the interpretation that recognizable epithelial and sarcoma-like components in sarcomatoid carcinoma originate from the same stem cell.

Q54

Carcinoma with osteoclast-like giant cells contains malignant multinucleated giant cells.

Q55

Squamous cell carcinoma of the breast is a subtype of phylloides tumor.

Q56

Inflammatory breast carcinoma refers to ordinary ductal carcinoma with a marked inflammatory host reaction.

Q57

The presence of dermal lymphatic permeation is a sign of an ominous prognosis in breast carcinoma.

Q58

Paget's disease is an eczema-like lesion of the nipple and areola associated exclusively with infiltrating ductal carcinoma.

Q59

Mucin stain is almost always positive in Paget's disease.

Q60

The classic type of invasive lobular carcinoma is characterized by the presence of small, relatively uniform tumor cells growing singly in Indian file and in concentric fashion around lobules involved by in situ lobular neoplasia.

Q61

Any invasive tumor associated with lobular carcinoma in situ should be considered invasive lobular carcinoma.

Q62

The main morphologic difference between invasive ductal and lobular carcinoma is the small size of the cells and the uncohesiveness seen in lobular carcinomas.

Q63

Myoblastoid carcinoma is a proposed synonym for lipid-rich carcinoma.

Q64

Most cases of signet ring cell carcinoma are regarded as variants of lobular carcinoma.

Q65

Tubulolobular carcinoma is associated with a higher incidence of multifocality and positive axillary nodes than is pure tubular carcinoma.

Q66

Mixed ductal and lobular carcinomas are very common, comprising 30% of all breast carcinomas.

Q67

Microinvasive breast carcinoma is defined by any carcinoma in situ showing one or more areas of stromal invasion not surpassing 1 mm in diameter.

Q68

Most medullary carcinomas and intraductal comedocarcinomas are ER/PR negative, whereas most mucinous carcinomas are positive.

Q69

HER2/*neu* is an oncogene that encodes a transmembrane glycoprotein with tyrosine kinase activity, which belongs to the family of epidermal growth receptors.

Q70

FISH confirmation of immunostaining for Her2/*neu* is required only if the stain is 1+ positive.

Q71

HER2/*neu* overexpression is found in nearly all cases of high-grade (comedo-type) DCIS, in 20–30% of invasive ductal carcinomas, and in a smaller percentage of invasive lobular carcinomas.

Q72

The degree of local invasion is generally greater in invasive ductal than invasive lobular carcinoma.

Q73

Nipple invasion is present in 23–31% of all clinically detectable invasive carcinomas.

Q74

Distant breast carcinoma metastases are seen most commonly in the skeletal system, lung and pleura, liver, ovary, adrenal gland and central nervous system.

Q75

When a single enlarged axillary lymph node is involved by metastatic non-lymphoid tumor in the presence of clinically and radiologically normal breast and no evidence of tumor elsewhere, the most likely diagnosis is metastatic breast carcinoma or melanoma.

Q76

The term 'micrometastases' is applied to a microscopic cluster of metastatic cells within a lymph node that are not larger than 2 mm.

Q77

The most widely used clinical staging system for breast carcinoma is the one adopted by both the International Union against Cancer (UICC) and the American Joint Commission on Cancer Staging and End Result Reporting (AJC).

Q78

When conservative surgery is employed, microscopic evaluation of the surgical margins is not of crucial value as every lumpectomy is followed by radiation therapy.

Q79

At present, 5 years of tamoxifen therapy for early-stage hormone receptor-positive breast carcinoma is the standard adjuvant endocrine therapy.

Q80

Radiation therapy of breast carcinoma may result in bizarre nuclear changes, the formation of giant tumor cells, naked nuclei and abnormal mitotic figures.

Q81

Chemotherapy can induce striking vacuolization of the tumor cells as well as the atrophy of terminal ductal units.

Q82

Women who are over 50 years of age have a significantly better prognosis than those under 50.

Q83

The diameter of the primary tumor is one of the strongest predictive factors for the incidence of nodal metastases and survival rate.

Q84

Classic lobular carcinoma has worse clinical outcome than NOS infiltrating ductal carcinoma.

Q85

The Nottingham Modification of the Bloom–Richardson system for microscopic grading of breast carcinoma is applicable only to infiltrating ductal carcinomas.

Q86

Tumors with an absence of inflammatory reaction at the periphery have a lesser degree of nodal metastases and a better prognosis.

Q87

The correct way of counting mitoses in infiltrating ductal carcinoma is to start in the center of the tumor, including 10 high-power fields in the same area.

Q88

Expression of HER2-*neu* identifies a subset of patients with a poor prognosis, particularly when lymph nodes are involved.

Q89

Patients with estrogen receptor-positive tumors have a longer disease-free survival than the others.

Q90

For prognostic purposes, the best grouping system for axillary lymph node status is: negative nodes, one to four positive, and five and more positive.

Q91

Local recurrence is a sign of an ominous prognosis.

Salivary and sweat gland-type tumors

Q1

Embryologically, the breast is a modified salivary gland and therefore it is not surprising that a small proportion of benign and malignant tumors of the breast have an appearance analogous to that of tumors of the salivary glands.

Q2

Adenoid cystic carcinoma of the breast can show focal sebaceous differentiation.

Q3

Cases of sclerosing adenosis with a great predominance of myoepithelial cells and presenting in the form of multifocal microscopic lesions have been designated myoepitheliosis.

Q4

Adenomyoepithelioma is a benign lesion with no metastatic potential and occasional local recurrence.

Stromal tumors and tumor-like conditions

Q1

Phylloides tumor occurs in the same age group as breast carcinoma, with a median age of 45.

Q2

Microscopically the two key features of phylloides tumor are stromal hypercellularity and epithelial atypia.

Q3

Tumors with the configuration of fibroadenomas having a cellular stroma without atypical features concentrated in the periductal areas are consistent with benign phylloides tumor.

Q4

The epithelial component of malignant phylloides tumors always has features of carcinoma.

Q5

The cytologically malignant phylloides tumor has metastasizing potential.

Q6

Periductal stromal tumor is a new entity that has features of both phylloides and stromal sarcoma.

Q7

Radiation therapy is a risk factor for developing angiosarcoma.

Q8

Angiosarcomas of the breast are usually high-grade sarcomas.

Q9

Stromal sarcoma is the generic term given to malignant breast tumors thought to arise from the specialized stroma of this organ but lacking the epithelial component of a phylloides tumor.

Lymphoid tumors and tumor-like conditions

Q1

Primary breast lymphomas are nearly always of non-Hodgkin's type and are usually composed of B cells.

Q2

Primary breast lymphomas are bilateral in 25% of cases.

QUESTIONS

Other primary tumors and tumor-like conditions

Q1

Granular cell tumor is a benign lesion that can mimic malignancy both grossly and clinically.

Q2

Fibromatosis occurring during childbearing age is in general more cellular than that seen after the menopause.

Q3

Pseudoangiomatous stromal hyperplasia (PASH) represents a localized form of stromal overgrowth with hormonal pathogenesis.

Metastatic tumors

Q1

Renal cell carcinoma, endometrioid carcinoma and pancreatic adenocarcinoma are the most common sources of metastatic disease to the breast.

Q2

In children, the most common malignant tumor to metastasize to the breast is rhabdomyosarcoma.

Breast disease in children and adolescents

Q1

The most common pathologic condition of the breast between puberty and 20 years of age is fibroadenoma.

Q2

Virginal hypertrophy is massive unilateral or bilateral enlargement due mostly to stromal and lobular proliferation.

Q3

Carcinoma of the infantile breast is very rare, and most cases are of mucinous type.

Breast diseases in males

Q1

Cases of gynecomastia have been reported in type-1 neurofibromatosis.

Q2

Idiopathic non-hormonal gynecomastia is usually unilateral.

Q3

Lobules are never seen in gynecomastia.

Q4

There is a close histogenic link between solitary fibrous tumor, spindle cell lipoma and myofibroblastoma of the breast.

Q5

An increased incidence of male breast carcinoma is seen in Southeast Asia.

Q6

The incidence of positivity for estrogen receptors is lower in male breast carcinoma than in females.

Q7

Metastatic carcinoma to the male breast usually originates from the prostate, is almost always seen following estrogen therapy, and is often bilateral.

Normal anatomy

A1. True
These units are easily observed on microscopic slides. **(p. 1764)**

A2. True
TDLU has a distinct lobular configuration. **(p. 1764)**

A3. False
The epithelium is lined by a two cell-type lining, the inner epithelium and the outer myoepithelial cells. **(p. 1764)**

A4. False
Myoepithelial cells react with S-100, P-cadherin, smooth muscle actin, calponin and caldesmon. **(p. 1765)**

A5. True
The epidermis of the nipple and areola resembles that of the skin elsewhere, except for the presence of basally located clear cells known as Toker's cells, which are related histogenetically to Paget's disease. **(p. 1765)**

A6. True
These changes can mimic carcinoma. **(p. 1766)**

A7. False
Clear cell change within the lobules or ducts is clinically insignificant and shows no association with lupus (SLE). **(p. 1766)**

Ectopia, inflammatory and related lesions

A1. False
Ectopic breast tissue is typically identified along the 'milk line' that runs from the axilla to the inguinal region, the most common sites being the chest wall and the vulva. **(p. 1767)**

A2. True
Most of the cases are seen in premenopausal parous women and probably represent a localized response to components of stagnant colostrum. **(p. 1767)**

A3. False
Fat necrosis is associated with a history of trauma or is secondary to mammary duct ectasia/fibrocystic disease with large cyst formation. **(p. 1768)**

A4. True
Sometimes the lymphocytic infiltrate is accompanied by a stromal infiltrate of epithelioid cells that can lead to a mistaken diagnosis of invasive carcinoma or granular cell tumor. Lymphocytic mastitis can result clinically in a palpable mass; most cases are associated with diabetes (hence the proposed name diabetic mastopathy), but can also occur in association with intraductal carcinoma. **(p. 1768)**

A5. True
The lesion is composed of typical granulomas and can be mistaken clinically for advanced breast carcinoma. **(p. 1769)**

A6. False
Breast infarct can complicate a large variety of conditions, including anticoagulant therapy, intraductal papilloma, fibroadenoma, phylloides tumor, syphilis and Wegener's granulomatosis. **(p. 1769)**

Benign proliferative breast disease

A1. True
Microscopically, morphologic variations in fibroadenoma are plentiful, including hyalinization, multinucleated stromal giant cells, the presence of mature fat, smooth muscle and cartilage, prominent myxoid changes, infarcts, apocrine metaplasia, sclerosing adenosis, squamous metaplasia and lactational changes. **(p. 1770)**

A2. False
Malignant transformation of fibroadenoma is very rare (only 0.1%), and the large majority are epithelial in situ lesions. Sarcomatous transformation of the stroma is an even rarer phenomenon. **(p. 1772)**

A3. True
Microscopically, a close packing of uniform small tubules lined by single layer of epithelial cells and an attenuated layer of myoepithelial cells is seen. **(p. 1773)**

A4. True
Papillomas can give rise to a bloody nipple discharge and may be palpable in a subareolar location, rarely exceeding 3 cm in diameter. **(p. 1773)**

A5. False
Intraductal papillomas are complex, cellular and arborizing structures with nearly always absent necrosis and the presence of two cell types, myoepithelial and epithelial. **(p. 1773)**

A6. True

Immunohistochemical markers for myoepithelial cells may highlight the absence of this component in ductal carcinoma or atypical ductal hyperplasia. **(p. 1774)**

A7. False

Nipple adenoma is a variant of intraductal papilloma involving the terminal portion of the galactophorous ducts. **(p. 1775)**

A8. True

This is a variant of intraductal papilloma involving the terminal portion of the galactophorous ducts. **(p. 1775)**

A9. True

Adenosis represents glandular epithelial proliferation only. **(p. 1776)**

A10. False

The importance of this well-known form of adenosis that occurs at an average age of 30 years is mainly because of the high likelihood of its being misdiagnosed as carcinoma. The gross appearance of the lesion, with its multinodular configuration and increased resistance during dissection, is quite reminiscent of invasive carcinoma. **(p. 1776)**

A11. True

Sclerosing adenosis with an extensive stromal fibrosis can often mimic invasive ductal carcinoma. **(p. 1776)**

A12. False

This form of adenosis has small uniform glands and open lumina containing an eosinophilic secretion distributed in an irregular fashion. **(p. 1777)**

A13. True

Microglandular adenosis is also known as microglandular hyperplasia. **(p. 1777)**

A14. True

Fibrocystic disease can simulate the clinical, radiographic, gross and microscopic appearances of carcinoma. **(p. 1779)**

A15. False

This is the most important and troublesome component because of its possible relationship to carcinoma and the fact that it is responsible for most difficulties in the differential diagnosis between fibrocystic disease and carcinoma. **(p. 1780)**

A16. True

These features are most helpful in identifying the benign nature of this proliferation. **(p. 1780)**

A17. True

Collagenous spherulosis is characterized by the presence of intraluminal clusters of eosinophilic collagen-rich spherules that arise in the spaces between epithelial and myoepithelial cells. **(p. 1782)**

A18. False

This is a group of lesions characterized by small size, a stellate shape and a central fibrous core, and are usually seen in the context of fibrocystic disease. **(p. 1782)**

A19. True

The most important aspects of the sclerosing ductal lesion are the differential diagnosis and the possible relationship with ductal carcinoma. **(p. 1783)**

A20. True

Quantitative requirements for diagnosis of ADH have been proposed in that the lesion should measure less than 2 mm in aggregate or be present in two spaces. **(p. 1786)**

Carcinoma

A1. False

Breast carcinoma is the most common malignant tumor in the USA and northern Europe, and the leading cause of carcinoma death in women. **(p. 1787)**

A2. False

Asia and Africa show a very low incidence of breast carcinoma. **(p. 1787)**

A3. True

It has been proposed that the common denominator for most of these factors is strong and/or prolonged estrogen stimulation operating on a genetically susceptible background. **(p. 1788)**

A4. False

These are *BRCA1* and *BRCA2*, located on chromosomes 17q and 13q-12-13, respectively. **(p. 1788)**

A5. True

The product of *BRCA1* is a cell-regulated phosphoprotein that can be detected immunohistochemically. **(p. 1788)**

A6. False

50% of carcinomas are identified in the upper outer quadrant. **(p. 1789)**

A7. True

Multicentricity, defined by the presence of carcinoma in a breast quadrant other than the one containing the dominant mass, was detected in 13.4% of all breast carcinoma cases in one large study. **(p. 1789)**

A8. False

Extremely small tumors (1–2 mm) can be detected with this technique, which relies primarily on the presence of calcifications. **(p. 1789)**

A9. False
The incidence of calcifications in breast carcinoma is 50–60%, and in benign breast disease 20%. **(p. 1789)**

A10. True
However, aspiration of nipple secretions has limited diagnostic value and is used mostly for screening purposes. **(p. 1791)**

A11. True
In experienced hands this technique is highly reliable in tumor diagnostics. **(p. 1791)**

A12. False
In differentiating DCIS from invasive carcinoma and DCIS from atypical ductal hyperplasia FNA has very limited value. **(p. 1791)**

A13. True
This is based on the fact that core biopsy allows evaluation of both cytologic and architectural features, that it may provide a definitive diagnosis of invasive carcinoma, and also that it allows the identification of microcalcifications. **(p. 1793)**

A14. True
This is especially difficult in cases of lobular carcinoma made up of lymphocyte-like tumor cells. **(p. 1793)**

A15. True
These parameters show significant prognostic value. **(p. 1794)**

A16. False
Only intraductal papillary carcinoma originates in large ducts. Other DCIS subtypes are believed to originate in the TDLU (terminal ductal–lobular unit). **(p. 1795)**

A17. True
Comedocarcinoma may reach a large size – over 5 cm – and shows a high grade of cytologic atypia (grade 3). **(p. 1795)**

A18. False
The term EIC is proposed for tumors in which the intraductal component comprises 25% or more of the tissue examined. **(p. 1796)**

A19. True
Grossly, in situ papillary carcinoma may present as a well circumscribed mass. **(p. 1796)**

A20. False
The features of papillary carcinoma are uniform epithelial cells, the presence of one cell type only (lack of myoepithelial cells), nuclear hyperchromasia and high mitotic activity, lack of apocrine metaplasia, scanty or absent stroma, and lack of benign proliferative disease in the adjacent breast. **(p. 1796)**

A21. True
These clear globoid cells, which are immunoreactive for GCDFP-15 and negative for smooth muscle actin, should not be confused with myoepithelial cells and should not lead to an erroneous diagnosis of intraductal papilloma. **(p. 1797)**

A22. False
Papillary carcinomas arise de novo. **(p. 1797)**

A23. True
The micropapillary DCIS shows microscopic evidence of elongated epithelial projections projecting into the glandular lumen. **(p. 1798)**

A24. False
The cystic hypersecretory DCIS is characterized by cystic formations induced by the abundant secretory material; it deserves mention because of the ease with which it can be confused with a benign process. **(p. 1798)**

A25. True
The original assumption was that this represents a secondary extension of ductal carcinoma into the lobule. The evidence suggests that this phenomenon represents instead a variation in the growth pattern of DCIS within the lobule as a part of TDLU. **(p. 1799)**

A26. False
E-DCIS is often associated with adjacent intraductal papillomas with pagetoid involvement by the carcinoma. **(p. 1799)**

A27. True
In addition, the high-grade form of DCIS also shows P-cadherin expression. **(p. 1800)**

A28. False
If left untreated, DCIS will inevitably progress to an invasive carcinoma of similar morphologic features. **(p. 1800)**

A29. True
LCIS is multicentric in approximately 70% of cases and bilateral in 30–40%. **(p. 1800)**

A30. True
In the typical case, atypia, pleomorphism, mitotic activity and necrosis are minimal or absent, and there is some lack of cohesiveness among the tumor cells. **(p. 1800)**

A31. False
This change has been referred to as mural or pagetoid, but Paget's disease practically never occurs in LCIS. **(p. 1801)**

A32. True
The diagnosis of LCIS should be made only in cases in which the cellular proliferation has resulted in the formation of solid nests that have expanded the lobules. **(p. 1801)**

A33. True
Immunohistochemically, the tumor cells show positivity for keratin, EMA and milk fat globule antigen. **(p. 1801)**

A34. False
Approximately 20–30% of patients will develop invasive carcinoma, a risk about 8–10 times higher than for a control population. **(p. 1802)**

A35. True
Grossly the typical case is firm, poorly circumscribed and gritty; however, relatively circumscribed softer tumors can be seen as well (particularly medullary carcinomas). Tumors that are particularly hard because of the amount of fibrous stroma were traditionally referred to as 'scirrhous carcinoma.' **(p. 1802)**

A36. False
Glands are usually appreciated in infiltrating ductal carcinoma; however, tumor cells can also grow in diffuse sheets, well-defined nests, cords or individual cells. Glandular/tubular differentiation can be barely detectable or altogether absent. **(p. 1802)**

A37. False
Lymph vessel invasion is the most common type of invasion. It may be difficult to distinguish from artifactual tissue retraction. Perineural invasion is also commonly seen. **(p. 1804)**

A38. True
Surprisingly, 10–45% of all breast carcinomas show positivity for S-100, which is a marker for neural and melanocytic cells. This is a fact to remember in the differential diagnosis of tumors metastatic to axillary lymph nodes. **(p. 1804)**

A39. True
However, in the study by Fisher et al. the amount of mucin was marked and moderate in only 19% and slight in 34%, and in 47% there was no detectable mucin. **(p. 1804)**

A40. True
The clues to the diagnosis are the haphazard arrangement of the glands in the stroma with an absence of any organoid configuration; frequent invasion of the fat at the periphery; the cellular nature of the stroma; irregular and often angulated glands; open lumina with basophilic secretion; apocrine 'snouts' in the apical cytoplasm; the formation of trabecular bars; lack of myoepithelial cells; lack of basement membrane; and occurrence in two-thirds or more of cases of typical intraductal carcinoma in ducts within or outside the lesion, nearly always low grade in type. **(p. 1805)**

A41. False
It is tubular carcinoma that shows a high incidence of multricentricity, a history of bilateral breast carcinoma and a family history of breast carcinoma. Cribriform carcinoma is invasive ductal carcinoma closely related to tubular carcinoma, with an excellent prognosis. **(p. 1805)**

A42. False
The mucin content of mucinous ductal carcinomas is almost exclusively extracellular. Microscopically, the classic mucinous carcinoma is described as small clusters of malignant cells 'floating in the sea of mucin.' Signet ring cell carcinomas, even if technically speaking regarded mucinous tumors, are excluded from the group of pure mucinous ductal carcinomas. **(p. 1806)**

A43. True
The incidence is 2–4%. However, it has been shown that death from this tumor can occur 12 years or more after therapy. **(p. 1807)**

A44. True
The tumor is grossly well circumscribed and can therefore be mistaken for a benign process. **(p. 1807)**

A45. True
Such infiltrate represents a reaction of the host to the neoplasm. **(p. 1808)**

A46. False
They are usually negative for estrogen receptors but show a striking positivity for S-100. **(p. 1808)**

A47. False
The prognosis of medullary carcinoma is slightly better than that for NOS invasive ductal carcinoma when strict criteria for diagnosis of medullary carcinoma are applied. Often, the term medullary carcinoma has been misused for highly cellular breast carcinomas that behave in an aggressive fashion. **(p. 1808)**

A48. False
Apocrine change per se is a benign change and is most often associated with fibrocystic disease and other benign entities in the breast. However, focal apocrine change can be detected in up to 10% of ordinary carcinomas. **(p. 1809)**

A49. False
It is a rare form of carcinoma seen primarily in children, but can also occur in adults. **(p. 1809)**

A50. False
Only a minority of cases are associated with an intraductal component and mucin secretion. **(p. 1810)**

A51. True
Even a small proportion of ductal carcinoma in situ can stain positive with neuroendocrine markers. **(p. 1810)**

A52. True
On the whole, the behavior of metaplastic carcinoma seems to be more aggressive than that of ordinary invasive ductal-type carcinoma. **(p. 1811)**

A53. True
Immunohistochemically, the sarcoma-like elements of metaplastic tumors have usually acquired vimentin positivity but occasionally still retain epithelial markers. **(p. 1811)**

A54. False
All the available evidence suggests that the osteoclast-like elements are non-neoplastic histiocytic in nature and that they form from the fusion of mononuclear precursors. **(p. 1812)**

A55. False
Phylloides tumors may contain a squamous component, but squamous cell carcinoma of the breast is an extremely rare variant that is considered a variant of metaplastic carcinoma. **(p. 1812)**

A56. False
Inflammatory carcinoma was originally used in a clinical sense for a type of breast carcinoma in which the entire breast was reddened and warm, with widespread edema of the skin, simulating the appearance of mastitis. An 'inflammatory' clinical appearance almost always corresponds to dermal lymphatic permeation, and vice versa. **(p. 1813)**

A57. True
The presence of dermal lymphatic permeation by tumor cells is a sign of ominous prognosis whether the clinical appearance is that of inflammatory carcinoma or not. **(p. 1813)**

A58. False
If a definitive mass can be palpated beneath the diseased nipple the tumor will be invasive in over 90% of cases. However, if there is no palpable lesion 66% of cases will be associated with intraductal carcinoma. **(p. 1813)**

A59. False
Mucin staining may or may not be positive. Immunohistochemically cells are positive for EMA, CEA, CK7 and GCDFP-15, and Her-2/*neu*. They are negative for S-100. **(p. 1814)**

A60. True
Gland formations are not seen, and desmoplastic reaction is marked as well as lymphohistiocytic infiltration. **(p. 1815)**

A61. False
In order to call carcinoma a lobular carcinoma it has to have morphological features appropriate for this carcinoma. Ductal carcinomas can be associated with lobular carcinomas in situ, and vice versa. **(p. 1816)**

A62. True
In many cases the distinction between these two entities is difficult and to a large extent subjective. **(p. 1816)**

A63. False
Myoblastoid carcinoma is a proposed synonym for histiocytoid carcinoma. **(p. 1816)**

A64. True
Signet ring cell carcinoma shows cytoarchitectural features that are similar to those of lobular carcinoma, such as small cell size, uniformity and dissociation, and therefore is considered a variant of lobular carcinoma. **(p. 1817)**

A65. True
Tubulolobular carcinoma has a morphological and immunohistochemical profile intermediate between those of ductal and lobular carcinoma. **(p. 1817)**

A66. False
Mixed ductal and lobular carcinomas are actually very rare. **(p. 1817)**

A67. True
This definition is correct, but its application is not always straightforward owing to irregular nesting of carcinoma in situ and undefined separation of epithelium and stroma. **(p. 1818)**

A68. True
Not much correlation exists between the cytoarchitectural type of breast carcinomas and the presence of hormone receptors. However, it has been established that most medullary carcinomas and intraductal comedocarcinomas are ER/PR negative, whereas most mucinous carcinomas are positive. **(p. 1818)**

A69. True
Its overexpression can be measured by FISH or immunohistochemistry. **(p. 1819)**

A70. False
FISH confirmation is needed only if the staining is strongly positive (3+) or completely negative. Staining patterns in between (including 1+ and 2+) need to be reverted for FISH confirmation. **(p. 1819)**

A71. True
HER2/*neu* is usually positive in high-grade tumors. Its overexpression is a very good predictor of response to Herceptin, but not a very good predictor of response to chemotherapy or overall survival. **(p. 1819)**

A72. False
It is the reverse: the degree of local invasion is generally greater in lobular carcinoma, presumably aided by the lack of E-cadherin in the tumor cells. **(p. 1820)**

A73. True
The large majority of these are located less than 2.5 cm from the nipple. **(p. 1820)**

A74. True

Carcinomatous meningitis is a particularly devastating pattern of metastatic spread. **(p. 1820)**

A75. True

In 90% of cases the metastatic lesion will be metastatic breast carcinoma or metastatic melanoma. **(p. 1821)**

A76. True

Smaller clusters composed of just a few cells are reported under the term 'isolated tumor cells.' **(p. 1822)**

A77. True

It is based on the TNM system (Tumor, Nodes, Metastases). **(p. 1822)**

A78. False

Radiation therapy is often used as a postoperative adjunct; however, microscopic evaluation of margins is of crucial value, as the likelihood of ipsilateral recurrences and distant metastases is related to the vicinity and amount of carcinoma at the margins. **(p. 1822)**

A79. True

The decision as to whether to give chemotherapy or hormonal therapy to node-negative patients depends on a variety of clinical and pathologic parameters. **(p. 1823)**

A80. True

Extensive tumor necrosis may also develop, which is later surrounded by a thick fibrous wall. **(p. 1823)**

A81. True

However, in most instances the changes do not affect the histological grading of the carcinoma. **(p. 1823)**

A82. False

Women who are younger than 50 have significantly better prognosis than those over 50. Relative survival declines after age 50 and is particularly low in older women. **(p. 1824)**

A83. True

It has been pointed out that size determination has a greater prognostic significance when measured microscopically than grossly. **(p. 1824)**

A84. False

There is no significant prognostic difference between ordinary invasive ductal and invasive lobular carcinoma. A variant of lobular carcinoma associated with an extremely bad prognosis is signet ring cell carcinoma. **(p. 1824)**

A85. False

The microscopic grading system of breast carcinoma was conceived largely for invasive ductal carcinoma NOS, but it can also be applied to the other special types of ductal carcinoma and lobular carcinoma. **(p. 1825)**

A86. True

Obviously, these considerations do not apply to the specific case of medullary carcinoma. **(p. 1825)**

A87. False

The periphery of the tumor is usually the most mitotically active area, and therefore mitoses are to be counted only at the periphery of the tumor, with 10 high-power fields counted in the same area. **(p. 1825)**

A88. True

It also correlates with the grade of the tumor, but loses much of its independent prognostic significance in multivariate analysis. **(p. 1826)**

A89. True

However, the difference in long-term prognosis is minimal. **(p. 1826)**

A90. False

The most significant prognostic feature for breast carcinoma is status of the lymph nodes. It has been determined that patients with no lymph node metastases do much better than those with metastatic nodes. In the group with metastases patients with fewer than four positive nodes have a better survival rate than those with four and more. Therefore, the correct grouping is: no positive nodes, one to three positive nodes, and four or more positive nodes. **(p. 1826)**

A91. True

In one series of 60 patients with ipsilateral chest wall recurrence and no detectable distant metastases all died of metastatic carcinoma. **(p. 1827)**

Salivary and sweat gland-type tumors

A1. False

The breast is actually modified sweat gland; however, a close analogy exists between sweat and salivary glands, and therefore it is not surprising that a small proportion of benign and malignant tumors of the breast have an appearance analogous to tumors of the salivary glands. **(p. 1827)**

A2. True

Such differentiation indicates the potential to differentiate into skin adnexal structures. **(p. 1828)**

A3. True

Myoepithelial cells stain positive for calponin and smooth muscle actin. **(p. 1828)**

A4. True

Adenomyoepithelioma is a small, firm, well-circumscribed nodule composed of polygonal cells with clear cytoplasm, arranged in nests that are sometimes centered by gland-forming epithelial cells. It has no metastatic potential and only a few reported cases recurred locally. **(p. 1828)**

Stromal tumors and tumor-like conditions

A1. True
Phylloides tumor is rare in patients younger than 25, but occasionally it can occur in young adults and even adolescents. **(p. 1829)**

A2. False
Microscopically the two key features of phylloides tumor are stromal hypercellularity and the presence of benign glandular elements. It is the amount and appearance of stromal component that determines whether a breast neoplasm should be called fibroadenoma or phylloides tumor. **(p. 1829)**

A3. True
Very few of these patients are younger than 25 years of age, in striking contrast to the age distribution of fibroadenoma. **(p. 1829)**

A4. False
In most cases of malignant phylloides tumors the epithelial component is not neoplastic, but it can be quite proliferative and atypical. Very rarely, the features of either ductal or lobular carcinoma will be present. **(p. 1831)**

A5. True
The incidence of metastases ranges from 3% to 12%. **(p. 1831)**

A6. True
It contains epithelial structures as phylloides does, but lacks the phylloides leaf-like architectural structure. **(p. 1831)**

A7. True
Following radiation therapy for carcinoma of the breast the overlying skin can develop a variety of vascular proliferations, ranging from lymphangioma-like nodules to angiosarcomas. **(p. 1832)**

A8. False
The appearance within one lesion may vary from that of a highly undifferentiated solid neoplasm to one that is extremely bland cytologically. **(p. 1832)**

A9. True
Most of those spindle cell tumors have features of fibrosarcoma. **(p. 1833)**

Lymphoid tumors and tumor-like conditions

A1. True
There are exceptional examples of T-cell lymphomas reported. Hodgkin's lymphoma of the breast usually represents secondary involvement in stage IV. **(p. 1833)**

A2. True
Every fourth case of primary breast lymphoma is bilateral. **(p. 1832)**

Other primary tumors and tumor-like conditions

A1. True
Granular cell tumor is usually small but can reach a size of 10 cm or more. Grossly, it is firm, homogeneous and white or grayish yellow. Cells contain eosinophilic granular cytoplasm that shows positivity for S-100. **(p. 1835)**

A2. True
Such cases are also more infiltrative, aggressive, and prone to local recurrence. **(p. 1835)**

A3. True
PASH is usually seen in women of childbearing age and is progesterone sensitive. **(p. 1836)**

Metastatic tumors

A1. False
Malignant melanoma, lung, ovary, kidney and stomach tumors are the most common sources of metastatic disease to the breast. **(p. 1836)**

A2. True
In children, rhabdomyosarcoma, particularly of the alveolar type, is a common tumor that metastasizes to the liver. **(p. 1836)**

Breast disease in children and adolescents

A1. True

Fibroadenomas are exceptional before puberty. **(p. 1836)**

A2. False

Virginal hypertrophy is massive unilateral or bilateral enlargement due mostly to stromal and ductal proliferation. There is little or no lobular proliferation at all. **(p. 1837)**

A3. False

Most cases of infantile and childhood breast carcinomas are so-called 'juvenile secretory' in type. **(p. 1837)**

Breast diseases in males

A1. True

Gynecomastia before age 25 is usually related to hormonal pubertal changes, whereas after that age it can be related to cirrhosis, medication, hormonally active tumors or type-1 neurofibromatosis. **(p. 1838)**

A2. True

Idiopathic non-hormonal gynecomastia is usually unilateral, with the left breast involved more commonly, whereas hormone-induced gynecomastia tends to be bilateral. **(p. 1838)**

A3. False

Lobules as well as pseudoangiomatous stromal hyperplasia and focal squamous metaplasia can be seen in gynecomastia. **(p. 1838)**

A4. True

Their morphological appearances are very similar, containing uniform bland-looking spindle cells haphazardly arranged in fascicles separated by broad bands of hyalinized collagen. **(p. 1838)**

A5. False

An increased incidence of male breast carcinoma is seen in some Arab countries, where the incidence reaches 10%. The incidence of male breast carcinoma in the USA is 1%. **(p. 1839)**

A6. False

The incidence of positivity for estrogen receptors is higher in male breast carcinoma than in females. **(p. 1839)**

A7. True

Some cases have been confused with primary breast carcinoma, but immunohistochemical staining for prostate-specific antigen (PSA) may be helpful in the differential diagnosis. **(p. 1839)**

21 Lymph nodes

Normal anatomy

Q1

In a normal lymph node both the cortex and the medulla represent B zones, whereas the paracortex represents a T zone.

Q2

Primary follicles appear as round aggregates of lymphocytes and are characterized by the presence of germinal centers.

Q3

Germinal centers are composed of follicular center cells, macrophages and follicular dendritic cells, and are surrounded by a mantle of small B lymphocytes.

Q4

Expansion of the paracortex is indicative of humoral antibody production, whereas proliferative germinal centers always signify a cell-mediated immunologic reaction.

Lymph node evaluation

Q1

In the evaluation of generalized lymphadenopathy, as a rule the surgeon should submit for pathologic examination the most accessible lymph nodes, such as those in the inguinal area.

Q2

The surgeon performing a biopsy of intra-abdominal nodes or large cervical or axillary masses should require a frozen section biopsy to obtain a specific diagnosis at this point.

Q3

The specimen should be received fresh in the laboratory immediately after excision, bisected as soon as it is received, and sampled for appropriate analysis.

Q4

Core needle biopsy is particularly useful for the evaluation of primary lymphoid disorders.

Q5

Cytologic diagnosis of low-grade malignant lymphoma is accurate in more than 90% of cases.

Q6

Ultrastructural examination of lymph nodes has very limited significance in the evaluation of primary lymphoid disorders, but it can be of use in some specific diseases, such as Langerhans' cell histiocytosis and various metastatic tumors.

Q7

The Southern blot hybridization procedure is used to assess the size of rearranged fragments using a radiolabeled DNA hybridization probe specific for DNA sequences in or around the constant region.

Q8

Clonal antigen receptor gene rearrangement is absolutely specific for a neoplastic process.

QUESTIONS

Primary immunodeficiencies

Q1

The many varieties of primary immunodeficiency can be broadly divided into two major categories according to the type of the immunologic deficit: humoral and cell-mediated.

Q2

In primary immunodeficiencies of the humoral type the thickness of the paracortical area is greatly diminished.

Patterns of hyperplasia

Q1

From a topographic and functional standpoint the major patterns of reactive lymphoid proliferation are segmental and global.

Q2

This is a typical histologic appearance of reactive follicles.

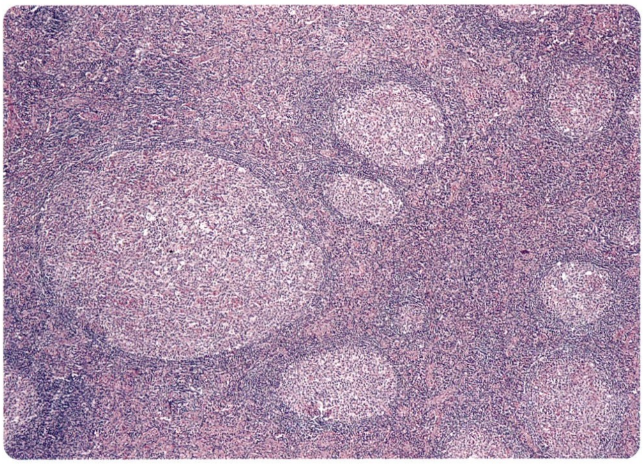

Fig. 21.1

Q3

Progressively transformed germinal centers are the morphologic expression of a distinctive type of follicular hyperplasia.

Q4

The main differential diagnosis of progressively transformed germinal centers is with nodular sclerosis Hodgkin's lymphoma.

Q5

Regressively transformed germinal centers are particularly prominent and numerous in Castleman's disease.

Q6

The diffuse form of paracortical hyperplasia is characteristic of dermatopathic lymphadenitis and nodal reactions to malignancy.

Q7

The cells present in the sinus represent an admixture of histiocytes and sinus lining cells.

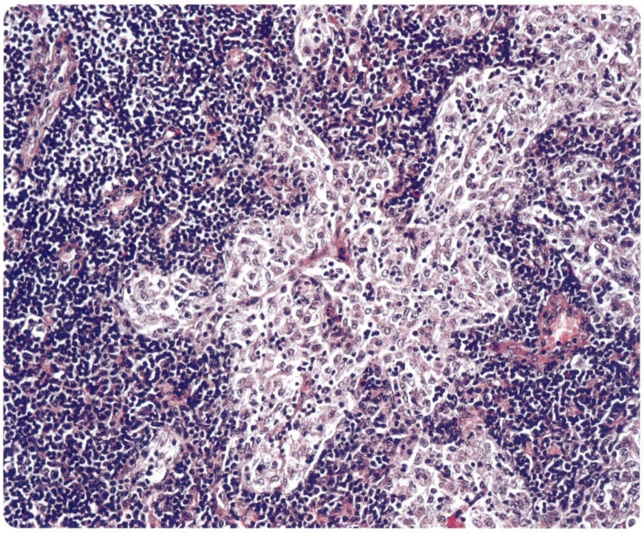

Fig. 21.2

Q8

The etiology of granulomatous lymphadenitis can be obtained by standard microscopic examination, but bacteriologic analysis is not important.

Q9

Monocytoid B-cell hyperplasia occurs most frequently in toxoplasmosis.

Q10

Plasmacytoid monocytes are a subtype of T cells.

Q11

The term polykaryocyte is used for a type of multinucleated giant cell found in lymphoid tissues.

Inflammatory/hyperplastic diseases

Q1

The typical case of acute nonspecific lymphadenitis should always be biopsied to exclude a malignant process.

Q2

Suppurative lymphadenitis is characteristic of Kikuchi's lymphadenitis.

Q3

Most patients with necrotizing lymphadenitis (Kikuchi's lymphadenitis) are young women with a persistent, painless cervical lymphadenopathy of modest dimensions that may be accompanied by fever.

Q4

The general features of chronic lymphadenitis are small granulomas composed mainly of epithelioid cells, with scattered Langhans' giant cells and lymphocytes.

Q5

The most common location of clinically apparent lymphadenopathy involved by tuberculosis is the axillary region.

Q6

In the United States, caseating granulomatous disease in a cervical lymph node of a child unaccompanied by pulmonary involvement is most frequently caused by *Mycobacterium tuberculosis*.

Q7

Sarcoidosis is more common in whites than in blacks, and the most common affected organs are the bone marrow and spleen.

Q8

Erythema nodosum often precedes pulmonary sarcoidosis, and functional hyperparathyroidism is found almost invariably in this disease.

Q9

The basic lesion of sarcoidosis is a small granuloma composed mainly of epithelioid cells, with scattered Langhans' giant cells and lymphocytes.

Q10

An asteroid body in the cytoplasm of a multinucleated giant cell is specific for sarcoidosis.

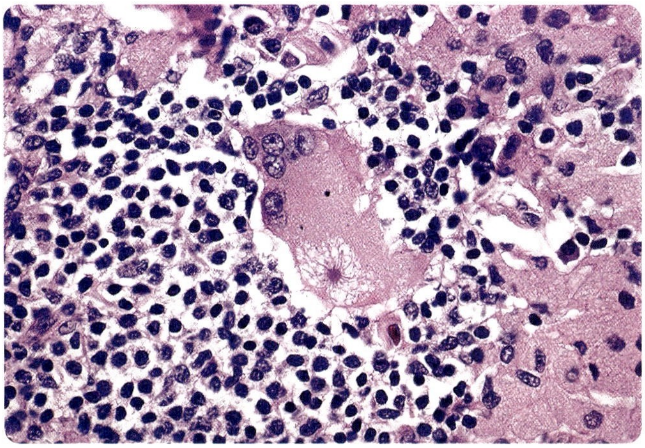

Fig. 21.3

Q11

The Kveim test is positive in all cases of sarcoidosis.

Q12

The most important fungal lymphadenitis is histoplasmosis.

Q13

Toxoplasmic lymphadenitis (Piringer–Kuchinka lymphadenitis), in its most typical form, involves the posterior cervical nodes of young women.

Q14

Microscopically, the typical triad of toxoplasmic lymphadenitis is constituted by marked follicular hyperplasia, small granulomas composed almost entirely of epithelioid cells, and distension of marginal and cortical sinuses by monocytoid B cells.

Q15

The lymph node sinuses appear dilated and prominent in this picture.

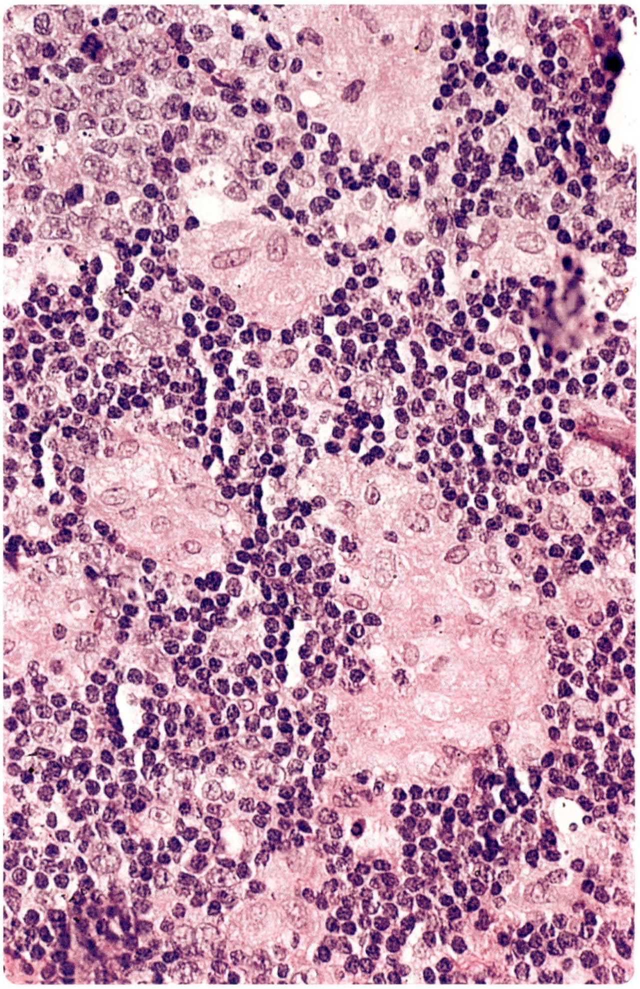

Fig. 21.4

Q16

Generalized lymphadenopathy is a common finding in primary and tertiary syphilis.

Q17

Mesenteric lymphadenitis is characterized by accumulation of large, pale, rounded histiocytes with granuloma formation.

Q18

In the lymphadenitis produced by *Yersinia enterocolitica*, small granulomas and abscesses are commonly present.

Q19

Cat-scratch disease is characterized by a primary cutaneous lesion and enlargement of regional lymph nodes, usually axillary or cervical.

Q20

The early lesions of cat-scratch disease have histiocytic proliferation and follicular hyperplasia, intermediate lesions have granulomatous changes, and late lesions have abscesses of various sizes.

Q21

The agent of cat-scratch disease is *Chlamydia trachomatis*.

Q22

A history of handling rabbits suggests the diagnosis of tularemia, bacterial disease produced by *Francisella tularensis*.

Q23

The most common clinical manifestation of brucellosis is lymphadenopathy.

Q24

The lymph node abnormalities in AIDS patients include mycobacterial and other opportunistic infections, Kaposi's sarcoma, malignant lymphoma and florid reactive hyperplasia.

Q25

The term chronic lymphadenopathy syndrome has been defined as an unexplained enlargement of nodes of at least 3 months' duration at two or more extrainguinal sites in an individual at risk for AIDS.

Q26

The etiologic agent of classic infectious mononucleosis is EBV, and the diagnosis should be confirmed by lymph node biopsy.

Q27

Microscopically, nodes and other lymphoid organs affected by infectious mononucleosis are characterized by effacement of the architecture; infiltration of the trabecula, capsule and perinodal fat; and the marked proliferation of immunoblasts, immature plasma cells and mature plasma cells ('polymorphic B-cell hyperplasia').

Q28

Microscopically, the changes of postvaccinial lymphadenitis are characterized by follicular hyperplasia and small granulomas composed almost entirely of epithelioid cells.

Q29

Mucocutaneous lymph node syndrome, also known as Kawasaki's syndrome, is caused by EBV.

Q30

The microscopic appearance of lupus lymphadenitis may be indistinguishable from that of Kikuchi's disease, but immunophenotyping should resolve the issue in most cases.

Q31

Most patients with rheumatoid arthritis have generalized lymphadenopathy at some time during their illness. The microscopic appearance may be quite similar to that of the hyaline–vascular type of Castleman's disease.

Q32

The hyaline vascular type of Castleman's disease is characterized by a diffuse plasma cell proliferation and marked vascular proliferation in the interfollicular tissue.

Q33

The solitary form of Castleman's disease is characterized by a round, well-circumscribed mass located most commonly in the spleen.

Q34

The hyaline–vascular type of Castleman's disease is usually asymptomatic, whereas the plasma cell type is often associated with fever, anemia, elevated erythrocyte sedimentation rate, hypergammaglobulinemia and hypoalbuminemia.

Q35

POEMS syndrome (Polyneuropathy, Organomegaly, Endocrinopathy, M-protein and Skin changes) is sometimes seen in association with multicentric Castleman's disease.

Q36

Evidence of clonal rearrangement for immunoglobulin and T-cell receptor genes has been found in cases of solitary Castleman's disease.

Q37

Angioimmunoblastic lymphadenopathy is currently regarded as a form of peripheral T-cell lymphoma, which occurs almost exclusively in adults and elderly individuals and is characterized clinically by fever, anemia, polyclonal hypergammaglobulinemia and generalized lymphadenopathy.

Q38

The lymph node changes of angioimmunoblastic lymphadenopathy are characterized by obliteration of the nodal architecture by a polymorphic cellular infiltrate and by an extensive proliferation of finely arborizing vessels of the caliber of postcapillary venules.

Q39

Antiepileptic drugs derived from hydantoin can result in a hypersensitivity reaction manifested by hepatomegaly, splenomegaly, localized lymphadenopathy and leukopenia.

Q40

Dermatopathic lymphadenitis is a form of nodal hyperplasia usually secondary to a generalized dermatitis, particularly those with exfoliative features.

Q41

Follicular hyperplasia is a characteristic feature of dermatopathic lymphadenitis.

Q42

Rosai–Dorfman disease presents in its most typical form as massive, painless bilateral lymph node enlargement in the neck associated with evidence of clonal rearrangement of T-cell receptor genes.

QUESTIONS

Q43

Histiocytes in this picture have within their cytoplasm intact lymphocytes, a feature that has been designated as emperipolesis or lymphocytophagocytosis.

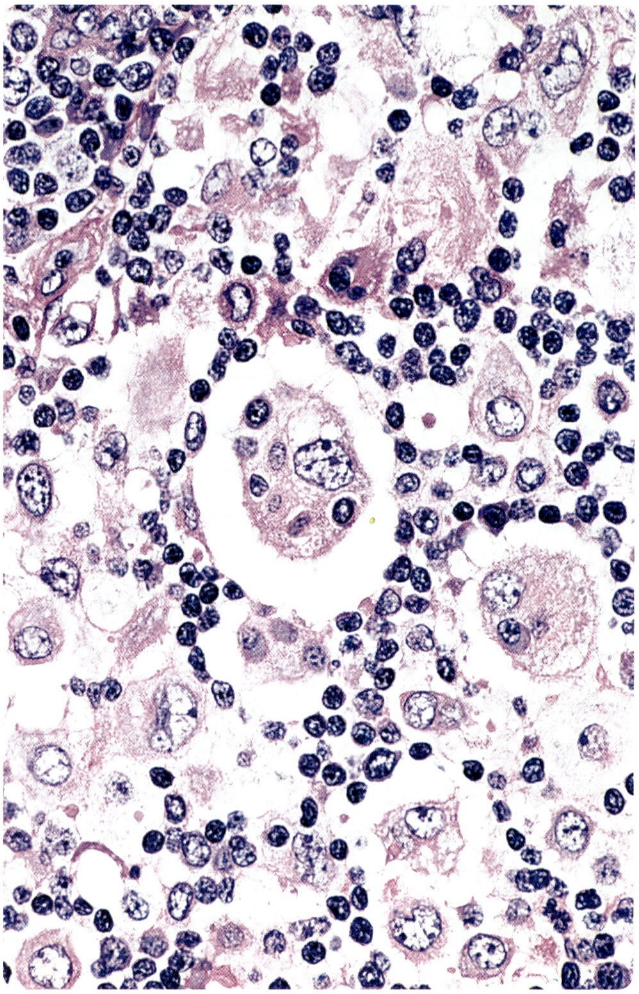

Fig. 21.5

Q44

Ultrastructurally, in Rosai–Dorfman disease the histiocytes located in the sinuses contain a highly characteristic Birbeck's granule.

Q45

Rosai–Dorfmann disease is positive for S-100 protein and CD1a, in contrast to Langerhans' cell histiocytosis, which is negative for CD1a.

Q46

Scattered Langerhans' cells are normally present in the skin, lymph nodes, thymus and other organs; therefore the identification of a few cells in one of these sites is not necessarily indicative that the patient has Langerhans' cell histiocytosis.

Q47

Langerhans' cell histiocytosis can present as solitary or multiple lesions in one organ system (bone being the most common) or as disseminated disease.

Q48

Erdheim–Chester disease is histiocytosis of unknown etiology involving mainly the liver, spleen and lymph nodes.

Q49

Kimura's disease is a malignant disorder that usually presents as a generalized lymphadenopathy.

Q50

Chronic granulomatous disease is the result of a genetically determined enzymatic defect of lymphocytes and plasma cells.

Q51

Microscopically, chronic granulomatous disease is characterized by granulomas with necrotic purulent centers.

Q52

Lipophagic granuloma is defined as a collection of mononuclear and multinuclear giant cells, both types exhibiting a cytoplasmic foamy appearance and lacking a significant participation of other cell types.

Q53

Whipple's disease can result in marked enlargement of mesenteric lymph nodes and the formation of numerous granulomas with necrotic purulent centers.

Malignant lymphoma

Q1

Malignant lymphoma is the generic name given to tumors of lymphocytes and histiocytes.

Q2

Hodgkin's lymphoma is characterized by a monomorphic appearance of the tumor tissue, similar to most other malignant lymphomas.

Q3

In almost all cases of Hodgkin's lymphoma EBV genomes have been identified in Reed–Sternberg cells.

Q4

Except for the very early stages, lymph nodes involved by Hodgkin's lymphoma are typically enlarged, hard and nodular, with a homogeneous appearance.

Q5

The classic Reed–Sternberg cell, as seen in all subtypes of classic Hodgkin's lymphoma, is a large cell with abundant weakly acidophilic or amphophilic cytoplasm, which may appear homogeneous or granular and which lacks a pale zone in the Golgi area. The nucleus is bilobed or polylobed, so that the cell appears binucleated or multinucleated.

Q6

The Reed–Sternberg cells in these images are by themselves diagnostic for Hodgkin's lymphoma.

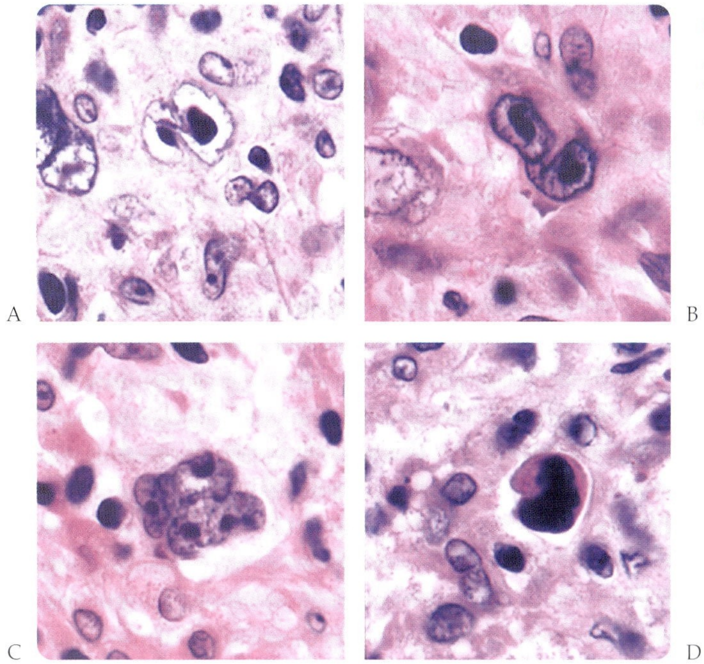

Fig. 21.6

Q7

The requirement for the presence of classic Reed–Sternberg cells, which is absolute for the initial diagnosis of Hodgkin's lymphoma, can be lessened somewhat in subsequent biopsies from patients with documented Hodgkin's lymphoma.

Q8

The immunocytochemical profile of the Reed–Sternberg cell is characterized by positivity for CD30, CD15 and CD45 in all cases.

Q9

The REAL/WHO classification describes four major types of Hodgkin's lymphoma: nodular sclerosis, lymphocyte predominance, lymphocyte depletion, and mixed cellularity.

Q10

In nodular lymphocyte-predominant Hodgkin's lymphomas the predominant cell is a small B lymphocyte. The lymph node architecture is partially or totally effaced, and the infiltrate has a variously pronounced nodular pattern of growth.

Q11

The classic Reed–Sternberg cell is a hallmark of nodular lymphocyte-predominant Hodgkin's lymphomas.

Q12

L&H cells express the pan-B-cell markers but are consistently negative for T-cell markers. They may express CD30 or EMA, and they generally lack CD15 expression.

Q13

Lacunar cells are pathognomonic for nodular sclerosis Hodgkin's lymphoma.

Q14

Cases of nodular sclerosis Hodgkin's lymphoma showing a lack of lacunar cells have been referred to as the syncytial, sarcomatoid or sarcomatous variant.

Q15

In mixed cellularity Hodgkin's lymphoma, a large number of eosinophils, plasma cells and atypical mononuclear cells are admixed with classic Reed–Sternberg cells, which tend to be numerous. Focal necrosis may be present, but fibrosis should be minimal or absent.

Q16

The lymphocyte-rich type of Hodgkin's lymphoma is characterized by the presence of Reed–Sternberg cells scattered against a nodular (most commonly) or diffuse background largely composed of small lymphocytes and practically devoid of eosinophils and neutrophils.

Q17

The lymphocyte depletion group of Hodgkin's lymphoma includes two morphologically different subtypes, designated 'diffuse fibrosis' and 'reticular'.

Q18

The microscopic typing of Hodgkin's lymphoma should always be made on examination of a biopsy obtained before the start of treatment.

Q19

Hodgkin's lymphoma may present in a variety of ways, the most common being fever, night sweats and loss of weight.

Q20

The typical patient with nodular lymphocyte-predominant Hodgkin's lymphoma is a child with involvement of the inguinal lymph node, spleen, liver and bone marrow.

Q21

Lymphocyte depletion of Hodgkin's lymphoma is characteristically present in the neck and/or mediastinum of young females.

Q22

The diagnosis of Hodgkin's lymphoma should be questioned for any lymphoma involving Waldeyer's ring, the skin and the gastrointestinal tract, especially if this happens to be the first manifestation of the disease.

Q23

Most cases of Hodgkin's lymphoma begin in the mediastinum and spread from there to lymph nodes and to extranodal sites.

Q24

Splenic involvement is thought to represent a critical stage in the spread of Hodgkin's lymphoma and is an early manifestation of blood vessel dissemination.

Q25

Patients treated for Hodgkin's lymphoma, in contrast to those treated for non-Hodgkin's lymphoma, are not at increased risk for the development of a second tumor later in life.

Q26

Clinical stage remains the most important prognostic parameter in Hodgkin's lymphoma, although the differences between the various stages have greatly diminished. Only stage IV disease and constitutional symptoms continue to present a serious therapeutic problem.

Q27

In the United States there is a bimodal distribution of small lymphocytic lymphoma, with a peak at 15–40 years and a second, smaller peak in the seventh decade.

Q28

The architecture of the node in small lymphocytic lymphoma is massively and monotonously effaced by a population of small round lymphocytes with clumped chromatin, inconspicuous nucleoli, barely visible cytoplasm and scanty mitotic activity.

Q29

Immunohistochemically, small lymphocytic lymphomas are usually reactive for T cell-related antigens CD3, CD5 and CD43.

Q30

In addition to the well-differentiated lymphocytes, cases of small lymphocytic lymphoma show an admixture of larger cells (prolymphocytes and paraimmunoblasts) with vesicular nuclei and prominent nucleoli, singly or in small aggregates that simulate germinal centers.

Q31

Transformation of a small lymphocytic lymphoma (or a chronic lymphocytic leukemia) into a blastic, histiocytic or large cell neoplasm on a background of chronic lymphocytic leukemia has been traditionally known as Richter's syndrome and is accompanied by a precipitous decline in the clinical course.

Q32

The serum findings of macroglobulinemia can be associated with a microscopic picture of plasma cell myeloma.

Q33

The Dutcher bodies in this figure are cytoplasmic immunoglobulin inclusions.

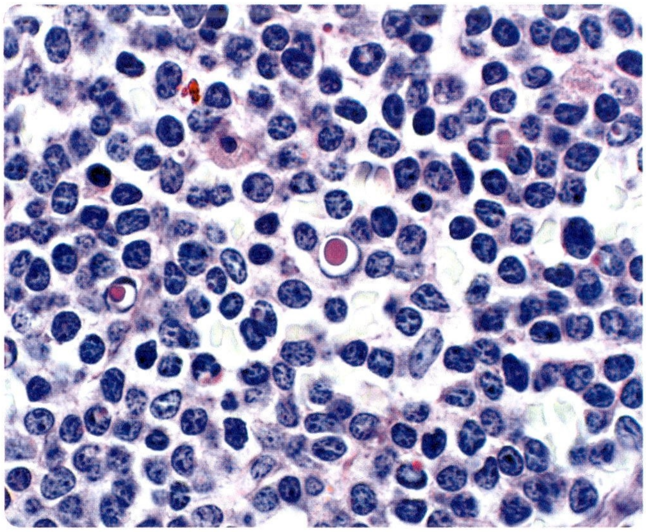

Fig. 21.7

Q34

Tumors producing IgM globulin or 'heavy chains' have the anatomic distribution and cytologic appearance of plasma cell myeloma.

Q35

Follicular (nodular) lymphoma is a B-cell neoplasm that comprises up to 40% of all adult non-Hodgkin's lymphomas in the United States, but in other countries the relative incidence is much lower.

Q36

Grossly and at low-power examination, the most distinctive feature of follicular lymphoma is the nodular pattern of growth.

Q37

The cytologic composition of the neoplastic nodules of follicular lymphoma is characterized by a mixture in different proportions of small and large lymphoid cells, both of which resemble their normal follicular counterparts.

Q38

Immunohistochemically, the tumor cells of follicular lymphoma express pan-B antigens such as CD20 and CD79a in addition to CD5 and CD43; CD10 is usually negative.

Q39

Depending on the relative proportion of small and large cells, follicular lymphomas are subdivided into three categories.

Q40

In the bone marrow, follicular lymphoma tends to have a central location.

Q41

The low-power appearance of mantle cell lymphoma is largely that of a diffuse lymphoma, although there may be a suggestion of nodularity accentuated by the occasional presence of small germinal center-like structures.

Q42

The tumor cells of mantle cell lymphoma are always positive for CD5.

Q43

Mantle cell lymphoma is a low-grade neoplasm with a current overall 5-year survival rate of over 75%.

Q44

Marginal zone B-cell lymphoma is a family of low-grade B-cell lymphoma that includes monocytoid B-cell lymphoma, low-grade lymphoma of mucosa-associated lymphoid tissue (MALT-lymphoma) and splenic marginal zone lymphoma.

QUESTIONS

Q45

Compared to most other types of lymphoma, diffuse large B-cell lymphoma has a greater tendency for extranodal presentation.

Q46

Diffuse large B-cell lymphoma in this picture is characterized by an admixture of cleaved and non-cleaved large cells.

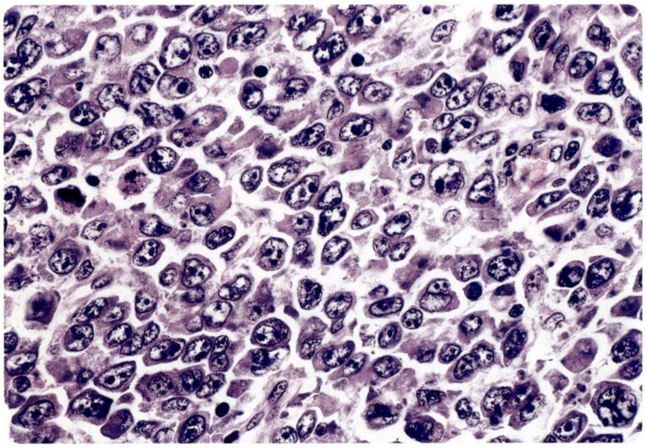

Fig. 21.8

Q47

In the T cell/histiocyte-rich type of diffuse large B-cell lymphoma the neoplastic T-cell population is overshadowed by reactive histiocytes.

Q48

Peripheral (post-thymic) T-cell lymphoma is an extremely heterogeneous group of lesions, many of them occurring primarily at extranodal sites.

Q49

At the molecular level, most peripheral T-cell lymphomas exhibit clonal rearrangements of the immunoglobulin heavy chain gene.

Q50

Clinically, two types of anaplastic large cell lymphoma are recognized: a systemic form (which may affect nodes or extranodal sites, including skin) and a primary cutaneous form (without extracutaneous involvement at the time of presentation).

Q51

Microscopically, anaplastic large cell lymphoma has a polymorphic appearance, with a variable admixture of neutrophils, lymphocytes, histiocytes and large highly atypical cells showing marked pleomorphism. The nuclei of these cells are often horseshoe shaped and multiple, and nucleoli are prominent.

Q52

Immunohistochemically, the tumor cells of anaplastic large cell lymphoma are by definition ALK positive and C20 positive.

Q53

Lymphoblastic lymphoma most often occurs in adults. On CT scanning a large mediastinal mass is seen in almost all cases.

Q54

Permeation of the wall of blood vessels in a targetoid fashion is a characteristic feature of lymphoblastic lymphoma.

Q55

Immunohistochemically, it has been shown that the majority of cases of lymphoblastic lymphoma are of B-cell lineage.

Q56

Burkitt's lymphoma is a high-grade malignant lymphoma composed of germinal center B cells which can present in three clinical settings: endemic, sporadic and immunodeficiency-associated. Burkitt's lymphomas (especially of the endemic form) harbor latent EBV genomes.

Q57

Microscopically, the pattern of growth of Burkitt's lymphoma is nodular, composed of large and cleaved cells, with low mitotic activity.

Q58

Immunohistochemically, it has been shown that virtually all cases of Burkitt's lymphoma are of B-cell lineage.

Q59

The occurrence of two different and well-delineated varieties of lymphoma in a single anatomic site or mass is known as discordant lymphoma.

Q60

Malignant histiocytosis affects any age group but has a predilection for older men. Bone marrow and brain involvement is common, but hepatomegaly is infrequent.

Q61

Malignant histiocytosis is a disease with low malignant potential and a very good prognosis. Overall survival with modern chemotherapy is more than 90%.

Q62

Patients with genetically determined immune deficiencies have an increased incidence of malignant tumors, especially lymphomas. This includes ataxia–telangiectasia, Wiskott–Aldrich syndrome, X-linked lymphoproliferative syndrome, common variable immunodeficiency and severe combined immunodeficiency syndrome.

Q63

The incidence of lymphoma is increased in recipients of all types of organ transplant as a direct or indirect result of the induced immunosuppression.

Q64

Patients with HIV infection are at a high risk for developing malignant tumors, principally Hodgkin's lymphoma.

Q65

Autoimmune diseases are not characterized by an increased incidence of lymphoma.

Lymph node inclusions

Q1

This is a picture of a cervical lymph node. The finding of ductal structures is a sign of metastatic carcinoma.

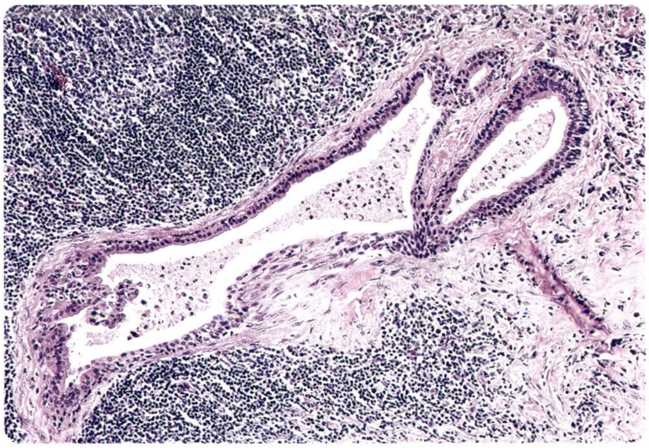

Fig. 21.9

QUESTIONS

Other non-neoplastic lesions

Q1

Adipose metaplasia of lymph nodes is a very rare finding. Differential diagnosis from well-differentiated liposarcoma can be very difficult.

Q2

Vasculitis involving the lymph nodes may be seen in a large number of disorders: polyarteritis nodosa, Henoch–Schönlein purpura, Wegener's granulomatosis, systemic lupus erythematosus, drug hypersensitivity and mucocutaneous lymph node syndrome.

Q3

Two types of malignancy that have been occasionally found to undergo extensive and sometimes massive infarct-type necrosis when involving lymph nodes are malignant lymphoma and metastatic malignant melanoma.

Q4

Hyaline material in the stroma of lymph nodes in this picture is rare in the aortoiliac region, so the possibility of an underlying malignancy should be suspected.

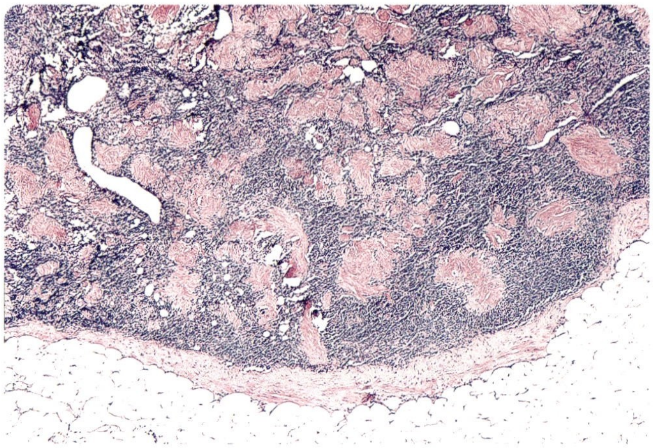

Fig. 21.10

Tumors of the cells of the accessory immune system

Q1

The accessory immune system includes two major categories of cell: antigen-presenting cells (dendritic cells) and antigen-processing cells (macrophages).

Q2

Dendritic follicular cells are associated with the T zones of the nodes. They have complex cell prolongations that interdigitate with each other, but desmosomes are absent. Immunohistochemically, they are reactive for S-100 protein.

Q3

Langerhans' cells, also known as littoral cells (particularly in the spleen), are characterized by macrophagic properties. They also have endothelial features, and therefore exhibit reactivity for CD31.

Q4

Dendritic follicular cell tumor often presents as a solitary mass in a cervical lymph node, but can involve other lymph node groups and a large variety of extranodal sites. The behavior is that of a malignant tumor, with local recurrence and distant metastases to sites such as the liver and lung.

Q5

The microscopic appearance of interdigitating dendritic cell tumor can be indistinguishable from that of dendritic follicular cell tumor. The diagnosis is dependent on the immunohistochemical profile.

Vascular tumors and tumor-like conditions

Q1

Kaposi's sarcoma of the lymph nodes may be associated with typical skin lesions or develop in their absence.

Other primary tumors and tumor-like conditions

Q1

Mastocytosis never involves the lymph nodes except in patients with HIV infection.

Q2

Traditionally, acute myeloid leukemia has been referred to as granulocytic sarcoma or chloroma when it appears as a tumor mass in a lymph node or some other location outside the bone marrow.

Q3

Hemorrhagic spindle cell tumor with amianthoid fibers is a distinctive benign neoplasm that occurs preferentially in inguinal lymph nodes.

Q4

Inflammatory pseudotumor of lymph nodes is always a generalized disease characterized by a bulky mediastinal mass without clinical symptoms.

Q5

Inflammatory pseudotumor of lymph nodes (and spleen) seems to be a different entity from its homonym in the soft tissue, lung and other sites.

Q6

Lymph node metastases are common with carcinomas, malignant melanomas and germ cell tumors and rare with sarcomas and central nervous system tumors. It is very rare for soft tissue sarcomas to present initially as a lymph node metastasis. The outstanding exception is alveolar rhabdomyosarcoma.

Q7

Features favoring lymphoma in contrast to metastatic carcinoma are focal nodal involvement, definite nesting, extensive necrosis, a predominantly sinusal distribution, and solid tumor plugs in lymphatic vessels.

Q8

The metastatic carcinomas that most closely simulate a malignant lymphoid process are nasopharyngeal lymphoepithelioma and lobular carcinoma of the breast.

Q9

Of the conventional special stains, only the reticulin stain may help in the differential diagnosis between metastatic carcinoma and lymphoma.

Q10

The large majority of tumors metastatic to upper cervical lymph nodes originate from the thyroid.

Q11

Midcervical nodes containing papillary carcinoma are always examples of metastatic thyroid carcinoma.

Q12

Most carcinomas metastatic to supraclavicular lymph nodes originate in the lung or breast. Other sources of metastases to this nodal group, particularly if located on the left side, are carcinoma of the stomach, pancreas, prostate and testis.

Q13

The large majority of metastatic tumors in axillary nodes of adult females are breast carcinoma and malignant melanoma.

Q14

Inguinal nodes are often the recipients of carcinomas from the internal abdominal organs and testis.

Normal anatomy

A1. True

Both cortex and medulla represent B zones and are therefore associated with a humoral type of immune response. The paracortex is the zone situated between the cortex and the medulla, which contains the mobile pool of T lymphocytes responsible for cell-mediated immune responses. **(p. 1878)**

A2. False

Primary follicles lack germinal centers. In contrast, secondary follicles appear following antigenic stimulation and are characterized by the presence of germinal centers. **(p. 1878)**

A3. True

The cells present in germinal centers are B lymphocytes known as follicular center cells (centroblasts and centrocytes, or small and large cleaved and non-cleaved cells), macrophages and follicular dendritic cells. **(p. 1878)**

A4. False

Expansion of the paracortex is indicative of cell-mediated immunity, whereas proliferative germinal centers are indicative of humoral immunity. **(p. 1878)**

Lymph node evaluation

A1. False

Not all lymph nodes are ideally suited for histologic evaluation of systemic lymphadenopathy. For example, inguinal nodes should be avoided because of the high frequency of chronic inflammatory and fibrotic changes present in them. Whenever possible, the largest lymph node in the region should be biopsied. Small superficial nodes may show only nonspecific hyperplasia, whereas a deeper node of the same group may show diagnostic features. **(p. 1879)**

A2. False

The surgeon should require a frozen section biopsy to be certain that the tissue is representative and not to obtain a specific diagnosis at this point. **(p. 1879)**

A3. True

The portion to be embedded in paraffin can be placed in 10% buffered formalin or, preferably, in B5 or analogous mercury-containing fixative. The alcohols and xylenes should be changed frequently. **(p. 1879)**

A4. False

Core needle biopsy is adequate for the diagnosis of metastatic carcinoma but is rarely used for the evaluation of primary lymphoid disorders. **(p. 1879)**

A5. False

The cytologic diagnosis of malignant lymphoma can be made in only 50–75% of cases, the accuracy being greatest in the high-grade lesions. Fine needle aspiration has proved to be most useful for the selection of a representative node for biopsy, for the diagnosis of recurrent lymphoma, for staging the extent of the disease, and for monitoring treatment. **(p. 1879)**

A6. True

The role of ultrastructural examination in the evaluation of primary lymphoid disorders is very limited since the advent of immunocytochemical and genetic molecular techniques. **(p. 1879)**

A7. True

Genetic rearrangement can be detected by Southern blot or polymerase chain reaction (PCR). **(p. 1886)**

A8. False

Clonal antigen receptor gene rearrangement is not absolutely specific for neoplasia, but it can be confidently used for the staging or detection of relapse in lymphoid cases with an established diagnosis. **(p. 1887)**

Primary immunodeficiencies

A1. False

Primary immunodeficiencies can be divided into three categories: humoral, cell-mediated, and due to defects in phagocytes and other cells of the accessory immune system. **(p. 1887)**

A2. False

In primary immunodeficiencies of the humoral type, cortical reactive centers and medullary plasma cells are scanty or absent. In diseases of cell-mediated immunity, the thickness of the paracortical area is greatly diminished. **(p. 1888)**

Patterns of hyperplasia

A1. False
From a topographic and functional standpoint the major patterns of reactive lymphoid proliferation are follicular/nodular, interfollicular/paracortical, diffuse, sinusal and mixed. **(p. 1888)**

A2. True
Reactive follicles vary considerably in size and shape; their margins are sharply defined and surrounded by a mantle of small lymphocytes; the follicles are composed of an admixture of small and large lymphoid cells with irregular nuclei; mitoses are numerous; and phagocytosis of nuclear debris by histiocytes is prominent. **(p. 1888)**

A3. True
These germinal centers are large and contain numerous small lymphocytes, the borders are indistinct, and the interphase between the center of large lymphoid cells and the cuff of small lymphocytes is blurred. However, residual 'starry sky' macrophages are present. **(p. 1888)**

A4. False
The main differential diagnosis is with nodular lymphocyte-predominant Hodgkin's lymphoma. **(p. 1888)**

A5. True
Regressively transformed germinal centers are small, practically devoid of lymphoid cells, and composed of follicular dendritic cells, vascular endothelial cells, and hyalinized PAS-positive intercellular material. **(p. 1889)**

A6. False
Expansion of the paracortical (interfollicular) region can be nodular or diffuse. The nodular form is characteristic of dermatopathic lymphadenitis and of nodal reactions to malignancy. The diffuse form is a feature of viral lymphadenitis and drug reactions, and of immunoblastic proliferations in general. **(p. 1890)**

A7. True
The sinuses appear dilated and prominent in various disorders. The most common is sinus hyperplasia (sinus histiocytosis, sinus catarrh), seen in nodes draining infectious or neoplastic processes and characterized by an increased number of macrophages in the lumen. **(p. 1890)**

A8. False
In most cases a combination of clinical, morphologic and bacteriologic data is necessary to determine the etiology of the granulomas. **(p. 1890)**

A9. True
Monocytoid B-cell hyperplasia has also been seen in many other reactive disorders, such as cat-scratch disease, infectious mononucleosis, AIDS and autoimmune disorders. **(p. 1892)**

A10. False
Plasmacytoid monocytes belong to the macrophage/monocyte series. **(p. 1893)**

A11. True
The Warthin–Finkeldey giant cell of measles is the paradigm for polykaryocytes. These cells may be found in lymph nodes in association with many reactive and neoplastic disorders. **(p. 1893)**

Inflammatory/hyperplastic diseases

A1. False
The typical case of acute nonspecific lymphadenitis is rarely biopsied. Microscopically, the general features are sinus dilatation, accumulation of neutrophils, vascular dilatation, and edema of the capsule. **(p. 1893)**

A2. False
Suppurative lymphadenitis is a feature of staphylococcal infections, lymphogranuloma venereum, cat-scratch disease and many other infections. **(p. 1893)**

A3. True
Kikuchi's lymphadenitis is generally benign and self-limited. Microscopically, the affected nodes show focal, well-circumscribed paracortical necrotizing lesions. There are abundant karyorrhectic debris, scattered fibrin deposits, and collections of large mononuclear cells. Plasma cells and neutrophils are very scanty, in contrast to plasmacytoid monocytes, which are often numerous. **(p. 1894)**

A4. **False**
Chronic lymphadenitis is characterized by follicular hyperplasia; prominence of postcapillary venules; increased numbers of immunoblasts, plasma cells and histiocytes; and fibrosis. **(p. 1894)**

A5. **False**
The most common location is the cervical region ('scrofula'), where a draining sinus that communicates with the skin ('scrofuloderma') may form. **(p. 1895)**

A6. **False**
It is most frequently caused by atypical mycobacteria. Microscopically, the host reaction may be indistinguishable from that of tuberculosis, but often the granulomatous response is overshadowed by suppurative changes. **(p. 1895)**

A7. **False**
The most common affected organs in sarcoidosis are the lung, lymph nodes, eyes, skin and liver, and the disease is more common in blacks. **(p. 1895)**

A8. **True**
Erythema nodosum often precedes or accompanies other manifestations of sarcoidosis. Functional hypoparathyroidism is the rule, although a few cases of sarcoidosis coexisting with primary hyperparathyroidism have been reported. **(p. 1895)**

A9. **True**
Langhans' giant cells are smaller and have fewer nuclei than those typically seen in tuberculosis. Necrosis is either absent or limited to a small central fibrinoid focus. **(p. 1895)**

A10. **False**
Asteroid bodies, like Schaumann bodies and calcium oxalate crystals, are sometimes found in the cytoplasm of giant cells. None of these inclusions is specific for sarcoidosis. From a pathologic standpoint the diagnosis of sarcoidosis is always one of exclusion. **(p. 1896)**

A11. **False**
The Kveim test for sarcoidosis is an intradermal reaction that occurs following inoculation with an extract of human spleen involved with the disease. It is positive in 60–85% of patients with sarcoidosis, and the number of false positive results is small. **(p. 1897)**

A12. **True**
Other fungal diseases known to result in lymphadenitis are blastomycosis, paracoccidioidomycosis, coccidioidomycosis and sporotrichosis. **(p. 1897)**

A13. **True**
Toxoplasmosis, one of the most common parasitic infections of humans and other warm-blooded animals, is caused by the protozoan parasite *Toxoplasma gondii*. **(p. 1897)**

A14. **True**
If the diagnosis of toxoplasmic lymphadenitis is suspected from the microscopic pattern, it should be confirmed serologically. **(p. 1897)**

A15. **False**
There are no sinuses on this picture of toxoplasmosis. These are small non-caseating granulomas composed of epithelioid cells, which is almost pathognomonic for toxoplasmosis. **(p. 1898)**

A16. **False**
Generalized lymphadenopathy is a common finding in secondary syphilis, whereas localized node enlargement can be seen in the primary and tertiary stages of the disease. **(p. 1898)**

A17. **False**
Mesenteric lymphadenitis is a benign, self-limited disease characterized by capsular thickening and edema, an increase of immunoblasts and plasma cells in the cortical and paracortical regions, dilatation of sinuses with accumulations of large lymphocytes within, and germinal center hyperplasia. **(p. 1899)**

A18. **False**
This is unusual in infections caused by *Yersinia enterocolitica*, but in the lymphadenitis produced by *Yersinia pseudotuberculosis*, small granulomas and abscesses are commonly present. **(p. 1900)**

A19. **True**
The primary lesion of cat-scratch disease is a red papule in the skin at the site of inoculation, usually appearing between 7 and 12 days after contact. **(p. 1900)**

A20. **True**
These abscesses are very suggestive of the diagnosis because of their pattern of central, sometimes stellate, necrosis with neutrophils, surrounded by palisading histiocytes. **(p. 1900)**

A21. **False**
The agent of cat-scratch disease is a coccobacillary pleomorphic extracellular bacterium, *Bartonella henselae*. **(p. 1900)**

A22. **True**
The diagnosis of tularemia is supported by a rise in hemagglutinin titers. **(p. 1901)**

A23. **False**
The most common clinical manifestations of brucellosis are fever, hepatomegaly and splenomegaly. Lymphadenopathy is uncommon and, when present, usually of modest dimensions. **(p. 1901)**

A24. True

Florid reactive hyperplasia is the most common lymph node abnormality in AIDS patients. In many cases the reactive germinal centers show a feature termed follicle lysis, characterized by invagination of mantle lymphocytes into the germinal centers. Some lymph nodes in AIDS patients may show advanced lymphocyte depletion, with or without abnormal (regressively transformed) germinal centers. **(p. 1901)**

A25. True

Overall, up to a quarter of patients have developed AIDS on follow-up. **(p. 1902)**

A26. False

In most instances the presumptive clinical diagnosis of infectious mononucleosis is confirmed by examination of the peripheral blood and serologic evaluation without need of a lymph node biopsy. **(p. 1902)**

A27. True

Features of importance in the differential diagnosis from lymphoma include the predominantly sinusal distribution of the large lymphoid cells, follicular hyperplasia with marked mitotic activity and phagocytosis, an increase in the number of plasma cells, and vascular proliferation. **(p. 1902)**

A28. False

The changes are those of a diffuse or nodular paracortical expansion, with mixed cellular proliferation consisting of eosinophils, plasma cells and a large number of immunoblasts. The presence of numerous immunoblasts scattered among the lymphocytes is the most important histologic feature of postvaccinial hyperplasia. **(p. 1903)**

A29. False

It is a febrile disorder of unknown etiology that usually affects children, characterized by fever, cervical lymphadenopathy, pharyngeal and conjunctival inflammation, and erythematous skin rashes. **(p. 1904)**

A30. False

The lymph node changes in lupus erythematosus are generally of a nonspecific nature and consist of moderate follicular hyperplasia associated with increased vascularization and scattered immunoblasts and plasma cells. The immunophenotype of lupus lymphadenitis is nonspecific. **(p. 1904)**

A31. False

The microscopic appearance of rheumatoid arthritis may be similar to that of the plasma cell type of Castleman's disease. **(p. 1905)**

A32. False

Microscopically, two major categories of Castleman's disease have been described: hyaline–vascular and plasma cell. The hyaline–vascular type is characterized by large follicles with marked vascular proliferation and hyalinization of their abnormal germinal centers. Tight concentric layering of lymphocytes at the periphery of the follicles results in an onion-skin appearance. The plasma cell type of Castleman's disease is characterized by a diffuse plasma cell proliferation in the interfollicular tissue, sometimes accompanied by numerous Russell bodies. **(p. 1905)**

A33. False

From the point of view of clinical presentation, Castleman's disease has been divided into the solitary form, characterized by a round, well-circumscribed mass located most commonly in the mediastinum, and the multicentric or systemic form, which presents with generalized lymphadenopathy and may also involve the spleen. The treatment of solitary Castleman's disease is surgical excision, which has been found to result in rapid regression of the associated abnormalities whenever present. **(p. 1905)**

A34. True

The long-term prognosis of systemic Castleman's disease is poor; the disease tends to persist for months or years, and to result sometimes in renal or pulmonary complications. **(p. 1905)**

A35. True

The multicentric or systemic form of Castleman's disease is nearly always of the plasma cell type. **(p. 1905)**

A36. False

It has been found in cases of systemic Castleman's disease together with copies of the EBV genome, no such features having been detected in the solitary form of the disease. **(p. 1905)**

A37. True

Some cases of angioimmunoblastic lymphadenopathy show clonal populations of B cells in addition to a clonal population of T cells. **(p. 1908)**

A38. True

Angioimmunoblastic lymphadenopathy is a systemic disease with lesions in the lymph nodes, spleen, liver, bone marrow and skin. **(p. 1909)**

A39. False

Hypersensitivity reactions to drugs derived from hydantoin are manifested by skin rash, fever, generalized lymphadenopathy (mainly cervical) and peripheral eosinophilia. The changes disappear if the drug is discontinued. **(p. 1910)**

A40. True
It may occur in any skin disorder in which itching and scratching are prominent; this includes inflammatory dermatoses such as psoriasis and neoplastic diseases such as mycosis fungoides. **(p. 1911)**

A41. False
Dermatopathic lymphadenitis is characterized by marked pale widening of the paracortical zone occupied by histiocytes, Langerhans' cells and interdigitating dendritic cells. **(p. 1911)**

A42. False
Molecular studies of involved tissue have failed to show evidence of clonality, in keeping with their presumed reactive nature. Most cases occur during the first or second decade of life associated with fever, leukocytosis, elevated erythrocyte sedimentation rate, and polyclonal hypergammagloblinemia. **(p. 1911)**

A43. True
Although not specific, this is a constant feature of Rosai–Dorfman disease and is therefore of great diagnostic significance. **(p. 1912)**

A44. False
Ultrastructurally, the histiocytes located in the sinuses have extensive pseudopodia and lack Birbeck's granules. **(p. 1912)**

A45. False
Rosai–Dorfmann disease is positive for S-100 but negative for CD1a, in contrast to Langerhans' cell histiocytosis, which is positive for both S-100 protein and CD1a. **(p. 1913)**

A46. True
The infiltrate should have a sizeable number of these cells before such a diagnosis is entertained. **(p. 1914)**

A47. True
The term Letterer–Siwe disease was used in the past for the systemic form occurring in infants, and Hand–Schüller–Christian disease for the less widespread and more indolent type seen in older children and adults. **(p. 1914)**

A48. False
The most common sites of Erdheim–Chester disease are the central nervous system, bones and lung. **(p. 1915)**

A49. False
Kimura's disease is an inflammatory disorder of unknown etiology that usually presents as a mass lesion in the subcutaneous tissue of the head and neck region or the major salivary glands, often associated with regional lymphadenopathy. **(p. 1915)**

A50. False
It is an enzymatic defect of granulocytes and monocytes. **(p. 1916)**

A51. True
Chronic granulomatous disease closely simulates the appearance of cat-scratch disease. **(p. 1916)**

A52. True
By far the most common situation in which this occurs is represented by the incidental microscopic finding of periportal and mesenteric nodes in asymptomatic individuals, probably the result of mineral oil ingestion. **(p. 1916)**

A53. False
Whipple's disease is characterized by the presence of lipophagic granulomas; granulomas with necrotic purulent centers have been reported in cat-scratch disease, atypical mycobacteriosis, tularemia and chronic granulomatous disease. **(p. 1917)**

Malignant lymphoma

A1. False
Malignant lymphoma is the generic name given to tumors of the lymphoid system, and specifically of lymphocytes and their precursor cells, whether of T, B or null phenotypes. Although traditionally tumors presumed to be composed of histiocytes and other cells of the accessory immune system have also been included in the category of malignant lymphoma, it would seem more appropriate to regard them separately for both conceptual and practical reasons. **(p. 1917)**

A2. False
Hodgkin's lymphoma is a type of malignant lymphoma in which Reed–Sternberg cells are present in a 'characteristic background' of reactive inflammatory cells of various types, accompanied by a variable degree of fibrosis. **(p. 1917)**

A3. False
EBV genomes have been identified in up to half of cases, particularly in the mixed cellularity subtype, in young patients, and/or in developing countries. **(p. 1918)**

A4. False
The gross appearance of lymph nodes involved by Hodgkin's lymphoma is somewhat dependent on the microscopic subtypes. The consistency varies from soft to hard depending on the amount of fibrosis. Some degree of nodularity is often appreciated, particularly in the nodular sclerosis form. Except for lymphocyte-predominant Hodgkin's lymphoma, the cut surface of the node has a more heterogeneous appearance than in most non-Hodgkin's lymphomas. **(p. 1918)**

A5. True

In the most typical example of the Reed–Sternberg cell the two nuclear lobes face each other (mirror image), resulting in the oft-cited 'owl's eye' appearance. Cells with this set of features but lacking nuclear lobation have been referred to as mononuclear variants of Reed–Sternberg cells or Hodgkin's cells. **(p. 1918)**

A6. False

The Reed–Sternberg cell of Hodgkin's lymphoma needs to be distinguished from other multinucleated cells, e.g. megakaryocytes, pleomorphic immunoblasts in infectious mononucleosis and other viral diseases, neoplastic cells from a variety of epithelial and mesenchymal tumors, and some malignant lymphomas of non-Hodgkin's type. In all of these disorders it is of the utmost importance to examine not only the putative Reed–Sternberg cells but also the background against which they are situated. The more cytologically atypical the lymphoid population, the less likely the diagnosis of Hodgkin's lymphoma. **(p. 1919)**

A7. True

Under these circumstances the presence of a polymorphic infiltrate with atypical mononuclear cells but not classic Reed–Sternberg cells in a biopsy of bone marrow, liver or some other organ can be taken as evidence of involvement by Hodgkin's lymphoma. **(p. 1919)**

A8. False

CD15 is expressed in over 80% of cases; the pattern may be paranuclear, diffuse cytoplasmic, and/or corresponding to the cell membrane. CD30 is found in approximately 90% of cases, but CD45 (LCA) is expressed in less than 10%. **(p. 1920)**

A9. False

In the REAL/WHO scheme currently in use only two major categories are recognized: the nodular subtype of lymphocyte predominance and the classic Hodgkin's lymphoma. **(p. 1921)**

A10. True

The nodularity may be so pronounced as to simulate on low power the appearance of follicular lymphoma; however, the nodules of nodular lymphocyte-predominant Hodgkin's lymphomas are more irregular in size and staining quality, and the admixture of lymphocytes and epithelioid cells gives them a mottled appearance. **(p. 1922)**

A11. False

Classic Reed–Sternberg cells are absent in nodular lymphocyte-predominant Hodgkin's lymphomas. Instead there is a variable but usually large number of a type of Reed–Sternberg cell (the L&H cell or 'popcorn' cell) characterized by a folded, multilobed nucleus with smaller nucleoli. **(p. 1922)**

A12. True

Nodular lymphocyte-predominant Hodgkin's lymphoma is a κ light chain-restricted monotypic B-cell neoplasm that arises from germinal center cells at the centroblastic stage of differentiation. **(p. 1923)**

A13. False

Nodular sclerosis Hodgkin's lymphoma is characterized in its fully developed stage by broad collagen bands separating the lymphoid tissue in well-defined nodules, the presence of classic Reed–Sternberg cells, and a variant known as lacunar or cytoplasmic. Lacunar cells can also be seen in mixed-cellularity Hodgkin's lymphoma and even in reactive disorders. **(p. 1924)**

A14. False

In the syncytial variant lacunar cells form sheets and cohesive nests, particularly around areas of necrosis, to the point that a mistaken diagnosis of large cell non-Hodgkin's lymphoma, carcinoma, germ cell tumor or thymoma can be made. **(p. 1925)**

A15. True

A case exhibiting lymphocyte predominance or mixed cellularity will be diagnosed as nodular sclerosis if bands of fibrous tissue are present. A case with a marked predominance of lymphocytes will be categorized as mixed cellularity if there are numerous Reed–Sternberg cells. **(p. 1925)**

A16. True

The main differential diagnosis is with nodular lymphocyte-predominant Hodgkin's lymphoma and is based primarily on the presence of cells with the typical morphologic and immunohistochemical features of Reed–Sternberg cells. **(p. 1925)**

A17. True

In the diffuse fibrosis subtype the number of lymphocytes and other cells progressively decreases as the result of heavy deposition of collagen fibers. The reticular subtype is characterized by a very large number of diagnostic Reed–Sternberg cells among atypical mononuclear cells and other elements. **(p. 1925)**

A18. True

Radiation therapy and chemotherapy result in focal necrosis, fibrosis and profound nuclear aberrations, features that may render a proper pathologic evaluation impossible. **(p. 1926)**

A19. False

The most common presentation of Hodgkin's lymphoma is painless enlargement of superficial (usually cervical) lymph nodes. Fever, night sweats and loss of weight (so-called 'B symptoms') occur in approximately 25% of cases; their presence influences the clinical staging. Pruritus is also frequent. **(p. 1928)**

A20. False
The typical patient is a man in his 40s with involvement of the high cervical nodes. This microscopic form practically never involves the spleen, liver or bone marrow except when it changes to a more aggressive histologic pattern. **(p. 1928)**

A21. False
The lymphocyte depletion group, which comprises less than 5% of all cases of Hodgkin's lymphoma, may present in adults or elderly patients as a febrile illness with pancytopenia or lymphocytopenia, hepatomegaly, abnormal liver function tests and no peripheral lymphadenopathy, or it may manifest the usual clinical presentation of Hodgkin's lymphoma. Mediastinal involvement is the rule in nodular sclerosis, inconstant in mixed cellularity and lymphocyte depletion, and exceptional in nodular lymphocyte predominance. **(p. 1928)**

A22. True
Most of these cases are examples of non-Hodgkin's lymphoma with Reed–Sternberg-like cells. A diagnosis of Hodgkin's lymphoma also should be viewed with suspicion if it presents as a complication of a natural immune deficiency, immunosuppression or other immune diseases. **(p. 1928)**

A23. False
Most cases of Hodgkin's lymphoma begin in lymph nodes and spread by involvement of the adjacent lymph node groups. **(p. 1928)**

A24. True
The approximate number of tumor nodules present in the spleen should be indicated because of their relation to the prognosis; specifically, it should be stated whether there are five or more. It is not important to subclassify the disease in the spleen into the specific type. **(p. 1928)**

A25. False
Patients treated for Hodgkin's lymphoma (particularly those in the pediatric age group) are at increased risk for the development of a second tumor, including breast carcinoma, soft tissue sarcoma and malignant mesothelioma. **(p. 1929)**

A26. True
A large mediastinal mass (more than one-third of the maximum intrathoracic diameter), multiple nodules in the spleen, or multiple extranodal sites of involvement are unfavorable prognostic factors. The latter relates directly to the staging and is of great prognostic importance. **(p. 1929)**

A27. False
Small lymphocytic lymphoma occurs preferentially in the middle-aged and elderly. The symptoms are scanty, the evolution is prolonged and the survival is very good. **(p. 1932)**

A28. True
The distribution of the disease is usually diffuse, but on occasions it is confined to the marginal zone, perifollicular or interfollicular regions surrounding benign lymphoid follicles, the latter pattern being referred to as interfollicular small lymphocytic lymphoma. **(p. 1932)**

A29. False
Small lymphocytic lymphomas are nearly always of B-cell type, so they are usually positive for CD20 and negative for CD3. They are usually positive for CD5, CD23 (in contrast to mantle cell lymphoma) and CD43. **(p. 1933)**

A30. True
These formations (known as proliferative centers, growth centers or pseudofollicles) have no prognostic significance. **(p. 1934)**

A31. True
Fever, increasing lymphadenopathy, weight loss and abdominal pain are frequent, sometimes accompanied by hepatomegaly and splenomegaly. **(p. 1934)**

A32. True
Macroglobulinemia can also be associated with small lymphocytic lymphoma, small lymphocytic lymphoma with plasmacytic differentiation and large cell lymphoma. **(p. 1935)**

A33. False
Dutcher bodies are intranuclear immunoglobulin inclusions. **(p. 1936)**

A34. False
Such tumors have the anatomic distribution and cytologic appearance of malignant lymphoma, whereas most of those secreting IgG globulin or a light chain are clinically and microscopically classifiable as plasma cell myeloma. **(p. 1936)**

A35. True
Most cases occur in elderly individuals. It is very unusual under 20 years of age and relatively uncommon in blacks. **(p. 1937)**

A36. True
With progression of the disease this distinct nodularity becomes blurred, and eventually most of the proliferation acquires a diffuse pattern. **(p. 1937)**

A37. True
The small cells have been variously referred to as germinocytes, centrocytes, poorly differentiated lymphocytes and small cleaved follicular center cells. The large cells are two or three times the size of normal lymphocytes; over the years they have been designated germinoblasts, centroblasts, histiocytes, large (cleaved or non-cleaved) follicular center cells, large lymphoid cells and lymphoblasts. **(p. 1937)**

A38. False

The tumor cells of follicular lymphoma express pan-B antigens and CD10 in most cases, but CD5 and CD43 are usually negative. **(p. 1939)**

A39. True

Patients in the first category are often asymptomatic, usually have generalized disease and have a good prognosis, to the point that some authors advise against aggressive treatment for them. Tumors in the third category are more commonly localized at the time of presentation but run a more aggressive clinical course and are more likely to lose their nodular pattern of growth and become diffuse. The prognosis of tumors in the second category is intermediate between these two, but closer to the first. **(p. 1940)**

A40. False

The bone marrow infiltrates tend to have a paratrabecular location. In the spleen, it tends to affect the B-derived lymphoid follicles located eccentrically in the white pulp. In the liver, the infiltrate is predominantly periportal. In the skin, there is an extensive dermal infiltrate without particular relation to vessels or adnexae. **(p. 1942)**

A41. True

Most of the small lymphocytes are similar to those of small lymphocytic lymphoma, but others show slightly irregular and indented nuclear contours approaching those seen in small cleaved cell follicular lymphoma. Two commonly seen morphologic features of mantle cell lymphoma are hyalinized blood vessels and a scattering of epithelioid histiocytes, the former representing an important diagnostic clue and the latter sometimes resulting in a starry-sky appearance. **(p. 1943)**

A42. False

The tumor cells of mantle cell lymphoma are always positive for immunoglobulins and B cell-associated antigen, but CD5 expression is not always present. **(p. 1944)**

A43. False

The median survival of mantle cell lymphoma is approximately 3–5 years. As a group, it is characterized by more widespread disease and a slower response to chemotherapy than follicular lymphoma. The blastic variant has a more aggressive clinical course. **(p. 1945)**

A44. True

Monocytoid B-cell lymphoma is a tumor of small to medium-sized lymphocytes with round or slightly indented nuclei and relatively abundant clear cytoplasm, usually located in lymph nodes. Low-grade lymphoma of mucosa-associated lymphoid tissue is a neoplasm in which the cell population – all of small size – has been described as including small round lymphocytes, monocytoid B cells, cells with slightly irregular nuclei (centrocyte-like), plasmacytoid cells and plasma cells. Splenic marginal zone lymphoma is characterized by involvement of the marginal zone of the spleen. **(p. 1945)**

A45. True

Approximately 40% of cases present in extranodal sites, such as the digestive system, skin and skeletal system. **(p. 1946)**

A46. False

This is the immunoblastic type of diffuse large B-cell lymphoma. In this form, the predominant tumor cell has the appearance of an immunoblast: a large vesicular nucleus with a prominent central nucleolus and thick nuclear membrane and deeply staining amphophilic and pyroninophilic cytoplasm with a distinct nuclear hof. **(p. 1948)**

A47. False

The tumor cells are B cells (not T cells) and may represent less than 10% of the entire cell population. The majority are reactive T cells and histiocytes. **(p. 1948)**

A48. True

They include mycosis fungoides and Sézary syndrome, NK/T-cell lymphoma (nasal type), enteropathy-type T-cell lymphoma, hepatosplenic T-cell lymphoma, subcutaneous panniculitis-like T-cell lymphoma, Lennert's lymphoma and anaplastic large cell lymphoma. **(p. 1950)**

A49. False

Most peripheral T-cell lymphomas exhibit clonal rearrangements of the β T-cell receptor gene, with a minority showing rearrangement of the γ or δ T-cell receptor genes. Approximately 10% of peripheral T-cell lymphomas show clonal rearrangements of the immunoglobulin heavy chain gene in addition to clonal rearrangements of the β T-cell receptor gene. **(p. 1951)**

A50. True

The systemic form can involve sites such as the bone marrow, bone, respiratory tract and gastrointestinal tract. It can occur in children or adults and is rather aggressive. The cutaneous form occurs predominantly in adults and has an indolent course, with some of the individual lesions regressing spontaneously. **(p. 1951)**

A51. True

It is characteristic for these tumor cells to form in a cohesive fashion and to involve preferentially the lymph node sinuses. **(p. 1952)**

A52. False

Not all cases of anaplastic large cell lymphoma express ALK protein. The tumor cells are CD30+ (Ki-1) positive and there is also consistent positivity for EMA, interleukin (IL)-2 receptor, clusterin, cadherins and galectin-3. Pan-lymphoid and some T cell-related markers are found in approximately half of cases; B-cell markers are absent or, rather, not allowed. In other words, if they are found in a lesion with the morphologic features of anaplastic large cell lymphoma, the lesion is taken out of that category and placed into that of an anaplastic variant of large B-cell lymphoma. **(p. 1952)**

A53. False

Lymphoblastic lymphoma is seen primarily in children and adolescents, but it also occurs in adults. In approximately half of the cases there is a mediastinal mass in the thymic region. The clinical course of the untreated disease is extremely aggressive, with rapid multisystem dissemination, a leukemic blood picture, and death after a few months. **(p. 1953)**

A54. True

The neoplastic cells have scanty cytoplasm and a nucleus that has a round contour (instead of the angulated shape typical of follicular lymphoma) but which on close examination shows the presence of delicate convolutions resulting from multiple small invaginations of the nuclear membrane. The chromatin is finely stippled, and nucleoli are inconspicuous. Mitotic activity is extremely high. **(p. 1953)**

A55. False

Approximately 80–85% of lymphoblastic lymphomas show T-cell markers. In approximately 15–20% of cases the tumor cells express B-cell rather than T-cell markers. Yet other lymphoblastic lymphomas lack both T- and B-cell features. **(p. 1954)**

A56. True

In all three forms peripheral lymphadenopathy is rare and, when present, is usually limited to a single group. Bone marrow involvement is common in the late stage of the disease, but leukemic manifestations are very rare. **(p. 1954)**

A57. False

Microscopically, the pattern of growth of Burkitt's lymphoma is usually diffuse, although early cases may show preferential involvement of germinal centers. The tumor cells are small (10–25 μm) and round. Mitoses are numerous, and a prominent 'starry sky' pattern is the rule, although by no means pathognomonic. **(p. 1955)**

A58. True

They express immunoglobulins (predominantly IgM), invariably associated with heavy and light chain restriction. B cell-specific antigens (such as CD19, CD20 and CD22) and B cell-associated antigens (such as CD24 and HLA-DR) are present. Most cases also feature CD10. They are negative for the activation markers CD25 and CD30. In contrast to lymphoblastic lymphoma, they do not express terminal deoxynucleotidyl transferase (TdT). **(p. 1955)**

A59. False

This combination is called composite lymphoma; the occurrence of two different types of lymphoma at separate anatomic sites has been referred to as discordant lymphoma. **(p. 1957)**

A60. False

The disease is most frequent among children and young adults. Fever, lymph node enlargement and constitutional symptoms appear early in the course of the disease. Hepatomegaly, splenomegaly and skin involvement are also common. In some patients, pulmonary symptoms dominate the clinical presentation. Common laboratory findings are anemia, leukopenia and thrombocytopenia. There is also elevation of serum ferritin levels. **(p. 1958)**

A61. False

Most cases were rapidly progressive and fatal, two-thirds of the patients dying within the first months after diagnosis. At autopsy, widespread organ involvement was found, usually without the formation of large masses but rather tumor growing diffusely in the interstitium. **(p. 1958)**

A62. True

Lymphomas arising in Wiskott–Aldrich syndrome were of the non-Hodgkin's type (predominantly large B-cell lymphomas with immunoblastic features) presenting as localized extranodal masses, whereas those arising in patients with ataxia–telangiectasia were of both Hodgkin's and non-Hodgkin's types, with a more conventional organ distribution. **(p. 1959)**

A63. True

Skin tumors, malignant lymphomas, Kaposi's sarcoma and cervical carcinoma are the most common neoplasms. The frequency of lymphoma has been estimated to be 350 times higher than in the age-matched general population. Virtually all cases of post-transplant lymphoproliferative disorders harbor EBV genomic DNA and RNA. **(p. 1959)**

A64. False

They are at a high risk for developing Kaposi's sarcoma and non-Hodgkin's lymphoma. The incidence of Hodgkin's lymphoma does not seem to be unduly increased, but the disease presents several differences from that seen in the immunocompetent population. Almost all cases are clinical stage III or IV at presentation, with frequent involvement of unusual sites such as the liver and skin; spread often occurs in a non-contiguous fashion; there is a predominance of unfavorable histologic subtypes; Reed–Sternberg cells and their variants are more numerous and more atypical; there is an increased number of non-lymphoid stromal cells; and there is a much higher incidence of presence of the EBV genomes in Reed–Sternberg cells. **(p. 1960)**

A65. False

Acquired diseases of the immune system in which an increased incidence of lymphoma has been recorded include rheumatoid arthritis, Sjögren's syndrome, Hashimoto's thyroiditis and other autoimmune diseases. **(p. 1960)**

Lymph node inclusions

A1. False

Inclusions of various types of benign tissue can occur within lymph nodes. Lack of awareness of this phenomenon can lead to a mistaken diagnosis of metastatic carcinoma. These include the following: salivary gland tissue, squamous epithelium, thyroid follicles, decidual reaction, müllerian-type epithelium, nevus cells, mesothelial cells and breast tissue. Salivary gland inclusions composed of ductal structures and acini are an extremely common finding in high cervical nodes. **(p. 1961)**

Other non-neoplastic lesions

A1. False

Adipose metaplasia of lymph nodes is very common. When extensive it may lead to the formation of large masses, up to 10 cm or more in diameter. These nodes are sometimes referred to as lipolymph nodes; the external iliac and obturator groups are the sites most commonly involved. **(p. 1963)**

A2. True

Some nodes otherwise showing the typical features of angioimmunoblastic lymphadenopathy may also show extensive vasculitis. Obliterative vasculitis is often seen in syphilitic lymphadenitis. **(p. 1963)**

A3. True

Therefore thorough examination of the infarcted node, the extranodal region and other nodes submitted is mandatory in order to exclude a concomitant or underlying malignancy. A thorough immunohistochemical study is also in order. The possibility of an underlying malignancy should be suspected if the infarcted node is markedly enlarged. **(p. 1964)**

A4. False

Hyaline material sometimes accumulates in the stroma of lymph nodes. This finding is very frequent in nodes of the aortoiliac region. Because of its homogeneous eosinophilic appearance it can be confused with amyloid. It should also be distinguished from the hyaline material deposited in nodes in cases of hemorrhagic spindle cell tumor with amianthoid fibers. The presence of this hyaline material has no clinical significance. **(p. 1964)**

Tumors of the cells of the accessory immune system

A1. True

The dendritic cells belong to the group of non-lymphoid elements classically designated as reticulum cells, which have been divided into more or less well-defined subtypes on the basis of location, enzyme histochemical, ultrastructural and immunohistochemical features. These are dendritic follicular cells, interdigitating dendritic cells, Langerhans' cells, fibroblastic reticulum cells, macrophages and sinus lining cells. **(p. 1965)**

A2. False

The aforementioned characteristics belong to interdigitating dendritic cells. Dendritic follicular cells are associated with the B zones of the node, and specifically with the germinal centers. Ultrastructurally, they have complex cell prolongations joined by complex desmosomes. Immunohistochemically, they exhibit reactivity for CD21, CD35, Ki-M4p, Ki-FDRC1p, CNA 42, fascin, Ki-M9, estrogen receptor α, epidermal growth factor receptor and the low-affinity nerve growth factor receptor. **(p. 1965)**

A3. False

Langerhans' cells are characterized by immunoreactivity to S-100 protein and CD1a, and the presence of Birbeck's granules at the ultrastructural level. Littoral cells, also known as sinus lining cells, have macrophagic properties and endothelial features. **(p. 1965)**

A4. True
The pattern of spread resembles that of a soft tissue sarcoma more than that of a malignant lymphoma. Intra-abdominal neoplasms tend to be particularly aggressive. Recurrent and metastatic lesions may show increased atypia and pleomorphism. **(p. 1966)**

A5. True
The tumor cells are positive for CD45RB, S-100 protein and the macrophage marker CD68, but negative for CD21 and CD35. Its behavior seems more aggressive than that of dendritic cell tumors. **(p. 1968)**

Vascular tumors and tumor-like conditions

A1. True
Microscopically, the involved nodes show proliferation of spindle cells separated by slit-like spaces containing red blood cells. **(p. 1970)**

Other primary tumors and tumor-like conditions

A1. False
Mastocytosis of the diffuse (systemic) type often involves lymph nodes, resulting in a partial or complete effacement of the architecture by a monotonous proliferation of round or polygonal cells. Special techniques that allow the identification of mast cells include Giemsa, metachromatic stains, chloroacetate esterase, and immunohistochemical demonstration of tryptase, CD117 and the adhesion molecule CD44/HCAM. **(p. 1971)**

A2. True
Clues to the diagnosis include a patchy or sinusal type of nodal involvement, sometimes associated with a single-file pattern of infiltration in the capsule; fine granularity of the cytoplasm; and the presence of eosinophilic myelocytes. **(p. 1971)**

A3. True
The main microscopic features are the proliferation of bland-looking spindle cells, sometimes in a palisading fashion; extensive foci of recent and old hemorrhage; and giant rosette-like collections of collagen fibers (so-called amianthoid fibers). **(p. 1973)**

A4. False
The disease may be localized or affect several lymph node groups, and may be accompanied by fever, anemia, elevated erythrocyte sedimentation rate and hypergammaglobulinemia. **(p. 1973)**

A5. True
The latter group, which can follow an aggressive clinical course and is accompanied by a balanced chromosomal translocation involving the *ALK* gene, is now regarded as a neoplastic process and has accordingly been renamed inflammatory myofibroblastic tumor. **(p. 1973)**

A6. True
Other sarcomas that have a greater than average tendency to metastasize to regional nodes are embryonal rhabdomyosarcoma, angiosarcoma, epithelioid sarcoma and synovial sarcoma. **(p. 1974)**

A7. False
The aforementioned features favor metastatic carcinoma. Features favoring lymphoma are the presence of focal nodularity within the tumor not induced by fibrosis, and diffuse permeation of walls of veins (as opposed to tumor thrombi) and adipose tissue if an extranodal component is present. The types of malignant lymphoma most likely to be misdiagnosed as metastatic carcinoma are anaplastic large cell lymphoma, large cell lymphoma with sclerosis resulting in prominent nesting, large cell lymphoma with a predominantly sinusal pattern of growth, nodular sclerosis Hodgkin's lymphoma with a concentration of large mononuclear variants of Reed–Sternberg cells around areas of necrosis, and signet ring lymphoma. **(p. 1975)**

A8. True
The first may masquerade clinically and pathologically as Hodgkin's lymphoma because of its common presentation in a young adult with painless unilateral cervical lymphadenopathy and the presence of a polymorphic population (including eosinophils) on microscopic examination. The second may be confused with malignant lymphomas of one type or another. **(p. 1976)**

A9. False
Reticulin stains have only limited value in this differential diagnosis. In general, positivity for the mucin stain will establish the diagnosis of adenocarcinoma. The presence of abundant glycogen and/or diastase-resistant mucosubstances in the cytoplasm of a large cell tumor on PAS staining will also rule out, for all practical purposes, a diagnosis of lymphoma. **(p. 1978)**

A10. False

They originate from the upper aerodigestive tract. Sites well known for harboring small, clinically undetectable primaries in the presence of cervical adenopathy are the nasopharynx and the retrotonsillar pillar. **(p. 1979)**

A11. False

They are usually examples of metastatic thyroid carcinoma, a possibility that becomes a virtual certainty in the presence of psammoma bodies. However, these papillary tumors may also originate from the salivary gland, ovary or thymus. Squamous cell carcinomas in lymph nodes of this region usually arise in the upper aerodigestive tract, particularly the pharynx and larynx. **(p. 1979)**

A12. True

Supraclavicular nodes involved by intra-abdominal carcinomas are sometimes referred to as Virchow's or Troisier's nodes. **(p. 1979)**

A13. True

Lung carcinoma should also be considered, especially in older patients with a smoking history. **(p. 1979)**

A14. False

They are often the recipients of carcinomas from the external genital organs (usually evident on clinical examination) or malignant melanomas of the lower extremities, but only rarely from the internal abdominal organs (ovary, uterine cervix, anal canal) and even less commonly from the testis, unless direct extension to the scrotal skin has occurred. **(p. 1979)**

22 Spleen

Normal anatomy

Q1

Hematopoiesis (erythrocytes, granulocytes, megakaryocytes, lymphocytes and macrophages) and reservoir (storage or sequestration of platelets and other formed elements) are not important functions of the spleen in normal adult humans.

Q2

The white pulp is made up of T and B lymphocytes, the former located in the periarteriolar lymphoid sheath and the latter eccentrically to this sheath in the form of primary lymphoid follicles.

Q3

Biopsy of the spleen should be performed in all patients with a bleeding tendency. In the majority of patients aspiration cytology will not be of diagnostic help, so core needle biopsy should be performed.

Rupture and splenectomy

Q1

The two most common reasons for rupture of the normal spleen are hemolytic anemia and immune thrombocytopenic purpura.

Q2

Following traumatic rupture, splenic tissue may implant in the form of encapsulated nodules on the peritoneal surface, the abdominal wall, and even within the pleural cavity, lung parenchyma and brain, a process known as splenosis.

Q3

The diseases most commonly associated with spontaneous rupture of the spleen are infectious mononucleosis, malaria, typhoid fever, subacute bacterial endocarditis, peliosis lienis, malignant lymphomas, leukemias, and primary non-lymphoid splenic neoplasms.

Q4

Rupture of the spleen with resulting hemoperitoneum is the most frequent cause of death in infectious mononucleosis.

Q5

Splenectomy performed in adults for traumatic rupture of the spleen results in an increased incidence and severity of infections.

Q6

Overwhelming infection may occur days to years after removal of the spleen; it begins abruptly, frequently lacks an identifiable focus, and usually progresses rapidly despite appropriate antibiotic therapy, resulting in a mortality of 50–80%.

Congenital anomalies and cysts

Q1

An accessory (supernumerary) spleen usually measures more than 4 cm in diameter, and it is always a solitary lesion in contiguity with the tail of the pancreas.

Q2

Congenital absence of the spleen (asplenia) is associated in more than 80% of cases with malformations of the heart, nearly always involving the atrioventricular endocardial cushion and the ventricular outflow tracts.

Q3

This is a picture of a typical epithelial (primary) cyst, characterized by its glistening inner surface with marked trabeculation. In contrast to pseudocysts (false or secondary cysts) trabeculation is always present.

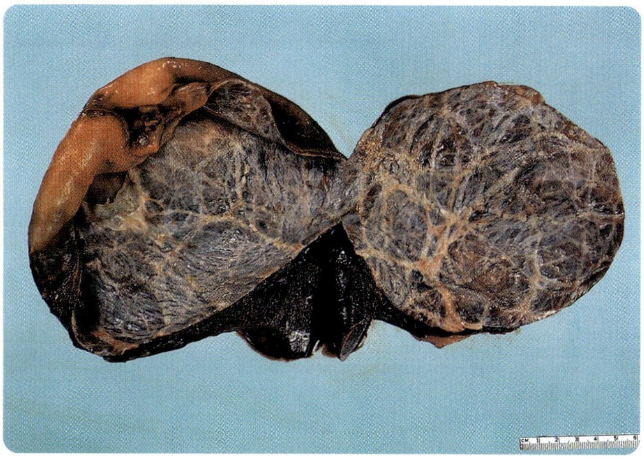

Fig. 22.1

Inflammation

Q1

Reactive follicular hyperplasia may be caused by measles and typhoid fever. Diffuse lymphoid hyperplasia can be the result of infection (particularly viral), graft rejection, or a component of angioimmunoblastic lymphadenopathy.

Q2

The presence of splenic granulomas in patients with lymphoma is an indication per se that the spleen is involved by tumor.

Hypersplenism and other non-neoplastic disorders

Q1

Hypersplenism (dysplenism) is the generic term used for the group of disorders in which the removal of hematopoietic elements by the spleen increases to a pathologic degree.

Q2

Immune (idiopathic) thrombocytopenic purpura is caused by the presence of an antiplatelet IgG, which is produced largely in the spleen.

Q3

The presence of foamy macrophages in the spleen is pathognomonic for immune thrombocytopenic purpura.

Q4

The most important pathologic change of thrombotic thrombocytic purpura is the presence of thrombi in arteries and arterioles without associated inflammation.

Q5

The best therapy for hereditary spherocytosis is steroid or immunosuppressive therapy.

QUESTIONS

Q6

Congestive splenomegaly is a direct consequence of portal hypertension. It may be caused by cirrhosis (by far the most common pathogenesis); thrombosis of hepatic veins (Budd–Chiari syndrome); thrombosis of the splenic veins; or occlusive thrombosis, cavernous transformation (recanalized thrombosis), sclerosis, or stenosis of the portal vein.

Q7

Most reported cases of peliosis of the spleen (peliosis lienis) have occurred in patients with radiation injury.

Tumors and tumor-like conditions

Q1

Metastatic carcinoma is by far the most common malignant tumor involving the spleen. Malignant melanoma and carcinoma of the lung, breast, stomach, large bowel, pancreas and liver are the most common types found.

Q2

Primary splenic lymphoma is defined as a neoplasm restricted only to the spleen. The most common type is marginal zone lymphoma.

Q3

Morphologic features favoring a B-cell phenotype of primary splenic lymphoma are epithelioid histiocytic reaction, tumor confinement to the periarteriolar lymphoid sheath and marginal zone, and clear cell or polymorphous cytologic features.

Q4

Secondary splenic involvement by tumor is particularly common in low-grade lymphomas, such as small lymphocytic lymphoma, lymphoplasmacytoid lymphoma, mantle cell lymphoma, follicle center lymphoma and marginal zone B-cell lymphoma.

Q5

This image represents polypoid growth of malignant lymphoma cells beneath the endothelium of a trabecular vein. This is a useful diagnostic sign for large B-cell lymphoma of the spleen.

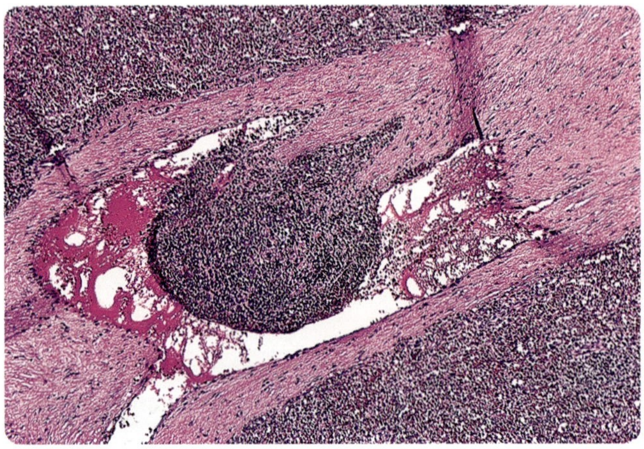

Fig. 22.2

Q6

Patients with localized splenic non-Hodgkin's lymphoma seem to have the same rate of survival as other stage I non-Hodgkin's lymphoma patients.

Q7

Marginal zone B-cell lymphoma of the spleen usually presents with splenomegaly, anemia, weight loss, and involvement of the bone marrow and liver.

Q8

Hepatosplenic γ/δ T-cell lymphoma typically occurs in young females and has a favorable prognosis.

Q9

The most common type of Hodgkin's lymphoma in the spleen is mixed cellularity.

Q10

Any type of leukemia can involve the spleen, the location for all types being predominantly the red pulp.

Q11

Hairy cell leukemia is a specific subtype of B-cell malignancy characterized by diffuse and usually marked enlargement of the spleen without the formation of nodules, except in the very early stages of the disease.

Q12

Hairy cell leukemia is very aggressive disease, usually without involvement of lymph nodes in the splenic hilum.

Q13

Myelofibrosis is characterized by an enlarged spleen with signs of congestion, hemosiderosis, and a paucity of lymphoid follicles.

Q14

The diagnosis of mastocytosis depends on the identification of mast cells, which usually appear as small clusters embedded in fibrous tissue, accompanied by a variable number of eosinophils, lymphocytes or histiocytes.

Q15

Angiosarcoma is the most common primary vascular tumor of the spleen.

Q16

This is a picture of inflammatory pseudotumor of the spleen. Spindle cells of myofibroblastic appearance are admixed with various types of inflammatory cell.

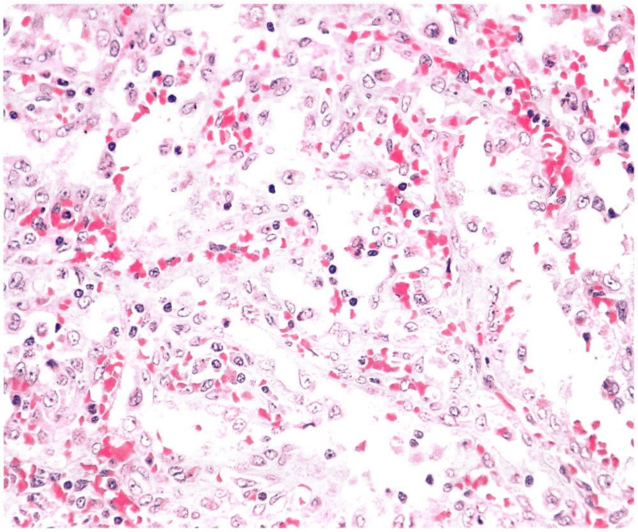

Fig. 22.3

Q17

Microscopically, inflammatory pseudotumor is composed of variable mixture of lymphocytes, plasma cells, eosinophils, histiocytes and spindle cells, the latter having an immunotype that has been interpreted as myofibroblastic.

Normal anatomy

A1. True

Important functions of the spleen in normal adult humans are phagocytosis (removal of particulate matter, red blood cell destruction, pitting and erythroclasis) and immunity (trapping and processing of antigen, 'homing' of lymphocytes, lymphocyte transformation and proliferation, and antibody production). **(p. 2019)**

A2. True

These lymphoid follicles contain germinal centers, particularly in children. **(p. 2019)**

A3. False

Biopsy is rarely attempted because of the possibility of hemorrhage and the preconceived notion that the biopsy will not be of diagnostic help. The procedure should not be performed on patients with a bleeding tendency. Aspiration cytology and core needle biopsy gave similar diagnostic yields, except for malignant lymphoma, in which core needle biopsy has proved superior. **(p. 2019)**

Rupture and splenectomy

A1. False

Blunt trauma to the abdomen and surgical intervention within the abdominal cavity are the two most common factors responsible for rupture of the normal spleen. In most instances hemoperitoneum is an immediate consequence, leading to an emergency splenectomy. **(p. 2020)**

A2. True

Some nodules are poorly developed architecturally, but others show a full complement of red and white pulp, resulting in an appearance similar to that of accessory spleen. **(p. 2020)**

A3. True

In every case of ruptured spleen without a history of trauma or in which the trauma seems insignificant, a careful microscopic study should be performed in order to rule out these possibilities. **(p. 2020)**

A4. True

This complication usually occurs from 10 to 21 days after the onset of the disease. **(p. 2020)**

A5. False

Splenectomy performed in adults for traumatic rupture of the spleen usually does not result in sequelae of any significance. Conversely, an increased incidence and severity of infections have been reported following splenectomy in young children. **(p. 2020)**

A6. True

Because of this, an attempt is now made to save splenic function in children by repair of the laceration or by partial splenectomy. If a total splenectomy is necessary a spleen autotransplant has been recommended. **(p. 2020)**

Congenital anomalies and cysts

A1. False

It may be solitary or multiple, usually measures less than 4 cm in diameter, and has a gross and microscopic appearance similar to that of the parent organ. Its most common location is the hilum of the spleen, and it is sometimes seen in contiguity with the tail of the pancreas. **(p. 2020)**

A2. True

Anomalies of the blood vessels, lung and abdominal viscera also are frequent. **(p. 2020)**

A3. False

Grossly, it is very difficult, if not impossible, to distinguish this lesion from a pseudocyst. Microscopically, the wall is lined by columnar, cuboidal (mesothelial-like) or squamous epithelium, whereas pseudocysts lack an epithelial lining. **(p. 2021)**

Inflammation

A1. True

Reactive follicular hyperplasia also occurs in a chronic form in a large number of infectious diseases, including AIDS, and in immune-mediated diseases such as idiopathic thrombocytopenic purpura, acquired hemolytic anemia, rheumatoid arthritis (including Felty's syndrome) and the systemic form of Castleman's disease, as well as in hemodialyzed patients. **(p. 2022)**

A2. False

Sarcoid-like granulomas can be seen in the spleen of patients with Hodgkin's lymphoma and, less commonly, non-Hodgkin's lymphoma or hairy cell leukemia, with or without involvement of the spleen by tumor. **(p. 2023)**

Hypersplenism and other non-neoplastic disorders

A1. True

Any of the cellular elements of the blood may be affected, singly or in combination. Thus neutropenia, thrombocytopenia, hemolytic anemia or pancytopenia may all be present. **(p. 2024)**

A2. True

The antibody-coated platelets have a short lifespan because they are rapidly removed by the cells of the reticuloendothelial system, particularly in the spleen and liver. Occasionally, thrombocytopenic purpura is seen as a manifestation of lupus erythematosus, viral infection, drug hypersensitivity, chronic lymphocytic leukemia or Hodgkin's lymphoma. **(p. 2024)**

A3. False

Foamy macrophages can be found in the spleens of patients with idiopathic thrombocytopenic purpura, but they also occur, as an incidental finding without clinical significance, in the malpighian follicles of normal individuals. They have also been described in Gaucher's disease, Niemann–Pick disease, Tay–Sachs disease, chronic granulomatous disease, thalassemia and hyperlipemic states. **(p. 2024)**

A4. True

Other changes include hyperplasia of B-cells and germinal centers, periarteriolar concentric fibrosis, hemosiderin-laden macrophages, hemophagocytosis and extramedullary hematopoiesis. **(p. 2025)**

A5. False

Hereditary spherocytosis is the hematologic disease that most benefits from splenectomy. The clinical cure rate is almost 100%, although the intrinsic red cell abnormality persists. In acquired hemolytic anemia, splenectomy is usually reserved for cases that cannot be controlled by steroid or immunosuppressive therapy. **(p. 2025)**

A6. True

Cases of portal hypertension accompanied by congestive splenomegaly in which no apparent cause is discernible either in the liver or in the hepatic or portal veins are referred to as idiopathic portal hypertension. **(p. 2025)**

A7. False

Most cases have occurred in patients with wasting diseases, such as tuberculosis and carcinomatosis, or in patients who have received anabolic–androgenic steroids. They have also been seen in association with chronic leukemia and following liver transplantation. **(p. 2026)**

Tumors and tumor-like conditions

A1. False

The most common malignant tumor involving the spleen is malignant lymphoma. **(p. 2027)**

A2. False

Primary splenic lymphoma is restricted to the spleen and hilar lymph nodes. The majority of cases are large cell lymphoma of B-cell immunophenotype, which can present as 'macronodular' nodules, 'micronodular' nodules, and as diffuse red pulp infiltration. **(p. 2027)**

A3. False

These are characteristics of a T-cell phenotype of primary splenic lymphoma. Morphologic features favoring a B-cell phenotype are multiple discrete nodules in the white pulp, large coalescing nodules, the coexistence of small lymphocytic lymphoma, and plasmacytoid features. **(p. 2027)**

A4. True

Splenic small lymphocytic lymphoma usually presents grossly and microscopically as nodules measuring a few millimeters in diameter, with preferential involvement of the white pulp. A nodular pattern of growth is common to several types of lymphoproliferative disease of the spleen and its presence should not be equated with a diagnosis of follicle center lymphoma. **(p. 2028)**

A5. False

This is a useful diagnostic sign for small lymphocytic lymphoma. Clues to the diagnosis in such cases include prominent enlargement and coalescence of follicles; the presence of a marked expansion of their mantle zone; germinal centers that are absent, inconspicuous or overrun by small cells; and clusters of small lymphoid cells protruding beneath the endothelium of trabecular veins. The latter can also be seen in adults with infectious mononucleosis. **(p. 2028)**

A6. True

The prognosis is directly related to the microscopic type and the clinical stage, in the sense that it is distinctly better for small lymphocytic tumors and for stage I and II disease. **(p. 2029)**

A7. True

Grossly, the splenic involvement manifests itself through miliary expansion of the white pulp. Histologically, there are nodular lymphoid infiltrates composed of small lymphocytes similar to mantle cells, with a component of larger cells with irregular nuclei and pale cytoplasm located towards the periphery of the nodules. **(p. 2029)**

A8. False

It typically presents with hepatosplenomegaly, fever and weight loss in young males, and carries a poor prognosis. The neoplastic infiltration involves the cords and sinuses of the spleen, and intrasinusoidal compartments of the liver and bone marrow. **(p. 2030)**

A9. False

The most common type is nodular sclerosis, but others may be seen as well. The spleen is the most common site of extranodal organ involvement by Hodgkin's lymphoma, but primary Hodgkin's lymphoma of the spleen is extremely rare. **(p. 2030)**

A10. True

The earliest involvement is in the cords, with secondary spillage into the sinuses. The most common types are chronic lymphocytic leukemia, prolymphocytic leukemia, chronic myelocytic leukemia and hairy cell leukemia. **(p. 2030)**

A11. True

Microscopically, hairy cell leukemia is a disease of the red pulp, which shows diffuse infiltration by a monotonous population of small mononuclear cells with very scanty mitotic activity and practically no phagocytosis. The distinctive enzyme histochemical feature of the disease is the presence of tartarate-resistant acid phosphatase. **(p. 2031)**

A12. False

The lymph nodes in the splenic hilum are often involved, the pattern of permeation being interfollicular. Splenectomy is the treatment of choice, and long survivals are common. **(p. 2032)**

A13. True

The results of splenectomy are not spectacular, but in some cases a moderate improvement has been noted. **(p. 2032)**

A14. True

The diagnosis is confirmed by staining the cytoplasmic granules with metachromatic dyes, with Leder's chloroacetate esterase reaction, or by the immunohistochemical demonstration of tryptase, chymase, carboxypeptidase, CD68 and CD117 (c-*kit*). **(p. 2033)**

A15. False

Hemangioma is the most common primary tumor of the spleen. Angiosarcoma is the most common malignant primary non-lymphoid tumor of the spleen. **(p. 2034)**

A16. False

This is a picture of littoral cell angioma. Microscopically, it is composed of anastomosing vascular channels resembling splenic sinuses. These channels have irregular lumina, often featuring papillary projections and cyst-like spaces. **(p. 2034)**

A17. True

An analogy has been drawn between this lesion and inflammatory pseudotumor of soft tissue, a lesion now generally regarded as neoplastic and redesignated inflammatory myofibroblastic tumor. However, whereas the latter is characterized by expression of ALK kinase and is unassociated with EBV, inflammatory pseudotumor of the spleen is ALK negative and often positive for EBV-encoded RNA with in situ hybridization tests. **(p. 2037)**

23 Bone marrow

Biopsy procedure and processing of specimen

Q1

Trephine biopsy of the bone marrow is the most reliable method for assessing marrow cellularity following the administration of antineoplastic drugs, and in assessing the status of engraftment following bone marrow transplantation.

Q2

Severe thrombocytopenia is a contraindication to marrow biopsy.

Q3

Particle sections are of limited value in marrow disorders that are accompanied by fibrosis; these frequently result in inadequately aspirated specimens. Nevertheless, any particles obtained in a marrow aspirate should be processed for histologic examination.

Q4

Immunohistochemistry with a wide range of antibodies can be performed with excellent results on most paraffin-embedded specimens.

Q5

Bone marrow fibrosis is usually a secondary phenomenon; the most common causes are metastatic tumor and malignant lymphoma.

Q6

The length of a biopsy specimen should be less than 1 cm, otherwise the results of immunohistochemistry will not be satisfactory.

Q7

Optimally, when interpreting a trephine biopsy the pathologist should examine the trephine imprints, bone marrow aspirate, blood smears and other pathology specimens. Clinical data are not helpful for interpretation of the biopsy specimen.

Normocellular bone marrow

Q1

Assessment of marrow cellularity must take into account the age of the patient because the amount of hematopoietic tissue in bone marrow from normal individuals varies with age.

Q2

The immediate subcortical area of the bone marrow may normally be more hypercellular than the deeper medullary areas.

Alterations in cellularity, necrosis and inflammation

Q1

Aplastic or hypoplastic marrow, referred to as aplastic anemia, occurs in both acquired and congenital forms.

Q2

This is a bone marrow section from a 7-year-old girl with idiopathic acquired aplastic anemia. Hematopoietic cells are almost totally absent. The blood findings in aplastic anemia are characterized by varying degrees of pancytopenia.

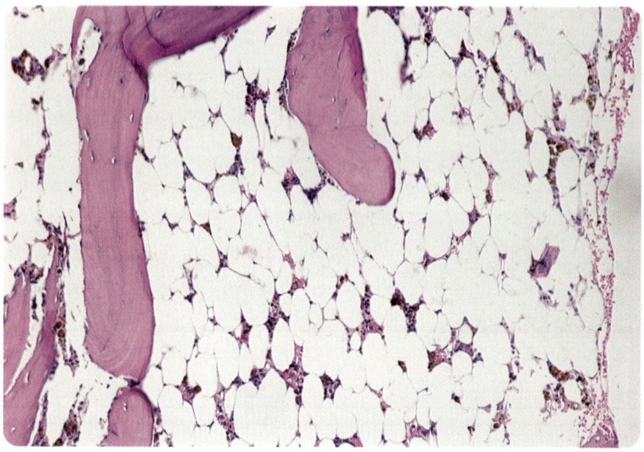

Fig. 23.1

Q3

Hypoplastic marrow may be encountered in some newly diagnosed cases of acute leukemia and myelodysplastic syndromes. Morphologically, it is impossible to distinguish these disorders from true aplastic anemia.

Q4

Hyperplasia of one or more myeloid cell lines may be found in several benign hematologic disorders, such as megaloblastic and sideroblastic anemias, hemolytic anemias and immune thrombocytopenia.

Q5

Gelatinous (serous) transformation is a degenerative change of the marrow caused by drugs or viral diseases.

Q6

Osteopetrosis is an uncommon disorder in which the bone trabeculae are markedly thinned, resulting in increased marrow space with hyperplasia in hematopoietic tissue.

Q7

Bone marrow necrosis unrelated to chemotherapy or radiation therapy occurs occasionally in patients with acute leukemia, malignant lymphoma and metastatic tumor.

Q8

In approximately 80% of cases with bone marrow granulomas no etiologic basis for the lesions is identified.

Q9

Typical granuloma formation may not be present in the marrow of some immunosuppressed patients with disseminated fungal or mycobacterial disease.

Q10

Nonspecific inflammatory alterations in the marrow from patients with a variety of systemic disorders are characterized by changes in both the vascular structures and the parenchyma.

Q11

The terms tumor myelopathy and myelitis have been applied to the specific marrow changes that are observed in patients with multiple myeloma.

Q12

Marrow biopsies from patients with AIDS have been generally reported to be hypocellular. Nonspecific findings include decreased lymphocytes, plasma cells and erythroid hyperplasia with all stages of maturation.

Q13

Lymphocytic aggregates of uniform size occur in the marrow of a relatively low percentage of patients with AIDS. These are randomly distributed, with a preferential paratrabecular distribution, composed primarily of large lymphocytes.

Q14

Marrow biopsies from patients with AIDS may have a numerous abnormal megakaryocytes with sparse cytoplasm and 'naked' megakaryocyte nuclei. This finding is specific for AIDS.

Leukemias and related disorders

Q1

The diagnosis and classification of the acute leukemias are optimally established from examination of Romanowsky-stained blood and bone marrow smears in conjunction with appropriate cytochemical techniques and chromosome analysis.

Q2

In a small minority of patients, particularly older individuals, acute myeloid leukemia and, rarely, acute lymphoblastic leukemia may present with a hypocellular marrow (i.e. hypoplastic or hypocellular acute leukemia).

Q3

The trephine biopsy provides the only accurate assessment of marrow cellularity and is of considerable importance in monitoring changes following treatment for leukemia. Regeneration of fat cells is followed by regeneration of normal hematopoietic cells in the successfully treated patient.

Q4

Acute panmyelosis with myelofibrosis (acute myelofibrosis) is distinguished from chronic idiopathic myelofibrosis by an abrupt onset, little or no red cell poikilocytosis, absence of or minimal splenomegaly, and a rapid clinical course.

Q5

Myeloid sarcoma is a special variant of malignant lymphoma characterized by myelofibrosis and a sarcomatous appearance.

Q6

The myelodysplastic syndromes are basically disorders of ineffective myelopoiesis with hyperplastic marrows and cytopenias, frequently pancytopenia with or without an increase in blasts.

Q7

This is a marrow biopsy from an adult with refractory anemia with excess blasts-2 (RAEB-2). The marrow is hypercellular with occasional foci of immature myeloid cells in the central marrow in non-paratrabecular and non-perivascular locations. This finding is known as abnormal localization of immature precursors (ALIP).

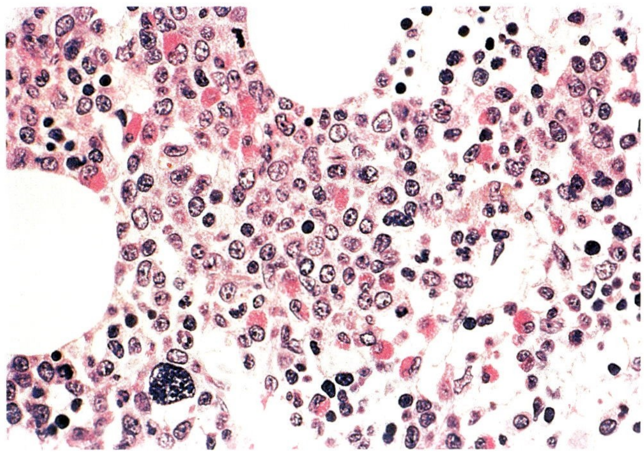

Fig. 23.2

Q8

Precise classification of the myelodysplastic syndromes is based principally on the evaluation of bone marrow biopsy. Marrow smears are not helpful for precise classification of these syndromes.

Q9

The de novo 5q– syndrome is a myelodysplastic syndrome that occurs primarily in older women who present with a macrocytic anemia, with normal to increased platelet counts and usually prolonged survival.

Q10

The therapy-related acute leukemias and myelodysplastic syndromes occur in patients who have been treated with chemotherapy, radiation therapy or both for a variety of malignant and non-malignant conditions.

Q11

Chronic myeloid leukemia is generally characterized by an elevated leukocyte count with more than 20% of myeloblasts in the blood and marrow smears.

Q12

Treatment with the tyrosine kinase inhibitor imatinib mesylate (Glivec) induces hematologic remission in a high percentage of patients with chronic myeloid leukemia in the chronic and accelerated phases of the disease.

Q13

The neutrophil alkaline phosphatase is decreased in almost all patients with polycythemia vera.

Q14

The 'spent phase' of polycythemia vera is characterized by a decrease in red cell mass and the development of myelofibrosis with a marked increase in reticulin fibers, collagenous fibrosis and abnormal megakaryocytes.

Q15

Essential thrombocythemia is an aggressive disorder characterized by splenomegaly and hypercellular bone marrow due to panhyperplasia of myeloid cells, principally erythroid precursors and megakaryocytes.

Q16

Chronic idiopathic myelofibrosis (agnogenic myeloid metaplasia) is a clonal myeloproliferative disease of undetermined etiology characterized by myeloid cell proliferation and reactive fibrosis.

Q17

The most important distinguishing biologic feature between chronic idiopathic myelofibrosis and chronic myeloid leukemia is the presence of the Philadelphia chromosome or molecular evidence of the *bcr-abl* hybrid gene in the hematopoietic cells.

Q18

The prefibrotic stage of chronic idiopathic myelofibrosis is marked by variable degrees of reticulin and/or collagen fibrosis; the marrow varies from hypo- to hypercellular. Expansion of the bone trabeculae may be present.

Q19

The majority of patients with chronic idiopathic myelofibrosis have an estimated median survival of 3–5 years from the onset of disease.

Q20

The morphology of the proliferating lymphocytes in chronic lymphocytic leukemia and well-differentiated lymphocytic lymphoma is the same and the two disorders are considered by the WHO as different manifestations of the same process.

Q21

Patients with chronic lymphocytic leukemia with focal, interstitial, or a combination of focal and interstitial involvement are predominantly in high clinical stages.

Q22

Richter's syndrome is the occurrence of a pleomorphic lymphoma in a patient with a prior history of B-chronic lymphocytic leukemia or another low-grade B-cell lymphoproliferative disorder, such as plasmacytoid lymphoma.

Q23

Prolymphocytic leukemia occurs primarily in younger individuals and is characterized by a predominant proliferation of mature lymphocytes. The patient usually has massive peripheral lymphadenopathy without splenomegaly.

Q24

Hairy cell leukemia is a chronic lymphoproliferative disorder of B-cell origin that manifests primarily in blood, marrow and spleen. There is a male preponderance.

Q25

In the majority of patients with hairy cell leukemia the marrow is hypercellular. The involvement may be diffuse or partial; the diffuse type is more common.

Q26

Hairy cell leukemia variant is a lymphoproliferative disorder usually presenting with a pancytopenia and lymphocytes with morphologic characteristics of centrocytes.

Q27

This is a bone marrow biopsy from a patient with splenic lymphoma with villous lymphocytes showing a paratrabecular, poorly demarcated aggregate of lymphocytes.

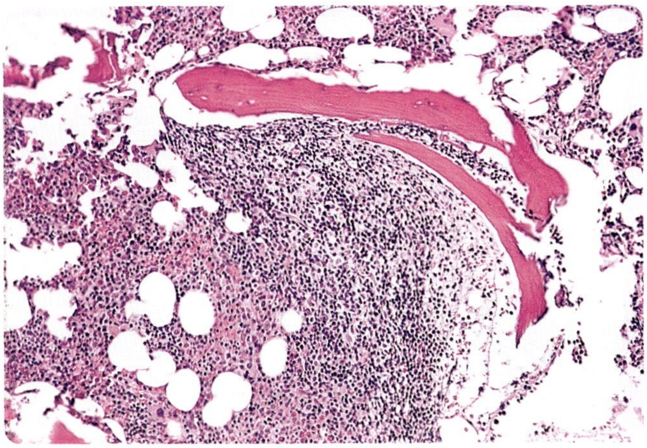

Fig. 23.3

Q28

A small number of patients with splenic lymphoma with villous lymphocytes and concurrent hepatitis C infection will undergo remission of the lymphoma following treatment of the hepatitis C with interferon-α_{2b} and the disappearance of hepatitis C RNA.

Non-Hodgkin's lymphoma

Q1

The incidence of marrow involvement in non-Hodgkin's lymphoma is higher in the low-grade lymphomas than in many of the high-grade lymphomas.

Q2

The focal paratrabecular pattern occurs exclusively in follicular center cell lymphomas.

Q3

The intrasinusoidal pattern of bone marrow involvement may occur most frequently with follicular lymphoma.

Q4

The cytopathology of the lesions in marrow sections usually parallels the cytologic characteristics in the lymph node; this is particularly true for follicular lymphoma.

Q5

There is no relationship between a diffuse or follicular pattern in the lymph node and the presence of focal or diffuse lesions in the marrow.

Q6

Peripheral T-cell lymphoma is characterized by a high incidence of marrow involvement at the time of initial diagnosis.

Q7

The large cell type is the most frequent cytologic pattern in the marrow lesions of peripheral T-cell lymphoma.

Q8

The mixed cell and large cell/immunoblastic types of peripheral T-cell lymphoma usually have an associated polycellular infiltrate consisting of histiocytes, plasma cells, eosinophils and neutrophils.

Q9

Polymorphous reactive lymphoid hyperplasia of the bone marrow has many histopathologic features similar to peripheral T-cell lymphoma, including a heterogeneous population of lymphocytes with intermixed plasma cells, immunoblasts, eosinophils, endothelial cells and epithelioid histiocytes.

Q10

Hodgkin's disease in the marrow may appear similar to the lesions of peripheral T-cell lymphoma. The presence of classic Reed–Sternberg cells and the lack of atypia in the lymphocyte population is evidence of Hodgkin's disease.

Q11

Genotypic studies to determine T-cell clonality are not helpful in distinguishing peripheral T-cell lymphoma in marrow biopsies or other tissues from the disorders considered in the differential diagnosis, because it cannot be done on fixed, paraffin-embedded tissue.

Q12

Sézary syndrome is a lymphoproliferative disorder of T-helper lymphocytes related to mycosis fungoides and characterized by erythroderma and abnormal lymphoid cells in the blood.

Q13

Large granulated T-cell lymphocytic leukemia usually presents with lymphadenopathy and frequently severe anemia. Most patients have hepatomegaly, but splenomegaly never occurs.

Q14

The lesions of angioimmunoblastic T-cell lymphoma contain varying proportions of immunoblasts and plasmacytoid monocytes. Plasma cells and neutrophils are very scanty, a feature of diagnostic importance.

Q15

This is a bone marrow smear from a patient with aggressive NK cell leukemia/lymphoma. The lymphoma cells have relatively abundant cytoplasm containing numerous coarse azurophilic granules.

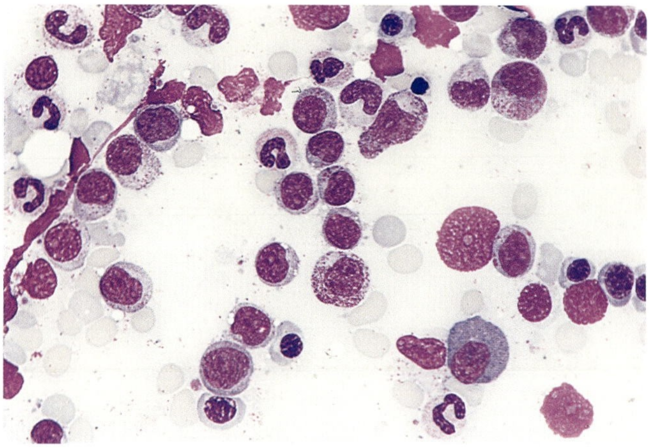

Fig. 23.4

Lymphoma/leukemia

Q1

The 'starry sky' appearance characteristic of lymph nodes in Burkitt's lymphoma is almost always present in bone marrow biopsies.

Q2

Acute lymphoblastic leukemia is distinguished from lymphoblastic lymphoma on the basis of the percentage of lymphoblasts in the marrow.

Benign lymphocytic aggregates

Q1

Unusually large benign lymphocytic aggregates may occur in the marrow of patients with diseases related to the immune system, such as AIDS and rheumatoid arthritis.

Q2

A preferential paratrabecular margination of a lymphoid infiltrate is characteristic for benign lesions.

Hodgkin's lymphoma

Q1

The incidence of marrow involvement in Hodgkin's lymphoma is highest in the lymphocyte-predominant type.

Q2

Marrow involvement in Hodgkin's lymphoma is not associated with clinical symptoms.

Q3

The histopathologic classification of Hodgkin's lymphoma should not be based on examination of involved bone marrow because of different manifestations of the disease in lymph node and bone marrow tissue.

Q4

The presence of Reed–Sternberg cells or mononuclear variants is of critical importance to the recognition of Hodgkin's lymphoma in marrow, and a definitive diagnosis should not be established without their identification on the appropriate cellular background.

Histiocytic disorders

Q1

If the morphologic characteristics of a marrow lesion suggest a histiocytic disorder, appropriate cytochemical, immunologic, cytogenetic and molecular studies should be performed. The diagnosis is essentially one of exclusion.

Q2

The malignant histiocyte should be reactive with antibodies to myeloperoxidase, glycophorine and lectin.

Q3

The hemophagocytic syndromes are triggered by a variety of causes, including viral infections and some T-cell and B-cell lymphomas.

Q4

The evidence of phagocytic activity in patients with hemophagocytic syndromes may be less prominent in sections than in smear preparations.

Q5

Marrow involvement in Langerhans' cell histiocytosis (histiocytosis X) is frequently present and immunohistochemistry is not necessary to establish the correct diagnosis.

QUESTIONS

Plasma cell dyscrasias

Q1

This is a picture of bone marrow showing essentially normal architecture and interstitial infiltration by myeloma cells.

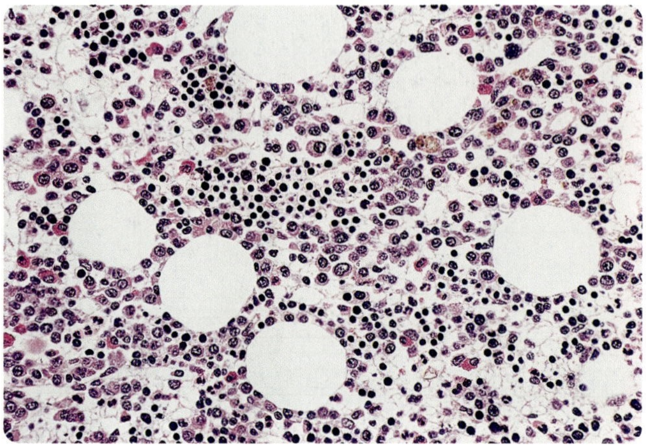

Fig. 23.5

Q2

The more mature the type of myeloma cell, i.e. plasmacytic and less than 20% marrow replacement, the more favorable is the prognosis.

Q3

An anaplastic evolution of myeloma may occur, and some of these cases have the histopathologic features of immunoblastic lymphoma. The cells in immunoblastic lymphoma usually express pan-B cell antigens; the plasma cells in approximately 80% of cases of myeloma do not express pan-B cell antigens. All clinical and laboratory findings should be considered.

Q4

Patients with plasma cell leukemia have a lower incidence of organomegaly than those with other forms of myeloma, and the disease is usually associated with a favorable prognosis.

Q5

Osteosclerotic myeloma is a form of plasma cell dyscrasia characterized by sclerotic bone lesions and progressive demyelinating polyneuropathy.

Q6

The only independent risk factors for progression of monoclonal gammopathy of undetermined significance to an overt myeloma are the concentration of the serum monoclonal protein at diagnosis and the type of monoclonal protein.

Q7

Solitary plasmacytomas are more frequent in females than males and have a peak incidence in childhood.

Q8

Plasmacytomas are generally divided into two broad groups based on location: plasmacytoma of bone and extramedullary or soft tissue plasmacytoma.

Q9

The patient with a solitary plasmacytoma usually has a lower hemoglobin level and hypercalcemia.

Q10

Lymphoplasmacytic lymphoma (Waldenström's macroglobulinemia) is characterized by hyperglobulinemia, increased serum viscosity, and a proliferation of lymphocytes in hematopoietic tissue as well as other organs.

Q11

The peripheral blood of patients with lymphoplasmacytic lymphoma shows a leukemic picture in approximately 30% of cases; the predominant cells are small lymphocytes or a mixture of small lymphocytes and plasmacytoid lymphocytes.

Q12

Intranuclear inclusions, frequently referred to as Dutcher bodies, are diagnostic for lymphoplasmacytic lymphoma.

Q13

Weakness, fatigue, fever and lymphadenopathy are common symptoms of the heavy chain diseases.

Systemic mastocytosis

Q1

Systemic mastocytosis usually occurs in combination with urticaria pigmentosa but may present in patients without cutaneous involvement.

Q2

The blood findings of systemic mastocytosis may include eosinophilia, anemia and leukocytosis, or leukopenia, thrombocytopenia and pancytopenia.

Q3

The mast cell lesions in bone marrow sections may be focal or diffuse. Focal lesions are always paratrabecular.

Q4

Patients with systemic mastocytosis have an increased incidence of myeloproliferative disorders.

Q5

The mast cells in mastocytosis are always very typical and there is no difficulty in recognizing their origin. Because of this, special stains are not necessary for diagnosis.

Metastatic tumors

Q1

Sarcomas have a relatively low incidence of marrow metastasis in adults.

Q2

This is a picture of bone marrow from a patient with chronic idiopathic myelofibrosis.

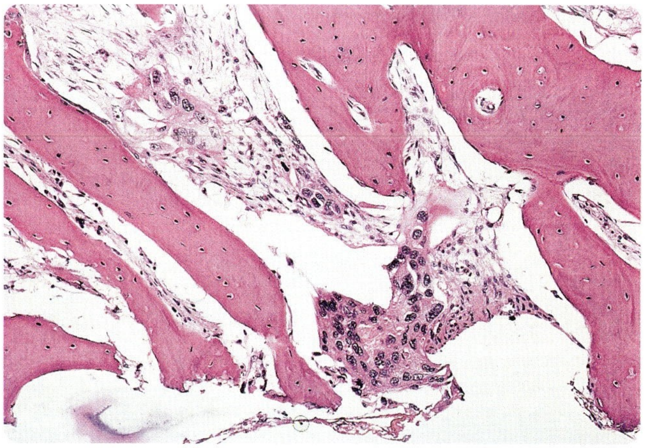

Fig. 23.6

Lipid storage diseases

Q1

The characteristic diagnostic morphologic feature of Gaucher's disease is the presence of foam cells; the cytoplasm is filled with clear vacuoles of varying sizes.

Q2

In contrast to Gaucher's disease, which is characterized by three major clinical types, there is only one clinical type of Niemann–Pick disease, characterized by nervous system involvement.

Bone marrow transplantation

Q1

Infection is a major cause of peritransplant morbidity and, in some cases, mortality in patients with bone marrow transplantation.

Q2

Megakaryocytes are usually the first hematopoietic type of cell to be reconstituted following bone marrow transplantation.

Biopsy procedure and processing of specimen

A1. True
Its greatest utility is in the evaluation of patients with malignant lymphoma, acute leukemias, myeloproliferative disorders, myelodysplastic syndromes, metastatic tumor, granulomatous disorders, myelofibrosis, aplastic anemia and plasma cell dyscrasias. **(p. 2047)**

A2. False
Severe thrombocytopenia is not a contraindication to marrow biopsy, but whenever a marrow biopsy is performed careful attention should be directed to preventing hematoma formation by applying an adequate pressure bandage to the biopsy site after the procedure. **(p. 2048)**

A3. True
Assessment of cellularity, determination of the extent of marrow involvement by neoplastic processes, and the relationship of lesions to marrow structures such as bone trabeculae and vasculature can be accurately assessed only in trephine biopsies. **(p. 2048)**

A4. True
Paraffin embedding is the preferred method for the routine processing of bone marrow biopsies. Plastic embedding offers some advantages over the paraffin method, such as excellent cytology and the ability to perform numerous histochemical reactions. **(p. 2048)**

A5. True
Fibrosis also occurs relatively frequently in the evolution of chronic myeloproliferative disorders, such as chronic myeloid leukemia and polycythemia vera. **(p. 2048)**

A6. False
Optimally, the biopsy specimen should be at least 1.5 cm in length and free of distortion caused by crushing or other damage. **(p. 2048)**

A7. False
Knowledge of the patient's clinical history, hematology profile, immunoelectrophoretic studies and radiographic findings may be of considerable importance and may greatly facilitate the interpretation of the biopsy specimen. **(p. 2049)**

Normocellular bone marrow

A1. True
In the first three decades of life more than half of the marrow is composed of hematopoietic cells. From the fourth to the seventh decade there is relative stabilization of the number of hematopoietic cells; beginning in the eighth decade there is a renewed decrease. **(p. 2052)**

A2. False
The subcortical area of the bone marrow may normally be hypocellular. Specimens that contain a substantial amount of subcortical marrow may be inadequate for estimating cellularity. In addition, the immediate paratrabecular areas may be preferentially hypocellular. **(p. 2052)**

Alterations in cellularity, necrosis and inflammation

A1. True
Acquired aplastic anemia may be idiopathic or result from known exposure to drugs, chemicals, viral infections or ionizing radiation. Fanconi's anemia is a syndrome of familial hypoplastic anemia. **(p. 2053)**

A2. True
In the most severe form of aplastic anemia the intertrabecular marrow space is occupied predominantly by adipose tissue with scattered lymphocytes, plasma cells, tissue mast cells and hemosiderin-laden macrophages. In less severe processes there is an increased amount of fat tissue and scattered small collections of erythroblasts, granulocytes and megakaryocytes. **(p. 2053)**

A3. False
These can generally be distinguished from true aplastic anemia by the population of blasts and immature granulocytes, in contrast to the mature lymphocytes, plasma cells and tissue mast cells in aplastic/hypoplastic marrows. The use of anti-CD34 is an additional aid in identifying blast cells. **(p. 2054)**

A4. True
One of the major problems in the evaluation of marrow from patients with benign disorders is that the proliferating erythroblasts or other myeloid cells may be misinterpreted as a leukemic proliferation; examination of the blood and marrow smears will prevent the possibility of this type of error. **(p. 2054)**

A5. False

It is an epiphenomenon associated with extreme malnourishment and weight loss and is reversible with resolution of the nutritional problem. The etiology is somewhat age related: anorexia nervosa, AIDS and acute febrile illnesses are the most common factors in young individuals, alcoholism and lymphomas in middle age, and carcinomas, lymphomas and congestive heart failure in older individuals. It is characterized by atrophy of fat cells and hematopoietic cells and the accumulation of serous fluid in the interstitium. **(p. 2054)**

A6. False

The diagnostic features of osteopetrosis include marked thickening of the bone trabeculae and a marked reduction in the medullary cavity. The decreased marrow hematopoiesis leads to extramedullary hematopoiesis with splenomegaly and a leukoerythroblastic blood picture. **(p. 2055)**

A7. True

In the early stages of necrosis the nuclei show pyknosis and karyorrhexis, and the cells have a granular appearance; this is followed by karyolysis. In advanced stages all cell outlines disappear, and the marrow space is replaced by an amorphous, granular eosinophilic debris. **(p. 2055)**

A8. True

The etiologic bases include fungi, *Mycobacterium tuberculosis, Mycobacterium avium intracellulare*, sarcoidosis, *Mycoplasma pneumoniae*, and viral infections such as infectious mononucleosis. Granulomas may also be found in patients with Hodgkin's disease and non-Hodgkin's lymphomas with or without marrow involvement by the lymphoma. Perivascular granulomas may be related to hypersensitivity states. **(p. 2056)**

A9. True

Marrow biopsies from patients with AIDS may contain scattered macrophages with acid-fast bacilli in the absence of granuloma formation. An increased number of macrophages with or without evident phagocytosis is sufficient reason to perform special stains for microorganisms. **(p. 2057)**

A10. True

These systemic disorders include acute infection, malignancy, connective tissue disease and immune disorders, most notably AIDS. **(p. 2059)**

A11. False

These terms have been applied to the nonspecific marrow changes observed in a high percentage of patients with malignant lymphoma. Such changes include edema of the vessel walls, plasma cell and mast cell proliferations in the adventitia, protein deposits adjacent to the vessels, patchy edema, depressed erythropoiesis, and increased granulopoiesis and megakaryocytopoiesis. **(p. 2059)**

A12. False

Bone marrow biopsies in this group of patients are usually hypercellular, although normocellular and hypocellular specimens may be observed. Nonspecific findings include marrow damage, increased plasma cells, myelodysplasia, serous degeneration, lymphocytic infiltration, increased reticulin and 'naked' megakaryocytic nuclei. **(p. 2059)**

A13. False

Lymphocytic aggregates of varying size occur in the marrow of a relatively high percentage of patients with AIDS. These are randomly distributed without preferential paratrabecular distribution; in some cases the lesions appear to be preferentially perisinusoidal. They are composed primarily of small lymphocytes, some of which may have irregularly shaped nuclei. There are usually associated plasma cells, histiocytes and increased vascular structures; eosinophils may be increased. **(p. 2059)**

A14. False

This finding is not specific for AIDS and may be present in other disorders, including the myeloproliferative diseases. **(p. 2060)**

Leukemias and related disorders

A1. True

Although smears and imprint preparations are generally superior to sections in classifying the majority of cases of acute leukemia, there are some types of acute leukemia that are accompanied by fibrosis or with unusual morphologic patterns in which the bone marrow sections are more informative than the bone marrow smears. **(p. 2060)**

A2. True

In the majority of cases of acute leukemia the marrow is markedly hypercellular because of the proliferation of leukemic cells, with replacement of normal hematopoietic cells. **(p. 2061)**

A3. True

The erythroid cells are usually the first to recover and frequently manifest dyserythropoietic changes as the result of chemotherapeutic drugs. The regeneration of the erythroid cells is followed in sequence by that of the granulocytes and megakaryocytes. **(p. 2062)**

A4. True

In acute panmyelosis with myelofibrosis there is hyperplasia of all three myeloid cell lines. The megakaryocytes may be particularly conspicuous; there may be considerable size variation, from very small megakaryocytes with non-lobulated nuclei to large cells with bizarre nuclear shapes. The nuclear chromatin is usually finely stippled, in contrast to the megakaryocytes in chronic idiopathic myelofibrosis in which the chromatin is more dense. **(p. 2063)**

A5. False

Myeloid sarcoma is an unusual variant of myeloid malignancy in which there is an extramedullary tumor mass composed of either myeloblasts alone or myeloblasts and more mature neutrophils. The tumor may occur as an isolated finding or may be associated with acute myeloid leukemia, chronic myeloid leukemia, chronic idiopathic myelofibrosis, hypereosinophilic syndrome and polycythemia vera. **(p. 2065)**

A6. True

In a minority of cases the marrow is hypocellular. Seven major categories have been proposed in the World Health Organization classification of hematopoietic neoplasms: refractory anemia; idiopathic refractory sideroblastic anemia with unilineage dysplasia; refractory cytopenia with multilineage dysplasia; refractory anemia with excess blasts-1; refractory anemia with excess blasts-2; myelodysplastic syndrome, unclassified; and the isolated 5q– syndrome. **(p. 2066)**

A7. True

A finding referred to as abnormal localization of immature precursors (ALIP) is characterized by aggregates (three to five cells) and clusters (more than five cells) of myeloblasts and promyelocytes in central areas of the marrow tissue away from the endosteal surface of the bone trabeculae and vascular structures. **(p. 2067)**

A8. False

Although the precise classification of the myelodysplastic syndromes is based principally on the evaluation of blood and marrow smears, there are some forms of myelodysplastic syndrome in which the bone marrow biopsy findings are highly suggestive of a specific process. **(p. 2067)**

A9. True

The marrow biopsy usually shows increased normal-sized to slightly smaller megakaryocytes, many with hypolobulated nuclei. **(p. 2067)**

A10. True

Two major forms have been recognized: alkylating agent/radiation-related type and topoisomerase II inhibitor-related type. **(p. 2067)**

A11. False

It is characterized by an elevated leukocyte count with basophilia, decreased neutrophil alkaline phosphatase, and the presence of the Philadelphia chromosome and/or molecular evidence of the *bcr-abl* hybrid gene in the hematopoietic cells. The number of myeloblasts in the blood and marrow smears in the chronic phase does not usually exceed 5%. The finding of more than 20% of myeloblasts in the blood and marrow smears denotes a blast transformation of chronic myeloid leukemia. **(p. 2068)**

A12. True

The hematologic remission is accompanied in most cases by morphologic normalization or near normalization of the bone marrow. The normalization of the marrow may occur even with persistence of the Philadelphia chromosome, or evidence of the *abl-bcr* hybrid gene. **(p. 2069)**

A13. False

The neutrophil alkaline phosphatase is elevated or at the upper range of normal in most patients. The bone marrow is usually markedly hypercellular; the major diagnostic feature is an increased red cell mass, and there are usually splenomegaly and some degree of leukocytosis and thrombocytosis. **(p. 2070)**

A14. True

An additional complication in some patients is the occurrence of acute myeloid leukemia; the incidence is higher in patients treated with chemotherapy, ^{32}P or radiation, as opposed to those treated only with phlebotomy. **(p. 2070)**

A15. False

It is an indolent myeloproliferative disorder characterized by increased megakaryocytes and thrombocytosis. The marrow is usually normocellular for age, but may be hyper- or hypocellular. **(p. 2070)**

A16. True

It occurs primarily in adults: the average age at diagnosis is approximately 60 years. There is some degree of detectable hepatosplenomegaly caused by extramedullary hematopoiesis. **(p. 2071)**

A17. True

In addition, the neutrophil alkaline phosphatase is decreased in approximately 90% of patients with chronic myeloid leukemia, and is normal or increased in the majority of patients with idiopathic myelofibrosis. Marrow fibrosis in chronic myeloid leukemia is generally a late occurrence and its onset usually heralds a more aggressive evolution, unlike idiopathic myelofibrosis, in which marrow fibrosis is present to some extent from the start and is generally associated with a more prolonged clinical course. **(p. 2071)**

A18. False

The aforementioned description characterizes the fibrotic stage of chronic idiopathic myelofibrosis. The prefibrotic stage is characterized by hypercellularity for age; there is an increase in abnormal megakaryocytes and granulocytes. Erythroid precursors may be reduced. There is no or only a minimal increase in reticulin fibers. **(p. 2071)**

A19. True

A minor population of patients with this disorder has a more rapid course, with a median survival of approximately 2 years. **(p. 2073)**

A20. True

The diagnosis of B-cell chronic lymphocytic leukemia is usually established when there is a persistent absolute lymphocytosis in excess of 10 000. It is usually accompanied by some degree of lymphadenopathy and hepatosplenomegaly. The distinction between these two closely related entities is based on arbitrary criteria: if the marrow shows a pattern of infiltration by small lymphocytes and the absolute lymphocyte count in the blood is fewer than 5×10^9/L, the diagnosis of well-differentiated lymphocytic lymphoma is more appropriate. **(p. 2073)**

A21. False

They are predominantly in low clinical stages. The diffuse or focal and diffuse patterns generally occur in patients with advanced clinical stages. **(p. 2073)**

A22. True

The syndrome is usually characterized by an abrupt change in clinical course, with the onset of fever, weight loss, localized adenopathy, dysglobulinemia, and histopathologic evidence of a pleomorphic lymphoma frequently containing multinucleated giant cells. **(p. 2075)**

A23. False

Prolymphocytic leukemia occurs primarily in older individuals and is characterized by a predominant proliferation of immature lymphocytes referred to as prolymphocytes. The number of prolymphocytes in the blood usually exceeds 55% of lymphocytes and may be more than 90%. The patient with B-cell prolymphocytic leukemia usually has massive splenomegaly without prominent peripheral lymphadenopathy. **(p. 2076)**

A24. True

The age range is 20–80 years, with a median of approximately 50 years. Patients generally have cytopenia or pancytopenia and splenomegaly without prominent peripheral lymphadenopathy. **(p. 2076)**

A25. True

Hairy cells express light chain-restricted cytoplasmic and surface immunoglobulin and pan-B cell antibodies; CD20 (L26) and DBA44 are of considerable aid in evaluating the extent of the leukemic infiltrate and in assessing the effects of chemotherapy in paraffin-embedded biopsy sections. Hairy cells also contain tartrate-resistant acid phosphatase (TRAP), which is a useful diagnostic feature of the disease. **(p. 2077)**

A26. False

It usually presents with marked leukocytosis and lymphocytes with morphologic characteristics intermediate between hairy cells and prolymphocytes. In contrast to typical hairy cell leukemia, there is no associated neutropenia and monocytopenia. **(p. 2078)**

A27. True

High magnification of a lesion is characterized by a predominant population of small lymphocytes with scattered large cells having abundant cytoplasm and prominent nucleoli. Mitotic figures are usually sparse. **(p. 2079)**

A28. True

Patients with splenic lymphoma with villous lymphocytes, not infected with hepatitis C, do not respond to the same therapy. **(p. 2080)**

Non-Hodgkin's lymphoma

A1. True

Approximately 60–70% of cases of follicular center cell lymphoma have marrow involvement at the time of initial diagnosis, in contrast to 33% for T-immunoblastic lymphoma and 25% for B-immunoblastic lymphoma. Splenic marginal zone B-cell lymphoma has a very high incidence of involvement. Marrow involvement in MALT-lymphoma has been reported in approximately 20% of cases. **(p. 2080)**

A2. False

The diffuse and focal non-paratrabecular patterns may occur with all types of lymphoma of both B- and T-cell type. Follicular lymphomas may also involve the marrow in a focal non-paratrabecular pattern. Marrow biopsies from patients with mantle cell lymphoma and splenic marginal zone B-cell lymphoma may also show both focal paratrabecular and non-paratrabecular lesions. **(p. 2080)**

A3. False

It occurs most frequently with splenic marginal zone B-cell lymphoma and γ/δ T-cell lymphoma, in which it may be the predominant pattern of involvement. **(p. 2081)**

A4. False

This is true for T-cell lymphomas and Burkitt's lymphoma. In approximately 20–25% of lymphomas, predominantly follicular, there may be discordance between the predominant cell type in the lymph node and the predominant cell type in the marrow. In these cases, the marrow lesions usually consist of small cleaved cells and the lymph node findings are a mixed or large cell type; the converse occurs but is less common. **(p. 2082)**

A5. True

Cases in which the lymph node has a diffuse pattern of involvement, such as small lymphocytic lymphoma or chronic lymphocytic leukemia, may manifest as focal lesions in the marrow. Cases with a follicular pattern in the lymph node may manifest as diffuse marrow involvement. **(p. 2083)**

A6. True

The marrow lesions are diffuse in approximately 60% of involved cases and focal in 40%. The focal lesions are usually randomly distributed, in contrast to the preferential paratrabecular involvement in follicular center cell lymphomas. **(p. 2083)**

A7. False

The predominant cytologic pattern in the marrow lesions of peripheral T-cell lymphoma usually corresponds to the pattern in lymph node or other tissue biopsies and can generally be categorized into one of three primary histopathologic types: small lymphocytic, mixed cell, and large cell/immunoblastic. The mixed cell type is the most frequently encountered. **(p. 2085)**

A8. True

Epithelioid histiocytes are frequently noted, either in focal clusters or scattered throughout the lesions. The focal collections frequently have a granulomatous appearance. **(p. 2085)**

A9. True

Distinction between the focal lesions of peripheral T-cell lymphoma and the polymorphous reactive lymphoid lesions may not be possible on morphologic features alone. Markedly atypical cells with prominent nucleoli are more compatible with lymphoma. The size of the lesions is not always a reliable distinguishing feature: reactive lesions may show extensive marrow replacement, particularly in patients with AIDS. The lesions of peripheral T-cell lymphoma may be relatively small. **(p. 2085)**

A10. True

Multinucleated immunoblasts resembling Reed–Sternberg cells may be present in peripheral T-cell lymphoma; in these instances, review of lymph nodes and other tissue biopsies and immunologic studies is critical in distinguishing peripheral T-cell lymphoma from Hodgkin's disease. **(p. 2085)**

A11. False

Clonal rearrangement of one of the T-cell receptors is substantial evidence of a malignant process. The determination of clonality may be made on fresh aspirate or trephine biopsy specimens and fixed, paraffin-embedded tissue. **(p. 2086)**

A12. True

The leukocyte count may be normal or markedly elevated, with a high percentage of Sézary cells. The Sézary cells, as observed in Romanowsky-stained blood smears, have distinctive features. The nuclei of Sézary cells frequently have an unusual configuration that has been characterized as cerebriform. **(p. 2086)**

A13. False

Large granulated T-cell lymphocytic leukemia is an uncommon form of T-cell leukemia that usually presents with a modest lymphocytosis and frequently severe neutropenia. Approximately 50% of patients have splenomegaly, but lymphadenopathy is uncommon. **(p. 2086)**

A14. False
The lesions of angioimmunoblastic T-cell lymphoma contain varying proportions of lymphocytes, immunoblasts, plasma cells, histiocytes, neutrophils and eosinophils. Vascular proliferation, endothelial cells and fibroblasts are frequently identified. **(p. 2088)**

A15. True
The lymphoma cells are distinguished from neutrophil myelocytes by the lack of specific granules. **(p. 2089)**

Lymphoma/leukemia

A1. False
The 'starry sky' appearance is infrequently present in bone marrow biopsies. **(p. 2091)**

A2. True
If there are fewer than 25% lymphoblasts in the bone marrow the case is classified as lymphoma; if there are more than 25% the case is classified as leukemia. **(p. 2091)**

Benign lymphocytic aggregates

A1. True
Benign aggregates are usually few in number, well circumscribed, loosely structured, and contain histiocytes and plasma cells and frequently mast cells in addition to lymphocytes. The lymphocytes are usually small with generally round nuclei that have condensed chromatin and inconspicuous or no evident nucleoli. Vascular structures are frequently present. **(p. 2092)**

A2. False
A preferential paratrabecular localization of a lymphoid infiltrate is evidence for a diagnosis of lymphoma. A random distribution of lymphoid aggregates with an occasional aggregate juxtaposed to a trabecula has no diagnostic specificity, as this pattern may occur with benign or malignant lesions. **(p. 2092)**

Hodgkin's lymphoma

A1. False
It is approximately 10% in classic Hodgkin's mixed cellularity type and approximately 1% in lymphocyte-predominant and lymphocyte-rich classic Hodgkin's lymphoma. Nodular sclerosis has an incidence of approximately 3%. **(p. 2094)**

A2. False
Marrow involvement is significantly associated with B symptoms, bulky disease, involvement of lymph nodes both above and below the diaphragm, and negatively correlated with the diameter of a mediastinal mass. **(p. 2094)**

A3. True
Fibrosis is a common finding in Hodgkin's lesions in the marrow and is not limited to nodular sclerosis and lymphocyte-depletion types. **(p. 2094)**

A4. True
Definitive histopathologic criteria for the diagnosis of marrow involvement in Hodgkin's lymphoma include typical Reed–Sternberg cells on a cellular background characteristic of Hodgkin's lymphoma, or mononuclear Reed–Sternberg variants on a cellular background typical of Hodgkin's lymphoma if typical Reed–Sternberg cells are identified in other specimens. **(p. 2096)**

Histiocytic disorders

A1. True

Cell marker studies for B- and T-cell lineage should be performed to exclude poorly differentiated lymphomas. Poorly differentiated carcinomas and plasmablastic tumors must also be excluded. Because the macrophage is derived from the monocyte system it may be difficult in some instances to distinguish between what is termed malignant histiocytosis and what is monoblastic/monocytic leukemia. **(p. 2096)**

A2. False

It should be reactive with antibodies to lysozyme and CD68 and non-reactive to antibodies to T and B lymphocytes. There may be some degree of reactivity with antibody to S-100 protein. **(p. 2097)**

A3. True

Viruses associated with this disorder include cytomegalovirus, Epstein–Barr virus, adenovirus and parvovirus B_{19}. The process has been observed with bacterial and protozoan infections. **(p. 2097)**

A4. True

The marrow smears of patients with hemophagocytic syndromes contain numerous histiocytes, many showing evidence of phagocytosis of erythrocytes and precursors, platelets and granulocytes. **(p. 2097)**

A5. False

Marrow involvement is uncommon and usually associated with the multisystem, multifocal form of the disease. The marrow lesions may be focal, small and barely perceptible, or confluent and extensive, replacing large areas of a biopsy. Immunohistochemical reactions for S-100 protein and CD1a highlight the Langerhans' cell infiltrate. However, with some fixatives and decalcifying agents the reaction with antibody to CD1a may be suboptimal in bone marrow biopsies. **(p. 2098)**

Plasma cell dyscrasias

A1. True

In trephine sections the distribution of plasma cells may be focal, interstitial, diffuse, or a combination of these patterns. **(p. 2100)**

A2. True

The more immature or poorly differentiated the myeloma cells, i.e. plasmablastic, and the more extensive the marrow involvement (>50% replacement), the more unfavorable the prognosis. **(p. 2101)**

A3. True

The plasma cells in anaplastic myeloma are usually of the IgG or IgA heavy chain class, in contrast to B-immunoblastic lymphoma in which the cells are IgM. **(p. 2102)**

A4. False

These patients have a higher incidence of organomegaly and the prognosis is unfavorable. **(p. 2102)**

A5. True

A high percentage of patients with osteosclerotic myeloma have multiorgan involvement, including polyneuropathy, organomegaly, endocrinopathy and skin changes, the so-called 'POEMS syndrome.' **(p. 2102)**

A6. True

The risk for progression to myeloma or a related disorder at 10 years was 6% for an initial monoclonal protein of 0.5 g/dL or less, compared to 34% for an initial monoclonal protein of 3.0 g/dL. Monoclonal proteins of IgM or IgA type carry a higher risk of progression than IgG paraprotein. **(p. 2104)**

A7. False

They are more frequent in males and the peak incidence is in the sixth decade. **(p. 2104)**

A8. True

The solitary plasmacytoma of bone may occur in both flat and long bones; the most common site is the axial skeleton, particularly a vertebra. The most frequent sites of extramedullary or soft tissue plasmacytomas are the nasal fossa, maxillary sinus and nasopharynx. **(p. 2104)**

A9. False

The solitary plasmocytoma is characterized by a normal hemoglobin level and no hypercalcemia. **(p. 2105)**

A10. True

Hepatosplenomegaly, lymphadenopathy and neurologic abnormalities are frequent findings; anemia and hyperviscosity are commonly noted laboratory abnormalities. **(p. 2105)**

A11. True

A similar population of cells predominates in the bone marrow. Mature plasma cells, tissue mast cells and histiocytes may also be increased. In some cases plasma cells may predominate. **(p. 2106)**

A12. False

These inclusions, which are variably PAS positive, may be observed in other lymphomas, multiple myeloma and reactive proliferations, and are not diagnostic of lymphoplasmacytic lymphoma. **(p. 2106)**

A13. True

Hepatomegaly, splenomegaly and peripheral lymphadenopathy are each present in slightly more than half of the cases. Anemia, leukopenia and thrombocytopenia also occur frequently. **(p. 2106)**

Systemic mastocytosis

A1. True

The bone marrow is the most frequent site of non-cutaneous involvement in systemic mastocytosis. **(p. 2108)**

A2. True

The clinical symptoms are varied and include diarrhea, weakness, fractures, weight loss, arthralgia, flushing episodes and bronchospasm. **(p. 2109)**

A3. False

Focal lesions are more common and may be paratrabecular, perivascular, or randomly distributed. The paratrabecular lesions are frequently marked by a margination of the infiltrate along the endosteal surface of the bone structure or juxtaposition of a lesion to a bone spicule. The perivascular lesions may be associated with prominent medial and adventitial hypertrophy and collagen fibrosis. **(p. 2109)**

A4. True

The chronic myeloproliferative disorder occurring with systemic mastocytosis displays many features of chronic myelomonocytic leukemia or an unclassified chronic myeloproliferative disorder. **(p. 2110)**

A5. False

The mast cells may be very atypical and there may be considerable difficulty in recognizing their true nature. These cells may possess very abundant cytoplasm without evident granules, or have a fibroblastic appearance. Mast cell granules react with both toluidine blue and Giemsa stains. The primary distinction of mastocytosis from other disorders is based on the immunohistochemical demonstration of mast cells with antibody to mast cell tryptase. **(p. 2111)**

Metastatic tumors

A1. True

The tumors most frequently detected in bone marrow biopsies in adults are carcinoma of the breast, prostate, lung, stomach, colon, kidney and thyroid gland. **(p. 2112)**

A2. False

This is marrow from a patient with metastatic carcinoma with osteosclerotic reaction and foci of tumor cells. The approach to determining the site of origin of a metastatic tumor in a patient without a known primary lesion should be the same as for determining metastatic lesions in other sites. **(p. 2112)**

Lipid storage diseases

A1. True

The characteristic diagnostic morphologic feature of Gaucher's disease is the presence of Gaucher cells in the bone marrow, spleen, liver, lymph nodes and other organs. The cytoplasm has a characteristic fibrillary or striated pattern and is pale blue-gray in color. **(p. 2114)**

A2. False

The three major clinical types of Niemann–Pick disease are an acute neuronopathic form, a chronic form without nervous system involvement, and a chronic neuronopathic form. **(p. 2115)**

Bone marrow transplantation

A1. True

The major complications associated with bone marrow transplantation involve infection in the severely immunosuppressed host, graft rejection, and graft-versus-host disease. **(p. 2116)**

A2. False

Initially, foci of hematopoietic cells are usually unilineage and composed of tight clusters of erythroid precursors followed by aggregates of promyelocytes and myelocytes. Megakaryocyte reconstitution may lag behind the granulocytic and erythroid cells for prolonged periods. **(p. 2117)**

24 Bone and joints

Normal anatomy

Q1

Growing long bones have three distinct anatomic regions.

Q2

Osteoid is an unmineralized organic precursor matrix of bone.

Q3

Calvaria is formed through endochondral ossification.

Metabolic, inflammatory and non-neoplastic diseases

Q1

Osteoporosis represents a decreased mass of normally mineralized bone that can be reliably diagnosed by iliac crest bone biopsy.

Q2

Woven bone is a sign of a neoplastic process.

Q3

Foreign body giant cell reaction develops around a non-corrosive nail introduced into the medullary cavity of long bones for repair of fracture.

Q4

Osteomyelitis in young boys is most often caused by Gram-negative bacteria.

Q5

Chronic osteomyelitis may be accompanied by prominent periosteal proliferation and the formation of epithelium-lined sinuses extending deeply into the bone.

Q6

Aseptic bone necrosis in otherwise healthy person occurs most often because of the interruption of blood supply.

Tumors

Q1

In the diagnosis of bone sarcomas the microscopic appearance of the biopsy is the only parameter that determines the diagnosis.

Q2

Intense trauma of the bone in early childhood is associated with the development of a bone tumor in the adult life.

Q3

Aspirin can cure osteoid osteoma.

Q4

This recurrent bone tumor involving the spine most likely represents an osteoblastoma.

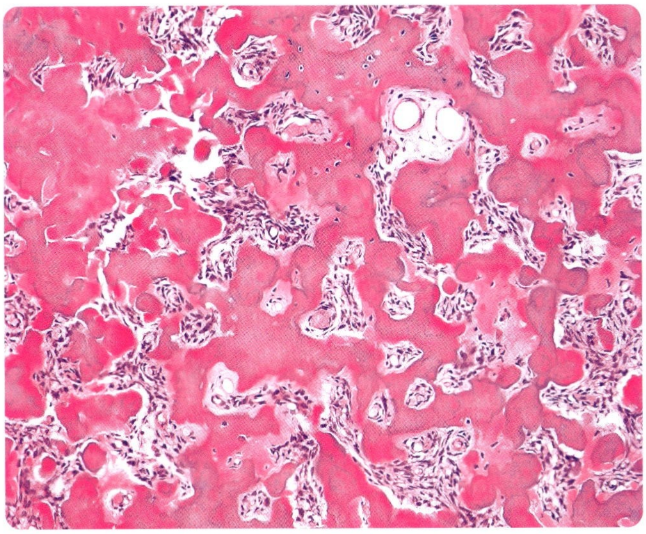

Fig. 24.1

Q5

A bone tumor arising in a metaphysis of lower femur in an 11-year-old boy with destruction of the cortex and elevation of the periosteum is most likely benign.

Q6

A malignant bone tumor with areas of fibroblastic chondroblastic differentiation and osteoid production is best diagnosed as osteosarcoma.

Q7

Conventional osteosarcomas have a characteristic 11;22 translocation, which is important for the diagnosis of this tumor.

Q8

Small cell osteosarcoma is characterized by a chromosomal translocation t(11;22)(q24;q12).

Q9

A slowly growing large lobulated mass around the knee joint with minimal cortical involvement and showing slightly atypical spindle cell tumor and irregularly shaped bone trabecules is characteristic of parosteal osteosarcoma.

Q10

Periosteal osteosarcoma is synonymous with parosteal osteosarcoma.

Q11

Post-chemotherapy tumor necrosis is the single most important prognostic parameter in conventional osteosarcoma of the extremities with no evidence of distant metastases at initial presentation.

Q12

A small expansile calcified tumor in the proximal phalanx of a hand is most likely an enchondroma, regardless of the age of the patient.

Q13

Multiple enchondromas associated with soft tissue hemangiomas (including spindle cell hemangioendotheliomas) carry no risk of malignant transformation.

Q14

Osteochondroma is the most common benign bone tumor.

Q15

A cellular tumor consisting of neoplastic chondroblasts, multinucleated osteoclast-like giant cells and chondroid matrix arising in the epiphysis of an 18-year-old man is most likely a chondroblastoma.

Q16

This tumor is most likely a chondromyxoid fibroma and it frequently recurs after a curettage.

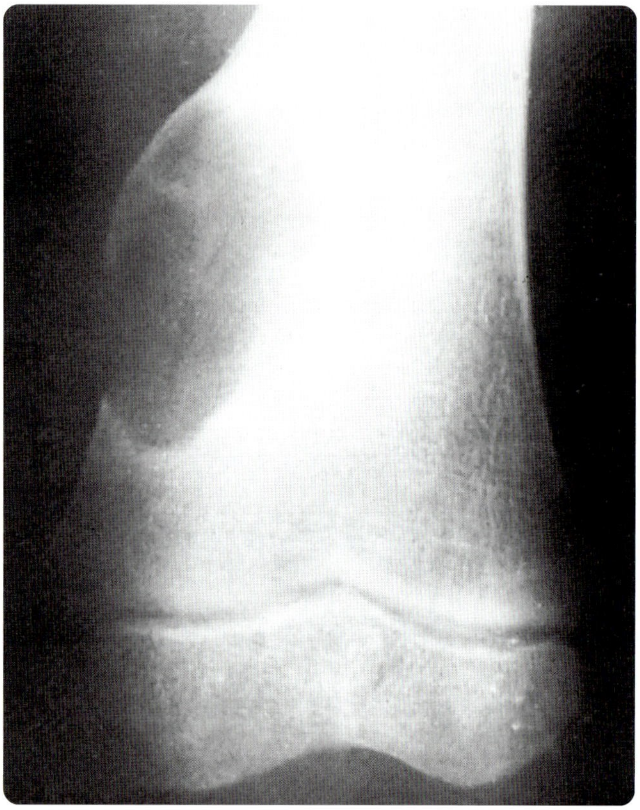

Fig. 24.2

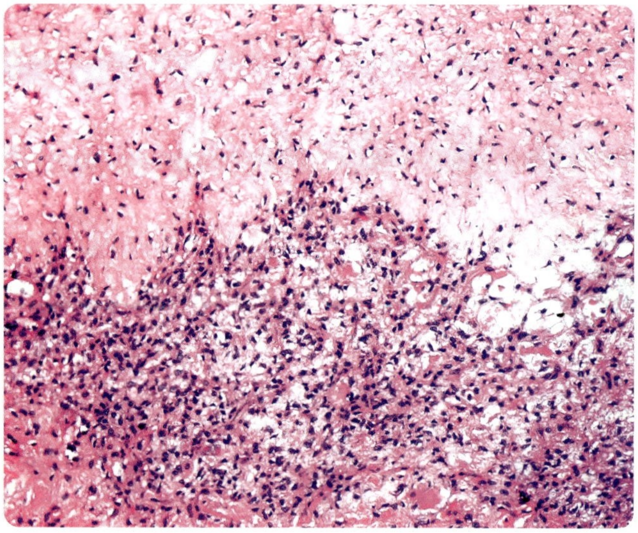

Fig. 24.3

Q17

Chondrosarcoma is distinguished from osteosarcoma by the lack of direct osteoid or bone formation by the tumor cells.

Q18

Cartilaginous tumor with a minor degree of cellular atypia but with the radiologic signs of aggressive growth is nevertheless benign.

Q19

Chondrosarcomas are positive for S-100 protein in immunohistochemical assays.

Q20

A dimorphic tumor in which areas of well-differentiated cartilage alternate with undifferentiated stroma composed of small cells positive for CD99 is best diagnosed as Ewing sarcoma.

Q21

An entirely lytic expansile lesion in the epiphysis, usually without peripheral bone sclerosis, or periosteal reaction in a 25-year-old appearing at the lower end of femur and causing a pathologic fracture, is most likely a giant cell tumor.

Q22

These figures illustrate the typical features of Ewing sarcoma involving the diaphysis of a long bone in a child.

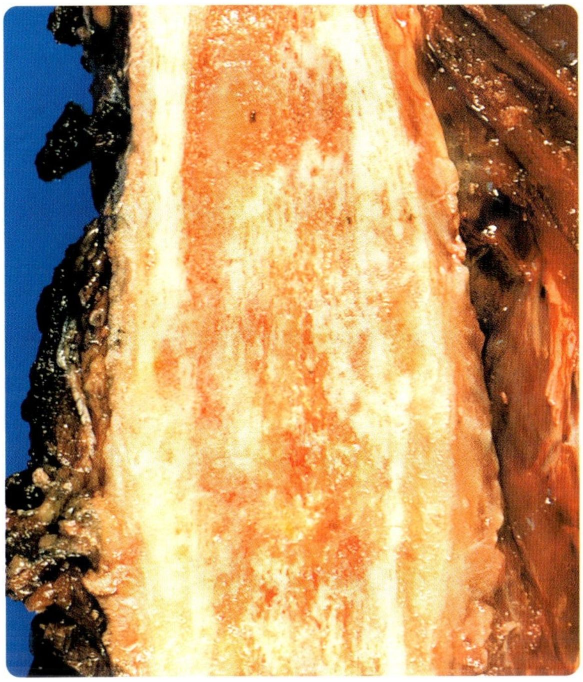

Fig. 24.4

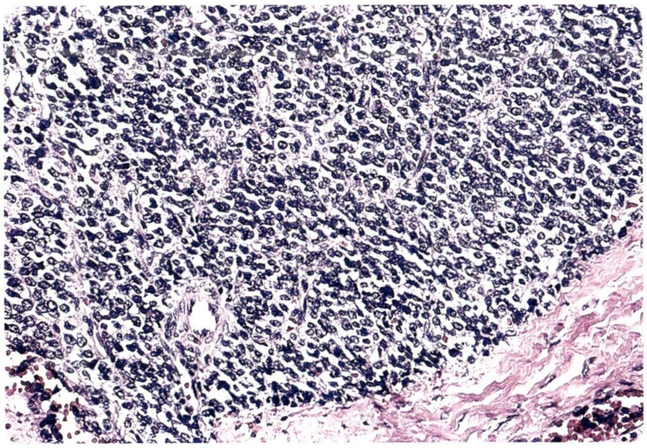

Fig. 24.5

Q23

The chromosomal translocation t11;22(q24;q12) can be used in primary diagnosis of Ewing sarcoma and is more reliable than the immunohistochemical reactivity with antibodies to CD99.

Q24

A jawbone tumor in a child showing diffuse growth of small cells with prominent nucleoli, numerous mitoses and a prominent starry sky pattern is consistent with PNET.

Q25

An epithelioid cell tumor of a bone with cells showing abundant acidophilic and vacuolated cytoplasm, a large vesicular nucleus (sometimes with prominent grooves), modest atypia and prominent myxoid stroma that is FVIII, CD31 and CD34 positive is best diagnosed as epithelioid hemangioendothelioma.

Q26

A lytic lesion of bone with mature adipose tissue dystrophic calcification, fat necrosis and hemorrhage is best diagnosed as marrow infarct.

Q27

Chordoma is a tumor of the sacrococcygeal area with symptoms of spinal cord compression that microscopically shows cords and lobules of cells with extensive myxoid stroma and positivity for cytokeratins, EMA and S100.

Q28

Cytokeratin expression in a lytic bone tumor of an adult is diagnostic of metastatic carcinoma.

Q29

An expansive lobulated tumor of the tibia that microscopically shows a biphasic mixture of small basaloid cells and an osteofibrous component is most likely a metastatic basal cell carcinoma.

Q30

Aneurysmal bone cyst is a reactive process due to the resorption of hemorrhage.

Q31

These figures show the typical features of benign fibrous histiocytoma of bone, also known as metaphyseal fibrous defect.

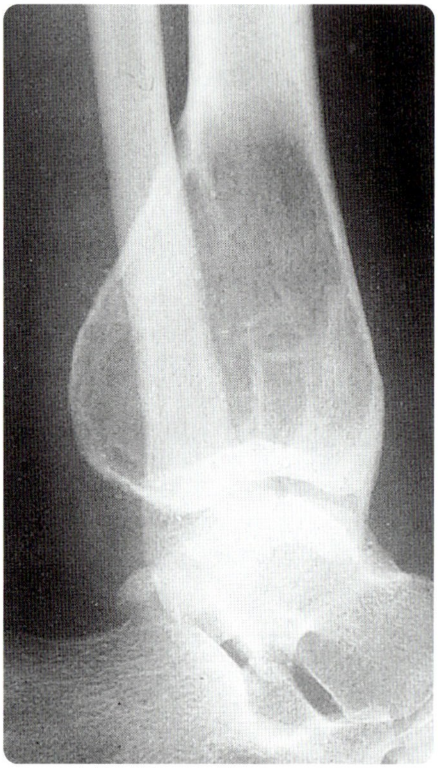

Fig. 24.6

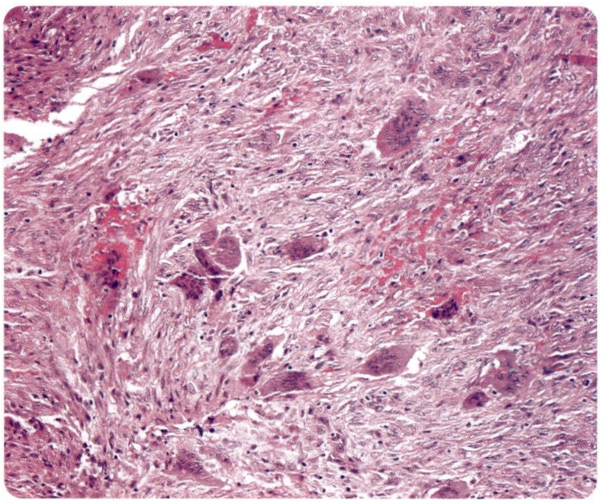

Fig. 24.7

Q32

Fibrous dysplasia may affect one or many bones.

Q33

Osteofibrous dysplasia is characterized by scattered bony spicules without osteoblast rimming and fibrous tissue of variable cellularity.

Q34

Juxtacortical osteosarcoma shows a maturational (zonal) pattern characterized by a central cellular area, an intermediate zone of osteoid formation, and a peripheral shell of highly organized bone.

Q35

This figure shows the typical microscopic features of Langerhans' histiocytosis presenting as an osteolytic bone lesion.

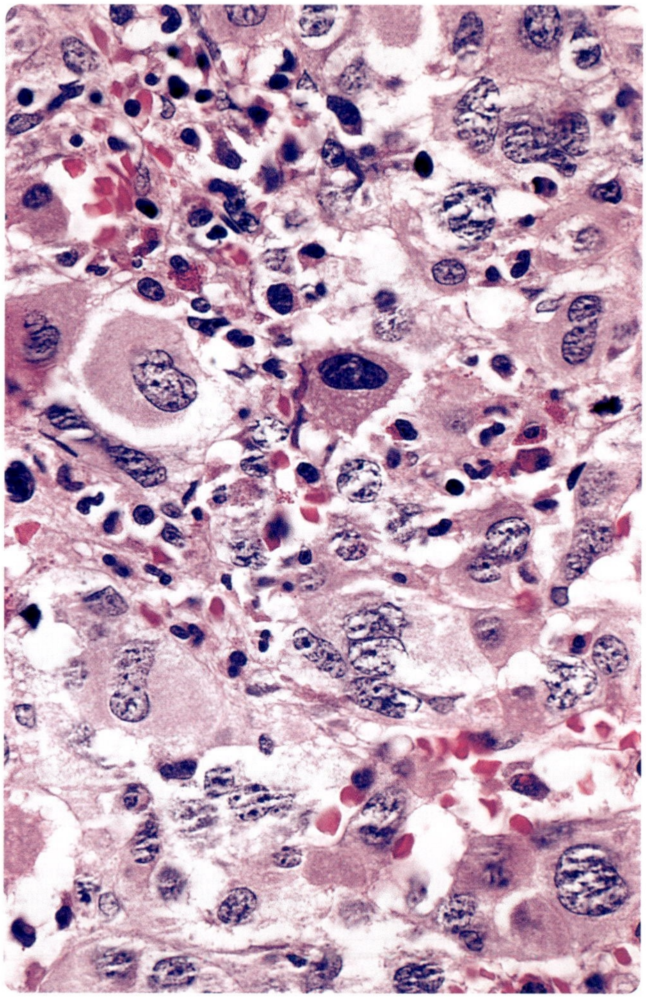

Fig. 24.8

Q36

A circumscribed soft tissue tumor found near the interphalangeal joint of a finger in a middle-aged otherwise healthy woman is most likely a giant cell tumor of the tendon sheath.

Q37

An ill-defined peri-articular mass around the knee joint composed of small histiocytes, foamy cells, hemosiderin-laden macrophages, and showing papillary projections is best diagnosed as diffuse-type giant cell tumor.

Q38

Synovial chondrosarcoma is an exceptionally rare entity that closely resembles synovial chondromatosis.

Q39

Synovial hemangioma most commonly presents in the knees of young males.

Normal anatomy

A1. True

The long bones are divided topographically into three regions: diaphysis, epiphysis and metaphysis. The diaphysis is the shaft. The epiphysis is at both ends of the bone and is partially covered by articular cartilage. The metaphysis is at the junction of the diaphysis and epiphysis. **(p. 2137)**

A2. True

It is an acidophilic material (on H&E staining) composed of a mixture of collagenous (mainly type I) and non-collagenous proteins and mucopolysaccharides. **(p. 2138)**

A3. False

Skull bones such as the calvaria are formed through membranous ossification, whereas the long bones of the extremities are formed through endochondral ossification. **(p. 2138)**

Metabolic, inflammatory and non-neoplastic diseases

A1. True

In osteoporosis both the osteoid and the calcium salts are lost from the bones. The disease develops when an individual is unable to repair and maintain the mass of bone tissue that has been acquired through growth and maturation. It is reliably diagnosed by iliac crest bone biopsy. **(p. 2139)**

A2. False

In woven bone (fiber bone) there is a haphazard arrangement of collagen fibers within the matrix, which is best appreciated with reticulum stains or under polarized light. The formation of woven bone is the key criterion for the diagnosis of fibrous dysplasia, but it also appears in any condition associated with accelerated bone turnover, such as the callus of a healing fracture and osteitis fibrosa cystica. **(p. 2139)**

A3. False

These nails are separated from the medullary cavity by fibrous tissue that is continuous with the periosteum. No foreign body giant cell reaction is observed. **(p. 2140)**

A4. False

Osteomyelitis is in 70–90% of cases caused by coagulase-positive staphylococci. *Salmonella* is a well-known cause of osteomyelitis in persons who have sickle cell anemia. **(p. 2140)**

A5. True

Periosteal reaction may be prominent and is visible on X-ray examination. Sinuses originally formed from the extension of the skin into the area of inflammation may become discontinuous from the skin. They may become filled with keratin-containing debris, similar to epidermal inclusion cysts of the skin. **(p. 2142)**

A6. True

Bone necrosis is most often caused by ischemia related to fracture or dislocation. Thus it is usually called avascular, and as it is not related to infection it is also called aseptic. **(p. 2143)**

Tumors

A1. False

The five basic parameters of importance in this regard are the age of the patient, the bone involved, specific area within the bone (epiphysis, metaphysis or diaphysis; cortex, medulla or periosteum), radiographic appearance, and microscopic appearance. **(p. 2147)**

A2. False

This is an interesting myth perpetuated on all continents and in all nations (particularly among grandmothers). Trauma usually only calls attention to an already present advanced bone tumor. **(p. 2150)**

A3. False

The pain associated with osteoid osteoma is characteristically more intense at night, relieved by non-steroidal anti-inflammatory drugs such as aspirin, and eliminated by the excision of the lesion. **(p. 2149)**

A4. True

The differential diagnosis for tumors composed of plump osteoblastic cells forming osteoid includes osteoid osteoma, osteoblastoma and osteosarcoma. Osteoblastoma is closely related to osteoid osteoma both microscopically and ultrastructurally. It is distinguished from the latter by the larger size of the nidus and the absence or inconspicuousness of a surrounding area of reactive bone formation. Osteosarcomas usually show more pronounced nuclear atypia, bizarre tumor cells and necrosis. The distinction between benign and malignant tumors may be very difficult and the input of the radiologist is of great significance. **(p. 2149–2150)**

A5. False

Osteosarcoma is the most frequent primary malignant bone tumor, apart from hematopoietic malignancy. It usually occurs in patients between 10 and 25 years of age; there is a slight male predominance (1.5 : 1). Most osteosarcomas arising de novo are located in the metaphyseal area of the long bones, particularly the lower end of the femur, the upper end of the tibia and the upper end of the humerus. The large majority of osteosarcomas arise within the medullary cavity, from which they extend into the cortex and can elevate or perforate the periosteum. In the latter circumstance a radiographic sign known as Codman's triangle develops. This, although useful, is not specific for osteosarcoma or even for a malignant tumor: it can be produced by any lesion that elevates the periosteum, including hematoma. **(p. 2150–2152)**

A6. True

Morphologic variations in osteosarcoma are plentiful. The osteoid may be sparse or massive; the cartilage may be immature, mineralized or highly myxoid, but a malignant bone tumor should be designated as osteosarcoma whenever osteoid is seen unconnected with cartilage and being formed directly from the tumor cells. **(p. 2152)**

A7. False

Most if not all osteosarcomas contain clonal chromosomal abnormalities, but no specific translocation has been described. **(p. 2153)**

A8. False

This is a characteristic translocation seen in the majority of Ewing sarcomas, which need to be differentiated from small cell sarcomas, which do not harbor this translocation. **(p. 2154)**

A9. True

This infrequent variant occurs in a slightly older age group than the conventional variety. Microscopically, there is a disorderly pattern of well-formed bone, osteoid, occasional cartilage and a highly fibrous spindle cell stroma. The most important differential diagnosis is with myositis ossificans, which is distinguished mainly on the basis of its orderly pattern of maturation. If the features of a high-grade osteosarcoma are seen focally in what is otherwise a typical juxtacortical osteosarcoma, one should *not* make the diagnosis of parosteal osteosarcoma, but rather of a conventional sarcoma. This is referred to as 'dedifferentiation,' and is associated with a markedly decreased survival rate. **(p. 2156)**

A10. False

This tumor grows on the surface of long bones, accompanied by bone spicules arranged perpendicular to the shaft. Microscopically, the tumors are relatively high-grade osteosarcomas with a prominent cartilaginous component (Fig. 24.9). **(p. 2156)**

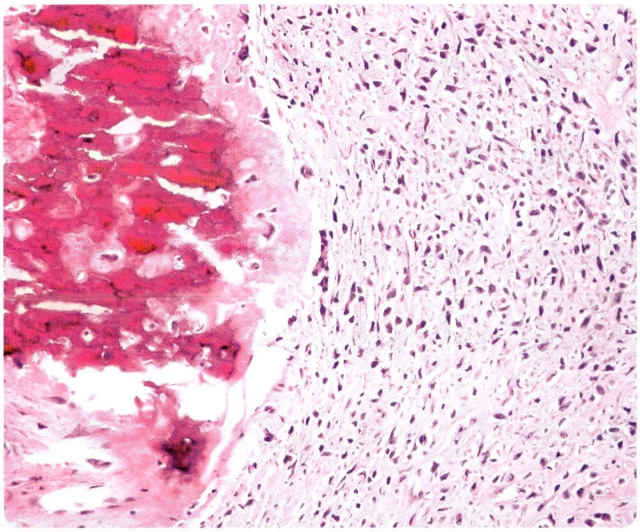

Fig. 24.9

A11. True

The presence of extensive tumor necrosis following chemotherapy is a good prognostic sign. **(p. 2157)**

A12. True

Enchondromas present in a wide range of ages. **(p. 2158)**

A13. False

Multiple enchondromas having a predominantly unilateral distribution are referred to as Ollier's disease, and multiple enchondromas in association with soft tissue hemangiomas (including spindle cell hemangioendotheliomas) as Maffucci's syndrome; both carry a significant risk of malignant transformation. **(p. 2158)**

A14. True

One of the most typical radiologic features is the fact that the lesions, when located in the metaphyses of long bones, grow out in a direction opposite to the adjacent joint. Characteristically there is a cap of cartilage covered by a fibrous membrane, which is continuous with the periosteum of the adjacent bone. The bulk of the lesion is made up of mature bone trabeculae located beneath the cartilaginous cap and containing normal bone marrow. In older lesions the cap thins out and may disappear altogether. **(p. 2159)**

A15. True

It is important to remember that several cases of chondroblastoma, microscopically indistinguishable from the rest, have behaved locally in an aggressive fashion, invading the soft tissues and developing tumor thrombi in lymph channels. Most of these aggressive tumors are located in the pelvis. **(p. 2162)**

A16. True

This tumor characteristically comprises hypocellular lobules with a myxochondroid appearance, separated by intersecting bands of highly cellular tissue composed of fibroblast-like spindle cells and osteoclasts. Local recurrence follows curettage of chondromyxoid fibroma in about 25% of cases. Cytogenetically, recurrent anomalies of 6q25 have been found. The most characteristic of these consist of the pericentrometric inversion inv(6)(p25q23). **(p. 2163)**

A17. True

Bone can be present in a bona fide chondrosarcoma, but this is non-neoplastic and probably originates from reabsorption of the tumor cartilage by a mechanism of endochondral ossification. **(p. 2166)**

A18. False

Correlation of the microscopic features with the clinical, and especially the radiographic, findings is essential. Large tumors of the long bones or ribs, or those that begin to grow rapidly over adolescence and reach a size of 8 cm or more, are almost invariably malignant. Minor degrees of atypia in the cartilaginous cells under these circumstances justify a diagnosis of chondrosarcoma. **(p. 2166)**

A19. True

Typically the antibody to S-100 protein stains both the nuclei and the cytoplasm of benign and malignant cartilaginous cells. **(p. 2166)**

A20. False

Mesenchymal chondrosarcoma is a specific variant of chondrosarcoma characterized microscopically by a dimorphic pattern in which areas of well-differentiated cartilage alternate with undifferentiated stroma. It can be confused with Ewing sarcoma, but it does not have the required 11;22 translocation. **(p. 2168)**

A21. True

Microscopically, the two main components of giant cell tumor are the so-called stromal cells and giant cells (Fig. 24.10). The giant cells are usually large and have over 20 or 30 nuclei, most of them arranged toward the center. They resemble osteoclasts. However, the mononuclear stromal cells are neoplastic. It is the only proliferating element in the lesion and the one exhibiting atypia in the rare cytologically malignant examples of this tumor. The natural history of giant cell tumor is that of a low-grade malignancy. In most reported series the incidence of clinical malignancy (expressed by uncontrollable local recurrence or metastases) has been in the range of 10%. **(p. 2169–2172)**

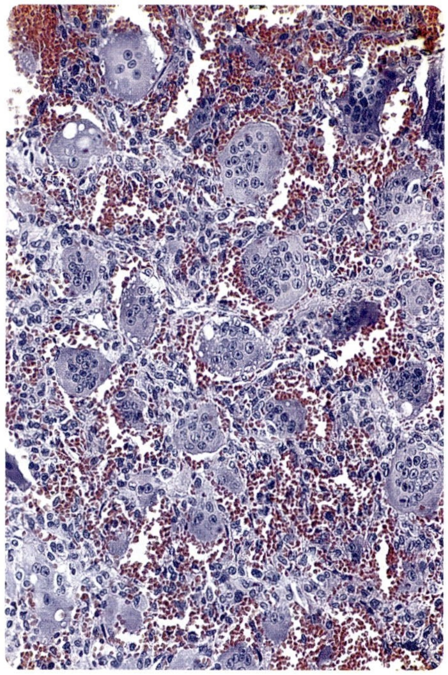

A

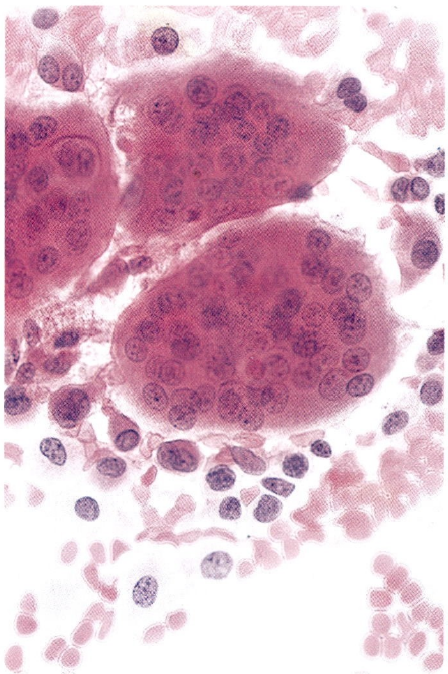

B

Fig. 24.10

A22. True

The tumor involves the diaphysis shows cortical thickening and widening of medullary canal and is composed of a monotonous population of small cells, which is typical for Ewing sarcoma. **(p. 2174)**

A23. True

Over 95% of Ewing sarcomas and PNETs show the typical chromosomal translocation t11;22(q24;q12), which results in the fusion of the *EWS* (Ewing's sarcoma) and *FLI* or *ERG* genes. CD99 (O13; HBA71; p30/32; MIC2) is a cell membrane protein coded by a gene located on the short arms of the X and Y chromosomes (pseudoautosomal gene) that is consistently expressed by the cells of ES/PNET (Fig. 24.11). It is, however, not pathognomonic for this family of tumors, inasmuch as expression of this marker has also been documented in embryonal rhabdomyosarcoma, other soft tissue sarcomas and lymphoblastic lymphoma. **(p. 2175–2176)**

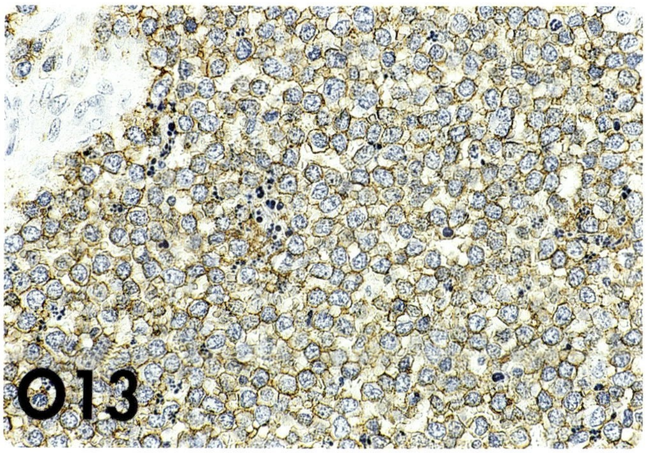

Fig. 24.11

A24. False

The picture is indicative of Burkitt's lymphoma. Immunohistochemistry for B-cell lineage expression and characteristic t(8;14)(q23;q21) translocation help establish the diagnosis. **(p. 1955)**

A25. True

Epithelioid hemangioendothelioma of bone is often multiple and may be associated with similar lesions in the skin or soft tissue, which are characteristically located in close proximity to the osseous foci (Fig. 24.12). The clinical course is protracted, especially for multicentric tumors; distant metastases are exceptional. A range of cytologic atypia exists in epithelioid vascular tumors of bone. Those exhibiting marked atypia (often accompanied by mitotic activity and necrosis) are better designated epithelioid angiosarcomas. **(p. 2180)**

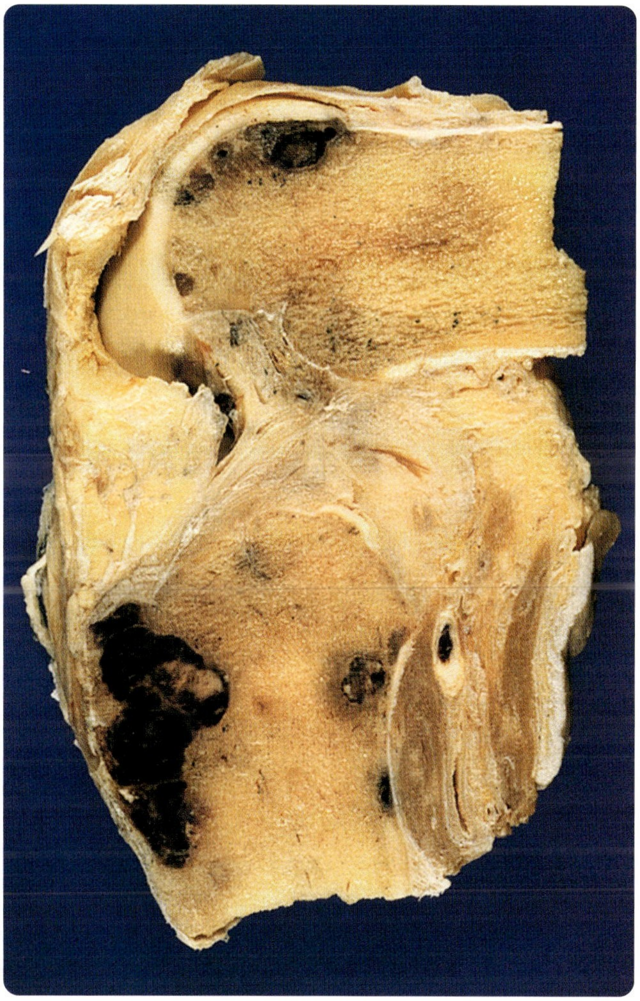

Fig. 24.12

A26. False

Lipoma of bone is a very rare tumor composed of mature adipose tissue devoid of hematopoietic elements. Older lesions have a tendency to calcify. **(p. 2182)**

A27. True

The differential diagnosis of tumors with a myxoid background in this location includes myxopapillary ependymoma, chondrosarcoma and metastatic (signet ring) adenocarcinoma. **(p. 2184)**

A28. False

Many bone and soft tissue tumors with epithelial phenotypes, such as synovial sarcoma, chordoma, adamantinoma of long bones and epithelioid sarcoma, express keratins. **(p. 2184–2185)**

A29. False

Although extremely rare, a primary bone tumor with this biphasic pattern is known as adamantinoma. Microscopically, several patterns of growth have been described. The most common consists of solid nests of basaloid cells with palisading at the periphery and sometimes a stellate configuration in the center. Less frequent forms have been described as spindle, squamoid and tubular; the latter closely simulates the appearance of a vascular neoplasm. The keratins expressed by adamantinoma are mainly 14 and 19, with lesser representation of keratins 5, 17, 7 and 13. **(p. 2186)**

A30. False

Aneurysmal bone cyst is a true neoplasm with established non-random cytogenetic aberrations (involving chromosome segments 17p11-13 and/or 19q22), irrespective of subtype. Aneurysmal bone cyst is seen usually in patients between 10 and 20 years of age. Radiographically, aneurysmal bone cyst shows eccentric expansion of the bone, with erosion and destruction of the cortex and a small peripheral area of periosteal new bone formation (Fig. 24.13). Neoplastic cells with the morphologic, ultrastructural and immunohistochemical features of fibroblasts, myofibroblasts and histiocytes form a spongy hemorrhagic mass (large spaces filled with blood are seen that do not have an endothelial lining). The differential diagnosis includes solitary bone cyst, giant cell tumor, hemangioma and telangiectatic osteosarcoma. **(p. 2188–2190)**

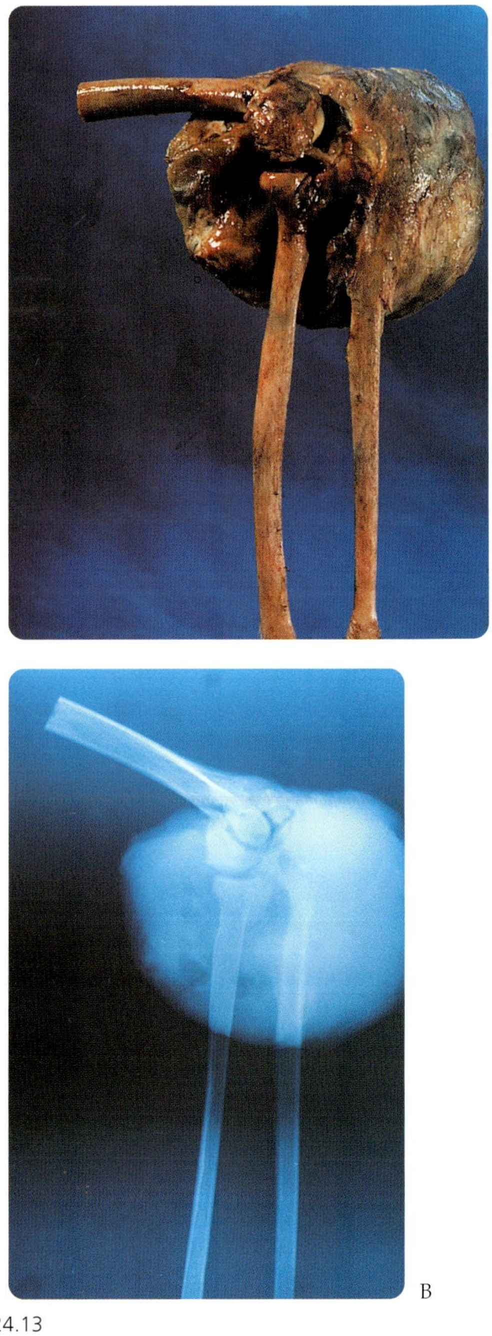

A

B

Fig. 24.13

A31. True

Benign fibrous histiocytoma of bone, also known as metaphyseal fibrous defect, is a synonymous distinctive lesion of bone that occurs in adolescents, most often in long tubular bones, particularly the upper or lower tibia or the lower femur. The other name for the same process is non-ossifying or non-osteogenic fibroma. Microscopically, it consists of cellular masses of fibrous tissue, often arranged in a storiform pattern. Scattered osteoclasts and collections of foamy and hemosiderin-laden macrophages are frequent. **(p. 2191)**

A32. True

This is a non-neoplastic condition that can present in two forms, monostotic and polyostotic. The less common polyostotic type is characterized by a unilateral distribution and is usually associated with endocrine dysfunction, precocious puberty in females, and areas of cutaneous hyperpigmentation (Albright's syndrome). Somatic mutation of the G protein underlies the disease in both forms. **(p. 2192–2193)**

A33. False

Osteofibrous dysplasia (fibro-osseous dysplasia, ossifying fibroma; Campanacci's lesion) is distinguished microscopically from fibrous dysplasia by the osteoblastic rimming of the bone trabeculae and the presence of lamellar bone, and radiographically by its cortical rather than medullary location. **(p. 2194)**

A34. False

This microscopic and radiologic zonation is characteristic of myositis ossificans, a reactive condition that may mimic osteosarcoma. **(p. 2195)**

A35. True

This osteolytic bone lesion consists of Langerhans' cells, other histiocytes, eosinophils and lymphocytes. Immunohistochemistry showed that the lesion contains CD1a and S-100-positive cells, confirming the diagnosis of Langerhans' cell histiocytosis. The differential diagnosis of Langerhans' cell histiocytosis of bone at the microscopic level includes osteomyelitis and the osseous manifestations of Rosai–Dorfman disease. **(p. 2196–2198)**

A36. True

Tendosynovial giant cell tumor (TSGCT, nodular tendosynovitis, fibrous histiocytoma of tendon sheath, xanthogranuloma, benign synovioma) is a common lesion that occurs more frequently in women than men, usually appearing in young and middle-aged persons. The lesion contains closely packed medium-sized polyhedral cells with a variable admixture of giant cells containing fat and hemosiderin. The great cellularity of this tumor, its variable pattern and the presence of mitotic figures may lead to an erroneous diagnosis of sarcoma. Nevertheless, a very rare malignant counterpart of this lesion has been described. The main differential diagnosis of TSGCT is epithelioid sarcoma. The presence of granuloma-like formations, necrosis, invasiveness, epithelioid features and keratin immunoreactivity favors the latter. **(p. 2206)**

A37. True

Pigmented villonodular synovitis is synonymous with diffuse type giant cell tumor. **(p. 2206)**

A38. True

Microscopically, the chondrocytes of primary synovial osteochondromatosis may show some degree of atypia and even binucleated forms, but this does not necessarily indicate malignancy. The distinction, which may be quite difficult, is based on the presence in the chondrosarcoma of obvious cytologic features of malignancy in the chondrocytes. **(p. 2208)**

A39. True

Most patients are young males and the knee is the most common site, followed by the elbows and fingers. The most common microscopic pattern is cavernous hemangioma. **(p. 2208)**

25 Soft tissues

Normal anatomy

Q1

Fibroblasts are reactive for vimentin and focally for actin.

Q2

Adipose tissue is divided into two major types: white fat and brown fat.

Q3

Brown fat cells are more prominent in infants than in adults.

Q4

Endothelial cells exhibit numerous pinocytotic vesicles, cytoplasmic microfilaments, specialized cell junctions, microvilli, continuous basal lamina, and Weibel–Palade bodies.

Q5

Endothelial cells exhibit reactivity for vimentin, factor VIII-related antigen (FVIII-RA, or more precisely von Willebrand factor), CD31, CD34, endothelin, FLI-1 and thrombomodulin.

Q6

Pericytes, smooth muscle cells and glomus cells are also part of the vasculature.

Q7

Schwann cells look somewhat similar to fibroblasts at the light microscopic level but are easily distinguished from them immunohistochemically because of their strong immunoreactivity for S-100 protein.

Q8

Perineurial cells are immunoreactive for epithelial membrane antigen (EMA) and Glut-1 and negative for S-100 protein.

Tumors

Q1

Most sarcomas arise from primitive multipotential mesenchymal cells, which in the course of neoplastic transformation undergo differentiation along one or more lines.

Q2

The prognosis of soft tissue tumors is independent of grading.

Q3

The French Federation of Cancer Centers Sarcoma Group grading system takes into account the grade of differentiation (1–3), number of mitoses (1–3) and the extent of necrosis (1–3) to assign grades I–III for most sarcomas.

Q4

The large majority of soft tissue sarcomas arise from malignant degeneration of pre-existing benign tumors.

Q5

A soft tissue mass in the hand or wrist of a child or adolescent, attached to a tendon and characterized by a diffuse fibroblastic growth in which spotty calcification occurs, is most likely a calcifying aponeurotic fibroma.

Q6

Giant cell fibroblastoma is a childhood equivalent of dermatofibrosarcoma protuberans.

Q7

A small tumor composed of spindle cells set in a loosely textured mucoid matrix of the upper extremities that grew rapidly (within a few weeks) and shows infiltrative margins is most likely malignant.

Q8

Proliferative fasciitis is a lesion similar to nodular fasciitis, characterized by the presence of a distinct population of large basophilic cells resembling ganglion cells.

Q9

Proliferative myositis is the designation for an intramuscular tumor that is histologically similar to proliferative fasciitis.

Q10

This figure shows the typical features of elastofibroma, a benign, poorly circumscribed tumor-like condition involving almost exclusively the subscapular region of elderly individuals.

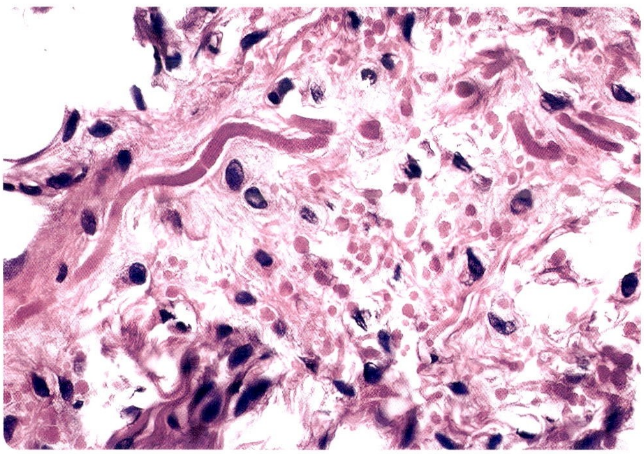

Fig. 25.1

Q11

A solitary fibrous tumor of the pleura and mediastinum is a mesothelial neoplasm arising in pleural and non-pleural sites.

Q12

Fibromatosis coli is a benign site-specific fibromatosis that affects infants before the age of 6 months.

Q13

Desmoid tumor is a neoplasm of the abdominal wall appearing exclusively in women during or following pregnancy.

Q14

Fibrosarcomas express vimentin and type I collagen but not smooth muscle markers, histiocytic markers or basal lamina components.

Q15

Congenital fibrosarcoma is genetically closely linked to congenital mesoblastic nephroma.

Q16

A tumor composed of spindled myofibroblasts, plasma cells, lymphocytes and eosinophils arising in the omentum of a 10-year-old child is most likely characterized by overexpression of ALK protein.

Q17

The differential diagnosis of a cellular spindle cell tumor of the sole is usually between fibromatosis, synovial sarcoma, malignant melanoma and Kaposi's sarcoma.

Q18

The association of soft tissue tumors, usually of the fibromatosis type, with multiple colonic polyposis and occasionally multiple osteomas is known as Gardner syndrome.

Q19

A tumor composed of fibroblastic cells arranged in fascicles that intersect each other at acute angles resulting in a herringbone appearance is always diagnostic of fibrosarcoma.

Q20

Pleomorphic sarcoma that does not show any specific phenotypic line of differentiation is best characterized as malignant fibrous histiocytoma (MFH).

Q21

Storiform–pleomorphic malignant fibrous histiocytoma is the rarest type of pleomorphic sarcoma.

Q22

Myxofibrosarcoma is synonymous with low-grade fibromyxoid sarcoma.

Q23

Most tumors with the inflammatory MFH pattern are dedifferentiated liposarcomas.

Q24

Angiomatoid fibrous histiocytoma (angiomatoid MFH) is an invariably fatal form of childhood malignant fibrous histiocytoma.

Q25

A localized tumor found between metatarsal bones and composed of distorted nerve with epineurial fibrosis is best described as Morton's neuroma.

Q26

Palisading of nuclei in a well-circumscribed soft tissue tumor is diagnostic of schwannoma.

Q27

Neurofibroma is synonymous with neurilemmoma (schwannoma).

Q28

Neurofibromatosis (von Recklinghausen's disease) is caused by loss-of-function mutations and deletions of the *NF1* gene.

Q29

Neurofibromatosis type 2 is as prevalent as type 1.

Q30

Perineurial cells are vimentin positive, EMA positive and S-100 negative and give rise to peripheral nerve sheath tumors.

Q31

Multiple myxoid nodules with the presence of plumper, epithelial-like cells and a distinct fascicular or plexiform arrangement characterize nerve sheath myxoma.

Q32

Diagnosis of malignant peripheral nerve sheath tumor (MPNST) should be the primary consideration in the presence of a malignant tumor of soft tissues composed of spindle cells: (1) when the tumor develops in a patient with type I von Recklinghausen's disease or (2) when the tumor is obviously arising within the anatomic compartment of a major nerve or in continuity with a neurofibroma.

Q33

The presence of metaplastic tissues such as cartilage, bone, muscle or blood vessels in a tumor suspicious for MPNST should argue strongly against this diagnosis.

Q34

Strong S-100 positivity is diagnostic of MPNST.

Q35

A tumor composed of an admixture of mature lipocytes and uniform spindle cells set against a mucinous and fibrous background is best described as myxoid liposarcoma.

Q36

A lipomatous tumor containing hyperchromatic multinucleated ('floret-like') tumor cells within the fibrous septa traversing the neoplasm invariably denotes sarcomatous change.

Q37

A well-differentiated lipomatous tumor located in the subcutis, with clusters of thick-walled capillaries often on the periphery of the neoplasm and with hyaline thrombi, is diagnostic of angiolipoma.

Q38

Lipoblastoma is distinguished from myxoid liposarcoma by the virtue of the young age of the patient, distinct lobulation, and the absence of giant cells or pleomorphic nuclei.

Q39

Hibernomas are distinguished from myxoid liposarcomas by distinct chromosomal rearrangements.

Q40

Lipoblast is a mononuclear or multinucleated cell with one or more cytoplasmic vacuoles that contain fat.

Q41

Myxoid and round cell liposarcoma belong to the same genetic entity and the latter is considered a poorly differentiated variant of the former.

Q42

Atypical lipomatous tumor category encompasses atypical lipoma and well-differentiated liposarcoma.

Q43

Dedifferentiated liposarcoma is the term used for the emergence of a non-lipogenic undifferentiated solid component within an atypical lipomatous tumor.

Q44

Hemangiomas are classified into capillary, cavernous and venous types based on the prevalent histologic pattern.

Q45

Papillary endothelial hyperplasia is a distinct intravascular papillary proliferation of anastomosing vascular channels and plump endothelial cells.

Q46

Spindle cell hemangioma is a tumor that combines the features of cavernous hemangioma and Kaposi's sarcoma illustrated here.

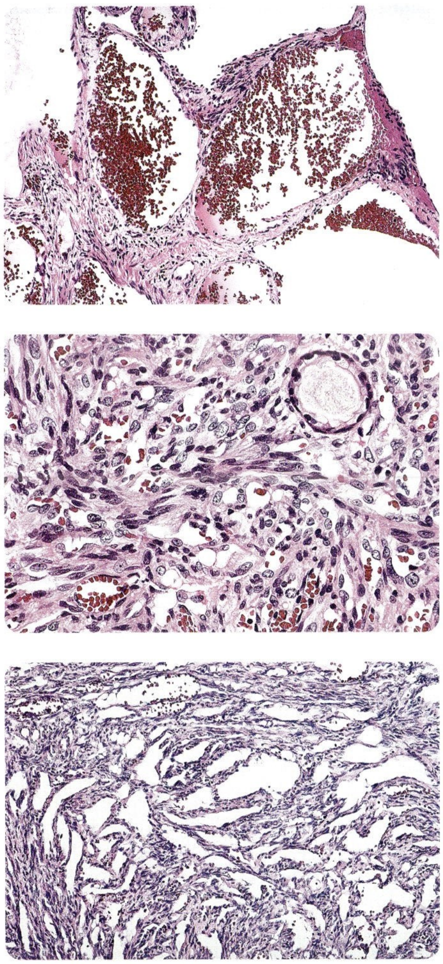

A B C

Fig. 25.2

Q47

Glomus tumors originate most often from the glomus coccygeum.

Q48

Hemangioendothelioma is a term used for vascular tumors of borderline malignancy.

Q49

The cells of epithelioid hemangioendothelioma are reactive for keratin.

Q50

This figure shows the freely anastomosing vascular channels lined by atypical endothelial cells that are diagnostic of angiosarcoma.

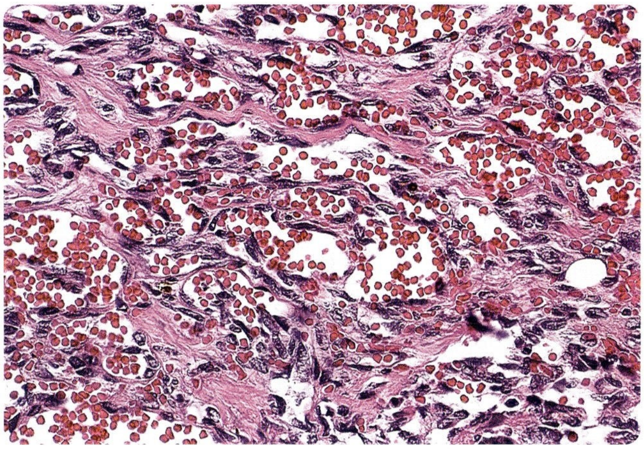

Fig. 25.3

Q51

Most soft tissue leiomyosarcomas are located in the extremities.

Q52

Pleomorphic rhabdomyosarcoma is the most common type of rhabdomyosarcoma.

Q53

Embryonal rhabdomyosarcoma is common in the head and neck region, particularly the orbit, nasopharynx, middle ear and oral cavity.

Q54

Alveolar rhabdomyosarcoma predominates in an older age group, frequently in the extremities, and has a distinctly worse prognosis than the embryonal variant.

Q55

Synovial sarcoma exhibits dual epithelial and mesenchymal differentiation.

Q56

The diagnosis of myxoma in a child should be seriously questioned.

Q57

Granular cell tumor arises exclusively in the tongue.

Q58

This tumor arising in the thigh of a young female with large cells having vesicular nuclei, prominent nucleoli, and a granular cytoplasm separated by fibrous tissue into well-defined nests is most likely an alveolar soft part sarcoma.

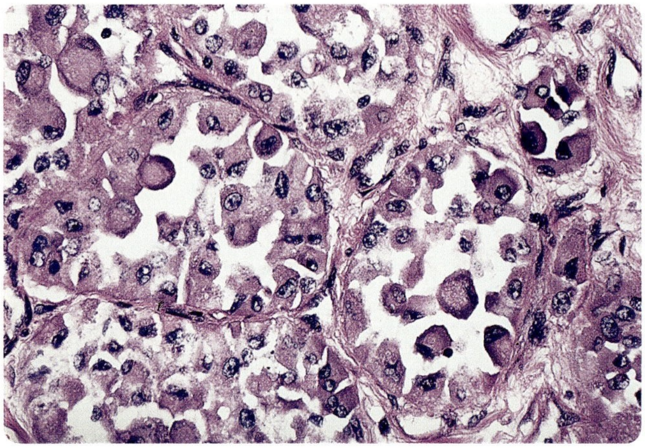

Fig. 25.4

Q59

A malignant tumor arising from large tendons of the foot and exhibiting immunoreactivity for S-100 protein and HMB-45 is most likely metastatic melanoma.

Q60

A necrotic tumor in the hand of a young man composed of nodules and clusters of deeply acidophilic (eosinophilic) epithelioid cells is probably a necrobiotic granuloma.

Q61

A small superficial lobulated tumor with an incomplete peripheral rim of bone and small and round cells with scanty atypia and few mitoses is typical of ossifying fibromyxoid tumor (OFMT).

Q62

A tumor composed of cells with deeply and homogeneously acidophilic cytoplasm and occasional lateral displacement of the nucleus (so-called rhabdoid cells) arises exclusively in the kidneys.

Q63

Parachordoma is a soft tissue tumor typically described adjacent to tendons, synovium and osseous structures within extremities.

Normal anatomy

A1. True
Like all other mesenchymal cells fibroblasts contain vimentin in intermediate filaments of their skeleton, and also have actin in microfilaments. They are responsible for the production of the various extracellular materials, including the many types of collagen. Their shape varies from spindle (especially when stretched along bundles of collagen fibers) to stellate (in myxoid areas). Myofibroblasts are modified fibroblasts that show features intermediate between fibroblasts and smooth muscle cells. **(p. 2238)**

A2. True
White fat is mainly located in the subcutaneous tissue, mediastinum, abdomen and retroperitoneum, and brown fat is concentrated in the interscapular region, neck, mediastinum, axillae and retroperitoneum. **(p. 2238)**

A3. True
Brown fat cells are more abundant in infants than in adults. In adults they are concentrated in the interscapular region, neck, mediastinum, axillae and retroperitoneum. **(p. 2238)**

A4. True
The Weibel–Palade body, a membrane-bound organelle, is thought to be specific to this cell type and shown to contain the von Willebrand factor. **(p. 2238)**

A5. True
Endothelial cells of normal lymph vessels show a much weaker staining for FVIII-RA than endothelial cells from blood vessels. **(p. 2238)**

A6. True
These cells are characterized ultrastructurally by cytoplasmic microfilaments exhibiting focal condensations, numerous pinocytotic vesicles and a thick continuous basal lamina. Immunohistochemically, they show reactivity for actin, vimentin and myosin; positivity for desmin is largely restricted to smooth muscle cells. **(p. 2238)**

A7. True
S-100 protein is a good marker for Schwann cells. **(p. 2239)**

A8. True
Peripheral nerves are formed by axons, Schwann cells, perineurial cells and fibroblasts. Most of the fibroblasts are located in the epineurium, which is the outer sheath of fully developed nerves. They are immunoreactive for CD34. Each nerve fascicle is surrounded by the perineurium. **(p. 2239)**

Tumors

A1. True
Traditionally, soft tissue sarcomas have been classified according to a histogenetic concept (e.g. fibrosarcoma as a tumor arising from fibroblasts, osteosarcoma as a tumor arising from osteoblasts, and so on). The acceptance of this alternative scheme does not require a change in terminology: a liposarcoma remains as such, but is now viewed not as a tumor arising from a lipoblast but as one exhibiting lipoblastic differentiation. **(p. 2239)**

A2. False
A relationship has been found between various microscopic grading systems and outcome, which in some cases is directly related to the histotype but in others it is applied within a given histotype. **(p. 2240)**

A3. True
The three-grade system is set up as follows: Grade I is defined as a total of 2 or 3 when summing the scores obtained for each of the three histologic criteria; Grade II represents a total of 4 or 5; Grade III represents a total of 6, 7 or 8. **(p. 2241)**

A4. False
The large majority of soft tissue sarcomas arise de novo, although the latter phenomenon may occur (as in neurofibromas). **(p. 2242)**

A5. True
Mitoses are scarce and atypical cytologic features are absent. Scattered osteoclast-like giant cells are frequently seen. Calcifying aponeurotic fibroma can be confused with rheumatoid nodule, schwannoma and fibromatosis. **(p. 2243)**

A6. True
Owing to their ultrastructural, immunohistochemical and molecular similarities these tumors are now considered a spectrum of the same neoplasm. The translocation t(17;22)(g22;g13) creating a fusion of the COLIA gene and PDGFB has been shown a consistent finding in DFSP and GCF. **(p. 2244)**

A7. False
One should strongly consider nodular fasciitis in the differential diagnosis. Small size, short duration, red blood cell extravasation, keloid-type collagen, and lack of markedly atypical cells are the main features favoring a diagnosis of nodular fasciitis. In other words, it is permissible for nodular fasciitis to be hypercellular, infiltrative and mitotically active, but not to have cells with large atypical hyperchromatic nuclei. **(p. 2244–2247)**

A8. True
Nodular fasciitis and its variants are characteristically located in the somatic soft tissues, but fasciitis-like lesions with a somewhat different morphologic appearance (even more sarcomatoid) can develop from the stromal tissue of a variety of organs, such as the bladder, prostate, vulva, vagina and cervix. **(p. 2244–2247)**

A9. True
Skeletal muscles of the shoulder, thorax and thigh are those most commonly affected. The hallmark of the lesion is the presence of very large basophilic cells with vesicular nuclei and very prominent nucleoli, resembling ganglion cells or rhabdomyoblasts. **(p. 2244–2247)**

A10. True
Microscopically, collagen bundles alternate with numerous acidophilic, refractive cylinders often containing a central dense core, both of which stain strongly with elastic stains. This lesion is not a true neoplasm but rather a reactive hyperplasia involving abnormal elastogenesis. **(p. 2247)**

A11. False
This soft tissue neoplasm is composed of a subset of fibroblast-like cells and is ubiquitous. Microscopically, the alternation of hyper- and hypocellular areas, the deposition of dense keloid-type collagen and the occurrence of hemangiopericytoma-like areas are the most distinguishing features. They are typically positive for CD34 and bcl-2; focal reactivity for muscle stains has been reported. Keratins are generally negative. **(p. 2248)**

A12. True
This is a type of fibromatosis that affects the lower third of the sternomastoid muscle and appears at birth or shortly thereafter. **(p. 2249)**

A13. False
Most soft tissue fibromatoses are in intimate contact with skeletal muscles (musculoaponeurotic fibromatosis). They tend to occur equally commonly in men and in other locations. **(p. 2250)**

A14. True
Fibrosarcomas react only with antibodies to vimentin and type collagen I. The presence of focal immunoreactivity for smooth muscle actin, laminin or collagen (not an unusual occurrence) should be taken to indicate incipient differentiation along myoid or possibly myofibroblastic lines. **(p. 2252–2254)**

A15. True
Congenital fibrosarcoma is an extremely cellular tumor characterized by rapid growth and extensive local invasion. It harbors the same chromosomal translocation t(12;15)(p13;q25) leading to *ETV6-NTRK3* as is seen in congenital mesoblastic nephroma. **(p. 2253)**

A16. True
Inflammatory myofibroblastic tumor is a distinctive entity occurring in the mesentery or retroperitoneum of children. ALK receptor tyrosine kinase overexpression results from a rearrangement in chromosome 2p23. **(p. 2254–2255)**

A17. True
Palmar fibromatosis is also known as Dupuytren's contracture, and plantar fibromatosis as Ledderhose's disease. These conditions occur predominantly in adults. Contracture of the fingers or toes is the leading clinical manifestation. Fibrosarcoma of the palmar and plantar areas is exceptional. **(p. 2249–2252)**

A18. True
In Gardner syndrome fibromatosis involving the intestinal wall (not an uncommon occurrence) needs to be distinguished from gastrointestinal stromal tumor (GIST). Fibromatosis seems to be CD117 negative, as opposed to bona fide GIST, which express this epitope. **(p. 2252)**

A19. False
Many other soft tissue tumors, particularly synovial sarcoma, liposarcoma, malignant fibrous histiocytoma and malignant peripheral nerve sheath tumor, often contain areas closely resembling fibrosarcoma. Only careful examination of different blocks of the tumor will provide the correct diagnosis in these instances. Immunohistochemically, the prototypical fibrosarcoma should have reactivity for vimentin and type I collagen, but not for smooth muscle markers, histiocytic markers or basal lamina components. **(p. 2252–2254)**

A20. True
Malignant fibrous histiocytoma (undifferentiated high grade pleomorphic sarcoma) is a diagram of exclusion and the possibility of other sarcomas, sarcomatoid carcinoma, melanoma and lymphoma must be ruled out. **(p. 2253)**

A21. False

Storiform–pleomorphic MFH is the prototypical and most common member of this group. Most cases occur in the deep soft tissues of the extremities in adults, with a peak in the seventh decade. The presence of highly pleomorphic tumor cells and a storiform pattern of growth are the two most important microscopic features. Inflammatory elements, such as lymphocytes, plasma cells and eosinophils, are usually mixed with the neoplastic cells. Metaplastic bone and cartilage formation may be present focally. Immunohistochemically, there is usually reactivity for vimentin, α_1-antitrypsin, α_1-antichymotrypsin, CD68, factor XIIIa, ferritin, and sometimes also focally for actin, desmin and lysozyme. **(p. 2257)**

A22. False

Low-grade myxofibrosarcoma (a variant of malignant fibrous histiocytoma) differs from low-grade fibromyxoid sarcoma by a more developed vascular pattern, a more myxoid matrix, greater nuclear atypia and the presence of cells resembling lipoblasts. **(p. 2258–2259)**

A23. True

In all likelihood inflammatory MFH is a pattern of growth rather than a specific tumor type, in the sense that the same microscopic appearance (i.e. intense neutrophilic infiltration in pleomorphic tumors associated with phagocytosis of neutrophils by the tumor cells) can be seen in otherwise typical liposarcomas, irradiated osteosarcomas and other undifferentiated tumors. **(p. 2260–2261)**

A24. False

Although this tumor was originally placed under the MFH umbrella, several studies have provided evidence to suggest a vascular or myoid nature. Also, immunoreactivity for desmin has been found in over half of the cases. Angiomatoid MFH is a low-grade malignant tumor that has a tendency for local recurrence and rarely metastasizes. **(p. 2261)**

A25. True

Morton's neuroma (metatarsalgia) can be regarded as a subtype of traumatic neuroma caused by repeated mild trauma to the region. Its typical location is the interdigital plantar nerve between the third and fourth toes. The lesion is more common in adult women. **(p. 2263)**

A26. False

Schwannoma (neurilemmoma) is a benign nerve sheath neoplasm that characteristically shows two distinctive patterns, designated A and B. The type A areas, which in small tumors comprise almost their entirety, are quite cellular, composed of spindle cells often arranged in a palisading fashion or in an organoid arrangement (Verocay bodies). In type B areas the tumor cells are separated by abundant edematous fluid that may form cystic spaces. Palisading of nuclei is not unique to schwannoma. It can also occur in leiomyoma, leiomyosarcoma, GIST, calcifying aponeurotic fibroma, and even in non-neoplastic smooth muscle (most commonly in the appendiceal wall). **(p. 2264–2266)**

A27. False

The gross, microscopic and ultrastructural features of neurofibroma, as well as its natural history, are distinct from those of schwannoma. As a rule, the tumors are not encapsulated and have a softer consistency than schwannoma. The more superficial tumors appear as small, soft, pedunculated nodules protruding from the skin (molluscum pendulum). Deeper tumors grow larger. Tumors resulting in diffuse tortuous enlargement of peripheral nerves are designated plexiform neurofibromas and are usually seen in the context of type I neurofibromatosis. Microscopically, neurofibromas are formed by a combined proliferation of all the elements of a peripheral nerve: axons, Schwann cells, fibroblasts, and (in the plexiform type) perineurial cells. In contrast to schwannomas, Verocay bodies, palisading of nuclei and hyaline thickening of the vessel wall are almost always absent in neurofibromas. Malignant transformation of neurofibromas should be suspected in the presence of frequent mitoses, overly expressed cell proliferation markers and the presence of p53 in many tumor cells. **(p. 2266–2269)**

A28. True

Multiple neurofibromas represent the most important component of the genetically determined disorder known as neurofibromatosis or von Recklinghausen's disease type I. This is one of the most common autosomal dominant diseases in humans, the prevalence being 1 in 2500–3300. In addition to neurofibromas, patients with type I von Recklinghausen's disease often have many other associated lesions, the most common being the café au lait spot. This consists microscopically of an increase in the amount of melanin in the epidermal basal layer and is sometimes seen overlying a neurofibroma. **(p. 2266–2269)**

A29. False

NF2 is genetically different from NF1, resulting from an alteration of a gene located on chromosome 22. It is characterized by the presence of a variety of neoplasms in the central nervous system, the most distinctive of which are bilateral acoustic schwannomas. NF2 is much less common than NF1, affecting 1 in 40 000 live births. **(p. 2269)**

A30. True

Perineuriomas are composed of extremely elongated cells arranged in parallel bundles, the appearance being not too dissimilar from that of neurofibroma or pacinian neurofibroma (Fig. 25.5). **(p. 2269–2270)**

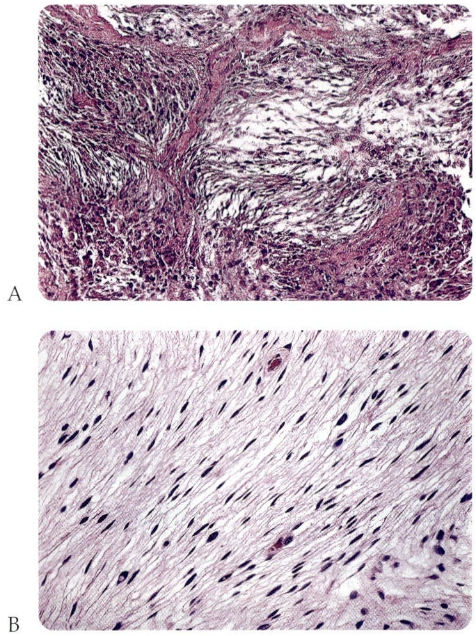

Fig. 25.5

A31. True

It seems likely that nerve sheath myxoma and the cutaneous tumor described as neurothekeoma are closely related. **(p. 2270)**

A32. True

In the absence of these circumstances the light microscopic diagnosis of MPNST is often only presumptive and dependent on a combination of features, none of which is diagnostic per se. They include: serpentine shape of the tumor cells; arrangement in palisades or whorls; a marked contrast between the deeply hyperchromatic nuclei and the pale cytoplasm ('punched-out nuclei'); perivascular concentration of tumor cells, with a plumper shape; epithelioid appearance of the endothelial cells of these vessels; the presence of large gaping vascular spaces, resulting in a hemangiopericytoma-like appearance; and geographic areas of necrosis, with tumor palisading at the edges. **(p. 2271–2275)**

A33. False

Metaplastic tissues such as cartilage, bone, muscle or blood vessels are present in approximately 15% of cases of typical MPNST. The most spectacular variant is characterized by the presence of well-developed skeletal muscle and has been dignified by the picturesque term malignant triton tumor. Glands, skeletal muscle and other tissues can coexist in the same tumor. **(p. 2271–2275)**

A34. False

Immunoreactivity to S-100 protein in MPNST tends to be focal and not particularly strong, except in the epithelioid variant of this tumor; therefore, the presence of strong and diffuse immunoreactivity for S-100 protein in a malignant spindle cell tumor with morphologic features suggestive of MPNST should raise the possibility of the alternative diagnosis of malignant melanoma, particularly if the lesion is located in the skin or a lymph node. **(p. 2271–2275)**

A35. False

One should consider first the diagnosis of a spindle cell lipoma. This is a benign fatty tumor characteristically located in the regions of the shoulder and posterior neck of adults. Features that assist in distinguishing it from myxoid liposarcoma include the absence of lipoblasts, the absence of a prominent plexiform vascular pattern and the presence of thick ('ropy') collagen bundles, and the great uniformity of the proliferating spindle cells. **(p. 2276)**

A36. False

Pleomorphic lipoma is a variant of spindle cell lipoma that contains multinucleated ('floret-like') giant cells. In some instances the border between pleomorphic lipoma and atypical lipoma is arbitrary. **(p. 2277)**

A37. True

These are well-circumscribed small tumors that occur shortly after puberty. They are often painful and characteristically multiple. Angiolipomas in which the vascular component predominates (cellular angiolipomas) can be confused with Kaposi's sarcoma or angiosarcoma. **(p. 2277–2278)**

A38. True

Lipoblastoma (well defined) and lipoblastomasis (diffuse lesion) almost exclusively affects infants and young children (below the age of 5 years). Cytogenetically, lipoblastoma/lipoblastomasis is often associated with rearrangements of 8q. **(p. 2278)**

A39. True

Cytogenetically, hibernomas are often associated with aberrations of 11q.13. Myxoid liposarcomas may contain areas of hibernoma-like cells. The typical most common cytogenetic change in myxoid/round cell liposarcoma is the translocation t(12;16)(q13;p11). **(p. 2279)**

A40. True

The common morphologic denominator of liposarcoma is the lipoblast. This appears as a mononuclear or multinucleated cell with one or more cytoplasmic vacuoles that contain fat. The nucleus may be pushed aside by a single large vacuole, resulting in a signet ring configuration, or it may remain centrally located but exhibit small indentations by multiple small vacuoles. This highly characteristic scalloped nuclear appearance can also be appreciated in specimens obtained from fine needle aspiration. **(p. 2280)**

A41. True

Myxoid liposarcoma is characterized by proliferating lipoblasts in different stages of differentiation, a prominent anastomosing capillary network, and a mucoid matrix rich in hyaluronidase-sensitive acid mucopolysaccharides. The presence of a delicate network of thin-walled vessels is an important feature in the differential diagnosis from myxoma and other myxoid tumors. In the round cell type the tumor cells are small and have a distinctly acidophilic cytoplasm. The presence among them of scattered lipoblasts establishes the diagnosis. Cytogenetically, myxoid and round cell liposarcoma are characterized by the reciprocal translocation t(12;16)(q13;p11), which results in the *TLS-CHOP* rearrangement. *CHOP* is a gene involved in adipocyte differentiation. **(p. 2280–2281)**

A42. True

The behavior of atypical lipomatous tumors is substantially different depending on their location: those situated in the somatic soft tissues may recur, but these recurrences are controllable so that there are no tumor-related deaths; however, those originating in the retroperitoneum have a very high incidence of recurrence (some of these recurrences having a 'dedifferentiated' appearance), and some patients die as a result. In view of these findings, and based on pragmatic criteria, the proposal has been made to use the term *atypical lipoma* for the former and *well-differentiated liposarcoma* for the latter. Cytogenetically, close to 80% of atypical lipomatous tumors (including the dedifferentiated examples) show marker ring and giant chromosomes, in stark contrast to lipomas of either ordinary or spindle/pleomorphic type. **(p. 2281–2283)**

A43. True

Microscopically, the dedifferentiated component is usually high grade, with an appearance reminiscent of fibrosarcoma or malignant fibrous histiocytoma. **(p. 2283–2284)**

A44. True

Capillary hemangiomas are made up of small vessels of capillary caliber and can occur in any organ. Cavernous hemangiomas are composed of larger vessels with cystically dilated lumina and thin walls. Large-vessel hemangiomas may be composed of vessels with the structure of veins (venous hemangiomas) or a combination of veins and arteries (racemose, cirsoid or arteriovenous hemangiomas). **(p. 2285–2287)**

A45. True

Intravascular papillary endothelial hyperplasia (Masson's hemangioma or Masson's lesion) is probably not a true neoplasm but an exorbitant organization and recanalization of a thrombus. It was first described by Masson in hemorrhoidal vessels as 'vegetant intravascular hemangioendothelioma' and nowadays commonly referred to as Masson tumor. **(p. 2287)**

A46. True

This vascular tumor was originally described as spindle cell hemangioendothelioma. It may present at any age, has a male preponderance, occurs preferentially in the dermis and subcutaneous tissue of the distal extremities, and combines histologically the features of cavernous hemangioma and Kaposi's sarcoma. **(p. 2288–2289)**

A47. False

The classic location of the glomus tumor is the subungual region, but it can occur elsewhere in the skin, soft tissues (particularly in the flexor surface of the arms and about the knee), nerves, stomach, nasal cavity and trachea. The glomus coccygeum is a normal structure located on the ventral side of the coccyx. Three microscopic types of glomus tumor have been recognized: solid, angiomatous and myxoid. The solid type can be confused with sweat gland tumor, melanocytic nevus or metastatic carcinoma. This is particularly the case when the tumor cells are very epithelioid and/or grow in an Indian-file fashion. The angiomatous type can have a diffuse quality, in the sense of looking like an angiomatosis with an increased number of glomus cells in the vessel wall. An oncocytic variant of glomus tumor, in which the cytoplasm of the glomus cells is packed with mitochondria, has also been described. Often the diagnostic relationship between tumor cells and blood vessels can be clearly seen only at the very periphery of the neoplasm. **(p. 2288–2290)**

A48. True

The preferred use of the term is for vascular tumors of an endothelial nature that occupy an intermediate position between benign hemangioma and full-blown angiosarcoma. **(p. 2292)**

A49. True

Epithelioid hemangioendothelioma is one of several related proliferative lesions of endothelial cells having as a common denominator an epithelioid or histiocytoid morphology, often accompanied by immunoreactivity for keratin. **(p. 2292)**

A50. True

Variations in the appearance of the neoplastic endothelial cells are great. Their shape ranges from very elongated to plump and epithelioid, and their size from small to giant, with the occasional development of multinucleated forms. The differential diagnosis of angiosarcoma includes hemangioma for the better-differentiated lesions, Kaposi's sarcoma for those with a predominantly spindle component, and carcinoma or amelanotic melanoma for the poorly differentiated types. Immunohistochemically and ultrastructurally, various endothelial markers can be demonstrated depending on the degree of differentiation; of these, CD31 is probably the most reliable. In the epithelioid variant of angiosarcoma, coexpression of keratin is common. **(p. 2293–2294)**

A51. True

Leiomyosarcoma of soft tissue is relatively rare. The differential diagnosis between leiomyoma and leiomyosarcoma of the soft tissues depends on a combination of gross and microscopic features. High mitotic activity is virtually diagnostic of malignancy. A diagnosis of leiomyosarcoma should also be strongly suspected for tumors that are overly large, necrotic or hemorrhagic, even if their mitotic count is low. **(p. 2298–2300)**

A52. False

It is actually the least common of the three forms of rhabdomyosarcoma (pleomorphic, embryonal and alveolar). **(p. 2301)**

A53. True

The large majority occur in children between the ages of 3 and 12 years, but they can also be seen in younger patients and in adults. Microscopically, the tumor cells are small and spindle shaped. A prognostically favorable variant of embryonal rhabdomyosarcoma is represented by the spindle cell type, which is composed of elongated spindle cells arranged in a fasciculated or storiform pattern. **(p. 2302–2303)**

A54. True

In the classic series reported by Enzinger, 92% of patients had died from widespread metastasis within the first 4 years after diagnosis. The lung and regional lymph nodes are the most common metastatic sites. Alveolar rhabdomyosarcomas are consistently associated with the translocation t(2;13) or t(1;13), which results in the gene fusions *PAX3-FKHR* and *PAX7-FKHR*, respectively. **(p. 2303–2306)**

A55. True

Immunohistochemically, there is strong reactivity for keratin in the epithelial areas and often in the spindle cells as well. Because normal or reactive synovial cells do not express keratin, the possibility has been raised that synovial sarcoma is not differentiating towards synovial structures, as traditionally believed, but towards true epithelium. Vimentin, EMA, CEA, calponin, HBME-1, and occasionally S-100 protein are also expressed by this tumor. In fact, it is not rare to find monophasic synovial sarcomas that are focally reactive for EMA but not keratin. It has also been found that a significant number of cases of synovial sarcoma are immunoreactive for CD99, the marker characteristically associated with Ewing sarcoma/PNET. In over 90% of cases synovial sarcoma exhibits the chromosomal translocation t(x:18)(p11.2;q11.2), which results in the fusion of the *SYT* gene on chromosome 18 with either *SSX1* (in two-thirds of cases) or *SSX2* (the other third) on chromosome X. **(p. 2309–2313)**

A56. True

Myxomas are rare neoplasms that have a mucoid, slimy gross appearance. They almost always occur in adults and are more common in females. Microscopically, a typical myxoma has a bland and hypercellular appearance throughout, mitotic activity is practically absent, and blood vessels are extremely scanty. The differential diagnosis of myxoma comprises two types of disease. The first is a group of neoplasms in which myxoid change can be a prominent secondary feature, such as liposarcoma, myxofibrosarcoma, chondrosarcoma, leiomyosarcoma, embryonal rhabdomyosarcoma, neurofibroma, nerve sheath myxoma/neurothekeoma and aggressive angiomyxoma. The second group of diseases from which myxoma should be distinguished is a variety of non-neoplastic disorders resulting in focal mucinous degeneration of the skin or soft tissues, such as nodular fasciitis, localized myxedema, mucous (myxoid) cyst, ganglion, follicular mucinosis (alopecia mucinosa), papular mucinosis and cutaneous focal mucinosis. **(pp. 2306–2309; 2315–2317)**

A57. False

It also arises in other locations, such as the skin, vulva, breast, larynx, bronchus, esophagus etc. Individual cells forming the tumor are large and their cytoplasm is highly granular (Fig. 25.6). Most granules are small and regular. **(p. 2317)**

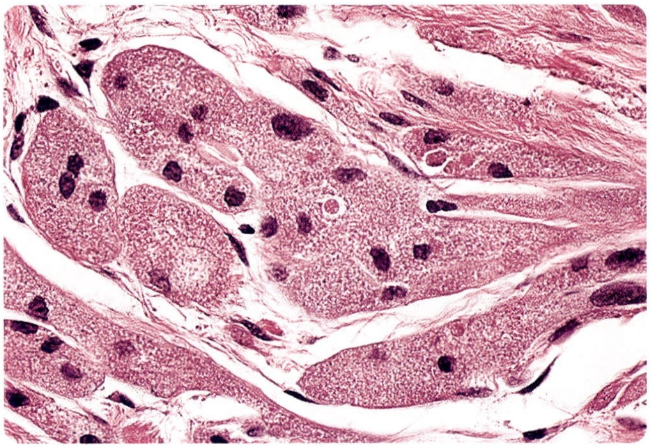

Fig. 25.6

A58. True

Alveolar soft part sarcomas most often involve the deep soft tissues of the thigh and leg. PAS stain sometimes demonstrates the presence of diastase-resistant intracytoplasmic needle-like structures. These are seen on electron microscopy as membrane-bound crystals with a periodicity of 58–100 nm, sometimes arranged in a cross-grid pattern (Fig. 25.7). This feature is of great diagnostic value in lesions that are controversial in nature. **(p. 2318–2320)**

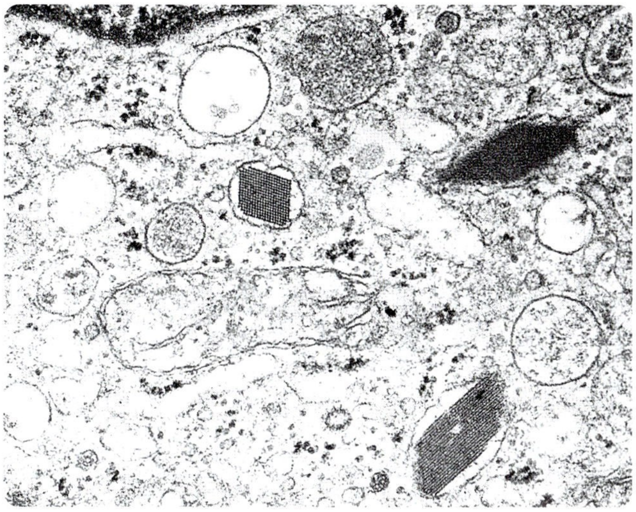

Fig. 25.7

A59. False

It is more likely an example of clear cell sarcoma of tendons and aponeuroses (malignant melanoma of soft parts). Clear cell sarcoma is associated with the chromosomal translocation t(12;22)(q13;q12). **(p. 2320)**

A60. False

Although rare, such presentation should raise suspicion of epithelioid sarcoma. Immunohistochemically, there is positivity for keratin, EMA, vimentin and CD34. Local recurrence is the rule, although it may take years for this to develop. Lymph node metastases are relatively common and constitute an ominous prognostic sign. **(p. 2321)**

A61. True

The behavior of this tumor is indolent, but local recurrences develop in a quarter of cases. **(p. 2323–2324)**

A62. False

Rhabdoid tumor of soft tissues exists; however, it is probably not a specific tumor entity but rather the expression of a 'rhabdoid' phenotype that can develop in a wide variety of tumor types, including epithelioid sarcoma, synovial sarcoma, intra-abdominal desmoplastic small cell tumor, rhabdomyosarcoma, malignant melanoma and various types of carcinoma. **(p. 2328)**

A63. True

This type of tumor may belong to a group of tumors showing differentiation toward myoepithelial cells, presumably connected to skin adnexae, which can occur either in a pure form (myoepitheliomas) or in association with glandular structures (mixed tumors). **(p. 2327–2328)**

26 Peritoneum, retroperitoneum and related structures

Normal anatomy

Q1

The peritoneal cavity is lined by mesodermally derived tissue mesothelium that contains cytokeratin intermediate filaments like all other epithelia.

Q2

Normal mesothelial cells react with antibodies to calretinin and thrombomodulin.

Inflammation and other non-neoplastic lesions

Q1

Pancreatitis typically produces chemical peritonitis and the peritoneal fluid does not contain bacteria.

Q2

Peritonitis complicating perforation of the stomach or intestines is caused by mixed bacterial infection.

Q3

Talcum powder can cause peritoneal granulomas that contain birefringent crystals visible microscopically under polarized light.

Q4

Solitary cysts of the peritoneum are lined by mesothelial cells.

Q5

The lesion called multicystic benign mesothelioma occurs more often in men than in women and is prone to malignant transformation.

Q6

Florid mesothelial hyperplasia in incarcerated inguinal hernial sacs is particularly common in children and may resemble malignancy.

Q7

Mesothelial hyperplastic reactive changes appear histologically as papillary projections or a tubular structure, but when solid mesothelial nests and psammoma bodies are found one should diagnose such lesions as malignant.

Q8

Nodular histiocytic/mesothelial hyperplasia presents in the form of grossly visible nodules that evoke a desmoplastic reaction and could be mistaken for mesothelioma.

Tumors

Q1

Benign mesotheliomas are usually small papillary structures found incidentally at laparoscopy.

Q2

Malignant mesotheliomas are almost all found in men with a history of asbestos exposure.

Q3

Malignant mesothelioma typically affects the visceral epithelium of the intestines but does not involve the mesenteric peritoneum.

Q4

Most malignant mesotheliomas are histologically biphasic and contain a carcinomatous and a sarcomatous component.

Q5

The deciduoid form of mesothelioma is found only in women and is not related to asbestos exposure.

Q6

Malignant mesotheliomas typically react with antibodies to carcinoembryonic antigen (CEA) and are thus indistinguishable immunohistochemically from adenocarcinomas of the intestine.

Q7

The most important indicator of malignancy of a mesothelioma is the invasion of fat or solid organs.

Q8

Intra-abdominal desmoplastic small cell tumor (DSCT) has a tendency to occur in the pelvis of adolescent and young adult males.

Q9

Intra-abdominal desmoplastic small cell tumor is composed of small blue cells showing typically marked nuclear pleomorphism, but lacking mitotic activity and stroma.

Q10

Intra-abdominal desmoplastic small cell tumor reacts with antibodies to keratin and calretinin and is thus a form of mesothelioma.

Q11

Pseudomyxoma peritonei is in most instances caused by a peritoneal seeding of primary mucin-producing tumors of the ovary.

Q12

Metastatic carcinoma represents the most common malignant tumor of the omentum.

Q13

Most retroperitoneal lymphomas are of T-cell origin.

Q14

Liposarcomas are the most common primary retroperitoneal soft tissue sarcomas.

Q15

Malignant fibrous histiocytomas (MFH) and leiomyosarcomas are the second and third most common malignant tumors of the retroperitoneum.

Q16

Retroperitoneal germ cell tumors in males may present as seminomas.

Q17

Most retroperitoneal malignant germ cell tumors in infants and children have the appearance of yolk sac tumor (endodermal sinus tumor).

Normal anatomy

A1. True

The peritoneal lining is mesodermal in origin but the mesothelial surface layer has all the typical epithelial features. Ultrastructurally the cells are interconnected with one another with tight junctions and desmosomes and the surface is covered with microvilli. Immunohistochemically it reacts with antibodies to cytokeratins. **(p. 2373)**

A2. True

Normal mesothelial cells and mesotheliomas react with the antibodies to calretinin, thrombomodulin, and also with antibodies to cytokeratins 5 and 6 and epithelial membrane antigen (EMA). They are negative for CEA and a variety of antibodies recognizing glycoproteins on adenocarcinomas. **(p. 2373)**

Inflammation and other non-neoplastic lesions

A1. True

Peritonitis in acute pancreatitis is caused by pancreatic juices that contain enzymes capable of destroying tissues (e.g. fat necrosis) and eliciting inflammation. **(p. 2374)**

A2. True

This type of peritonitis, usually called secondary peritonitis, is caused by the mixed bacterial flora that reside in the gastrointestinal tract. **(p. 2374)**

A3. True

Spilled talc causes multiple peritoneal granulomas that contain foreign body giant cells and hydrated magnesium silica crystals, which are birefringent under polarized light. **(p. 2375)**

A4. True

These cysts usually have a thin translucent wall and microscopically are lined by cuboidal or flattened mesothelial cells. **(p. 2375)**

A5. False

This lesion is almost exclusively found in the pelvis of women who have had previous surgery, pelvic inflammatory disease or endometriosis. The lesion therefore most likely represents multiple peritoneal inclusion cysts rather than a neoplasm. They tend to recur, but do not progress to malignant mesothelioma. **(p. 2376)**

A6. True

The mesothelial lining has a capacity to undergo hyperplasia if irritated. Thus it is no surprise that such hyperplastic reaction may be quite florid and may resemble neoplasia, especially in incarcerated or irritated hernias of children. **(p. 2377)**

A7. False

Mesothelial hyperplastic reactive changes may appear histologically as papillary projections, tubular structures or solid mesothelial nests, with scattered psammoma bodies. These lesions should not be considered malignant and must be distinguished from malignant mesotheliomas. **(p. 2377)**

A8. False

Nodular histiocytic/mesothelial hyperplasia is not visible on gross examination and is usually an incidental microscopic finding. It may be mistaken for mesothelioma or carcinoma, but it does not have the nuclear features of malignancy and does not evoke a desmoplastic response. **(p. 2377–2378)**

Tumors

A1. True

Benign mesotheliomas are usually small papillary tumors histologically reminiscent of choroid plexus. Many are most likely non-neoplastic but rather reactive. **(p. 2378)**

A2. False

Approximately 50% of mesotheliomas are found in persons with a history of asbestos exposure. Such patients have usually been heavily exposed to asbestos, unlike pleural mesotheliomas, which occur even after transient asbestos exposure. Even though there is a male preponderance, women are also affected. **(p. 2379)**

A3. False

The plaques and nodules of malignant mesothelioma are scattered over visceral and parietal peritoneum and also involve the mesenteric surfaces, causing shortening of the mesentery. **(p. 2379)**

A4. False

Most often malignant mesotheliomas consist of epithelial cells lining papillary structures and tubules. In other cases mesotheliomas are biphasic, and in addition to the epithelial component also have a sarcomatoid component. Some tumors show cartilaginous or other forms of stromal metaplasia. **(p. 2380)**

A5. False

So-called deciduoid mesothelioma is a rare variant that occurs in both women and men, and in some cases is like the mesothelioma related to asbestos. Deciduoid areas may be also found in otherwise typical tubulopapillary mesotheliomas. **(p. 2380)**

A6. False

CEA is rarely found in mesotheliomas. Immunohistochemistry is generally useful for distinguishing mesotheliomas from adenocarcinomas of the pleural cavity. The best immunohistochemical markers for mesothelioma are calretinin, *WT1* gene product, thrombomodulin and cytokeratin CK5/6. **(p. 2380–2382)**

A7. True

The invasion of fat or solid organs is the most important indicator of malignancy of a mesothelioma, and is useful for distinguishing it from reactive hyperplasia. Reactive hyperplasia shows no invasiveness and the proliferation occurs in a linear fashion on the free surface of the peritoneum. **(p. 2381)**

A8. True

DSCT has a predilection for males under the age of 35. The tumors show a predilection for the pelvis but may extend into the scrotum and involve the entire peritoneal cavity. **(p. 2382)**

A9. False

DSCT is typically composed of relatively uniform small round cells. The nuclei are hyperchromatic but monotonous. There is high mitotic activity. Nests of cells are enclosed in abundant fibrous stroma. **(p. 2382)**

A10. False

DSCT is a tumor that typically shows immunoreactivity with antibodies to epithelial markers (e.g. keratin), muscle markers (e.g. desmin) and neural markers (e.g. neuron-specific enolase). Usually it does not stain with antibodies to calretinin or thrombomodulin. It reacts with antibodies to *WT1* marker and carries a translocation of genes that are involved in the pathogenesis of Wilms' tumor and Ewing sarcoma, two tumors to which it shows also some microscopic similarity. **(p. 2384)**

A11. False

In most instances pseudomyxoma peritonei is a complication of a primary tumor in the appendix. **(p. 2386–2387)**

A12. True

Most of these metastases originate from primary malignant tumors of the ovary and gastrointestinal tract. **(p. 2388)**

A13. False

Most retroperitoneal lymphomas are of B-cell origin. They may cause extensive fibrosis and could be mistaken for idiopathic retroperitoneal fibrosis. **(p. 2394)**

A14. True

Liposarcomas and atypical lipomatous tumors (well-differentiated liposarcomas) are the most common soft tissue sarcomas of the retroperitoneum. Benign lipomas are very rare. Other adipose tumors are myolipomas and angiolipomas. **(p. 2396–2397)**

A15. True

All histologic variants of MFH are found. Leiomyosarcomas resemble those in other sites, but occasionally show granular cell changes and skeletal muscle differentiation. **(p. 2397)**

A16. True

Retroperitoneal germ cell tumors may be primary or may be metastases from a primary in the testis. Histologically these tumors may be classified as seminomas or other non-seminomatous germ cell tumors. **(p. 2399)**

A17. True

These yolk sac tumors may occur in a pure form or admixed with other germ cell tumor components. **(p. 2402)**

27 Cardiovascular system

Normal anatomy

Q1

The pericardium has two main parts: parietal and visceral.

Q2

Cardiac muscle fibers have centrally located nuclei.

Q3

The semilunar valves are covered with a layer of endothelium and consist of three layers: fibrosa, spongiosa and ventricularis.

Myocardial biopsy

Q1

The final diagnosis of idiopathic hypertrophic cardiomyopathy can be best made by transvascular biopsy of the myocardium.

Q2

Leukocytic infiltrates in myocardial biopsies are found only in myocarditis and are useful for distinguishing myocarditis from idiopathic dilated cardiomyopathy.

Q3

Amyloidosis is associated with hypertrophic cardiomyopathy.

Q4

Right ventricular dysplasia has a genetic basis.

Q5

In viral myocarditis the cellular infiltrates are most often composed of neutrophils.

Q6

Giant cell myocarditis occurs typically in the course of sarcoidosis.

Q7

Adriamycin cardiotoxicity is characterized by infiltrates containing numerous eosinophils.

Heart transplant

Q1

Heart transplants are best monitored by measuring the serum complement, and myocardial biopsy is indicated only when serologic studies are equivocal.

Q2

This transplant myocardial biopsy shows signs of mild rejection.

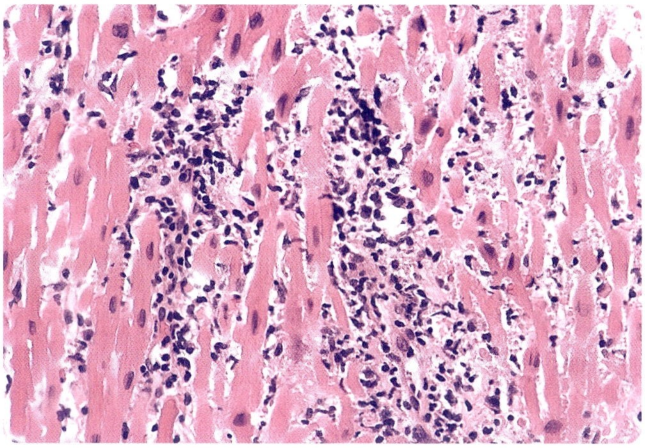

Fig. 27.1

Q3

Transplant vasculopathy involving large and medium-sized heart vessels is characterized by fibrinoid necrosis of the intima and leukocytic infiltrates.

Cardiac valves

Q1

For the proper evaluation of chronic cardiac valvular diseases macroscopic examination is usually more informative than microscopic examination.

Q2

Myxoid degeneration is common in mitral valves removed for floppy mitral valve disease.

Q3

Rupture of mitral chordae is seen only in patients who have mitral stenosis.

Q4

Bicuspid valves are the most common anomaly of the pulmonary valve.

Cardiac tumors

Q1

Myxomas are the most common primary heart tumors.

Q2

Sporadic myxomas typically occur in the right atrium of males under the age of 30.

Q3

Familial cardiac myxomas are part of the Carney syndrome.

Q4

Cardiac myxomas consist of polygonal or stellate cells surrounded by an abundant loose myxoid stroma.

Q5

Rhabdomyoma may be a congenital heart tumor that occurs in association with other abnormalities.

Q6

Among cardiac sarcomas, which are in general very rare tumors, the most common ones are angiosarcomas.

Q7

Most primary cardiac lymphomas have been reported in patients with AIDS and were classified as diffuse large cell type.

Q8

Malignant tumors with a marked tendency to metastasize to the heart by the hematogenous route are hepatocellular carcinomas.

Pericardium

Q1

Sarcoidosis may occasionally be diagnosed by pericardial biopsy.

Q2

Dense fibrosis and calcification in the pericardium may be a consequence of radiation therapy.

Q3

Florid mesothelial proliferation is much more common than mesothelioma, from which it must be distinguished.

Q4

The most common tumors metastasizing to the pericardium are primary carcinomas of the lung.

Arteriosclerosis

Q1

The spindle cells in atherosclerotic plaques are derived from fibroblasts and smooth muscle cells.

Q2

Aortic aneurysms caused by atherosclerosis are most often located in the ascending part of the thoracic aorta.

Q3

Cystic medial change is a manifestation of atherosclerosis of the aorta.

Q4

Patients with aortic aneurysms live longer than those who have aortic aneurysm resection.

Q5

The most common site of aneurysms on the extremities are the popliteal and femoral arteries.

Q6

Aortic dissection occurs most often in the abdominal aorta.

Q7

Dissections of the aorta are classified according to the location of the intimal tear and the extent of the dissection.

Q8

Thrombi occluding major arteries can be a consequence of fungal infection, especially by *Aspergillus* and *Mucor*.

Q9

Intestinal infarction may result from the occlusion of mesenteric arteries or veins.

Arteritis

Q1

Takayasu's disease has a predilection for the aortic arch and the major arteries originating from it.

Q2

Kawasaki's disease is a disease of infants and young children and may present with cardiac ischemia and the formation of coronary aneurysms.

Q3

Most aneurysms of the mesenteric arteries are related to infection.

Q4

Giant cell arteritis may present clinically as polymyalgia rheumatica.

Q5

Clinically, the most common form of vasculitis is the one involving small vessels.

Tumors

Q1

Primary tumors of the aorta or the pulmonary artery are almost invariably malignant.

Q2

Most malignant tumors originating in the inferior vena cava are angiosarcomas.

Q3

The disease known as systemic malignant angioendotheliomatosis is actually an angiotropic malignant lymphoma.

Normal anatomy

A1. True

Visceral pericardium covers the heart and is also called epicardium or serous pericardium; parietal pericardium forms the pericardial sac and is also called fibrous pericardium. Both parts are lined on the luminal side by a mesothelial layer. **(p. 2417)**

A2. True

Cardiac fibers (myocytes) have centrally located nuclei, in contrast to skeletal muscle cells which have subsarcolemmal nuclei. **(p. 2417)**

A3. True

Fibrosa is made of dense collagen, the spongiosa of proteoglycans, loosely arranged collagen and fibroblasts, and the ventricularis is rich in elastic fibers. **(p. 2417)**

Myocardial biopsy

A1. False

Idiopathic hypertrophic cardiomyopathy is characterized by myofiber disarray and hypertrophy and interstitial fibrosis. Unfortunately these changes are not diagnostic and may be found in several other heart diseases. Furthermore, the transvascular biopsy is less informative than septal myomectomy specimens or those obtained at thoracotomy or autopsy. **(p. 2418)**

A2. False

Infiltrates of leukocytes are found in approximately 50% of myocardial biopsies from patients who have idiopathic dilated cardiomyopathy, and are not pathognomonic of myocarditis. **(p. 2418)**

A3. False

In general terms cardiomyopathies are classified as dilated, hypertrophic or restrictive, and infiltrative. Amyloidosis of the heart is classified as infiltrative cardiomyopathy and can be diagnosed by myocardial biopsy. **(p. 2418)**

A4. True

Right ventricular dysplasia is a familial condition characterized by infiltration of the right ventricle with adipose and fibrous tissue and right ventricular failure. **(p. 2418)**

A5. False

Myocarditis caused by viruses is accompanied by infiltrates of lymphocytes and macrophages. The infiltrates of neutrophils are typically found in the early stages of myocardial infarction or in myocardial microabscesses that develop during bacterial sepsis. **(p. 2418–2419)**

A6. False

Giant cell myocarditis is an idiopathic condition characterized by destruction of cardiac myocytes by giant cells and T lymphocytes. It differs from sarcoidosis, which is characterized by the formation of granulomas in the heart. **(p. 2419)**

A7. False

Adriamycin cardiotoxicity is characterized by a loss of cross-striation of cardiac myocytes and homogeneous basophilic staining of their cytoplasm. There is very little or almost no inflammation. Eosinophils are usually found in eosinophilic myocarditis and various hypereosinophilic states. **(p. 2419)**

Heart transplant

A1. False

Endomyocardial biopsy is the most sensitive indicator of rejection and is routinely performed following heart transplantation. **(p. 2420)**

A2. False

This figure shows signs of moderate transplant rejection characterized by prominent infiltrates of lymphocytes and destruction of cardiac muscle fibers (myocytolysis). **(p. 2421)**

A3. False

Injury of the endothelium is typically followed by fibromuscular intimal proliferation, leading to narrowing of the vascular lumen. **(p. 2420–2421)**

Cardiac valves

A1. True
Naked eye examination, which may be complemented by X-ray examination, is usually more informative than microscopic examination of chronic valvular lesions. The clinical history is also essential and could provide critical information. **(p. 2422)**

A2. True
This myxoid degeneration results from the accumulation of glycosaminoglycans in the stroma of the valve. **(p. 2422)**

A3. False
Mitral stenosis is characterized in most cases by thickening, fusion and foreshortening of the chordae tendineae. In contrast, floppy mitral valves associated with mitral insufficiency are usually thin and elongated. Rupture of these chordae is seen in more than 50% of surgically removed floppy mitral valves. **(p. 2422)**

A4. True
Overall, congenital abnormalities account for 95% of pathologic changes involving the pulmonary valves, and most of those are bicuspid. **(p. 2422)**

Cardiac tumors

A1. True
Myxomas account for approximately 50% of all primary heart tumors. **(p. 2425)**

A2. False
Approximately 75% of all cardiac myxomas occur in the left atrium (86%), and are most often found in middle-aged women. **(p. 2425)**

A3. True
Cardiac myxomas occur in Carney syndrome, a genetically determined complex that also includes labial lentiginosis, eyelid and cutaneous myxomas, myxoid mammary fibroadenomas, adrenocortical nodular hyperplasia with Cushing's syndrome, and large calcifying Sertoli cell tumor of the testis. **(p. 2425)**

A4. True
These mesenchymal cells produce the acidic mucopolysaccharides that give the tumor its myxoid consistency. **(p. 2425)**

A5. True
Rhabdomyomas are typically seen in the first decade and many are congenital. Some patients have tuberous sclerosis and some have other congenital heart diseases. **(p. 2426)**

A6. True
Sarcomas of the heart are rare, but in this group angiosarcomas account for the most malignancy. Cardiac angiosarcoma is typically located in the atrium. Histologically it has the same features as angiosarcoma in other sites. **(p. 2428)**

A7. True
Primary lymphomas of the heart are very rare. Most were found in patients with AIDS and were classified as diffuse large cell type. **(p. 2429)**

A8. False
For no obvious reasons melanomas have a tendency to metastasize to the heart by the hematogenous route. Other tumors that have such a tendency are carcinomas of the kidney, lung and breast, choriocarcinomas and childhood rhabdomyosarcomas. **(p. 2430)**

Pericardium

A1. True
Sarcoidosis may cause granulomatous pericarditis, which can be diagnosed by pericardial biopsy. It must be distinguished from tuberculous pericarditis, which is rare today in the US. **(p. 2430)**

A2. True
Radiation therapy may induce constrictive pericarditis characterized by dense fibrosis and calcification and obliteration of the pericardial cavity. **(p. 2430)**

A3. True

Mesotheliomas of the pericardium are very rare, whereas mesothelial proliferation is quite commonly found in many forms of pericarditis. Florid mesothelial proliferation limited to the surface of the pericardium should therefore not be confused with mesotheliomas, which show the usual signs of malignancy and are invasive. **(p. 2431)**

A4. True

Lung cancer is the most common tumor metastasizing to the pericardium. The other tumors that tend to metastasize to the pericardium are breast carcinoma, malignant melanoma and lymphomas. **(p. 2431)**

Arteriosclerosis

A1. True

The spindle cells in atherosclerotic plaques are heterogeneous in nature, but most are derived from fibroblasts and smooth muscle cells. **(p. 2438)**

A2. False

Most atherosclerotic aneurysms are located in the abdominal aorta. **(p. 2438)**

A3. True

In most instances cystic medial change predisposing to aortic dissection is a consequence of atherosclerosis or hypertension. **(p. 2439)**

A4. False

The operative mortality today of patients with aortic aneurysms is significantly lower than the likelihood of rupture of the aneurysm without operation. **(p. 2439)**

A5. True

Aneurysms of the arteries of the extremities are rare except for the popliteal and femoral arteries. **(p. 2439)**

A6. False

Aortic dissection usually begins in the ascending part or the upper descending part of the thoracic aorta. **(p. 2440)**

A7. True

Aortic aneurysms are classified according to the location of the tear and the extent of dissection. Type I begin in the ascending aorta and extend beyond it; type II are confined to the ascending aorta; type III A begins in the descending and stops above the diaphragm; type IIIB begins in the descending aorta and extends below the diaphragm. **(p. 2440)**

A8. True

Aspergillus and *Mucor* tend to invade the vessel wall and cause thrombi. **(p. 2442)**

A9. True

Atherosclerosis of the mesenteric arteries or thromboemboli may cause acute mesenteric occlusion. Similarly, thrombi in the venous system may cause intestinal infarction, which is characterized by severe venous congestion. **(p. 2444)**

Arteritis

A1. True

The arch of the aorta and the brachiocephalic and carotid arteries are most often affected by this chronic granulomatous disease of unknown etiology. Clinically it may thus present as a 'pulseless disease,' or with symptoms pertaining to ischemia of the eyes and brain, and weakness or sensory defects in the upper extremities. **(p. 2447)**

A2. True

Kawasaki's disease is a disease of infants and young children of unknown etiology. It is thought to be an immune response to bacterial toxins that act as 'superantigens.' It affects arteries and the coronary arteries are often affected. Kawasaki's disease may be the cause of sudden death, cardiac ischemia or coronary aneurysms. **(p. 2448)**

A3. True

Most aneurysms of the mesenteric arteries are either mycotic (i.e. related to bacterial infection caused by septic emboli in bacterial endocarditis) or syphilitic. **(p. 2449)**

A4. True

Polymyalgia rheumatica, a common syndrome characterized by muscle pain and tenderness, involving mainly the muscles of the neck, shoulder and pelvic girdle, may be a manifestation of generalized giant cell arteritis. **(p. 2449)**

A5. True

In most instances the inflammation involves the small blood vessels of the dermis. It either represents a hypersensitivity reaction to drugs or bacterial antigens, or is part of a systemic autoimmune disease. **(p. 2449)**

Tumors

A1. True

Most tumors originating in the aorta or pulmonary veins are sarcomas. They may be classified histologically as fibrosarcoma, leiomyosarcoma, rhabdomyosarcoma etc. **(p. 2449)**

A2. False

Most malignant tumors of the inferior vena cava and other large veins are leiomyosarcomas. **(p. 2449)**

A3. True

Immunohistochemistry has shown that most of these malignant vascular lesions, previously thought to be primary vascular neoplasms, are actually malignant lymphomas. **(p. 2449)**

28 Neuromuscular system

CENTRAL NERVOUS SYSTEM

Normal anatomy

Q1

Cerebrospinal fluid is drained into the venous sinuses via arachnoid villi.

Q2

The contents of the posterior fossa include the cerebellum, pons, medulla and pulvinar.

Q3

The pineal gland is situated posterior to the roof (or 'tectum') of the midbrain.

Congenital abnormalities

Q1

Meningomyeloceles are more common than simple meningoceles.

Q2

Fifteen percent of encephaloceles exit the cranial cavity in the region of the occiput via defects in the posterior wall of the foramen magnum or occipital bone.

Q3

Neuroglial heterotopias of the nasal region can be composed of astrocytic, neuronal and meningeal cells enmeshed in fibrous tissue.

Q4

Ecchordosis physaliphora is a mass derived from notochordal remnants.

Q5

This figure shows a lesion that is often associated with tuberous sclerosis.

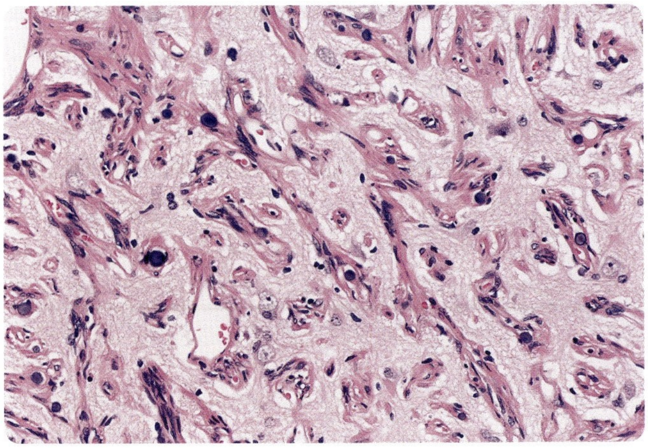

Fig. 28.1

Q6

The lining cells of colloid cysts of the third ventricle are immunohistochemically negative for transthyretin (prealbumin).

Q7

Within the neuraxis a common location for epidermoid cysts is the cerebellopontine angle, whereas dermoid cysts are more commonly seen within the cerebellar vermis.

Q8

Glioependymal cysts are most commonly situated in the spinal cord.

Q9

Arachnoid cysts are most commonly seen in the sylvian fissures.

Cerebrovascular disorders

Q1

The most reliable way to differentiate an infarct from a focus of demyelination is the predominance of foamy macrophages in the latter.

Q2

The most common cause of subarachnoid hemorrhage in adults is saccular, or 'berry,' aneurysm rupture.

Q3

Neoplastic intracranial aneurysm most commonly results from embolization of primary lung carcinoma to the cerebral vasculature.

Q4

Cavernous angiomas are defined as a back-to-back collection of blood-filled vessels comprised solely of fibrous tissue.

Q5

Primary angiitis of the CNS frequently presents with exclusive involvement of large vessels at the base of the brain.

Q6

Hemorrhage associated with cerebral amyloid angiopathy is usually seen in a lobar distribution.

Q7

The histologic hallmark of CADASIL is accumulation of a granular, basophilic, PAS-positive material in the tunica media of affected vessels.

QUESTIONS

Inflammatory diseases

Q1

The MRI scan depicted here is suspicious for a demyelinating pseudotumor.

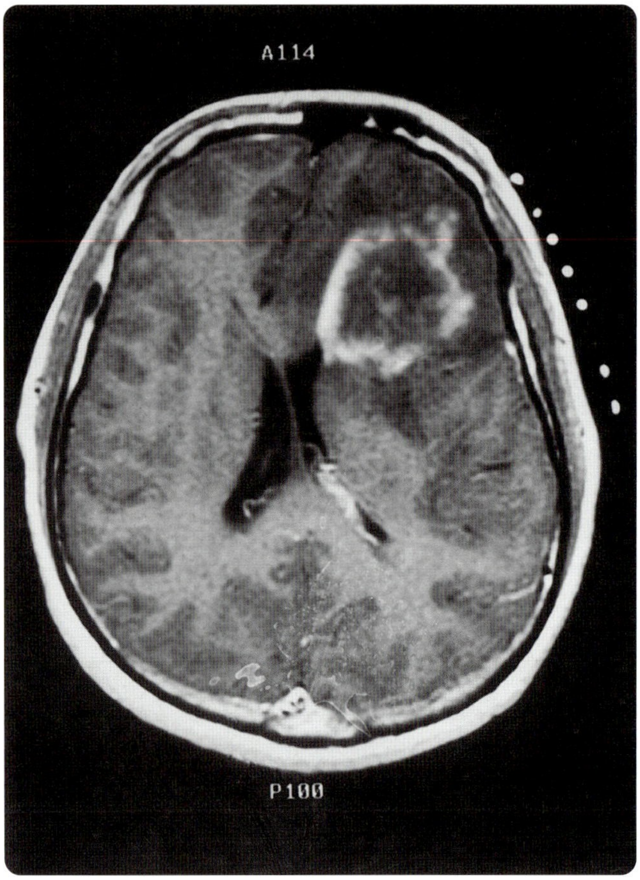

Fig. 28.2

Q2

Diffuse infiltration of macrophages is so rarely a feature of the untreated glioma as to virtually exclude this diagnosis.

Q3

Rasmussen's syndrome is an idiopathic panencephalitis of childhood.

Q4

Limbic encephalitis is usually a paraneoplastic phenomenon.

Q5

Rosai–Dorfman disease of the dura is usually clinically indistinguishable from meningioma.

Infectious diseases

Q1

Abscesses originating from an otitis can be encountered in the cerebellar hemispheres.

Q2

Hematogenous seeding of the CNS from distant foci of infection most often has its origin in chronic suppurating pulmonary disorders.

Q3

Only 40–50% of patients with brain abscesses present with fever.

Q4

'Daughter' abscesses tend to bud from the superficial aspects of cerebral abscesses.

Q5

Most epidural spinal abscesses evolve along the length of the anterolateral spinal cord.

Q6

Candida is the single most common CNS mycosis.

Q7

Neurocysticercosis can involve the ventricular system and basal cisterns in a distinctive pattern of infestation.

Q8

The pseudocysts of cerebral toxoplasmosis are filled with minute, PAS-positive tachyzoites.

Q9

Herpes simplex encephalitis demonstrates a predilection for the anteromedial temporal lobes, orbitofrontal cortex, insulae and cingulate gyri.

Q10

The oligodendroglial karyomegaly seen in progressive multifocal leukoencephalopathy (PML) reflects distension of the nucleus by a population of polyoma virus particles.

Q11

HIV-1 exhibits neuronal tropism within the nervous system.

Q12

A biopsy from a patient with progressive cognitive decline, generalized myoclonus and an electroencephalogram with a 'burst suppression' pattern of spike and wave complexes should be handled with special prion-control precautions by laboratory personnel.

Q13

For safety purposes, a brain biopsy specimen demonstrating a few scattered intracortical vacuoles should be given a diagnosis of 'probable CJD' until proved otherwise.

Primary tumors

Q1

Well-differentiated (WHO grade II) fibrillary astrocytic neoplasms typically present after age 40.

Q2

Diffuse fibrillary astrocytoma is most commonly seen in the cerebral hemispheres.

Q3

A brain biopsy demonstrating microcystic change and scattered calcospherites militates strongly against the diagnosis of astrocytoma.

Q4

The identification of either endothelial hyperplasia or focal coagulative tumor necrosis in an astrocytic neoplasm suffices for a diagnosis of glioblastoma multiforme by WHO criteria.

Q5

Vasculopathic changes, including ectasia, fibrinoid necrosis and obliterative mural fibroplasia are characteristic of glioblastoma multiforme.

Q6

Any cytokeratin cocktail immunohistochemical stain will suffice in distinguishing a primary astrocytic neoplasm from a metastatic carcinoma.

Q7

Events that abrogate p53 function commonly occur early in the evolution of fibrillary astrocytomas.

Q8

Oligodendrogliomas also usually display nuclear p53 immunoreactivity.

Q9

Pilocytic astrocytomas exhibit a decided predilection for the anterior optic pathway.

Q10

Classically associated with the juvenile pilocytic astrocytoma are the cytoplasmic structures known as Rosenthal fibers and eosinophilic granular bodies. These structures are simply morphologic variants of one another.

Q11

Pilocytic astrocytomas frequently display extensive infiltration of the adjacent subarachnoid space and leptomeninges.

Q12

Pilocytic astrocytomas not infrequently exhibit malignant degeneration if left untreated.

Q13

The principal differential diagnosis of a lesion represented on MRI as a cyst with a mural nodule includes pilocytic astrocytoma, pleomorphic xanthoastrocytoma and ganglioglioma.

Q14

Pleomorphic xanthoastrocytoma is characterized by an intricate pericellular pattern of reticulin deposition.

Q15

The malignant behavior of pleomorphic xanthoastrocytomas is suggested by the bizarre, multinucleated astrocytes seen in these tumors.

Q16

The periventricular 'candle gutterings' seen in tuberous sclerosis are essentially miniature subependymal giant cell astrocytomas.

Q17

The most frequent location for oligodendrogliomas is the brain stem.

Q18

Oligodendrogliomas are usually found to lie mainly within the cortex.

Q19

Under the microscope, oligodendrogliomas tend to exhibit a tendency to perineuronal tumor cell aggregation ('satellitosis').

Q20

Oligodendrogliomas can contain intensely GFAP-positive 'mini-gemistocytes.'

Q21

Immunolabeling for S-100 protein, membranous Leu7 (CD57) reactivity and expression of carbonic anhydrase C are reliable markers for use in diagnosing oligodendroglioma.

Q22

A four-tiered grading system has emerged for oligodendroglioma that essentially parallels the WHO classification of astrocytoma.

Q23

For oligodendroglioma, combined and isolated allelic losses involving chromosomes 1p and 19q are predictive of relatively prolonged patient survival.

Q24

Ependymomas tend to be diffusely infiltrating on neuroradiologic study.

Q25

A helpful cytological feature in diagnosing ependymoma is that tumor cell nuclei can exhibit longitudinal nuclear grooving.

Q26

Tanycytic ependymomas are typically encountered within the fourth ventricle.

Q27

CAM 5.2 immunohistochemistry is useful in distinguishing papillary ependymoma from choroid plexus papilloma.

Q28

The myxopapillary ependymoma is a morphologically distinctive ependymoma variant virtually restricted to the region of the conus medullaris and filum terminale.

Q29

Subependymoma is a benign (WHO grade I) neoplasm. However, some examples contain a subset of cells with conspicuously enlarged and atypical nuclei, modest mitotic activity and foci of coagulative necrosis. These findings are predictive of an aggressive course.

Q30

Astroblastoma usually presents as a mass in the cerebral hemisphere of a child, adolescent or young adult.

Q31

A near constant feature of chordoid glioma of the third ventricle is interstitial and perivascular infiltration by lymphocytes.

Q32

Gliomatosis cerebri is a rare condition in which large portions of the brain are permeated by neoplastic cells in such a manner as to suggest a transformative 'field effect' rather than the centrifugal spread of an initially localized glial tumor.

Q33

Pituicytoma is a very rare neoplasm of the sellar and suprasellar compartments.

Q34

Sarcomatous change has been estimated to occur in some 20% of glioblastomas.

Q35

The identification of an architecturally and cytologically distinct, GFAP-negative component is requisite to the segregation of true gliosarcoma from collagenized, spindle cell ('desmoplastic') glioblastomas.

Q36

Most choroid plexus papillomas come to attention during early childhood, displaying a predilection for the lateral ventricles.

Q37

Choroid plexus papillomas may evidence limited ependymal differentiation, signaled by foci in which tumor cells extend tapering, GFAP-immunoreactive cytoplasmic processes toward their fibrovascular cores.

Q38

In contrast to its benign counterpart, choroid plexus carcinoma more often presents in adults than in children.

Q39

The presence of neuronal multinucleation is suggestive of either a reactive process or a ganglion cell tumor.

Q40

Cytologic atypism, if sufficiently pronounced, constitutes grounds for the diagnosis of anaplastic ganglioglioma.

Q41

Ultrastructurally, the neoplastic neurons of ganglion cell tumors share with normal cortical neurons the presence of dense-core neurosecretory granules.

Q42

Desmoplastic infantile ganglioglioma is usually accorded a WHO grade II status, with tumors exhibiting a frankly malignant histologic appearance (e.g. conspicuous mitotic activity and necrosis with palisading) given a WHO grade III designation.

Q43

Central neurocytomas often exhibit labeling for the Hu and NeuN neuronal nuclear proteins.

Q44

Cerebellar liponeurocytoma is principally a tumor of childhood.

Q45

The depicted lesion, seen in a FLAIR MR sequence, is most consistent with an anaplastic oligodendroglioma.

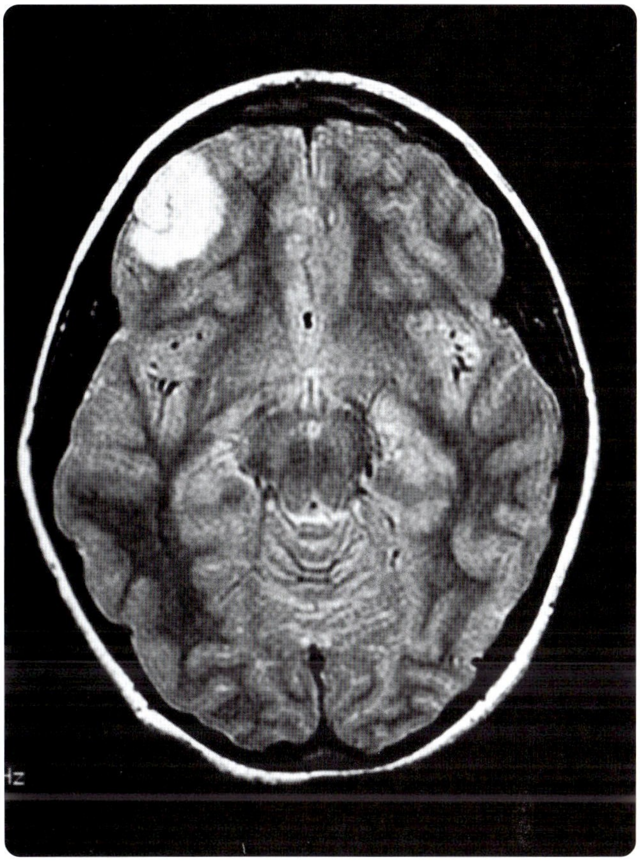

Fig. 28.3

Q46

The presence of the 'specific glioneuronal element' is required for the morphologic diagnosis of dysembryoplastic neuroepithelial (DNT).

Q47

Gangliogliomas often share with glioneuronal hamartomas the expression of CD34, restricted in the normal CNS to embryonic neural stem cells and endothelium.

Q48

Although dysplastic gangliocytoma of the cerebellum usually occurs in sporadic fashion, it is now recognized as a potential manifestation of Gorlin syndrome.

Q49

At least 75% of childhood medulloblastomas arise in the lateral cerebellar hemisphere.

Q50

The 'pale islands' of desmoplastic medulloblastoma constitute loci of concentrated immunoreactivity for synaptophysin.

Q51

Synaptophysin is a useful immunohistochemical stain in the differential diagnosis of medulloblastoma.

Q52

At present, the therapeutic approach to medulloblastomas is predicated solely on clinical variables.

Q53

Because of the invasive nature of surgical intervention, conventional radiotherapy is the first-line treatment for medulloblastoma in children under the age of 3.

Q54

On occasion, medulloblastoma metastasizes systemically. The most common metastatic site is the lung.

Q55

The most common genetic alteration associated with classic medulloblastoma involves abnormality of chromosome 22.

Q56

The diagnosis of neuroblastoma should be reserved for extracerebellar neoplasms of embryonal appearance that can be shown to differentiate solely along neuronal lines.

Q57

The atypical teratoid/rhabdoid tumor (AT/RT) is a highly aggressive neoplasm.

Q58

The *INI1* gene mutation on chromosome 22 is exclusively seen in relation to AT/RT.

Q59

Apart from manifestations of obstructive hydrocephalus owing to aqueductal compression, pineal parenchymal tumors can also present with disturbances of ocular motility resulting from pressure on the mesencephalic tectum.

Q60

The defining histologic feature of pineocytoma is the 'pineocytomatous rosette.'

Q61

Ultrastructural studies have demonstrated that the cytoplasmic processes elaborated by pineocytoma cells distinctly resemble those of native pineocytes in the tendency of microtubule-laden neurite-like cellular extensions to end as bulbous expansions containing clear vesicles of synaptic-type dense-core ('neurosecretory') vesicles and vesicle-crowned rodlets.

Q62

Males are more commonly afflicted by meningiomas than females.

Q63

Ionizing cranial irradiation confers a significant risk for subsequent meningioma development.

Q64

Overlying bony invasion by meningioma is indicative of a more aggressive course.

Q65

Meningotheliomatous variants of meningioma are characterized by a lobular microarchitecture and are populated by cells having delicate round or oval nuclei, inconspicuous nucleoli, lightly eosinophilic cytoplasm and indistinct cytoplasmic borders.

Q66

Transitional meningioma is so called because it is a hybrid of meningotheliomatous and fibrous meningioma.

Q67

Of particular diagnostic utility is the observation that a large majority of meningiomas exhibit (at least focally) membranous, as well as diffuse cytoplasmic immunolabeling for EMA.

Q68

A meningioma specimen is received which, upon microscopic examination, exhibits hypercellularity, cigar-shaped nuclei, and a patternless sheet-like cellular arrangement. These criteria in themselves allow the pathologist to designate the meningioma as 'atypical' (i.e. WHO grade II).

Q69

Laterally situated intracranial lipomas most often involve the seventh cranial nerve.

Q70

Solitary fibrous tumors (SFTs) are generally benign in appearance and clinical evolution.

Q71

Gross total resection of fibrosarcomas usually proves curative.

Q72

Intracranial variants of intravascular papillary endothelial hyperplasia (also known as Masson's vegetant intravascular hemangioendothelioma), which may evolve from pre-existing vascular malformations or develop within dural venous sinuses, have been known to regrow if subtotally excised.

Q73

Meningeal hemangiopericytomas, like meningiomas, exhibit a distinct predilection for women.

Q74

Meningeal hemangiopericytomas, like meningiomas, feature cells with nuclei containing intranuclear pseudoinclusions.

Q75

Meningeal hemangiopericytomas, like meningiomas, stain positively for epithelial membrane antigen (EMA).

Q76

Regrowth at the primary site despite seemingly complete initial resection is typical of meningeal hemangiopericytoma.

Q77

Schwannomas often assume a 'dumbbell' configuration.

Q78

Bilateral eighth-nerve schwannoma is a defining feature of neurofibromatosis type 2 (NF-2).

Q79

The majority of cases of primary central nervous system lymphoma (PCNSL) arise in the setting of AIDS.

Q80

Sporadic cases of PCNSL tend to have a different appearance on post-contrast MRI compared to AIDS-related PCNSL.

Q81

Intracranial masses in older adults that regress substantially with corticosteroid administration alone prior to biopsy are highly suspicious for PCNSL.

Q82

Most PCNSLs are high-grade non-Hodgkin's lesions of diffuse large cell type.

Q83

Most PCNSLs are B-cell neoplasms.

Q84

Given adequate time, most patients with PCNSL develop systemic lymphomatous infiltrates.

Q85

Patients with angiotropic lymphoma often present with neurologic dysfunction that reflects multifocal cerebral infarction resulting from occlusion of vascular lumina by malignant lymphoid cells.

Q86

Sharing with other extragonadal germ cell tumors a predilection for the midline, at least 80–90% of CNS examples arise along an axis extending from the suprasellar cistern and infundibulum to the pineal gland.

Q87

Intracranial germinoma demonstrates cytoplasmic immunolabeling for placental alkaline phosphatase (PLAP), α-fetoprotein (α-FP), and β-HCG.

Q88

The diagnosis of melanocytoma should be questioned if conspicuous nuclear atypia and pleomorphism is present.

Q89

Immunoreactivity for epithelial membrane antigen supports the diagnosis of melanocytoma.

Q90

Malignant melanomas of the CNS may present as diffuse leptomeningeal growths or discrete masses.

Q91

Primary paragangliomas of the craniospinal axis usually arise in the region of the cauda equina.

Q92

Paragangliomas of the CNS are histologically, ultrastructurally and immunophenotypically comparable to their systemic counterparts.

Q93

By definition, a chordoma is intraosseous.

Q94

Intradural chordomas share with their osseous counterparts expression of cytokeratins and EMA, both alien to the chondrosarcoma.

Q95

Von Hippel–Lindau disease is an autosomal dominant disorder caused by germline mutations of VHL, a tumor-suppressor gene localized to chromosome 3p.

Q96

Hemangioblastoma often constitutes a sharply circumscribed mural nodule, at times diminutive, in what is otherwise a smooth-walled cyst or, at spinal levels, syrinx.

Q97

The hemangioblastoma 'stromal cell' serves as a supporting structure for the neoplastic endothelial cells that make up the tumor.

Q98

The stromal cells of hemangioblastoma label for such endothelial markers as CD31 and CD34.

Q99

Like medulloblastoma, neuroblastoma and glioblastoma, hemangioblastoma follows an aggressive clinical course.

Secondary tumors

Q1

Colorectal carcinoma is the systemic cancer most likely to present initially as an intracerebral tumor.

Q2

Most metastases are located in the deep white matter.

Q3

With the provision of adequate tissue a confident diagnosis of metastatic carcinoma can often be made at the time of surgery by examination of smear or crush preparations.

Q4

Glial neoplasms of various types, including fibrillary astrocytomas, may be labeled by antibodies to cytokeratins (particularly the AE1/3 'cocktail') and, on occasion, EMA.

Peripheral nerve

Q1

The four types of preparation needed for a proper evaluation of a nerve specimen are: paraffin embedding after B5 fixation, teased nerve fibers, cryostat sections after 'quench' freezing in isopentane–liquid nitrogen, and plastic resin embedding for light and transmission electron microscopy.

Q2

Renaut bodies are most prominent during fetal life.

Q3

Unmyelinated nerve fibers tend to be larger, in order to accommodate the slower conduction speed in these fibers.

Q4

Wallerian degeneration is primarily a demyelinating process.

Q5

In the Guillain–Barré syndrome, a characteristic mechanism of demyelination is the stripping of myelin off the axon by invading macrophages.

Q6

The process depicted here can only be shown in cross-section.

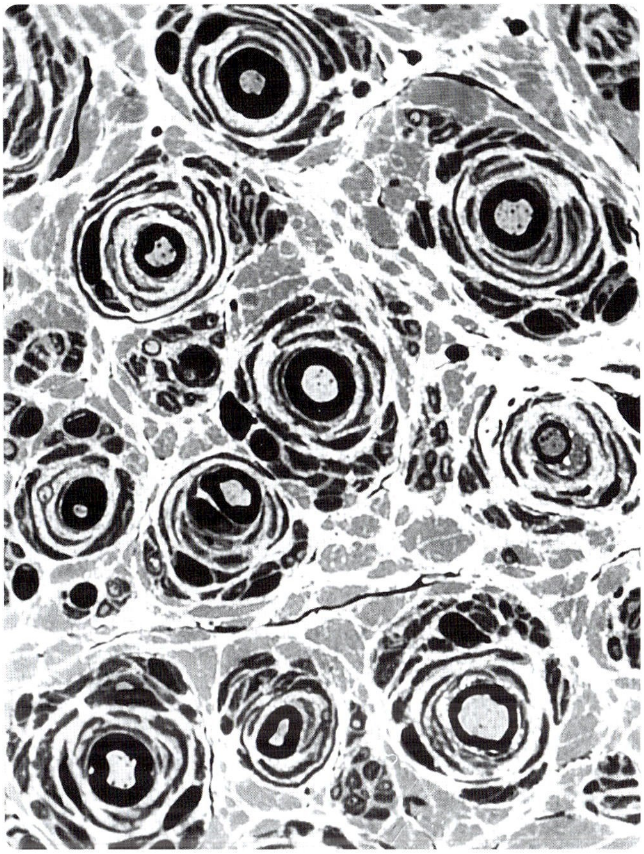

Fig. 28.4

Q7

Patients with Charcot–Marie–Tooth disease (CMT) develop weakness and wasting distally in the upper extremities, associated with areflexia and sensory loss. The lower extremities are involved at a later stage.

Q8

In Krabbe's globoid cell leukodystrophy, frozen sections of peripheral nerve examined under polarized light disclose birefringent 'Maltese crosses.'

Q9

In Guillain–Barré syndrome semithin sections of peripheral nerve show a hypercellular endoneurium.

Q10

The bacilli of *Mycobacterium leprae* are seen in more abundance on nerve biopsies demonstrating lepromatous as opposed to tuberculoid leprous neuritis.

Q11

Nerve biopsies showing perivascular aggregates of mononuclear cells without transmural inflammation and necrosis are not diagnostic of vasculitis.

Q12

The precursor protein of most types of familial amyloidotic polyneuropathy (FAP) has been identified as variant types of transthyretin.

Q13

All patients with peripheral neuropathy and IgM monoclonal gammopathy have IgM antibodies that bind to axons.

Q14

The ultrastructural finding of widely spaced myelin (WSM) is a unique feature of dysglobulinemic neuropathy.

Q15

Small, unmyelinated fibers are usually more severely affected in toxic-metabolic neuropathy.

Q16

Chronic treatment with chloroquine may cause axonal degeneration and demyelination.

Skeletal muscle

Q1

Up to 4% of muscle fibers in the normal adult fascicle may show internalization of the nuclei.

Q2

Ultrastructurally, the sarcomere's A band is darker than the I band.

Q3

With the ATPase reaction at pH 9.4, the type I fibers are pale and type II fibers are dark.

Q4

In an ATPase reaction at pH 9.4, a quadriceps muscle biopsy contains roughly one-third pale-staining fibers and two-thirds dark-staining fibers.

QUESTIONS

Q5
NADH-TR, succinic dehydrogenase, and cytochrome oxidase all stain type I fibers darker than type II fibers.

Q6
In Werdnig–Hoffman disease the markedly atrophic fibers have angulated contours.

Q7
Perifascicular fiber atrophy is typical of polymyositis.

Q8
The inclusions of inclusion body myositis (IBM) are slit-like intrasarcoplasmic rimmed vacuoles.

Q9
Duchenne's muscular dystrophy (DMD) is a defect in the intranuclear protein dystrophin, which is located on the short arm of the X chromosome (Xp12.2).

Q10
The clinical course of Becker's muscular dystrophy (BMD) is slightly more severe than that of DMD.

Q11
At least 25% of the fibers in central nuclear myopathy have centrally placed nuclei.

Q12
The inclusions in rod (nemaline) myopathy are best seen with modified Gomori trichrome as granular perinuclear deposits.

Q13
Periodic paralysis is related to abnormalities in the influx and efflux of calcium ions in muscle fibers.

Q14
Electron microscopy helps to distinguish acid maltase deficiency from other glycogenoses.

Q15
Mitochondrial myopathies are always maternally inherited.

Q16
Toxic reaction to chloroquine and hydroxychloroquine results in a vacuolar myopathy associated with proximal weakness.

CENTRAL NERVOUS SYSTEM

Normal anatomy

A1. True
When amassed into a grossly visible group these are called arachnoid, or pacchionian, granulations. **(p. 2462)**

A2. False
The pulvinar is a thalamic structure situated well above the tentorium cerebelli. The other structures mentioned are indeed nestled within the posterior fossa. **(p. 2462)**

A3. True
Labeled as the 'seat of the soul' by the 17th century scientist René Descartes, the pineal gland is now considered a neuroendocrine organ. **(p. 2462)**

Congenital abnormalities

A1. True
Furthermore, meningomyeloceles are usually associated with neurologic impairment, whereas meningoceles can often be repaired with no residual sequelae. **(p. 2463)**

A2. False
The occiput is the most common location of this anomaly, accounting for 80% of encephaloceles. **(p. 2464)**

A3. False
The inclusion of meninges rules out heterotopia in favor of encephalocele, as the presence of meningeal cells implies communication with the intracranial compartment. **(p. 2466)**

A4. True
Loosely translating from its Greek origin, the term ecchordosis physaliphora means 'bubble-like forms emerging from the notochord.' **(p. 2466)**

A5. False
This figure shows the typical features of meningioangiomatosis, which is not associated with tuberous sclerosis but with another phakomatosis: neurofibromatosis type 2. **(p. 2466)**

A6. True
Colloid cysts of the third ventricle are endodermal in origin, with a mucosa-type lining. Transthyretin is positive in choroid plexus-type cells. **(p. 2466)**

A7. True
In contrast to epidermoid cysts, dermoid cysts tend to be midline. **(p. 2467)**

A8. False
The most common location of glioependymal cysts is the paraventricular white matter of the frontal and parietal lobes. **(p. 2470)**

A9. True
They can also be seen in the cisterna magna, cerebellopontine angles, and, less commonly, in the suprasellar region and along the spinal neuraxis. **(p. 2470)**

Cerebrovascular disorders

A1. False
The principal histological difference between these two entities is the relative preservation of axons in demyelination. Infarcts, in contrast, exhibit indiscriminate cell death, with no axonal sparing. **(p. 2471)**

A2. True
For children, the most common cause of subarachnoid hemorrhage is trauma. **(p. 2471)**

A3. False
Neoplastic aneurysm formation most commonly results from embolization of cardiac myxomas. **(p. 2473)**

A4. True
A directly apposed arrangement of vessels, devoid of neuroglial tissue, is requisite for the diagnosis of cavernous angioma. **(p. 2474)**

A5. False

Small to medium-sized leptomeningeal and intracortical arteries are the most commonly involved vessels, sometimes with angiitis of the large vessels of the base of the brain as well. **(p. 2476–2477)**

A6. True

In contrast, hypertensive hemorrhages tend to occur in the basal ganglia. **(p. 2477)**

A7. True

Although the exact nature of this material is unknown, immunohistochemical staining with Notch 3 protein is usually positive. **(p. 2479)**

Inflammatory diseases

A1. True

This case is especially suspicious for demyelinating pseudotumor as the lesion appears to fan out from a ventricular angle. Additionally, a characteristic 'broken ring' profile of enhancement directly abuts a ventricular surface. **(p. 2480)**

A2. True

Identification of such cells should instead suggest a non-neoplastic necrotizing process such as organizing infarction or a demyelinating process. **(p. 2482)**

A3. False

Rasmussen's syndrome is defined as a unilateral hemispheric encephalitis. **(p. 2484)**

A4. True

Limbic encephalitis is usually a complication of small cell carcinoma of the lung. **(p. 2485)**

A5. True

Both Rosai–Dorfman disease and meningioma are contrast-enhancing lesions on MRI and can impose a mass effect. **(p. 2486)**

Infectious diseases

A1. True

The temporal lobes are another typical location of otitis-related cerebral abscesses. **(p. 2487)**

A2. True

Disorders such as lung abscesses and bronchiectasis lead the list of conditions predisposing to 'metastatic' CNS abscesses. **(p. 2488)**

A3. True

The more common signs and symptoms are those of an expanding intracranial mass, which brings malignant neoplasm and, on occasion, demyelinating disease into the differential diagnosis. **(p. 2488)**

A4. False

The capsular organization of an abscess wall is typically most advanced along the superficial, juxtacortical perimeter of brain abscesses. Thus, there is a tendency for the lesions to bud from their deep aspects, with a tendency to rupture into the ventricular system rather than the arachnoid space. **(p. 2489)**

A5. False

Anterior tethering of the dura to adjacent vertebral bodies presumably accounts for the fact that most spinal epidural abscesses are posteriorly or posterolaterally positioned. **(p. 2489)**

A6. False

Cryptococcus neoformans is the agent of a diffuse leptomeningitis that is the single most common CNS mycosis. **(p. 2490)**

A7. True

This pattern of involvement is known as racemose cysticercosis. The term 'racemose' means 'formed like a cluster of grapes.' Racemose cysticerci evacuated from the ventricles or subarachnoid space present as grape-like clusters of interconnected larval 'bladders.' **(p. 2492–2493)**

A8. False

Toxoplasma pseudocysts are filled with bradyzoites, named for their slow replicative cycles. Tachyzoites are the rapidly proliferating, crescentic protozoal forms that lie outside the pseudocysts and are primarily responsible for the tissue injury seen in cerebral toxoplasmosis. **(p. 2494)**

A9. True

This 'limbic' distribution supports the hypothesis that spread of the virus is by a transolfactory route. **(p. 2495)**

A10. True

Specifically, the JC polyoma virus is the infecting agent in virtually all cases of PML. **(p. 2497–2498)**

A11. **False**
HIV-1 is alone among viral encephalitogens in exhibiting no particular tropism for neuroectodermal cell types, its replication in the nervous system taking place largely within marrow-derived macrophages and microglia. **(p. 2501)**

A12. **True**
These are the classic clinical features of Creutzfeldt–Jakob disease. Special handling is required in suspected cases of CJD because routinely formalinized and paraffin-embedded specimens retain infectious transmissibility. **(p. 2502–2503)**

A13. **False**
Scattered vacuoles are a common artifact of surgical manipulation and should not automatically prompt a presumptive diagnosis of CJD. **(p. 2502)**

Primary tumors

A1. **False**
WHO grade II fibrillary astrocytomas typically present in the third or fourth decade of life and are decidedly uncommon after age 40 (beyond which, the overwhelming majority of fibrillary astrocytic tumors exhibit anaplastic histologic features or are frank glioblastomas). **(p. 2504)**

A2. **True**
Here they are characteristically centered in the white matter. **(p. 2504)**

A3. **False**
In fact, microcystic change and calcospherites are highly suggestive of a glial neoplasm. In contrast, the presence of foamy macrophages strongly favors a diagnosis of demyelinating disease or infarction. **(p. 2505)**

A4. **True**
Classic pseudopalisading necrosis is not required for the diagnosis. **(p. 2508)**

A5. **False**
The changes described are the hallmarks of radiation effect. Distinguishing radiation effect from tumor necrosis and vascular proliferation will keep the diagnostician from overgrading an astrocytic tumor. **(p. 2509)**

A6. **False**
Reactive and neoplastic astrocytes will often stain with the AE1/3 cytokeratin cocktail, as would the majority of metastatic carcinomas. However, immunostains for CAM5.2, CK7, CK20 and the non-cytokeratin epithelial marker BerEP4 are reliably negative in astrocytes. **(p. 2510)**

A7. **True**
Abnormal accumulation ('overexpression') of mutant p53 in this setting is often evidenced by nuclear immunolabeling of neoplastic cells for this protein. **(p. 2512–2513)**

A8. **False**
Mutations of p53 are uncommon in this tumor group. **(p. 2514)**

A9. **True**
In addition to the anterior optic pathway, pilocytic astrocytomas tend to occur in the cerebellum and third ventricular/hypothalamic region. **(p. 2514)**

A10. **False**
Many observers, noting that both Rosenthal fibers and eosinophilic granular bodies are composed of hyaline pink material, assume that they represent the same material in different shapes. This conclusion can be contradicted on ultrastructural grounds. Electron microscopy of Rosenthal fibers reveals them to be comprised of masses of granular, electron-dense material surrounded by glial filaments. Eosinophilic granular bodies, on the other hand, are made up of engorged lysosomes containing membranous debris. **(p. 2516)**

A11. **True**
Nevertheless, dissemination via the CSF is exceptional. **(p. 2517)**

A12. **False**
In fact, malignant degeneration is rare and appears to be iatrogenic when it does occur, with nearly all reported cases being associated with radiation therapy. **(p. 2517)**

A13. **True**
Interestingly, this same tripartite differential diagnosis is operational at the microscope when one encounters aggregated eosinophilic granular bodies. **(p. 2519)**

A14. **True**
This feature reflects the elaboration by tumor cells of encircling basal lamina material. **(p. 2520)**

A15. **False**
Despite their disturbing morphology, pleomorphic xanthoastrocytomas tend to behave in a relatively benign clinical fashion, gross total resection usually sufficing to achieve long-term tumor control. **(p. 2520)**

A16. True
These small, non-obstructive tumors are composed of outsized astrocytes aggregated in a fibrillary matrix prone to calcification. **(p. 2521)**

A17. False
Only exceptionally do oligodendroglial neoplasms arise below the tentorium. **(p. 2522)**

A18. False
Oligodendrogliomas are usually found to lie mainly within white matter at operation, but extension into the overlying cortex is the rule. **(p. 2522)**

A19. True
In this sense they recapitulate the tendency of normal oligodendrocytes to array themselves in the same manner. **(p. 2523)**

A20. True
Mini-gemistocytes differ from gemistocytic astrocytes most obviously by the smaller cellular and nuclear size of the former. **(p. 2523)**

A21. False
At present there is no immunocytochemical reagent that consistently and specifically identifies neoplastic cells as oligodendroglial. Immunolabeling for S-100 protein, membranous Leu7 (CD57) reactivity and expression of carbonic anhydrase C are characteristic, but shared by other tumor types. **(p. 2523)**

A22. False
Most neuropathologists use a two-tiered grading system for oligodendrogliomas, segregating them into WHO grade II and grade III. **(p. 2525)**

A23. True
Furthermore, this karyotypic signature identifies a subset of anaplastic oligodendroglial neoplasms that can be driven into chemotherapy-induced remissions of gratifying durability. **(p. 2525)**

A24. False
Ependymomas tend to be well circumscribed and contrast enhancing on neuroradiologic study. **(p. 2526)**

A25. True
Longitudinal nuclear grooves are optimally visualized in cytological preparations, a feature that can facilitate intraoperative diagnosis. **(p. 2527)**

A26. False
They are typically encountered at spinal levels. **(p. 2528)**

A27. True
CAM 5.2 is generally negative in ependymomas and diffusely positive in choroid plexus papillomas. **(p. 2529)**

A28. True
An origin in the cervicothoracic segments of the spinal cord is exceptional, an intracranial presentation exceedingly rare. **(p. 2529)**

A29. False
Once a diagnosis of subependymoma is made, these other histological features do not confer a worse prognosis and therefore do not warrant labeling the lesion with a higher grade than WHO grade I. **(p. 2531–2532)**

A30. True
Astroblastoma usually presents as a well-demarcated contrast-enhancing mass in this age group. **(p. 2532–2533)**

A31. True
Russell body-bearing plasma cells also infiltrate the interstitial and perivascular regions of this tumor. **(p. 2534)**

A32. True
Affected areas are typically expanded in a non-destructive ('pseudohypertrophic') fashion. **(p. 2535)**

A33. True
This neoplasm is believed to derive from specialized glial elements known as pituicytes, native to the neurohypophysis and infundibulum. **(p. 2535)**

A34. False
Sarcomatous change is seen in approximately 2% of glioblastomas. **(p. 2536)**

A35. True
The same holds for distinguishing true gliosarcomas from gliomas associated with a florid fibroblastic reaction by virtue of meningeal invasion. **(p. 2536)**

A36. True
Adult cases, by contrast, are situated more often in the fourth ventricle or its lateral recesses, some presenting as tumors of the cerebellopontine angle. **(p. 2538)**

A37. True
This finding presumably reflects the ontogeny of the plexus epithelium as a form of specialized ependyma, but choroid plexus papillomas do not elaborate the fibrillary glial 'stroma' characteristic of ependymomas – an important differential diagnostic feature. **(p. 2539)**

A38. False
The overwhelming majority of choroid plexus carcinomas present in infancy or childhood. The diagnosis of choroid plexus carcinoma in an adult must be regarded with considerable skepticism (regardless of tumor location, morphology or immunohistochemical characteristics) as this entity is vanishingly rare beyond childhood. **(p. 2539)**

A39. False
The neoplastic neurons of ganglion cell tumor can harbor more than one nucleus. Multinucleation of astrocytes, not neurons, can be seen in the context of a reactive process. **(p. 2540)**

A40. False

Anaplastic ganglioglioma is the designation appropriate to tumors densely populated by mitotically active glial cells (microvascular proliferation and necrosis may also be encountered), cytologic atypism alone, even if pronounced, not constituting grounds for this diagnosis. **(p. 2541)**

A41. False

The neoplastic neurons of ganglion cell tumors often harbor dense-core neurosecretory granules when examined under the electron microscope. This feature is generally foreign to native cortical neurons. Additional, and somewhat more specific (albeit inconstant), immunohistochemical evidence for the tumoral nature of a suspect neuronal population is intense and diffuse perikaryal labeling for chromogranin A, a reflection of dense-core granule formation. **(p. 2542)**

A42. False

Their proliferative small cell components notwithstanding, a most favorable prognosis attaches to cases amenable to gross total resection and so these peculiar tumors are always accorded WHO grade I status. **(p. 2545)**

A43. True

However, expression of chromogranin A and neurofilament protein seems restricted to the rare variant exhibiting transition to ganglion cell-like morphology. **(p. 2547)**

A44. False

To date, this tumor has been encountered only in adults, with a mean age at diagnosis of approximately 50 years. **(p. 2547)**

A45. False

Although the frontal lobe is a common location for an oligodendroglioma, it characteristically arises in the white matter and extends to the cortex. The depicted lesion is largely confined to the cortical ribbon. The lack of either mass effect or surrounding edema suggests that this lesion is a slow-growing mass, rather than one representing an aggressive anaplastic lesion. The diagnosis here is dysembryoplastic neuroepithelial tumor. **(p. 2548)**

A46. True

The 'specific glioneuronal element' is a multinodular proliferation of oligodendrocyte-like cells (OLCs) that appear to be arranged along bundled axons and ramifying capillaries that are separated by a myxoid matrix in which well-differentiated neurons seem to float. This constellation of morphologic features is required for the diagnosis of DNT. **(p. 2458)**

A47. True

However, glioneuronal hamartomas do not evidence the cellularity, pleomorphism or conspicuous inflammatory infiltration of the bona fide ganglioglioma. **(p. 2550)**

A48. False

Gorlin syndrome is associated with desmoplastic medulloblastoma. Dysplastic gangliocytoma of the cerebellum usually occurs in sporadic fashion, but it also has an association with Cowden syndrome. **(p. 2551–2552)**

A49. False

At least 75% of childhood medulloblastomas arise in the cerebellar vermis, with the relative proportion of laterally positioned, hemispheric examples increasing with age. **(p. 2552)**

A50. True

The 'pale islands' of desmoplastic medulloblastoma are regions of immunoreactivity for other neuron-associated cytoplasmic antigens as well, including class III β-tubulin and microtubule-associated protein 2. **(p. 2554)**

A51. True

The labeling of nearly all medulloblastomas (including those of thoroughly undifferentiated histologic aspect) for synaptophysin is a property that may be exploited to exclude from further consideration such potentially confounding lesions as the poorly differentiated fourth ventricular ependymoma, other anaplastic gliomas, and primary cerebellar lymphoma. **(p. 2555)**

A52. True

Children below the age of 3 years at diagnosis, individuals of any age with evident CSF dissemination, or patients with bulky residual disease after surgery do not fare as well. **(p. 2556)**

A53. False

The price exacted of childhood medulloblastoma survivors by conventional radiotherapy – growth failure, endocrinopathy, significant intellectual impairment, behavioral disturbances, and the induction of secondary neoplasms that include meningiomas, sarcomas and glioblastomas – makes surgery and chemotherapy more attractive therapeutic alternatives in these patients. **(p. 2556)**

A54. False

Skeletal deposits, often widespread, account for over 90% of systemic metastases. **(p. 2556)**

A55. False

Isochromosome 17q formation is the most common genetic alteration associated with classic medulloblastomas. Abnormality of chromosome 22 is associated with atypical teratoid/rhabdoid tumor. **(p. 2556)**

A56. True

By definition, these neuronal tumors appear outside the cerebellum. **(p. 2558)**

A57. True

Survival beyond 1 year is exceptional for patients with this tumor. **(p. 2560)**

A58. False

Although over 90% of AT/RTs assessed to date have demonstrated this mutation, *INI1* alterations also characterize a subset of choroid plexus carcinomas and select tumors phenotypically indistinguishable from medulloblastomas and supratentorial PNETs. However, one might be accused of merely playing a semantic game in separating INI1-mutated PNETs from AT/RTs of exclusively neuroepithelial appearance. **(p. 2561–2562)**

A59. True

A classic oculomotor disturbance related to a pineal mass is upwards gaze paresis, termed Parinaud's syndrome. **(p. 2563)**

A60. True

These rosettes are composed of neoplastic cells arrayed about a conspicuous anuclear meshwork of delicate, synaptophysin-immunoreactive cytoplasmic processes. These structures look like outsized versions of Homer Wright rosettes, but are often less regular in contour. **(p. 2563)**

A61. True

Vesicle-crowned rodlets are also known as synaptic ribbons, which are recognized as a distinctive feature of mammalian pineocytes consisting of closely apposed, bar-like osmiophilic densities measuring approximately 700 nm in length by 50 nm wide surrounded by clear vesicles 60 nm in diameter. **(p. 2563)**

A62. False

Females are afflicted more commonly than males (especially at spinal levels). **(p. 2564)**

A63. True

Furthermore, radiation-related lesions are more often multiple, histologically atypical and clinically aggressive than those arising in sporadic fashion. **(p. 2564)**

A64. False

Neither bony invasion nor induced hyperostosis of adjacent bone is cause for concern with regard to meningiomas. **(p. 2565)**

A65. True

The indistinct cytoplasmic borders of meningotheliomatous meningiomas have earned them the alternative name 'syncytial meningiomas.' **(p. 2565)**

A66. True

Transitional meningioma maintains the lobular arrangement of the meningotheliomatous meningioma, but evidences the tendency to cellular elongation and streaming seen in fibrous meningioma. **(p. 2566)**

A67. True

Immunolabeling for EMA is useful in confirming the diagnosis of meningioma because it is a feature foreign to hemangiopericytoma, the nerve sheath tumor other than the rare perineurioma, solitary fibrous tumor and other fibroblastic neoplasms. **(p. 2570)**

A68. False

Close, but no cigar-shaped nuclei. Atypical meningiomas are defined as containing four to 19 mitotic figures per 10 high-power microscopic fields. Alternatively, a meningioma can be called atypical if it exhibits at least three of the following features: hypercellularity; sheet-like growth; macronucleoli; small cell components with high nuclear/cytoplasmic ratio; and zones of necrosis. **(p. 2571)**

A69. False

Intracranial lipomas, when laterally positioned, typically involve the eighth cranial nerve and are usually mistaken for acoustic schwannomas on clinical evaluation. **(p. 2573)**

A70. True

Gross total resection of SFTs usually proves curative. **(p. 2574)**

A71. False

Symptomatic local recurrence is the rule even after gross total resection of circumscribed, superficially positioned fibrosarcomas, and patients with high-grade lesions usually die from their disease within several years of diagnosis. **(p. 2574)**

A72. True

This lesion has also occasionally proved fatal as a result of associated mass effects. **(p. 2575)**

A73. False

Meningeal hemangiopericytomas are not gender biased. **(p. 2575)**

A74. False

Lack of intranuclear pseudoinclusions in meningeal hemangiopericytoma helps to distinguish it from meningioma. **(p. 2575)**

A75. False

EMA positivity in meningioma and negativity in meningeal hemangiopericytoma is another helpful distinguishing feature. **(p. 2576)**

A76. True

However, this may take years to become clinically apparent. **(p. 2576)**

A77. True

The 'dumbbell' shape results when the schwannoma squeezes through an adjacent intervertebral foramen and expands into the paravertebral soft tissues. **(p. 2577)**

A78. True
NF-2 is an autosomal dominant disorder linked to mutations involving a gene localized to chromosome 22. **(p. 2577)**

A79. False
The predilection of PCNSL for victims of AIDS is firmly established, but the majority of afflicted patients suffer no predisposing illness. **(p. 2579)**

A80. True
Extensive central necrosis lends to many HIV-1-associated PCNSLs a 'ring'-enhancing radiologic appearance, whereas sporadic cases tend to have a homogeneous contrast-enhancing appearance. **(p. 2579)**

A81. True
Occasional lymphomas even seem to disappear transiently with corticosteroid treatment. **(p. 2579)**

A82. True
Although most PCNSLs are high-grade non-Hodgkin's lesions of diffuse large cell type, all major cytologic variants have been reported in this location. Follicular (nodular) lymphoid neoplasms, however, are foreign to the neuroparenchyma. **(p. 2580)**

A83. True
The overwhelming majority (>95%) of PCNSLs exhibit a B-cell immunophenotype. **(p. 2580)**

A84. False
Systemic lymphomatous infiltrates develop in no more than 10% of cases. **(p. 2582)**

A85. True
Progressive encephalopathy, dementia and stroke are common clinical presentations. **(p. 2582)**

A86. True
In fact, germ cell tumors are the most common neoplasms encountered in the pineal gland. **(p. 2583)**

A87. False
Pure germinoma demonstrates cytoplasmic immunolabeling (often membranous) for placental alkaline phophatase (PLAP) but not α-FP or β-HCG. **(p. 2583)**

A88. True
Candidates for the diagnosis of melanocytoma should not harbor macronucleoli, evidence conspicuous nuclear atypia or pleomorphism, contain more than the very occasional mitotic figure, or exhibit necrosis. **(p. 2585)**

A89. False
Melanocytomas, in contrast to meningiomas, are epithelial membrane antigen negative. **(p. 2585)**

A90. True
The diffuse leptomeningeal form is known as 'melanomatosis.' **(p. 2586)**

A91. True
Primary paragangliomas of the craniospinal axis most commonly present as delicately encapsulated intradural masses attached to the filum terminale. **(p. 2586)**

A92. True
However, some CNS paragangliomas depart from the classic arrangement of epithelioid tumor cells in cohesive nests ('zellballen') and instead display spindled cytology and vaguely storiform growth or a vasocentric, pseudopapillary architecture. **(p. 2587)**

A93. False
Although it is true that chordomas are usually destructive tumors of the clivus and sacrococcygeum, there are entirely extraosseous intradural variants that typically lie ventral to the brainstem. **(p. 2587)**

A94. True
This immunoprofile helps to distinguish chordoma from chondrosarcoma, which is negative for these markers. **(p. 2587)**

A95. True
Sporadic hemangioblastomas commonly harbor mutations of the VHL gene as well. **(p. 2587)**

A96. True
A clear demarcation from adjacent native tissues is typical of hemangioblastomas.

A97. False
The term 'stroma' is from the Greek word meaning 'bed.' Usually pathologists use the word 'stroma' to indicate the benign underlying supporting structure of the neoplastic cells within a tumor. Hemangioblastoma terminology is quirky in that 'stromal cell' refers to the neoplastic cell itself, which inhabits the interstices between ramifying vascular arcades and is recognized by a pale cytoplasm that is often foamy in appearance. **(p. 2588)**

A98. False
The cytogenesis of hemangioblastoma stromal cells is not a settled matter. They do not express an endothelial immunophenotype, but do produce vascular endothelial growth factor and other promoters of angiogenesis. **(p. 2589)**

A99. False
Despite the misleading '-blastoma' suffix, hemangioblastoma is a benign neoplasm that usually lends itself to curative resection. **(p. 2589)**

Secondary tumors

A1. False

Carcinomas of the lung are the systemic cancers most likely to present initially as intracerebral tumors, accounting for roughly half of all such cases and up to 85% of lesions exhibiting adenocarcinomatous histology. **(p. 2590)**

A2. False

Most metastases are relatively superficial in location, straddling the gray–white junction to involve both cerebral cortex (thus the high incidence of associated seizures) and digitate white matter. **(p. 2591)**

A3. True

The cellular cohesion of most epithelial neoplasms is preserved in smear or crush preparations. **(p. 2591)**

A4. True

The use of these markers may thus be hazardous in distinguishing between a metastatic epithelial lesion and an epithelioid glioma. It would appear that CAM 5.2, CK7, CK20 and Ber EP4 perform in a more discriminating fashion as epithelial markers in this regard. **(p. 2592)**

Peripheral nerve

A1. True

Unlike biopsies for most other tissues, more extensive technical preparation is required for both muscle and nerve specimens. **(p. 2625)**

A2. False

Renaut bodies are not seen during fetal life and seem to increase in number with age, particularly near or at entrapment sites, suggesting that repetitive trauma may play a role in their pathogenesis. **(p. 2626)**

A3. False

Myelinated nerve fibers vary in outside diameter from 2 to 18 mm. Nerve fibers of less than 2 mm in diameter are unmyelinated. **(p. 2627–2628)**

A4. False

In Wallerian degeneration the cardinal feature is degeneration of the axon, which induces disintegration of myelin. This occurs throughout the distal segment of nerve after transection. **(p. 2628)**

A5. True

Macrophage-mediated segmental demyelination is not unique to Guillain–Barré syndrome, it is also seen in chronic inflammatory demyelinating polyneuropathy (CIDP) and in anti-MAG neuropathy. **(p. 2628)**

A6. True

This is an electron microscopic picture of 'onion bulbs,' a term that refers to overlapping layers of Schwann cell processes and intervening collagen arranged in rings around longitudinally oriented nerve fibers. **(p. 2629 and 2633)**

A7. False

The lower extremities are the first to be involved by these symptoms. The upper extremities become involved later. **(p. 2631)**

A8. False

'Maltese crosses' are characteristic of another inherited lysosomal enzyme deficiency, Fabry's disease. **(p. 2635 and 2637)**

A9. True

The endoneurium appears hypercellular because of the presence of numerous debris-laden macrophages that surround denuded axons. **(p. 2637)**

A10. True

Lepromatous and tuberculoid leprosy represent the two ends of the histologic spectrum of leprous neuritis. Lepromatous leprosy is pluribacillary, whereas tuberculoid leprosy is paucibacillary. **(p. 2642)**

A11. True

This is because similar changes are demonstrable in inflammatory neuropathies. **(p. 2645)**

A12. True

Originally called prealbumin, transthyretin is an acronym for a serum transport protein that binds thyroxin and vitamin A (retinoic acid). **(p. 2647)**

A13. False

Approximately one half of patients with peripheral neuropathy and IgM monoclonal gammopathy have IgM antibodies that bind to myelin. The most prevalent antibody activity among these IgM proteins is directed against myelin-associated glycoprotein (MAG) and/or sulfate-3 glucuronyl paragloboside (SGPG). **(p. 2650)**

A14. True

WSM represents focal separation of the virtual extracellular space between myelin leaflets caused by the intrusion of anti-MAG antibodies. **(p. 2650-1)**

A15. **False**

Axonal degeneration of varying severity is the usual pathologic finding in the neuropathy caused by systemic metabolic disorders. Myelinated fibers of larger diameter are always more severely affected. **(p. 2652)**

A16. **True**

Chronic treatment with chloroquine, even when prophylactic doses are given, may cause neuromyopathy. Ultrastructurally, myeloid bodies and curvilinear structures are conspicuous in Schwann cells, pericytes, and smooth muscle cells of blood vessels. **(p. 2654)**

Skeletal muscle

A1. **True**

The rest of the nuclei are subsarcolemmal, i.e. directly beneath the cell membrane. **(p. 2663)**

A2. **True**

This is because the lighter I band has only actin filaments, whereas the darker A band consists of the interdigitation of both actin and myosin filaments. **(p. 2664)**

A3. **True**

Type I fibers are slow twitch and type II fibers are fast twitch. **(p. 2665)**

A4. **True**

In quadriceps biopsies, about two-thirds are type II (fast twitch). These will stain darkly in ATPase reaction at pH 9.4. **(p. 2665)**

A5. **True**

This is because these reactants are staining mitochondrial components, and mitochondria are far more abundant in type I fibers. **(p. 2665)**

A6. **False**

Unlike other forms of neurogenic atrophy that demonstrate angulated fibers, the atrophic fibers in Werdnig–Hoffman disease are relatively round. **(p. 2666)**

A7. **False**

Perifascicular fiber atrophy is typical of dermatomyositis. **(p. 2668)**

A8. **False**

Rimmed vacuoles, characteristically lined by hematoxyphilic granules, are seen in IBM, but the inclusions of IBM are intranuclear and intracytoplasmic congophilic filaments. **(p. 2668)**

A9. **False**

Although DMD is indeed associated with a defect of the gene encoding dystrophin on Xp12.2, this protein is not intranuclear. Rather, dystrophin forms an integral part of the skeletal muscle cell membrane. **(p. 2669)**

A10. **False**

The clinical course of BMD is less severe than that of DMD. **(p. 2671)**

A11. **True**

The nuclei characteristically display a perinuclear halo on light microscopy that corresponds ultrastructurally to an accumulation of mitochondria and other organelles around the central nuclei. **(p. 2672–2673)**

A12. **False**

The inclusions in this disease are best visualized with modified Gomori trichrome, but in a subsarcolemmal location. **(p. 2673–2674)**

A13. **False**

An abnormality in the influx and efflux of potassium ions is affected in periodic paralysis. **(p. 2674)**

A14. **True**

Unlike other glycogen storage diseases, some of the glycogen granules in acid maltase deficiency are bound within lysosomal membranes. **(p. 2676)**

A15. **False**

Some mitochondrial myopathies involve nuclear, rather than mitochondrial, genetic defects. For instance, certain nuclear genes encoding Krebs cycle enzymes will secondarily affect mitochondrial function and morphology. In such cases, the disorder can be paternally inherited. **(p. 2677)**

A16. **True**

These vacuoles are present mainly in type I fibers and contain PAS-positive and acid phosphatase-positive lysosomal inclusions. **(p. 2678)**

29 Pituitary gland

Normal anatomy

Q1

The adenohypophysis originates from a small ectodermal diverticulum of the stomodeum and thus differs from the neurohypophysis, which originates from the neural tube.

Q2

Corticotrophs (ACTH cells) represent 55–70% of all adenohypophysial cells in the normal pituitary.

Pituitary adenoma

Q1

Pituitary adenomas may synthesize and release hormones, and in about 70% of cases there is clinical and/or biochemical evidence of a characteristic hypersecretory syndrome.

Q2

The term pituitary apoplexy is reserved for those cases with an abrupt onset of headache, ocular deficits and altered consciousness.

Q3

In autopsy series pituitary microadenomas are detected in about one out of every 20 cases.

Q4

The use of reticulin stains in the identification of the tumor–gland interface is of little use, as both adenomas and normal gland harbor reticulin.

Q5

Serum level values of prolactin (PRL) above 200 ng/mL are considered diagnostic of PRL-secreting adenomas.

Q6

Endocrine amyloid is not an uncommon feature of PRL-producing adenomas.

Q7

Densely granulated GH cell adenoma and sparsely granulated GH cell adenoma are considered variants of the same tumor. Therefore, separation of the two types is clinically irrelevant.

Q8

All ACTH cell adenomas are functional.

Q9

The ultrastructural characteristics of the depicted cell are indicative of an ACTH cell adenoma.

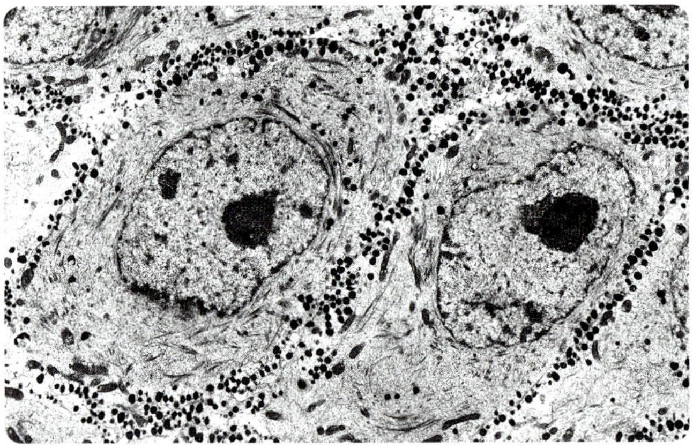

Fig. 29.1

Q10

Adenomas of TSH cell type are the least common pituitary tumor type.

Other lesions

Q1

Histologically, Rathke's cleft cysts are lined by predominantly columnar ciliated cells, rare goblet cells and adenohypophysial cells.

Q2

Most patients with craniopharyngioma are in their 70s and 80s.

Q3

Cystic craniopharyngiomas cannot be distinguished from epidermoid cysts occurring in the sellar region.

Q4

Pituitary granular cell tumors arise in the adenohypophysis, whereas pituicytomas arise from the infundibulum or neurohypophysis.

Q5

In xanthomatous hypophysitis the anterior pituitary is heavily infiltrated by granular to foamy histiocytes which are immunoreactive for CD68.

Normal anatomy

A1. True
The adenohypophysis originates from the stomodeum and is thus of ectodermal origin, whereas the neurohypophysis is an extension of the brain and originates from the embryonic neural tube. **(p. 2683)**

A2. False
Corticotrophs represent 15–20%. Somatotrophs (GH cells) account for 50% of all adenohypophysial cells; lactotrophs (prolactin-secreting cells) constitute 20%; thyrotrophs (TSH cells) constitute 5%; and gonadotrophs (FSH and LH cells) account for 10%. **(p. 2683)**

Pituitary adenoma

A1. True
It is also true that some patients present with insidious symptoms of hypopituitarism secondary to destruction of the normal gland or interference with the delivery of hypothalamic hormones. **(p. 2684–2685)**

A2. True
This uncommon but well-known neurosurgical emergency results from hemorrhage and necrosis in an adenoma. **(p. 2685)**

A3. False
Microadenomas are detected in about one-quarter of autopsies. **(p. 2685–2686)**

A4. False
The use of reticulin staining facilitates the identification of the tumor–gland interface. The reticulin network within the adenoma itself is disrupted, whereas the pituitary tissue at the periphery of the adenoma is compressed with condensation of the reticulin network. **(p. 2687)**

A5. True
Elevation of PRL serum levels up to 150 ng/m may be the result of a 'stalk effect,' which occurs when a mass impinges upon the pituitary stalk such that there is interference with the tonic inhibitory influence of hypothalamic dopamine upon prolactin-secreting cells of the pituitary. **(p. 2690)**

A6. True
Amyloid may be present in 'wisps' detectable only by electron microscopy both intracellularly and extracellularly, or seen in the formation of large extracellular spherules that are pathognomic for this type of neoplasm. **(p. 2690)**

A7. False
Although both types of GH cell adenoma are considered variants of the same tumor, separation of the two types is important because of a difference in prognosis. The densely granulated GH cell adenoma is a slow-growing, well-differentiated tumor that presents in older patients; after surgery it recurs less frequently. By contrast, the sparsely granulated type is larger at presentation, occurs in younger patients, is more aggressive, and is more likely to show invasive tendencies and recurrence. **(p. 2691–2692)**

A8. False
Most ACTH cell adenomas are functional, but some are hormonally silent masses. **(p. 2692)**

A9. True
The perinuclear concentric filamentous deposits are known as Crooke's hyalinization, a feature of ACTH cell adenoma. **(p. 2693)**

A10. True
TSH cell adenomas represent only 1% of all pituitary adenomas, with about 100 cases reported so far. **(p. 2694)**

Other lesions

A1. True
Foci of squamous differentiation are also demonstrable. **(p. 2697)**

A2. False
Most patients with craniopharyngioma are in the first or second decade of life, although some are in their 70s and 80s. The tumor has also been reported in fetuses and newborns. **(p. 2698)**

A3. False
Sometimes it is difficult to distinguish between these two entities. However, the presence of basal palisading and stellate reticulum favors a diagnosis of craniopharyngioma. **(p. 2700)**

A4. **False**

Both tumor types arise from the infundibulum or neurohypophysis. **(p. 2701)**

A5. **True**

As in granulomatous hypophysitis, the diagnosis of xanthomatous hypophysitis is made after the presence of acid-fast bacilli, spirochetes, other bacteria and fungi has been excluded. **(p. 2704)**

30 Eye and ocular adnexa

Normal anatomy

Q1

The eyelids contain sebaceous, apocrine and eccrine glands.

Q2

The conjunctiva contains melanocytes and mucin-secreting goblet cells.

Q3

The optic nerve is ensheathed in Schwann cell processes.

Eyelids

Q1

Chalazion represents a lipogranuloma that develops in and about a meibomian gland.

Q2

In general, malignant melanomas of the eyelid carry a favorable prognosis.

Q3

The so-called port-wine stain (nevus flammeus) may be associated with a choroidal hemangioma, glaucoma and a meningeal hemangioma, all on the ipsilateral side.

Lacrimal gland

Q1

Most neoplasms of the lacrimal gland characteristically displace the eye upward and temporally.

Orbit

Q1

Because it is a systemic disease, unilateral orbital involvement of hyperthyroidism with dysthyroid ophthalmopathy is virtually never seen.

Q2

In orbital involvement with Rosai–Dorfman disease the inflammatory pseudotumor is composed of large histiocytes (some exhibiting lymphocytophagocytosis), lymphocytes and plasma cells.

Q3

Adult orbital angiomas are typically soft, blue compressible tumors that diffuse throughout the orbit and often extend forward into the eyelids.

Q4

Microscopically, almost all optic gliomas are diffuse astrocytomas.

Q5

Exuberant arachnoidal hyperplasia in the setting of optic glioma can be confused with meningioma of the optic nerve.

Q6

The majority of patients with small lymphocytic proliferations localized to the ocular tissues have a dismal prognosis.

Conjunctiva

Q1

Dermoid tumors of the bulbar conjunctiva typically occur at the limbus, often encroaching on the cornea.

Q2

Pterygium extends into the cornea and is therefore a more important lesion than the pinguecula.

Q3

Ligneous conjunctivitis is a peculiar form of chronic pseudomembranous conjunctivitis that presents as a woody induration of the eyelids together with the formation of a pseudomembrane on the tarsal conjunctiva.

Q4

The propensity for the development of invasive melanoma in the setting of acquired conjunctival melanosis is directly related to the presence and degree of cellular atypia.

Cornea

Q1

Fuchs' corneal dystrophy is a term designating the endothelial decompensation that can occur some time after intraocular surgery, especially after cataract extraction.

Q2

The histopathology of early herpes simplex keratitis is characterized by infiltration of the posterior corneal stroma by lymphocytes and plasma cells.

Q3

Keratoconus usually becomes manifest in the sixth decade of life or thereafter.

Intraocular tissues

Q1

Unilateral congenital glaucoma may occur in von Recklinghausen disease or in the Sturge–Weber syndrome.

Q2

In tuberous sclerosis the most characteristic intraocular lesions are glial plaques and nodules in the nerve fiber layer of the retina.

Q3

Severe ocular trauma usually necessitates immediate enucleation.

Q4

Anterior synechiae, a possible sequela of choroiditis, is defined as adhesions between the iris and the lens.

Q5

Children having ocular infection with *Toxocara canis* usually have clinical evidence of systemic visceral larva migrans.

Q6

Phacoanaphylactic endophthalmitis is characterized by a granulomatous inflammatory reaction centered about an area of lens perforation.

QUESTIONS

Q7

Prophylactic enucleation of a phthisic eye is sometimes performed to obviate future sympathetic uveitis.

Q8

The essential feature of glaucoma is an unphysiologic state of increased intraocular pressure, caused in almost all cases by impaired outflow of aqueous humor.

Q9

Fig. 30.1 The process depicted here is most likely related to diabetes mellitus.

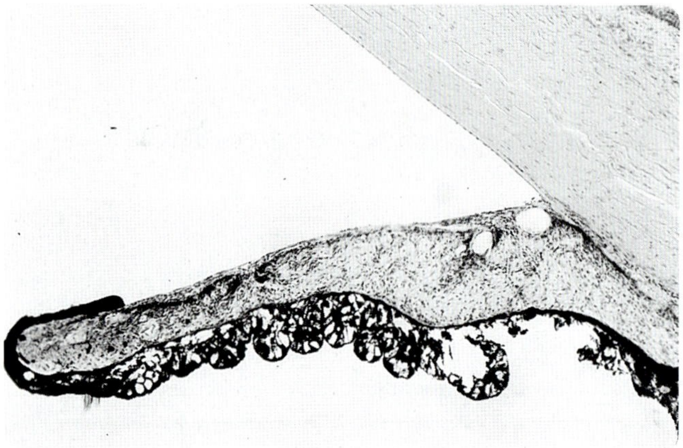

Fig. 30.1

Q10

Uveal melanomas are usually composed of a single cell type: spindle A, spindle B or epithelioid.

Q11

Although it is important for the pathologist to be aware of the cell type in distinguishing uveal melanomas from non-melanomas, cell type has no bearing on prognosis per se.

Q12

Because retinoblastoma is a tumor of childhood, this neoplasm rarely has enough time to develop necrosis.

Q13

The extent of optic nerve invasion by retinoblastoma should be reported with respect to whether the invasion ends anterior to, or posterior to, the lamina cribrosa of the sclera. Retrolaminar invasion should be further subdivided into lesions with or without resection line involvement.

Q14

Abnormalities of intraocular tissues are rarely present in patients with leukemia at autopsy.

Q15

Leiomyomas can develop in the ciliary body or the iris.

Normal anatomy

A1. True

The eyelids contain several types of accessory gland: sebaceous glands (glands of Zeiss and meibomian glands), apocrine glands (glands of Moll) and eccrine sweat glands. **(p. 2714)**

A2. True

The conjunctival epithelium is composed of two to five layers of columnar cells and also contains mucin-secreting goblet cells and melanocytes. **(p. 2714)**

A3. False

The optic 'nerve' is actually a CNS tract supported by oligodendroglia, not Schwann cells. Like the brain, the optic nerve is also surrounded by dura, arachnoid and pia mater. **(p. 2714)**

Eyelids

A1. True

Microscopically, the typical chalazion reveals multiple foci of granulomatous inflammation. In the center of many of the focal granulomas there is a small globule of fat, which in paraffin sections presents as an empty round to ovoid space. **(p. 2715)**

A2. False

Malignant melanomas of the eyelid carry a grave prognosis because they tend to metastasize early via the lymphatics and bloodstream. **(p. 2719)**

A3. True

In the Sturge–Weber syndrome port-wine stain can be associated with these other malformations. **(p. 2719)**

Lacrimal gland

A1. False

Most neoplasms of the lacrimal gland arise in the orbital lobe, where the gland is firmly attached to the orbital rim about the lacrimal fossa. The bone tends to restrict growth in its direction. Hence the enlarging tumor characteristically displaces the eye downward and nasally. **(p. 2721)**

Orbit

A1. False

Unilateral orbital involvement occurs with sufficient frequency in dysthyroid ophthalmopathy to warrant this condition always being considered in the differential diagnosis of orbital tumors. **(p. 2723)**

A2. True

Fibrosis can be very prominent as well. **(p. 2724)**

A3. False

This is a description of infantile orbital angioma. In adults orbital angiomas are usually encapsulated, situated close to the back of the eye, and can be surgically 'shelled' out. **(p. 2725)**

A4. False

Almost all optic gliomas are low-grade pilocytic astrocytomas, similar to those occurring in the cerebellum and in the region of the third ventricle. **(p. 2727)**

A5. True

The meningeal thickening seen in the setting of optic glioma can be accounted for by the combination of infiltrating tumor and reactive arachnoidal proliferation. **(p. 2727–2728)**

A6. False

The majority of patients with small lymphocytic proliferations localized to the ocular tissues enjoy an indolent clinical course and long survival, with only minimal therapeutic intervention. **(p. 2730)**

Conjunctiva

A1. True

Dermoid tumors of the bulbar conjunctiva are firm, localized, elevated opaque masses that usually occur at the limbus. **(p. 2730)**

A2. True

Pterygii can interfere with vision, so are often excised. Pingueculas are not in the line of sight and are therefore seldom excised. **(p. 2730–2731)**

A3. True

The cardinal histologic feature of ligneous conjunctivitis is the presence of large hyaline masses that may simulate amyloid. **(p. 2731)**

A4. True

The degree of melanocytic atypicality present in acquired conjunctival melanosis correlates with the likelihood of progression to melanoma. **(p. 2735)**

Cornea

A1. False

By definition, Fuchs' corneal dystrophy is a primary process with no apparent antecedent factors. When the endothelial decompensation occurs some time after intraocular surgery it is clinically referred to as aphakic bullous keratopathy. The clinical and histopathologic appearance is similar in both situations. **(p. 2736)**

A2. False

The histopathology of herpes simplex keratitis is characterized by infiltration of the anterior stroma by lymphocytes and plasma cells. In severe cases the posterior portion of the cornea is involved, with granulomatous reaction surrounding Descemet's membrane. **(p. 2736)**

A3. False

Keratoconus is a congenital ectasia of the central cornea that usually becomes manifest in the first decade of life. **(p. 2736)**

Intraocular tissues

A1. True

The increased intraocular pressure leads to retinal and optic nerve degeneration, corneal edema and scarring, and global enlargement. **(p. 2739)**

A2. True

Clinically these glial nodules may simulate a retinoblastoma. **(p. 2739)**

A3. False

Most injured eyes are removed at varying intervals because of secondary changes such as organization of hemorrhage, glaucoma, retinal detachment, infections, inflammation or complete atrophy (phthisis bulbi). **(p. 2740)**

A4. False

Anterior synechiae are defined as adhesions between the cornea and the iris, whereas posterior synechiae are adhesions between the iris and the lens. It is true that synechiae, both anterior and posterior, are possible sequelae of choroiditis. **(p. 2742)**

A5. False

Almost without exception, children who have had ocular infection have not had clinical evidence of systemic visceral larva migrans, and those who have had the systemic form have not had ocular lesions. Typically, a single migrating larva finds its way hematogenously into the eye and comes to rest in the vitreous or on the inner surface of the retina. **(p. 2743)**

A6. True

The process is believed to be the result of acquired hypersensitivity to lens protein. **(p. 2745)**

A7. True

Phthisic eyes are enucleated for several reasons, many because they are disfiguring and others because they become irritated as a result of periodic hemorrhages or bouts of uveitis. Some are enucleated for prophylactic reasons – the fear of sympathetic uveitis or malignant melanoma, either of which may develop long after the eye has become blind and phthisic. **(p. 2747)**

A8. True

Aqueous humor leaves the anterior chamber via the trabecular meshwork, which is present in the deep layers of the peripheral cornea, just in front of the anterior chamber angle. Blockage of this outflow is the usual cause of glaucoma. **(p. 2747)**

A9. True

This picture demonstrates rubeosis iridis with peripheral anterior synechiae in diabetes. A fibrovascular membrane covers the anterior surface of the iris. There is also marked diabetic vacuolization of pigment epithelial cells. These vacuoles have been demonstrated to contain glycogen and are related to the level of the blood glucose at the time of enucleation. **(p. 2750–2751)**

A10. False

It is rather unusual for these tumors to be composed of a single cell type. Mixtures of spindle A and B cells or mixtures of spindle and epithelioid cells are common. **(p. 2755)**

A11. False

Cell type is an extremely important parameter in the prognosis of uveal melanomas. There are no deaths with pure spindle A tumors. The 5-year survival rate is 66–75% for spindle B melanomas, 50% for mixed (spindle B and epithelioid) melanomas, and 25–33% for pure epithelioid melanomas. **(p. 2756)**

A12. False

The tumor tends to outgrow its blood supply, and irregular areas of necrosis are commonly observed. **(p. 2757)**

A13. True

The prognosis decreases with each of these levels of involvement. **(p. 2760)**

A14. False

Abnormalities of intraocular tissues are present in approximately 50% of patients with leukemia at autopsy. These are in the form of leukemic infiltrates and hemorrhages, particularly in the choroid and retina. **(p. 2760)**

A15. True

Some of these tumors are regarded as of possible neural crest origin and are designated mesectodermal leiomyomas. **(p. 2761)**

31 Ear

Normal anatomy

Q1

The outer auditory canal is covered by skin that differs little from the skin in other parts of the body.

Q2

The endolymphatic sac of the vestibular labyrinth is located partly in the petrous bone and partly within the dura.

Disease of the external ear

Q1

Ectopic salivary gland tissue is not uncommon in the external auditory canal.

Q2

Chondrodermatitis nodularis chronica helicis most often presents as an ulceration of the anthelix in young females.

Q3

Some lesions designated fibroepithelial papillomas or squamous papillomas of the external ears are most likely variants of seborrheic keratosis.

Q4

Basal cell carcinoma and squamous cell carcinomas are more common on the auricle than in the external auditory canal.

Q5

Squamous cell carcinomas of the external auditory canal are mostly of the adenoid (pseudoglandular) type and thus differ from squamous cell carcinomas on other parts of the face.

Q6

Squamous cell carcinomas of the external auditory canal have in general a better prognosis than those in the auricle.

Q7

Ceruminomas are adnexal tumors of the external auditory canal.

Q8

Adenoid cystic carcinoma has a tendency for perineural invasion.

Diseases of middle and inner ear

Q1

Inflammatory polyp, also known as otic polyp, is usually associated with perforation of the tympanic membrane.

Q2

Cholesteatoma consists predominantly of cholesterol crystals.

Q3

Otosclerosis produces changes in the temporal bone that are similar to those seen in Paget's disease, but these changes are not visible on surgically resected auditory ossicles.

Q4

Paragangliomas are the most common tumors of the middle ear.

Q5

Paragangliomas of the middle ear have a predilection for males.

Q6

Middle ear adenomas contain mucin and show neuroendocrine features.

Q7

Aggressive papillary middle ear tumor (APMET) is composed of clear cells and may resemble metastatic renal cell carcinoma.

Q8

Squamous cell carcinoma of the middle ear typically occurs in older patients with a history of chronic otitis media and hearing loss.

Q9

Rhabdomyosarcoma occurs almost exclusively in the elderly.

Q10

Primary tumors in the pharynx, salivary glands or central nervous system may involve the temporal bone and the inner and middle ear.

Normal anatomy

A1. True

Skin has the same structure in the auditory canal as elsewhere. It contains adnexal structures that include hair follicles, sebaceous glands and a special type of apocrine sweat gland (known as ceruminous glands), most of which are located in the outer third of this structure. **(p. 2771)**

A2. True

The intraosseous location accounts at least in part for the propensity of inner ear tumors to invade the petrous bone and extend into the cranial cavity. **(p. 2771 and 2777)**

Disease of the external ear

A1. True

Ectopic salivary gland tissue may be found in the external auditory canal and the middle ear. **(p. 2772)**

A2. False

Chondrodermatitis nodularis chronica helicis may occur in young persons and may involve the anthelix, but most often it is found as a round nodule covered with a crust on the helix of older persons. **(p. 2772)**

A3. True

Seborrheic keratosis commonly affects the external ear and may be mistaken for fibroepithelial or squamous papilloma. **(p. 2773)**

A4. True

Basal cell carcinomas and squamous cell carcinoma are more common on the sun-exposed parts of the ear than in the external auditory canal. In the auricle basal cell carcinoma predominates over squamous cell carcinoma, but in the external auditory canal the ratio is reversed. **(p. 2773)**

A5. False

Squamous cell carcinomas of the external ear are histologically indistinguishable from such tumors in other parts of the skin. Some tumors may be however of the adenoid (pseudoglandular), verrucous or spindle cell type. **(p. 2773)**

A6. False

Just the reverse is **true.** The better prognosis of auricular tumors is probably related to the earlier diagnosis of these tumors, compared to those in the external auditory canal. **(p. 2773)**

A7. True

The term is used for tumors presumably originating from the ceruminous glands in the external auditory canal. Four major categories are recognized: adenoma, benign mixed tumor, syringocystadenoma papilliferum and adenocarcinoma. **(p. 2774)**

A8. True

Like the adenoid cystic carcinoma of salivary glands, histologically identical tumors in the external ear canal have a tendency to spread along the nerves and metastasize to distant sites, such as the lungs and the brain. **(p. 2774)**

Diseases of middle and inner ear

A1. True

Otic polyps are usually a consequence of chronic otitis media and are typically associated with perforation of the tympanic membrane. **(p. 2775)**

A2. False

Cholesteatoma is typically a cyst bounded by keratinizing squamous epithelium and filled mostly with keratin squames and cell debris. Within the debris one may see cholesterol clefts surrounded by foreign body giant cells, but cholesterol is rarely if ever the most predominant component of these lesions. **(p. 2775)**

A3. True

The temporal bones shows Paget's disease-like woven bone with prominent cement lines. However, the material sent to pathology laboratories usually includes stapes head and crura, and these show no pathologic changes. **(p. 2775)**

A4. True

Paragangliomas originating from the glomus jugulare or glomus tympanicum are the most common tumors of the middle ear. **(p. 2775)**

A5. False

Paragangliomas of the middle ear have a predilection for females. They can be familial, bilateral, or associated with paragangliomas elsewhere. **(p. 2775–2776)**

A6. True

Middle ear adenomas are controversial lesions. However, because they show ultrastructural and immunohistochemical signs of neuroendocrine differentiation and thus have some features of carcinoids, it seem they should be regarded as amphocrine endocrine–exocrine tumors or adenocarcinoids of other sites. **(p. 2776)**

A7. True

APMET is a tumor composed of clear cells that form gland-like and papillary structures and may resemble renal cell carcinoma. It is probably closely related or even identical to the low-grade adenocarcinoma of probably endolymphatic sac origin (Heffner tumor). **(p. 2777)**

A8. True

An etiologic role for chronic otitis media has long been suspected. The tumors usually present with hearing loss, ear pain and discharge, which may be hemorrhagic. **(p. 2777)**

A9. False

Rhabdomyosarcoma of the middle ear is found almost exclusively in children. Microscopically, it can be of embryonal or botryoid type. **(p. 2777–2778)**

A10. True

In addition to these tumors that spread to the inner and middle ear locally, distant metastases can occur from primary tumors elsewhere, most often lungs, breast or kidney. **(p. 2778)**

32 Final comprehensive examination

This examination was constructed by the editors in the standard multiple choice format, i.e. for each question there is only one best answer. All major topics are covered. Some questions pertain to the theoretical aspects of surgical pathology, whereas others relate to macroscopic or microscopic or electron microscopic figures in the main textbook, testing the students' diagnostic skills. A brief explanation is given for each correct answer. Students who wish to study the material in greater detail are referred to the appropriate pages of the textbook for additional in-depth reading.

Instruction: Choose the one best answer.

Q1

Lymphocytic infiltrates of the thyroid associated with germinal center formation and hyperplasia of the follicular thyroid epithelium-lining follicles that have scalloped colloid is most consistent with the diagnosis of which thyroid disease?

A. Hashimoto's thyroiditis
B. Graves' disease
C. Lymphocytic thyroiditis
D. De Quervain's thyroiditis
E. Riedel's thyroiditis.

Q2

An enlarged nodular thyroid was found in a child known to have a genetic defect in iodine transport. What is the most likely diagnosis for this condition?

A. Agenesis of the thyroid
B. Familial C-cell hyperplasia
C. Dyshormonogenetic goiter
D. Endemic goiter
E. DiGeorge syndrome.

Q3

Which of the following thyroid tumors is most prone to undergo clear cell change?

A. Papillary carcinoma
B. Follicular carcinoma
C. Medullary carcinoma
D. Spindle cell anaplastic carcinoma
E. Hürthle cell tumor.

Q4

Many children exposed to high-dose radiation after the Chernobyl accident developed thyroid cancer. Which one of the following histologic types of carcinoma predominated in children exposed at a more advanced age?

A. Papillary carcinoma
B. Follicular carcinoma
C. Medullary carcinoma
D. Insular carcinoma
E. Anaplastic carcinoma.

Q5

Which of the following is the best diagnosis for this thyroid tumor?

A. Papillary carcinoma
B. Follicular carcinoma
C. Medullary carcinoma
D. Insular carcinoma
E. Anaplastic carcinoma.

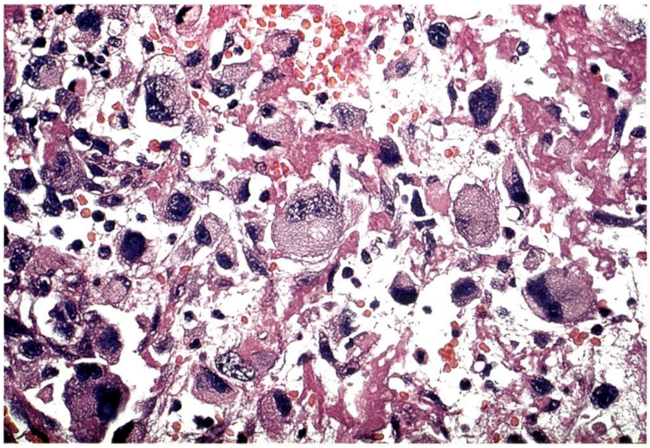

Fig. 9.2

Q6

Which one of the following hepatotropic viruses is the most likely underlying cause of these histology changes in a liver biopsy?

A. Hepatitis virus A
B. Hepatitis virus B
C. Hepatitis virus C
D. Hepatitis virus D
E. Hepatitis virus E.

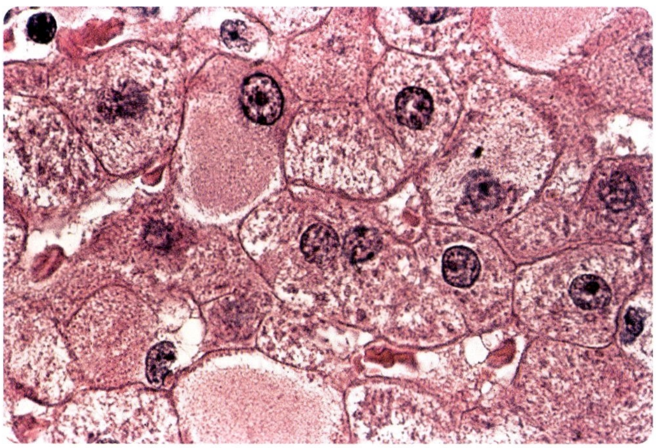

Fig. 13.4

Q7

Copper-rich granules were demonstrated by the rhodanine stain in hepatocytes at the periphery of nodules of a cirrhotic liver. Which of the following is the most likely underlying cause of the accumulation of copper in these hepatocytes?

A. Viral hepatitis B infection
B. Viral hepatitis C infection
C. Obstruction of bile flow
D. Alpha$_1$-antitrypsin deficiency
E. Alcohol abuse.

Q8

Which one of the following substances is the most common cause of macrovesicular steatosis of the liver in the US?

A. Ethanol
B. Tetracycline
C. Amiodarone
D. Valproate
E. Antiviral nucleoside analogs (e.g. filauridine).

Q9

Which of the following chronic liver diseases will most likely cause ductopenia, i.e. a loss of interlobular bile ducts?

A. Primary biliary cirrhosis
B. Alcoholic cirrhosis
C. Posthepatitic cirrhosis related to hepatitis virus B
D. Posthepatitic cirrhosis related to hepatitis virus C
E. Hemochromatosis.

Q10

Which of the following liver lesions is almost always found in young women who have used oral contraceptives?

A. Focal nodular hyperplasia
B. Liver cell adenoma
C. Fibrolamellar hepatocellular carcinoma
D. Trabecular liver cell carcinoma
E. Bile duct adenoma.

Q11

Which of the following subtypes of hepatocellular carcinoma has the best prognosis?

A. Clear cell carcinoma
B. Small cell carcinoma
C. Sarcomatoid carcinoma
D. Fibrolamellar carcinoma
E. Mixed hepatocarcinoma–cholangiocarcinoma.

Q12

This figure illustrates the histologic features of a nodular mass removed from the liver of an 18-month-old child. What is the most likely diagnosis for this lesion?

A. Biliary atresia
B. Biliary hamartoma
C. Mesenchymal hamartoma
D. Embryonal sarcoma of the liver
E. Hepatoblastoma.

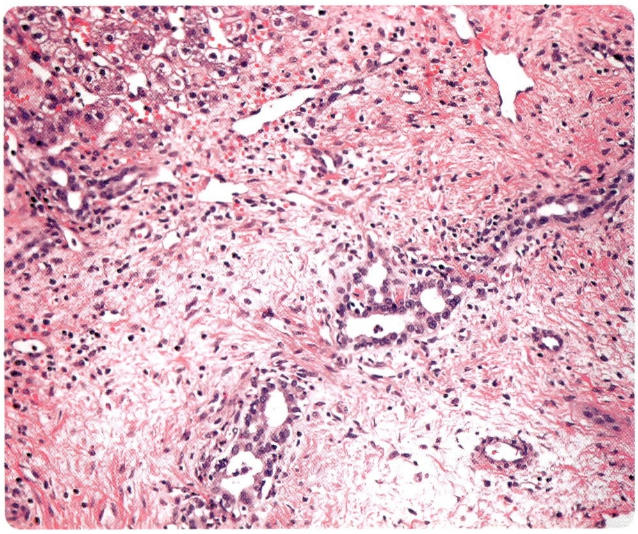

Fig. 13.5

Q13

What is the most common cause of obstructive jaundice in children beyond infancy?

A. Bile duct hamartoma (von Meyenburg complex)
B. Mesenchymal hamartoma
C. Choledochal cyst
D. Biliary atresia
E. Agenesis of the gallbladder.

Q14

Sclerosing cholangitis is most likely to be associated with which one of the following infections?

A. Viral hepatitis B
B. Viral hepatitis C
C. Human immunodeficiency virus infection
D. *Yersinia enteritidis* infection
E. *Entamoeba histolytica* infection.

Q15

Carcinoma of the extrahepatic bile ducts is most often located in which part of the extrahepatic biliary system?

A. Upper third of common bile duct
B. Middle third of common bile duct
C. Lower third of common bile duct
D. Cystic duct
E. None of the above – they show an even distribution along the entire system.

Q16

What is the most common malignant tumor of the extrahepatic bile ducts in children?

A. Adenocarcinoma
B. Carcinoid
C. Malignant lymphoma
D. Botryoid rhabdomyosarcoma
E. Metastatic carcinoma.

Q17

Which one of the following is the most common pathologic form of chronic pancreatitis?

A. Chronic calcifying pancreatitis
B. Groove pancreatitis
C. Lymphoplasmacytic sclerosing pancreatitis
D. Idiopathic duct-centric chronic pancreatitis
E. Chronic suppurative pancreatitis.

Q18

Pancreatic adenocarcinoma is in about 30% of cases accompanied by changes that do not usually occur in non-neoplastic conditions. Which one of the following changes is typically associated with pancreatic carcinoma and is not seen in chronic pancreatitis?

A. Squamous metaplasia
B. Pyloric gland metaplasia
C. Mucous hypertrophy
D. Proliferation of pancreatic endocrine cells
E. Atypia and papillary hyperplasia of ductal epithelium.

Q19

A spongy pancreatic tumor resembling infantile polycystic kidney was removed from an elderly woman. The microscopic features of this tumor are illustrated here. What is the best diagnosis?

A. Microcystic cystadenoma
B. Microcystic adenocarcinoma
C. Acinar cell adenoma
D. Acinar cell cystadenoma
E. Pancreatoblastoma.

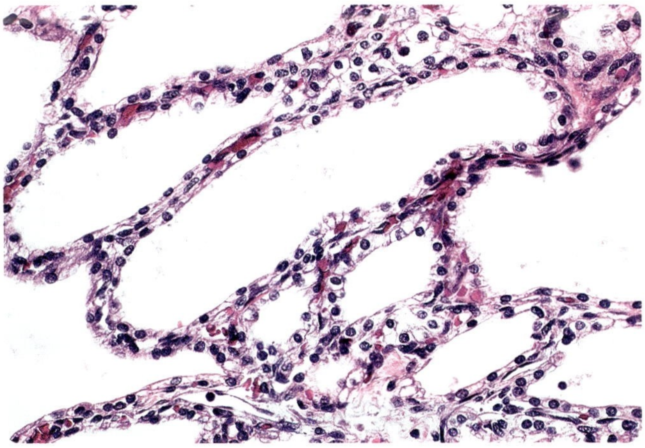

Fig. 15.11

Q20

This pancreatic tumor was removed from a 30-year-old man. Metastases were present in the regional lymph nodes. The tumor cells did not react with antibodies to chromogranin and synaptophysin, but were strongly reactive with antibodies to lipase. What is the most likely diagnosis?

A. Solid pseudopapillary tumor
B. Microcystic adenocarcinoma
C. Acinar cell adenoma
D. Acinar cell carcinoma
E. Pancreatoblastoma.

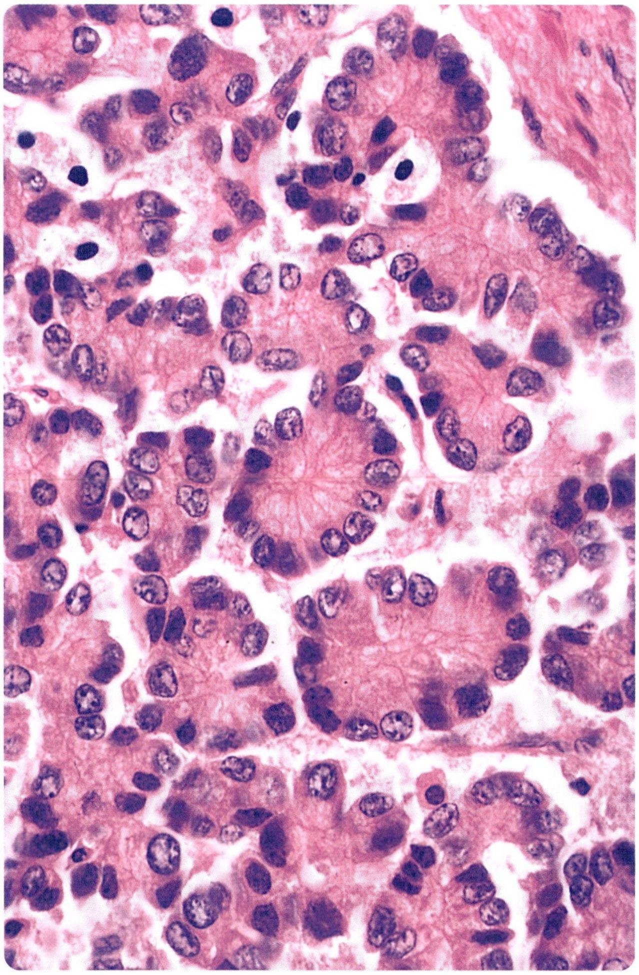

Fig. 15.12

Q21

In surgical pathology practice adrenocortical carcinomas are most often difficult to distinguish from which one of the following tumors?

A. Renal cell carcinoma
B. Transitional cell carcinoma
C. Prostatic adenocarcinoma
D. Breast carcinoma
E. Adenocarcinoma of the lung.

Q22

When attempting to distinguish adrenal cortical tumors from pheochromocytomas one may use a battery of immunohistochemical tests. Which of these markers listed here is expressed in adrenal medullary tumors and negative in adrenal cortical tumors?

A. Synaptophysin
B. Chromogranin
C. Vimentin
D. Keratin
E. Inhibin.

Q23

So-called spironolactone bodies (shown here) are typically found in which adrenal tumor after treatment with spironolactone?

A. Adrenal cortical adenoma with hyperaldosteronism
B. Adenoma with Cushing's syndrome
C. Adenoma with adrenogenital syndrome
D. Pheochromocytoma
E. Ganglioneuroma.

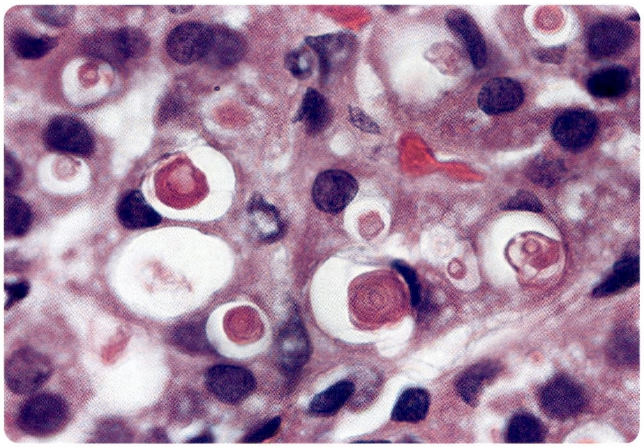

Fig. 16.11

Q24

Which adrenal tumor contains neurosecretory granules and synaptic endings visible on electron microscopy?

A. Adrenal cortical adenoma
B. 'Black adenoma'
C. Adrenal cortical adenocarcinoma
D. Pheochromocytoma
E. Neuroblastoma.

Q25

Mitosis–karyorrhexis index is useful for formulating the prognosis of which adrenal tumor?

A. Adrenal cortical adenoma
B. Schwannoma
C. Adrenal cortical adenocarcinoma
D. Pheochromocytoma
E. Neuroblastoma.

Q26

Immunohistochemically, sustentacular cells of pheochromocytoma typically react with the antibodies to which cell antigen?

A. Gastrin
B. Enkephalin
C. S-100 protein
D. Calbindin
E. Inhibin.

Q27

Which of the following renal diseases presents with nephritic syndrome and in the renal biopsy shows granular deposits of immunoglobulin G and complement along the capillary walls of glomeruli?

A. Minimal change glomerulopathy
B. Focal and segmental glomerulosclerosis
C. Membranous nephropathy
D. Diabetic nephropathy
E. Amyloidosis.

Q28

In which of the following diseases do the glomeruli stain with Congo red and contain fibrils that measure 8–10 nm in diameter when examined by electron microscopy?

A. Immunotactoid glomerulopathy
B. Focal and segmental glomerulosclerosis
C. Fibrillary glomerulopathy
D. Diabetic nephropathy
E. Amyloidosis.

Q29

This kidney biopsy was obtained from a man with a chronic liver disease. Which of the following liver diseases will most likely be the cause of these glomerular changes?

A. Alcoholic hepatitis
B. Chronic viral hepatitis C
C. Primary biliary cirrhosis
D. Hemochromatosis
E. Wilson disease.

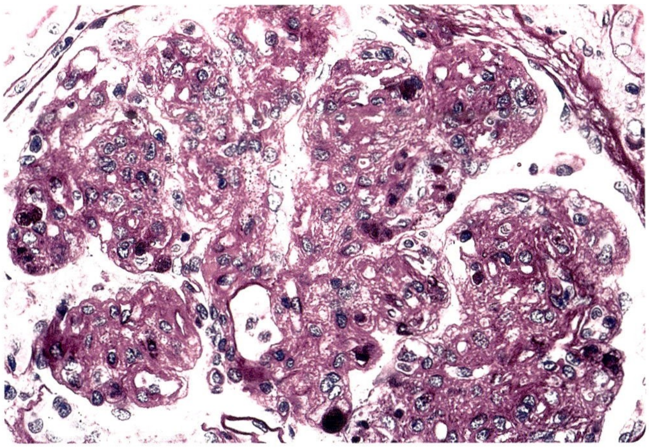

Fig. 17.4

Q30

This kidney biopsy was obtained from a 30-year-old man with recurrent hematuria and mild proteinuria. The arrow points to deposits most likely composed of which immunoglobulin?

A. IgA
B. IgD
C. IgG
D. IgE
E. IgM.

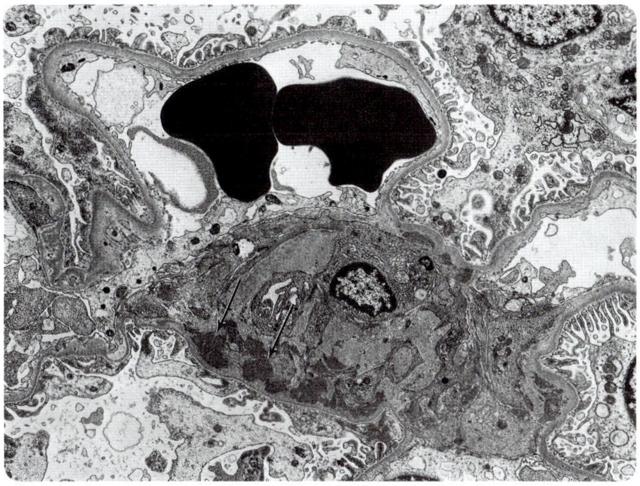

Fig. 17.5

Q31

A 2-year-old child was found to have a retroperitoneal tumor and lung metastases. What is the most likely diagnosis for this tumor?

A. Neuroblastoma
B. Wilms' tumor
C. Malignant pheochromocytoma
D. Ganglioneuroblastoma
E. Adrenal cortical carcinoma.

Q32

Which of the following cardiac diseases can usually be diagnosed by a biopsy of another, more accessible organ rather than the heart?

A. Idiopathic hypertrophic cardiomyopathy
B. Idiopathic dilated cardiomyopathy
C. Infiltrative cardiomyopathy
D. Loeffler endocarditis
E. Giant cell myocarditis.

Q33

Cardiac myxomas most often occur in which one of the following anatomic locations?

A. Right atrium
B. Left atrium
C. Right ventricle
D. Left ventricle
E. Sinus venosus.

Q34

Which of the following heart tumors is typically diagnosed in infants and children and may be congenital?

A. Rhabdomyoma
B. Myxoma
C. Pericardial mesothelioma
D. Angiosarcoma
E. Papillary fibroelastoma.

Q35

Temporal arteritis, also known as cranial arteritis and Horton's disease, is characterized by painful nodularity of arteries. Which of the following inflammatory cells are typically present in such lesions and are important for their microscopic diagnosis?

A. Eosinophils
B. Neutrophils
C. Plasma cells
D. Multinucleated giant cells
E. B lymphocytes.

Q36

This material was removed from a midline intracranial lesion located in the anterosuperior third ventricle. What is the most likely diagnosis?

A. Arachnoid cyst
B. Colloid cyst
C. Meningomyelocele
D. Craniopharyngioma
E. Cystic pituitary adenoma.

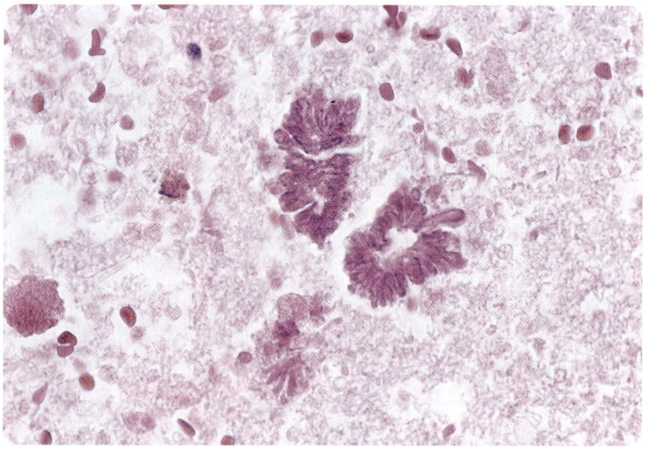

Fig. 28.5

Q37

Arteriovenous malformations are most often located in which part of the central nervous system?

A. Pons
B. Medullar oblongata
C. Cerebellum
D. Cerebral hemispheres
E. Cauda equina.

Q38

Which one of the following conditions represents the most common cause of non-traumatic peripheral lobar cerebral hematoma?

A. Granulomatous arteritis
B. Arteriovenous fistula
C. Cerebral amyloid angiopathy
D. Arteriovenous malformation
E. Capillary telangiectases.

Q39

Which of the following pathogens is the single most common cause of CNS mycosis?

A. *Aspergillus fumigatus*
B. *Cryptococcus neoformans*
C. *Pseudoallescheria boydii*
D. *Streptomyces griseus*
E. *Candida albicans*.

Q40

Which one of the following pathogens is the cause of progressive multifocal leukoencephalopathy?

A. Herpes simplex virus
B. Rabies virus
C. Human immunodeficiency virus
D. Measles virus
E. Polyoma JC virus.

Q41

Which tumor presents in children as 'psudohypertrophic' enlargement of the pons on neuroradiologic investigation?

A. Astrocytoma, diffuse fibrillary type
B. Oligodendroglioma
C. Ependymoma
D. Neurocytoma
E. Microglioma.

Q42

Microvascular hyperplasia characterized by disorderly proliferation of endothelial and myoepithelial cells of small blood vessels is typical of which intracranial tumor?

A. Meningioma
B. Pituicytoma
C. Craniopharyngeoma
D. Neurocytoma
E. Glioblastoma multiforme.

Q43

Which of the following glial tumors typically occurs in children and has a predilection for the cerebellum?

A. Pilocytic astrocytoma
B. Oligodendroglioma
C. Ependymoma
D. Neurocytoma
E. Glioblastoma multiforme.

Q44

This figure illustrates the microscopic features of a subarachnoid temporal lobe tumor removed from a 20-year-old man. The tumor was well demarcated, partially cystic, and contained superficially positioned contrast enhancing mural nodular components. What is the most likely diagnosis?

A. Pilocytic astrocytoma
B. Oligodendroglioma
C. Pleomorphic xanthoastrocytoma
D. Ganglioneuroma
E. Glioblastoma multiforme.

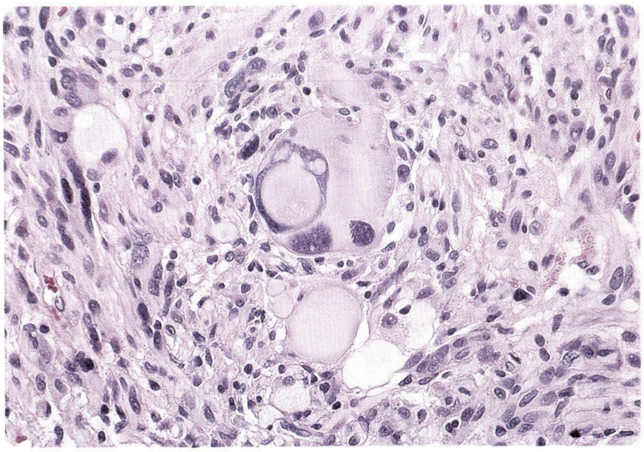

Fig. 28.6

Q45

Psammoma bodies are most likely to be found in which one of the following intracranial tumors?

A. Pilocytic astrocytoma
B. Meningioma
C. Ependymoma
D. Neurocytoma
E. Glioblastoma multiforme.

Q46

This electron micrograph shows the typical features of which intracranial tumor?

A. Schwannoma
B. Meningioma
C. Meningeal hemangiopericytoma
D. Neurocytoma
E. Medulloblastoma.

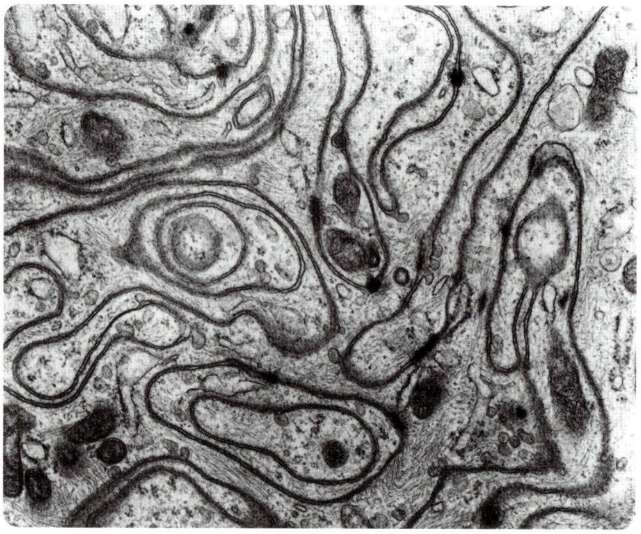

Fig. 28.7

Q47

This sural nerve biopsy show the typical features of which disease?

A. Guillain–Barré syndrome
B. Amyloidosis of the nerve
C. Polyarteritis nodosa
D. Hypertrophic neuropathy
E. Diabetic neuropathy.

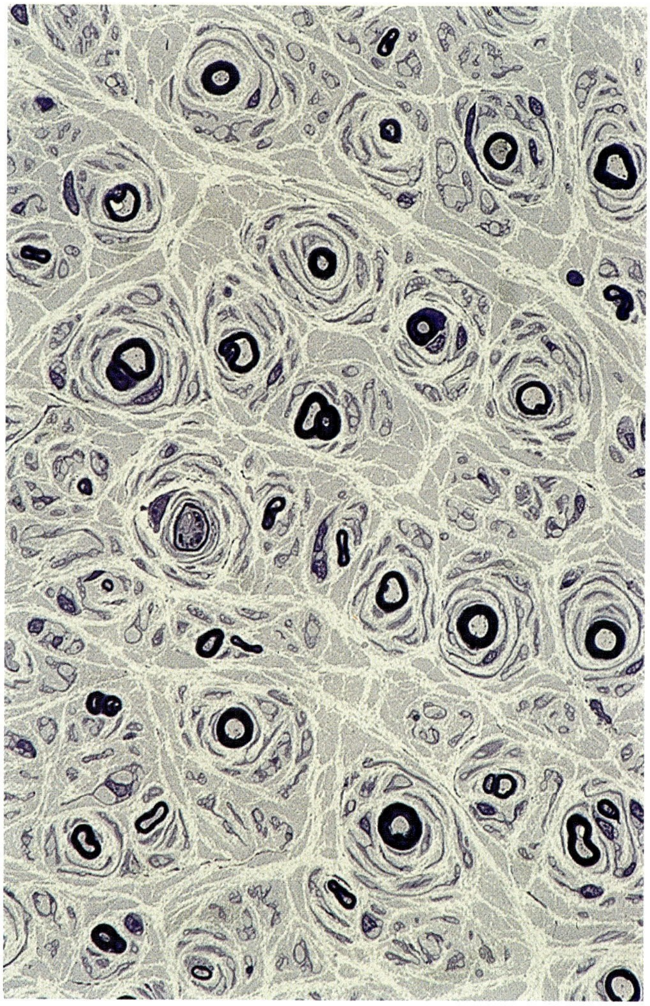

Fig. 28.8

Q48

This figure was prepared from a muscle biopsy treated by enzyme histochemistry, using the technique for the demonstration of succinate dehydrogenase. These changes are most consistent with which one of the following diagnoses?

A. Type I muscle atrophy
B. Type II muscle atrophy
C. Neurogenic atrophy with reinnervation
D. Werdnig–Hoffman disease
E. Duchenne muscular dystrophy.

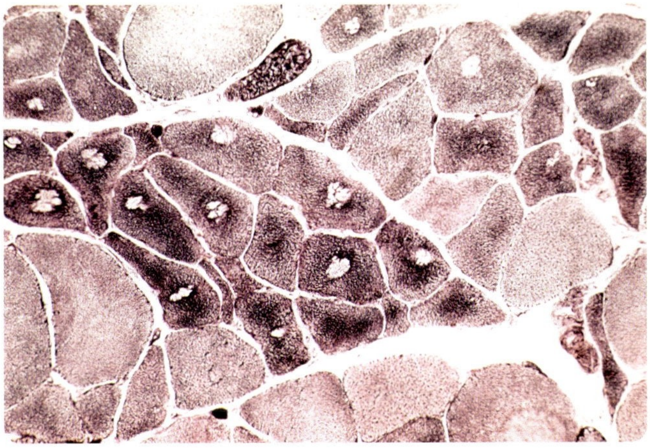

Fig. 28.9

Q49

This microphotograph illustrates the typical features of a sella turcica tumor removed from a 50-year-old woman. What is the most likely diagnosis?

A. Pituitary adenoma, solid growth pattern
B. Pituitary adenoma, papillary growth pattern
C. Pituitary adenoma, sinusoidal growth pattern
D. Pituitary adenoma, oncocytic type
E. Medulloblastoma.

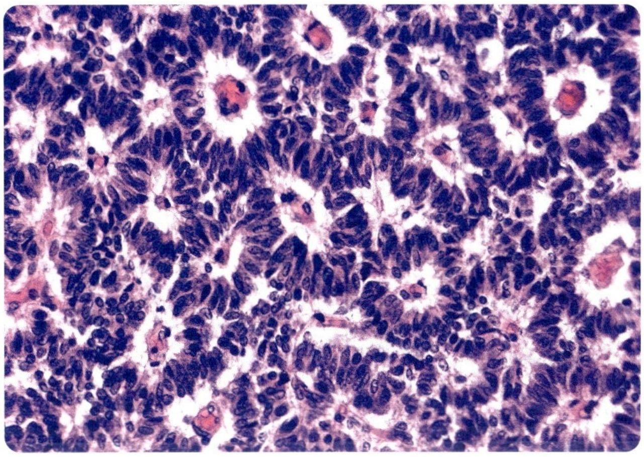

Fig. 29.2

Q50

Amyloid deposition and calcospherites, illustrated here, are most often found in which pituitary adenomas?

A. Corticotroph adenoma
B. Growth hormone secreting adenomas
C. Prolactinomas
D. TSH-secreting adenomas
E. Non-functioning oncocytomas.

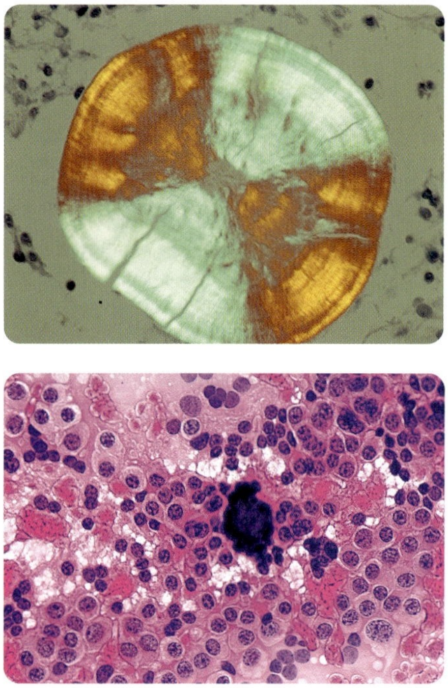

A

B

Fig. 29.3

Q51

This primary uveal tumor removed from the eye of a 60-year-old man was immunoreactive with antibodies to S-100 protein and unreactive with the antibodies to keratins. What is the most likely diagnosis?

A. Retinoblastoma
B. Medulloepithelioma
C. Melanoma
D. Basal cell carcinoma
E. Meningioma.

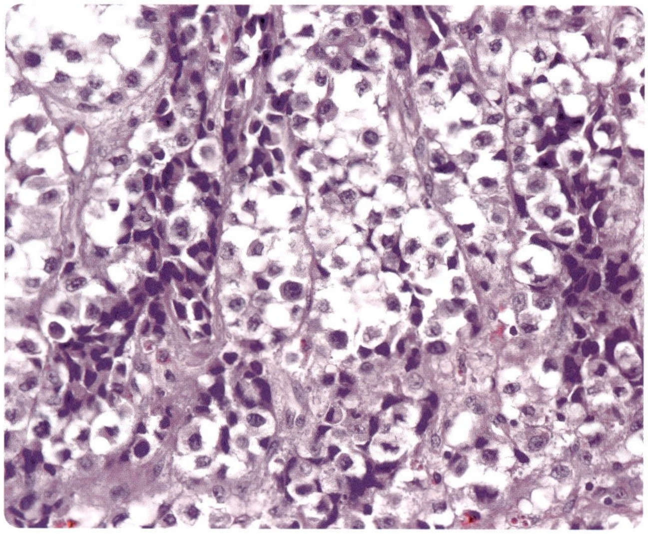

Fig. 30.2

Q52

Which one of the following intracranial tumors is most likely to be found in the middle ear?

A. Ependymoma
B. Glioblastoma multiforme
C. Oligodendroglioma
D. Medulloblastoma
E. Meningioma.

Q53

Leukocytoclastic vasculitis involving the skin, oral mucosa and conjunctiva is a typical histologic finding in which of the following diseases?

A. Crohn's disease
B. Behçet's disease
C. Riga–Fede disease
D. Melkersson–Rosenthal syndrome
E. Necrotizing sialometaplasia.

Q54

In the mouth, most squamous cells carcinomas in situ or early invasive squamous cell carcinomas are described clinically as:

A. Erythroplakia
B. Erythroleukoplakia
C. Leukoplakia
D. Ulceration
E. Papilloma.

Q55

These figures illustrate a salivary gland tumor found on the palate of a 35-year-old woman. Which of the following is the most likely diagnosis?

A. Benign mixed tumor
B. Basal cell adenoma
C. Adenoid cystic carcinoma
D. Polymorphous low-grade adenocarcinoma
E. Myoepithelioma.

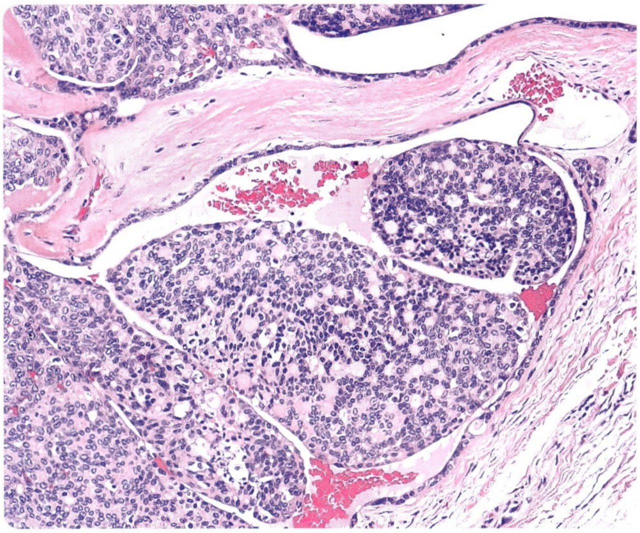

Fig. 5.1

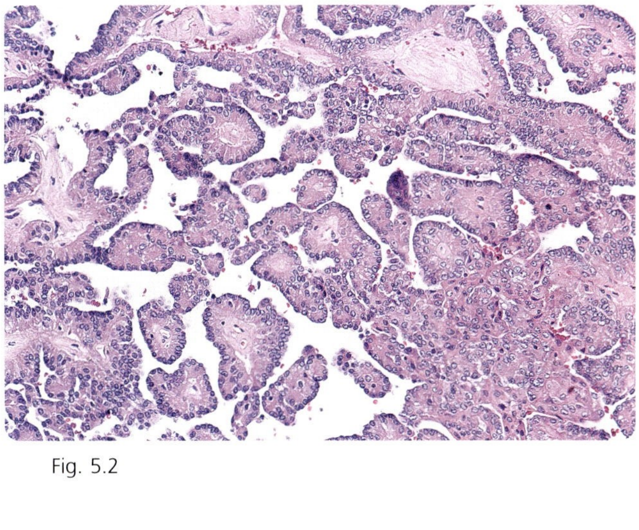

Fig. 5.2

Q56

Which one of the following is the most common jaw lesion composed of ostoclast-like multinucleated giant cells?

A. Central giant cell granuloma
B. Giant cell tumor of hyperparathyroidism
C. Cherubism
D. Aneurysmal bone cyst
E. Giant cell tumor (osteoclastoma).

Q57

This multilocular cystic tumor was diagnosed in a 17-year-old man. Which one of the following is the most likely diagnosis?

A. Adenoameloblastoma
B. Adenomatoid odontogenic tumor
C. Ameloblastic fibroma
D. Odontoma
E. Odontoameloblastoma.

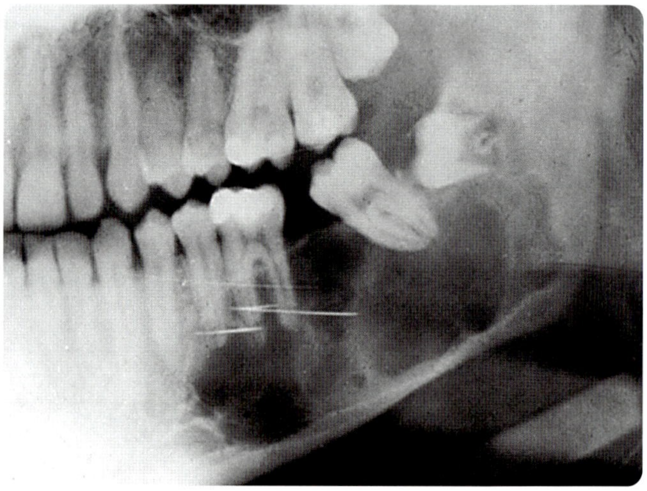

Fig. 6.1

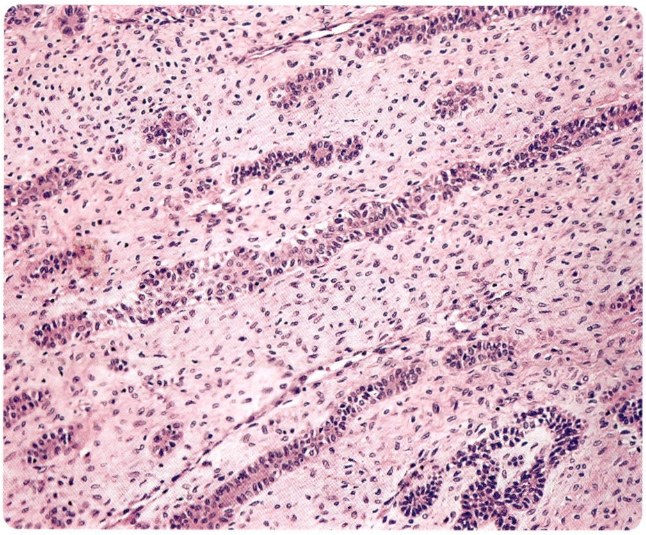

Fig. 6.2

Q58

Primary hyperparathyroidism is in over 80% of all cases associated with which one of the following lesions?

A. Solitary parathyroid adenoma
B. Multiple parathyroid adenomas
C. Parathyroid carcinoma
D. Parathyroid hyperplasia
E. Hypovitaminosis D.

Q59

This esophageal tumor was removed from a 60-year-old man. Which of the following is the most likely diagnosis?

A. Sarcomatoid carcinoma
B. Basaloid carcinoma
C. Small cell carcinoma
D. Myofibroblastic sarcoma
E. Leiomyosarcoma.

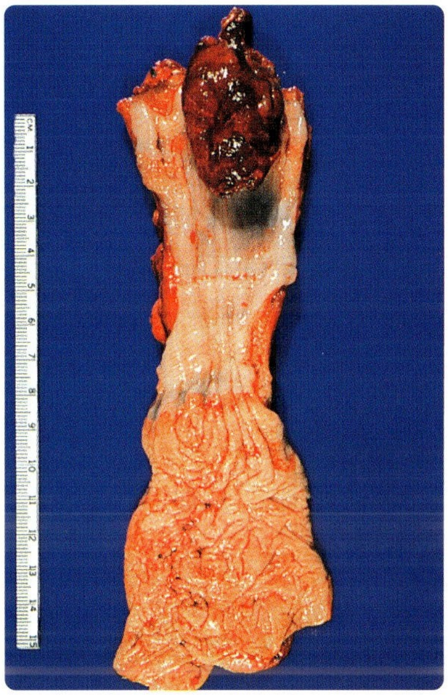

Fig. 11.1

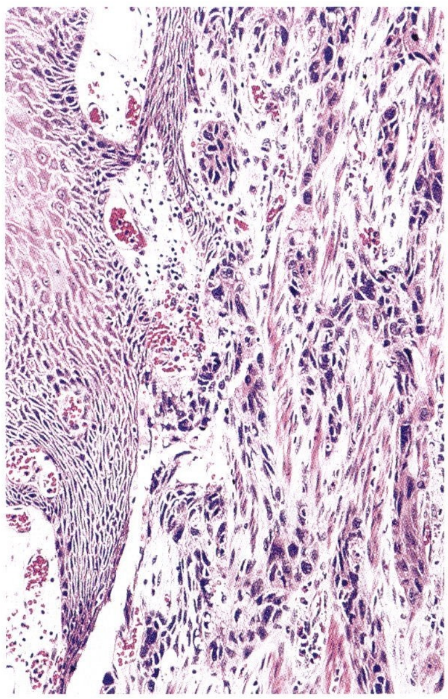

Fig. 11.2

Q60

Which of the following statements is true about type A or immune chronic gastritis?

A. It typically involves the pyloric antrum
B. It presents with hyperacidity of gastric contents
C. *Helicobacter pylori* are typically present in gastric glands
D. Serum contains high levels of gastrin
E. It is caused by allergy to foods.

Q61

Germline truncating mutations of the E-cadherin gene have been found in families with hereditary cancer of which type?

A. Squamous cell carcinoma of the esophagus
B. Gastric adenocarcinoma of the intestinal type
C. Gastric carcinoma of the diffuse type (signet ring carcinoma)
D. Gastric lymphoma
E. Gastrointestinal stromal tumor (GIST).

Q62

Which one of the following gastric tumors will most likely express Epstein–Barr virus gene transcripts?

A. Lymphoepithelioma-like carcinoma
B. Gastric adenocarcinoma of the intestinal type
C. Hepatoid adenocarcinoma
D. Adenosqumaous carcinoma
E. Gastrointestinal stromal tumor.

Q63

The gastric well-differentiated neuroendocrine tumors (WDNET) or carcinoids are most often composed of which cells?

A. Gastrin-producing cells
B. Enterochromaffin-like (ECL) cells
C. Secretin-secreting cells
D. Cholecystokinin-secreting cells
E. Somatostatin-secreting cells.

Q64

Which one of the following gastrointestinal tumors is related to the somatic mutation of a tyrosine kinase receptor (c-*kit*), and is best recognized with antibodies to CD117?

A. Leiomyosarcoma of the esophagus
B. Gastric adenocarcinoma of the intestinal type
C. Gastric carcinoma of the diffuse type (signet ring carcinoma)
D. Gastric lymphoma
E. Gastrointestinal stromal tumor (GIST).

Q65

AP12-MLT fusion, the result of t(11,18) translocation, was detected by FISH in a gastric lesion composed of lymphocytes showing cytologic atypical Dutcher bodies and lymphoepithelial lesions. These finding is most typical of which form of gastric lesion?

A. Pseudolymphoma
B. Intermediate/high-grade lymphoma, large B-cell type
C. Low-grade lymphoma of the MALT type
D. Burkitt's lymphoma
E. Macroglobulinemia.

Q66

Enteropathy-associated T-cell lymphoma is in most instances a complication of which disease?

A. Crohn's disease
B. Whipple's disease
C. Peutz–Jeghers syndrome
D. Celiac disease
E. Tropical sprue.

Q67

Enteroenteric fistulas are a common complication of which chronic intestinal disease?

A. Crohn's disease
B. Whipple's disease
C. Ulcerative colitis
D. Celiac disease
E. Intestinal angiodysplasia.

Q68

Gangliocytic paraganglioma is a distinct tumor that most often occurs in which part of the gastrointestinal tract?

A. Distal esophagus
B. Gastric fundus
C. Pyloric antrum
D. Distal duodenum
E. Rectum.

Q69

Pleomorphic adenomas (benign mixed tumors) occur most often in which anatomic location?

A. Parotid gland
B. Submaxillary gland
C. Sublingual gland
D. Soft palate
E. Hard palate and nose.

Q70

Which one of the following tumors is the most common malignant salivary gland tumor in children?

A. Acinic cell carcinoma
B. Adenoid cystic carcinoma
C. Mucoepidermoid carcinoma
D. Papillary adenocarcinoma
E. Salivary duct carcinoma.

Q71

Abscesses characterized by central, sometimes stellate necrosis with neutrophils, surrounded by a palisading of histiocytes are found in the axillary lymph nodes of a young man. What is the most likely diagnosis?

A. Tuberculosis
B. Sarcoidosis
C. Histoplasmosis
D. Cat-scratch disease
E. Brucellosis.

Q72

Which one of the following is the most common abnormality of lymph nodes in AIDS patients?

A. Mycobacterial infection
B. Kaposi's sarcoma
C. Hodgkin's lymphoma
D. Non-Hodgkin's lymphoma
E. Florid reactive hyperplasia.

Q73

This enlarged cervical lymph node was removed from a 30-year-old man. The lymph node architecture is totally or partially replaced by a nodular and diffuse infiltrate, consisting predominantly of small B lymphocytes, histiocytes, and large cells characterized by large nuclei and scant cytoplasm. One of these cells is present in the center of this picture. These cells did not react with antibodies to CD30 and CD15, but were strongly reactive with CD20. What is the best diagnosis for this tumor?

A. Anaplastic large cell lymphoma
B. Nodular sclerosis Hodgkin's lymphoma
C. Lymphocyte-rich Hodgkin's lymphoma
D. Nodular lymphocyte-predominant Hodgkin's lymphoma
E. T-cell-rich B-cell lymphoma.

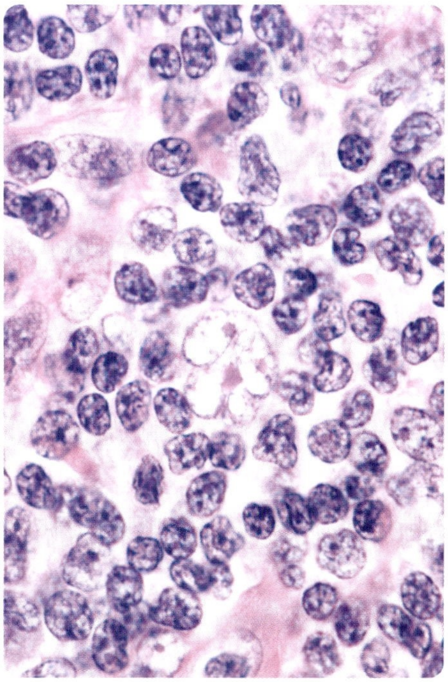

Fig. 21.11

Q74

Which one of the following lymphomas must be further subdivided into three categories depending on the relative proportion of small and large cells?

A. Nodular sclerosis Hodgkin's lymphoma
B. Small lymphocytic lymphoma
C. Follicular lymphoma
D. Marginal zone B-cell lymphoma
E. Diffuse large B-cell lymphoma.

Q75

Which one of the following metastatic carcinomas most closely simulates a malignant lymphoid process?

A. Nasopharyneal lymphoepithelioma
B. Cystadenoma lymphomatosum papilliferum
C. Lymphoepithelial cyst of pancreas
D. Ductal carcinoma of the breast
E. Medullary carcinoma of the breast.

Q76

Which one of the following diseases is most commonly associated with spontaneous rupture of the spleen?

A. Blunt trauma to the abdomen
B. Surgical intervention within the abdominal cavity
C. Castleman's disease
D. Infectious mononucleosis
E. Wiskott–Aldrich syndrome.

Q77

Which one of the following is the most common malignant tumor involving the spleen?

A. Metastatic carcinoma
B. Carcinosarcoma
C. Hemangioendothelioma
D. Angiosarcoma
E. Malignant lymphoma.

Q78

This figure shows a preparation from a very large spleen removed from a young man with hepatosplenomegaly, fever and weight loss. The neoplastic infiltration involves the cords and sinuses, and at the molecular level there is clonal rearrangement of the γ or δ chain of the T-cell receptor gene. What is the most likely diagnosis?

A. Hairy cell leukemia
B. Lymphoblastic lymphoma
C. Peripheral T-cell lymphoma
D. Hepatosplenic T-cell lymphoma
E. Anaplastic large cell lymphoma.

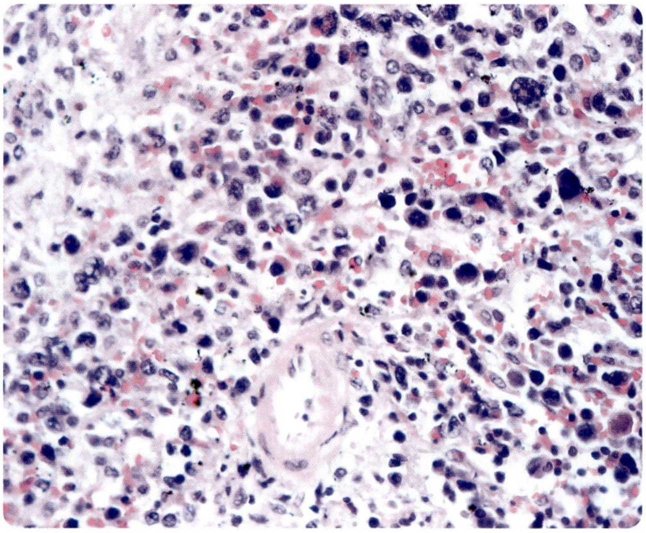

Fig. 22.4

Q79

Which is the most common subtype of Hodgkin's lymphoma in the spleen?

A. Nodular sclerosis
B. Lymphocyte rich
C. Lympocyte depletion
D. Nodular lymphocyte predominance
E. Mixed cellularity.

Q80

Which one of the following diseases is characterized by the presence of tartrate-resistant acid phosphatase?

A. Littoral cell angioma
B. Hairy cell leukemia
C. Lymphoblastic lymphoma
D. Hepatosplenic T-cell lymphoma
E. Anaplastic large cell lymphoma.

Q81

Which one of the following cells is most likely to be found between adipose tissue in the most severe form of idiopathic acquired aplastic anemia?

A. Erythroblasts and granulocytes
B. Erythroblasts and megakaryocytes
C. Granulocytes and megakaryocytes
D. Lymphocytes and plasma cells
E. Erythroblasts and myeloblasts.

Q82

Abnormal localization of immature precursors (ALIP) is most likely to be found in which one of the following diseases?

A. Hairy cell leukemia
B. Myelodysplastic syndromes
C. Myeloproliferative syndromes
D. Plasma cell dyscrasias
E. Malignant histiocytosis.

Q83

Which one of the following additional studies is most useful for the diagnosis of chronic myeloid leukemia?

A. Elevated leukocyte count
B. Hypercellularity of bone marrow
C. Molecular evidence of the *bcr-abl* hybrid gene in the hematopoietic cells
D. The number of myeloblasts in the blood and marrow smears
E. Immunohistochemical studies.

Q84

Which one of the following diseases could be found in a history of patient with Richter's syndrome?

A. Chronic lymphocytic leukaemia
B. Diffuse large B-cell lymphoma
C. Burkitt's lymphoma
D. Lymphoblastic lymphoma
E. Angioimmunoblastic lymphoma.

Q85

The central focus of well-differentiated lymphocytes is surrounded by lighter-staining cells which are reactive with α-antitrypsin, α-antichymotrypsin, CD68 and CD117 antibodies. Which one of the following is the most likely diagnosis?

A. Non-Hodgkin's lymphoma
B. Systemic mastocytosis
C. Plasma cell myeloma
D. Malignant histiocytosis
E. Fabry's disease.

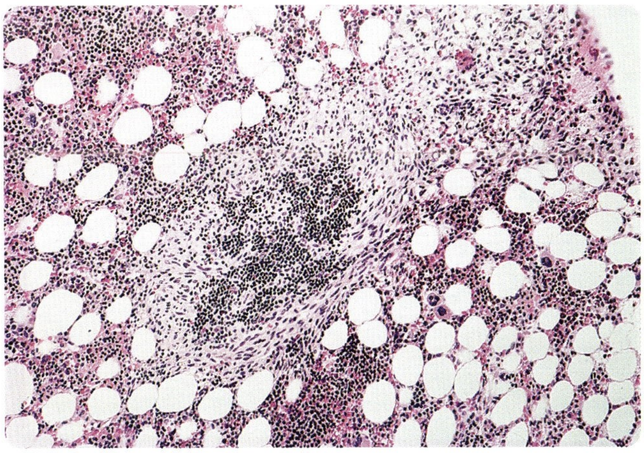

Fig. 23.7

Q86

Which one of the following pathogens is the single most common cause of osteomyelitis?

A. Coagulase-positive staphylococci
B. *Streptococcus*
C. *Mycobacterium tuberculosis*
D. *Proteus*
E. *Pseudomonas*.

Q87

Which one of the following anatomic sites is the most frequent location of osteosarcoma?

A. Metaphyseal area of the long bones
B. Metaphyseal area of the short bones
C. Diaphyses of the long bones
D. Epiphyses of the short bones
E. Flat bones.

Q88

Which one of the following tumors is associated with Ollier's disease?

A. Osteochrondroma
B. Chondroblastoma
C. Soft tissue hemangioma
D. Enchondroma
E. Chondrosarcoma.

Q89

This figure shows a preparation from a sacrococcygeal tumor removed from a 60-year-old man. Which one of the following is the most likely diagnosis?

A. Plasmacytoma
B. Chordoma
C. Chondroma
D. Chondrosarcoma
E. Osteochondroma.

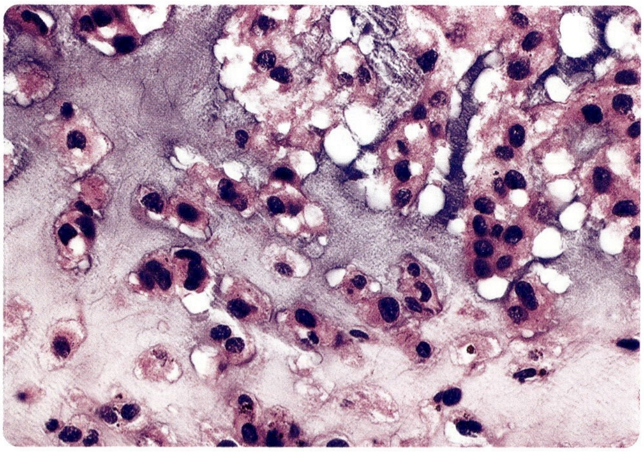

Fig. 24.14

Q90

This electron micrograph shows the typical features of which lesion?

A. Langerhans' cell histiocytosis
B. Rosai–Dorfman disease
C. Syringomyelia
D. Chordoma
E. Ewing sarcoma/PNET.

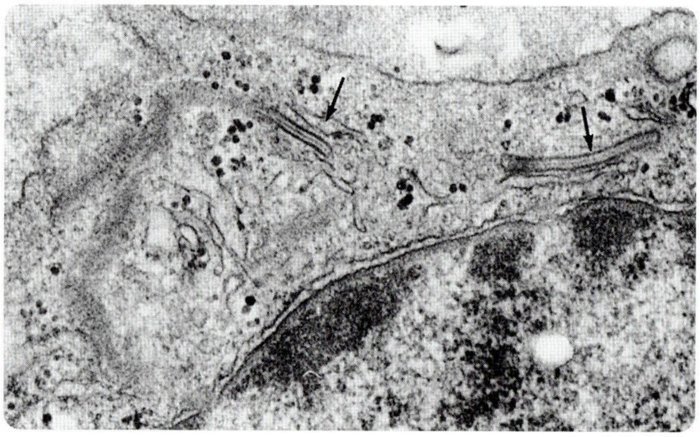

Fig. 24.15

Q91

Which one of the following lesions is caused by repeated mild trauma?

A. Amputation neuroma
B. Morton's neuroma
C. Palisaded encapsulated neuroma
D. Solitary circumscribed neuroma
E. Perineurioma.

Q92

Which of the following histologic subtypes is the most common form of liposarcoma?

A. Pleomorphic liposarcoma
B. Dedifferentiated liposarcoma
C. Spindle cell liposarcoma
D. Round cell liposarcoma
E. Myxoid liposarcoma.

Q93

Which one of the following sites is the classic location of the glomus tumor?

A. Extensor surface of the arms
B. Subungual region
C. Pelvis
D. Orbit
E. Oral cavity.

Q94

This picture of the common bile duct shows a concentration of tumor cells immediately beneath the epithelium ('cambium layer'). What is the most likely diagnosis?

A. Rhabdomyoma
B. Botryoid rhabdomyosarcoma
C. Pleomorphic rhabdomyosarcoma
D. Alveolar rhabdomyosarcoma
E. Sclerosing rhabdomyosarcoma.

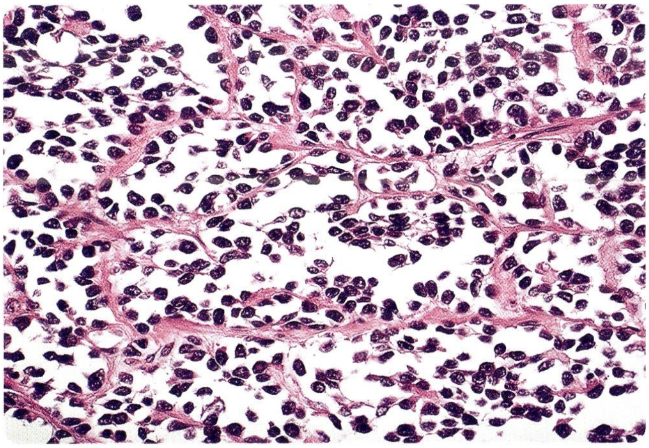

Fig. 25.8

Q95

Which one of the following soft tissue tumors is most commonly located on the extremities, particularly the hands and fingers?

A. Myxoma
B. Epithelioid sarcoma
C. Alveolar soft part sarcoma
D. Granular cell tumor
E. Liposarcoma.

Q96

Which of the following tumors displays simultaneous expression of epithelial, muscular and neural markers?

A. Intra-abdominal desmoplastic small cell tumor
B. Solitary fibrous tumor
C. Peritoneal angiosarcoma
D. Pseudomyxoma peritonei
E. Inflammatory myofibroblastic tumor.

Q97

Which one of the following is the most common primary site of origin of tumors that give rise to pseudomyxoma peritonei?

A. Ovary
B. Pancreas
C. Stomach
D. Appendix
E. Small intestine.

Q98

Which one of the following tumors is particularly prone to arise and grow in the perirenal region?

A. Malignant fibrous histiocytoma
B. Leiomyosarcoma
C. Adipose tissue tumor
D. Rhabdomyosarcoma
E. Solitary fibrous tumor.

Q99

This figure shows a preparation from a presacrococcygeal multiloculated cyst removed from a 50-year-old-man. Which of the following is the most likely diagnosis?

A. Tailgut cyst
B. Anal gland cyst
C. Teratoma
D. Cystic mucinous tumor
E. Cysts of müllerian origin.

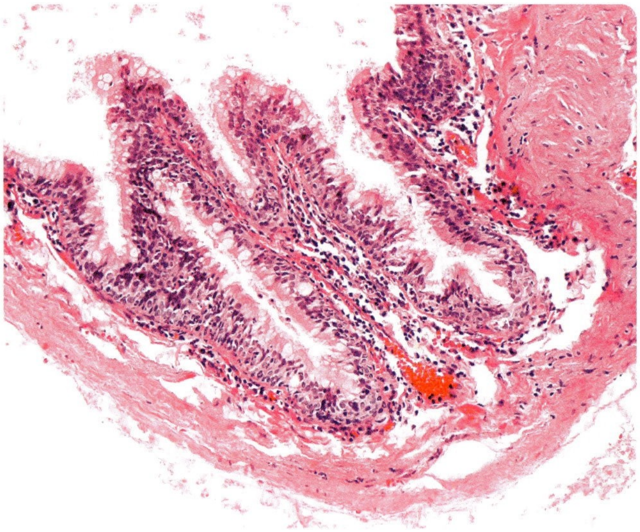

Fig. 26.1

Q100

Which one of the following is characterized by small openings in the intergluteal fold and a protrusion of hairs from such openings?

A. Immature teratoma
B. Pilonidal sinus
C. Hairy leukoplakia
D. Hair follicle hamartoma
E. Myxopapillary ependymoma.

Q101

Metastases to the vulva originate most often from carcinomas located in which one of the following primary sites?

A. Cervix
B. Endometrium
C. Lung
D. Kidney
E. Gastrointestinal tract.

Q102

This figure shows a preparation from a tumor of the uterine cervix removed from an elderly woman. What is the best diagnosis?

A. Endometrioid adenocarcinoma
B. Papillary serous carcinoma
C. Adenosquamous (mixed) carcinoma
D. Glassy cell carcinoma
E. Adenoid cystic carcinoma.

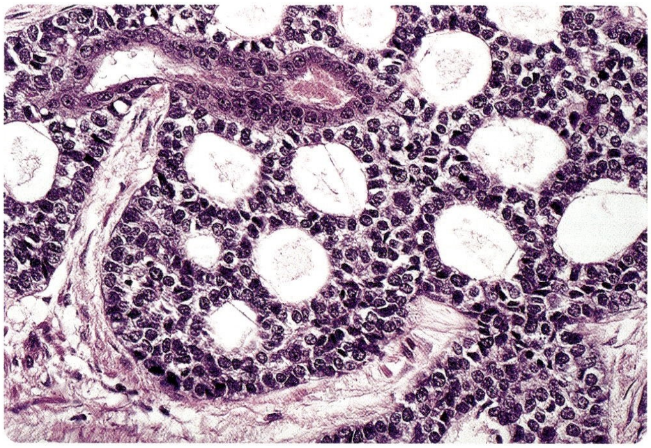

Fig. 19.1

Q103

Which one of the following forms of endometrial carcinoma has the worst prognosis?

A. Endometrioid adenocarcinoma
B. Adenoacanthoma
C. Secretory carcinoma
D. Papillary serous carcinoma
E. Ciliated carcinoma.

Q104

Which one of the following proteins is most likely to be elevated in the serum of patients with yolk sac tumor of the ovary?

A. α-Human chorionic gonadotropin
B. β-Human chorionic gonadotropin
C. α-Fetoprotein
D. α_1-Antitrypsin
E. Placental alkaline phosphatase.

Q105

Which of the following non-neoplastic lesions of the term placenta is the result of fetal renal agenesis?

A. Abnormally small placenta
B. Placenta accreta
C. Placenta circummarginata
D. Placenta circumvalata
E. Amnion nodosum.

Q106

Which one of the following is the most important diagnostic feature of sclerosing adenosis?

A. Architecture at low magnification
B. Architecture at high magnification
C. Foci of elastosis
D. Presence of apocrine metaplasia
E. Immunohistochemical features.

Q107

Which one of the following morphologic variants of ductal carcinoma in situ is classified as grade 3 on the basis of cytologic features?

A. Papillary
B. Comedocarcinoma
C. Solid
D. Cribriform
E. Micropapillary.

Q108

This figure shows a preparation from a tumor mass of the breast removed from a 50-year-old woman. What is the best diagnosis?

A. Radial scar
B. Microglandular adenosis
C. Tubular carcinoma
D. Classic (NOS) invasive ductal carcinoma
E. Invasive lobular carcinoma.

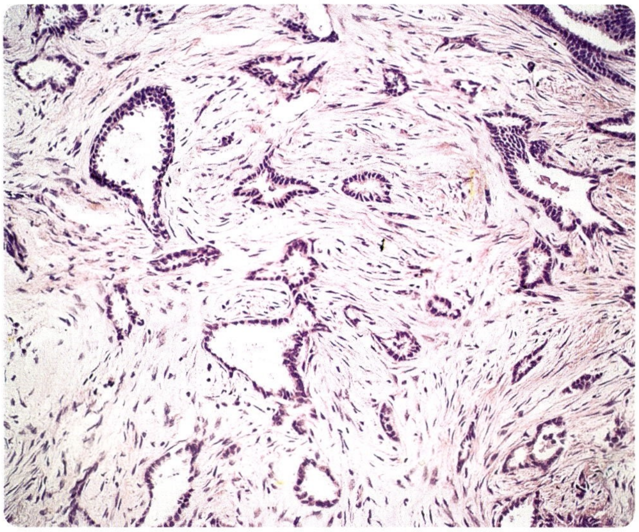

Fig. 20.1

Q109

Which one of the following tests is an excellent predictor of response to Herceptin?

A. Estrogen receptors
B. DNA ploidy
C. *BRCA-1* status
D. HER2/*neu*
E. *P53* and nm23.

Q110

Which one of the following breast tumors typically occurs in young women?

A. Malignant lymphoma
B. Angiosarcoma
C. Phylloides tumor
D. Invasive papillary carcinoma
E. Mucinous carcinoma.

Q111

Which one of the following dermatoses is characterized by Munro microabscesses?

A. Syphilis
B. Lyme disease
C. Psoriasis
D. Sarcoidosis
E. Lichen planus.

Q112

This figure shows a a skin biopsy following removal of a benign nevus. These changes are most consistent with which of the following diagnoses?

A. Bowen's disease
B. Squamous cell carcinoma
C. Basal cell carcinoma
D. Fibroepithelial tumor
E. Pseudoepitheliomatous hyperplasia.

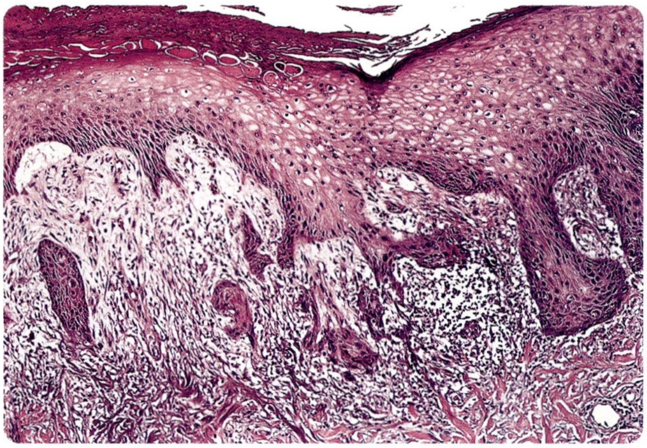

Fig. 4.25

Q113

Which one of the following tumors is characterized by solid nests of small basaloid cells which undergo abrupt keratinization, leading to the formation of 'ghost' and 'shadow' cells?

A. Pilomatrixoma
B. Basal cell carcinoma
C. Basosquamous (metatypical) carcinoma
D. Irritated seborrheic keratosis
E. Trichoepithelioma.

Q114

Which one of the following nevi is characterized by an ill-defined deep dermal proliferation of elongated and/or dendritic dermal melanocytes?

A. Spitz nevus
B. Blue nevus
C. Halo nevus
D. Cockarde nevus
E. Reed nevus.

Q115

Which one of the following forms of melanoma is usually not positive immunohistochemically for HMB-45 and Melan-A?

A. Acral lentiginous melanoma
B. Hutchinson's freckle
C. Desmoplastic melanoma
D. Balloon cell melanoma
E. Animal-type melanoma.

Q116

Invasive carcinoma of which part of the larynx has the best prognosis?

A. Glottic region
B. Supraglottic region
C. Transglottic region
D. Infraglottic region
E. Paraglottic region.

Q117

This lung was removed from a 60-year-old man. Which one of the following is the most likely diagnosis?

A. Abscess
B. Bronchiectasis
C. Bronchiolitis obliterans–organizing pneumonia
D. Chronic bronchitis
E. Emphysema.

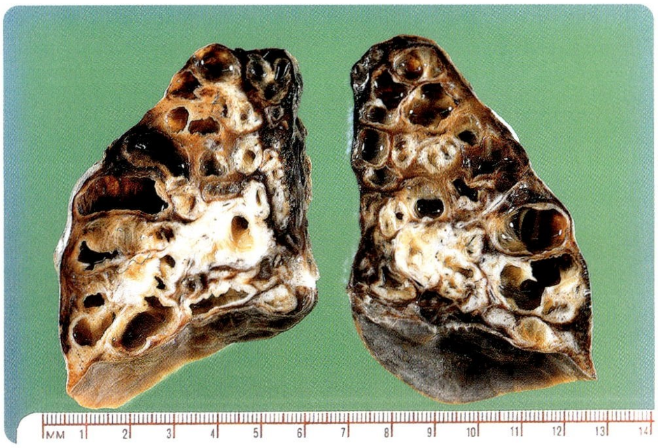

Fig. 7.9

Q118

Which one of the following pathogens is the most probable cause of the frothy alveolar exudates seen in this figure?

A. Cytomegalovirus
B. Herpes simplex
C. Adenovirus
D. *Pneumocystis carinii*
E. *Mycoplasma pneumoniae*.

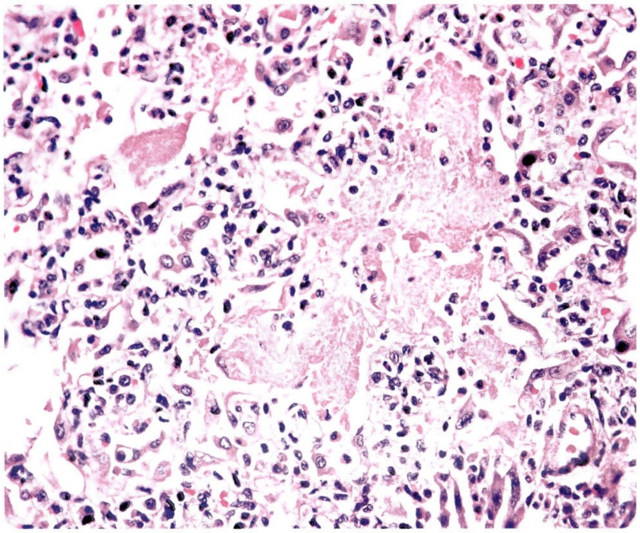

Fig. 7.10

Q119

Which one of the following forms of lung carcinoma presents grossly as gray-white foci of parenchymal consolidation?

A. Squamous cell carcinoma
B. Undifferentiated large cell carcinoma
C. Clear cell carcinoma
D. Bronchoalveolar carcinoma
E. Pulmonary blastoma.

Q120

Which one of the following lung tumors is characterized by diffuse positivity for HMB-45?

A. Adenoid cystic carcinoma
B. Mucoepidermoid carcinoma
C. Clear cell tumor
D. Epithelioid hemangioendothelioma
E. Small cell carcinoma.

Q121

Which one of the following thymic lesions is most often found in patients with myasthenia gravis?

A. Follicular hyperplasia
B. Sinus histiocytosis
C. Thymoma
D. Thymic carcinoma
E. Large cell lymphoma.

Q122

This figure shows a preparation from a large mediastinal mass which was largely solid, yellowish-gray and separated into lobules by connective tissue septa. What is the best diagnosis for this tumor?

A. Type A (spindle or medullary) thymoma
B. Type B1 (lymphocyte-rich or predominantly cortical) thymoma
C. Type B2 (cortical) thymoma
D. Type B3 (atypical) thymoma
E. Type AB (mixed) thymoma.

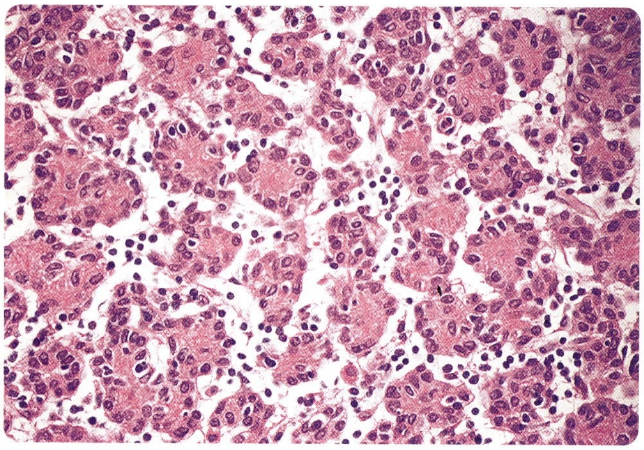

Fig. 8.4

Q123

This figure shows a biopsy of a solid, well-circumscribed but not encapsulated mediastinal mass. Which of the following is the most likely diagnosis?

A. Adenocarcinoma
B. Neuroblastoma
C. Yolk sac tumor
D. Carcinoid tumor
E. Thymoma.

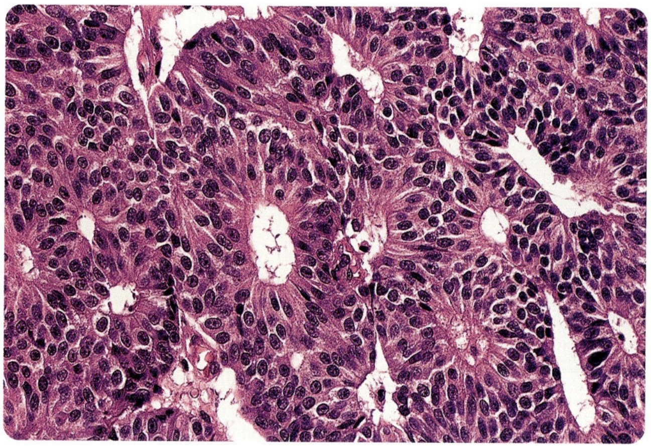

Fig. 8.5

Q124

Which one of the following is the most common primary neoplasm of the middle portion of the mediastinum?

A. Thymoma
B. Germ cell tumor
C. Malignant lymphoma
D. Malignant peripheral nerve sheath tumor
E. Liposarcoma.

Q125

Which one of the following tumors occurs most often in young women, frequently presenting as superior vena cava syndrome?

A. Lymphoblastic lymphoma
B. Mediastinal large cell lymphoma
C. Ganglioneuroma
D. Thymoma
E. Malignant peripheral nerve sheath tumor.

A1. B

Lymphocytic infiltrates of the thyroid associated with follicular hyperplasia and scalloping of the colloid are typical of Graves' disease. In lymphocytic thyroiditis the thyroid follicles are normal, and in Hashimoto's thyroiditis they are lined by oncocytic cells. In de Quervain's thyroiditis there are granulomas related to ruptured follicles. In Riedel's thyroiditis the thyroid follicles have been replaced by fibrous tissue, which may contain scattered lymphocytes and plasma cells. **(p. 523–524)**

A2. C

Genetic mutations interfering with normal synthesis of thyroid hormones include, among others, defects in iodine transport, unresponsiveness to TSH, abnormalities in thyroglobulin synthesis etc. These genetic defects cause dyshormonogenetic goiter characterized by nodular or diffuse enlargement of the thyroid. The follicles are lined by hyperplastic follicular cells displaying marked nuclear pleomorphism. **(p. 524)**

A3. E

Hürthle cell tumor has the highest propensity to undergo secondary clear cell change. This occurs as a result of vesicular swelling of the mitochondria. **(p. 548)**

A4. A

Papillary carcinoma predominated in children exposed to radiation at a later age, whereas follicular cancer predominated in children exposed at a younger age. **(p. 561)**

A5. E

This tumor is an anaplastic carcinoma of the thyroid, composed of giant cells. **(p. 552)**

A6. B

This figure shows 'ground-glass hepatocytes,' typical of chronic viral hepatitis B. The 'ground-glass areas' appear finely granular and paler than the cytoplasm of other hepatocytes, and in some cells it is separated from the membrane by a clear halo. **(p. 929)**

A7. C

Under normal circumstances copper is excreted in bile. The accumulation of copper in hepatocytes at the periphery of hepatic nodules of cirrhosis is most likely caused by biliary obstruction. **(p. 935)**

A8. A

Ethanol is one of the most common causes of macrovesicular steatosis, which may be associated focally with microvesicular steatosis. All the drugs listed here cause microvesicular steatosis. **(p. 937)**

A9. A

Ductopenia or paucity of interlobular bile ducts is a typical feature of advanced (stage 4) primary biliary cirrhosis, a disease characterized by immune destruction of bile ducts. Fibrous septa in other forms of cirrhosis usually contain numerous bile ducts. **(p. 949)**

A10. B

Liver cell adenoma has a striking predilection for females and is pathogenetically related to the use of oral contraceptives. **(p. 993)**

A11. D

Fibrolamellar hepatocellular carcinoma has the best prognosis: over half of all such carcinomas are resectable, and the cure rate is about 50%. The overall 5-year survival rate for other forms of hepatocellular carcinoma in the United States is only 3%. **(p. 1001)**

A12. B

This liver lesion is a mesenchymal hamartoma. Microscopically, it is composed of well vascularized mature connective tissue and elongated branching bile ducts. On first blush it is reminiscent of a breast fibroadenoma. **(p. 1011)**

A13. C

Choledochal cyst is the most common cause of obstructive jaundice in children beyond infancy, but it may also present in adulthood. **(p. 1037)**

A14. C

Human immunodeficiency virus infection may be associated with sclerosing cholangitis. The pathogenesis of sclerosing cholangitis is not known, but it is suspected that it might be related to infection with CMV or cryptosporidia, which occur at high rate in HIV-infected persons. **(p. 1043)**

A15. A

Approximately 50–70% of all carcinomas of the extrahepatic bile ducts are located in the upper third, including the hilum of the liver. **(p. 1049)**

A16. D

Botryoid rhabdomyosarcoma is the most common malignant tumor of the extrahepatic bile ducts in children. A few cases of this tumor have been described in adults. **(p. 1051)**

A17. A

In about 95% of cases chronic pancreatitis is pathologically classified as chronic calcifying pancreatitis. On gross examination it is nodular and misshapen, enlarged or atrophic, with foci of intraductal and intraparenchymal calcification. Microscopically, there is prominent perilobular and intralobular fibrosis, with dilatation of the ducts, squamous metaplasia, mucoprotein plugging and atrophy of acini. There are also foci of chronic inflammation. **(p. 1065)**

A18. E

Papillary hyperplasia and epithelial atypia are found in about a third of all cases of pancreatic adenocarcinoma, but are not found in chronic pancreatitis. Other changes listed here are associated at the same rate with neoplastic and non-neoplastic pancreatic lesions. **(p. 1071)**

A19. B

This microcystic tumor composed of low cuboidal cells with uniform round nuclei is a microcystic cystadenoma. The cells have optically clear cytoplasm, which contains glycogen. **(p. 1075–1076)**

A20. D

The tumor cells form acini and the tumor is thus best classified as acinar cell carcinoma. Immunohistochemistry with antibodies to chromogranin and synaptophysin gave negative results, which helped to exclude the diagnosis of islet cell tumor. As expected for acinar cell carcinomas, this tumor reacted with antibodies to lipase. **(p. 1081)**

A21. A

Adrenal cortical carcinomas and renal cell carcinomas resemble each other and it is often difficult to distinguish one from another. Likewise, it is difficult to distinguish adrenal cortical carcinomas from benign adrenal cortical adenomas and adrenal medullary tumors, such as pheochromocytoma. **(p. 1123)**

A22. B

Chromogranin is typically found in adrenal medullary tumors but is not present in adrenal cortical tumors. Inhibin, on the other hand, is positive in adrenal cortical tumors and is not found in adrenal medullary tumors. Vimentin and synaptophysin are found in both cortical and medullary tumors. Keratin may be found in adrenal cortical tumors. **(p. 1123)**

A23. A

Aldosterone-secreting tumors respond to treatment with spironolactone, forming concentric eosinophilic cytoplasmic bodies ('spironolactone bodies'). **(p. 1125)**

A24. E

Neuroblastoma contains neurosecretory granules and synaptic endings visible on electron microscopy. **(p. 1128)**

A25. E

Mitosis–karyorrhexis index (MKI) is useful for formulating the prognosis of neuroblastomas. It is calculated by counting karyorrhectic cells per 5000 tumor cells in random fields. A count of less than 100 is called low, 100–200 intermediate, and over 200 high. **(p. 1131)**

A26. C

Sustentacular cells typically react with the antibodies to S-100. **(p. 1138)**

A27. C

Membranous nephropathy presents with nephritic syndrome and shows granular deposits of immunoglobulin G and complement along the capillary walls of glomeruli. **(p. 1169)**

A28. E

In amyloidosis the glomeruli react with Congo red and contain fibrils that measure 8–10 nm on electron microscopy. **(p. 1181)**

A29. B

This figure shows the typical features of type I membranoproliferative glomerulonephritis, which may occur as a complication of chronic hepatitis C or B virus infection. **(p. 1191)**

A30. A

This renal biopsy shows osmiophilic deposits limited to the mesangial area. In a young adult with recurrent hematuria and mild proteinuria these findings are highly suggestive of IgA disease, and the deposits are thus most likely composed of IgA. **(p. 1195)**

A31. B

Metastases to the lung in a child with a retroperitoneal mass favors the diagnosis of Wilms' tumor over neuroblastoma and other adrenal tumors. On the other hand, metastases to the bones favor neuroblastoma, as Wilms' tumor rarely metastasizes to the bones. **(p. 1243)**

A32. C

Infiltrative cardiomyopathies such as those caused by amyloidosis or hemochromatosis are usually part of a systemic disorder and can be diagnosed indirectly by a biopsy of a more accessible organ. **(p. 2418)**

A33. B

Most cardiac myxomas occur in the left atrium, which contains 86% of sporadic and 62% of familial myxomas. **(p. 2425)**

A34. A

Cardiac rhabdomyomas are usually diagnosed during the first decade of life and many are congenital. **(p. 2426)**

A35. D

The nodules forming the typical lesions of temporal arteritis show partial destruction of the arterial wall and contain multinucleated giant cells. **(p. 2448)**

A36. B

This hyphae-like material was removed from a midline intracranial lesion represents degenerate nucleoproteins typically found in colloid cysts of the anterosuperior third ventricle. It is diagnostic of colloid cysts, allowing one to make the diagnosis in the proper clinical setting even without evidence of epithelium. **(p. 2467)**

A37. D

Arteriovenous malformations may occur in any part of the brain but are most often located in the hemispheric convexities in the distribution of the middle cerebral artery. **(p. 2475)**

A38. C

Cerebral amyloid angiopathy is the most common cause of peripheral lobar hematomas in the brain of the elderly. Such hematomas are located in the subarachnoid parts of the hemispheres, in contrast to hypertensive hematomas which typically involve the basal ganglia. **(p. 2477)**

A39. B

Diffuse leptomeningitis caused by *Cryptococcus neoformans* is the most common CNS mycosis. **(p. 2490)**

A40. E

Progressive multifocal leukoencephalopathy is caused by JC, a DNA polyoma virus. This virus is ubiquitous and usually causes brain lesions in persons who have defective cell-mediated immunity. **(p. 2497)**

A41. A

Brainstem gliomas causing 'pseudohypertrophic' enlargement of the pons on neuroradiologic investigation in children are most often histologically classified as astrocytomas of the diffuse fibrillary type. **(p. 2504)**

A42. E

Microvascular hyperplasia with heaped-up endothelial and myoepithelial cells is typically found in glioblastoma multiforme. It is related to mitogens released from tumor cells. **(p. 2508)**

A43. A

Pilocytic astrocytomas typically present in childhood or early adult life and are thus called 'juvenile pilocytic astrocytomas.' These tumors show a predilection for the cerebellum, third ventricle/hypothalamic region. **(p. 2514)**

A44. C

This tumor composed of bizarre multinucleated cells and spindle cells, typically located in the subarachnoid part of the temporal lobe of a young man, is a pleomorphic xanthoastrocytoma. These tumors tend to accumulate lipid, which accounts for the yellow color on gross examination, and the microvacuoles in the abundant cytoplasm of some tumor cells. **(p. 2530)**

A45. B

Calcifications in the form of psammoma bodies are a common feature of meningotheliomatous meningiomas. **(p. 2566)**

A46. B

This electron micrograph shows the well-developed interdigitating cytoplasmic processes of a meningioma. The tumor has abundant cytoplasm, which distinguishes it from tumors that have scant cytoplasm, such as neurocytoma, medulloblastoma or lymphoma. In contrast to hemangiopericytomas and schwannomas, which contain pericellular basement membranes, the cytoplasmic processes of this meningioma are not enclosed with basement membrane material. **(p. 2570)**

A47. D

This figure shows the typical onion bulbs of hypertrophic neuropathy. Such findings are characteristic of hereditary neuropathies such as Charcot–Marie–Tooth disease. **(p. 2631)**

A48. C

The muscle shows fiber type grouping and prominent target fibers, i.e. fibers that have a central pallor. These features are most consistent with denervation followed by reinnervation of the muscles. **(p. 2666–2667)**

A49. C

In general several growth patterns of pituitary adenoma are recognized, such as solid, papillary, sinusoidal or glandular. This microphotograph illustrates the typical features of a pituitary adenoma growing in a sinusoidal pattern, also called a trabecular growth pattern. **(p. 2687)**

A50. C

Amyloid deposition and calcospherites are relatively rare findings in pituitary adenomas, but are most often found in prolactinomas. **(p. 2689)**

A51. C

This figure illustrates the relatively nonspecific appearance of an epithelioid melanoma, which among other features shows cytoplasmic clearing. The intraocular location of the tumor, the large nuclei and prominent nucleoli and the positive staining with antibodies to S-100 protein (and other melanoma markers) had to be taken into consideration in the work-up of this tumor. **(p. 2755–2756)**

A52. E

Approximately 6% of all meningiomas arise from the surface of the petrous bone, from which they may invade into the middle ear. **(p. 2776)**

A53. B

Leukocytoclastic vasculitis involving the skin, oral mucosa and conjunctiva is a typical histologic finding in Behçet's disease. The cause of this disease is not known **(p. 250)**

A54. A

Most squamous cells carcinomas in situ or early invasive squamous cell carcinomas of the oral mucosa appear as velvety patches and are described clinically as erythroplakia. Only 10% of these lesions have a whitish component or appear as leukoplakia. **(p. 253)**

A55. D

These figures illustrate the microscopic features of a polymorphous low-grade adenocarcinoma. The tumors have in parts an orderly microglandular configuration and in other parts form papillae. The tumor can also have tubular, cribriform, solid and fascicular parts, not shown here. They occur most often on the palate of adult women. **(p. 261)**

A56. A

Central giant cell granuloma is by far the most common jaw lesion composed of osteoclast-like multinucleated giant cells. Its pathogenesis is not known. It is also known as reparative giant cell granuloma, a name suggesting that it results from the organization of minute or recurrent hemorrhages. **(p. 281)**

A57. C

This tumor is an ameloblastic fibroma. Typically they occur in young people, most of whom are under 21 years of age. The tumor is composed of a neoplastic fibrous stroma enclosing strips of ameloblastic epithelium, in contrast to adenoameloblastomas (also known as adenomatoid odontogenic tumor), which are composed of epithelial gland-like nests. **(p. 289)**

A58. A

Solitary parathyroid adenoma is the cause of primary hyperparathyroidism in over 80% of cases. It occurs in women and men in a ratio of 3:1, most often in the fourth decade. In 75% of cases it involves one of the lower parathyroid glands. **(p. 597 and 604)**

A59. A

This is a sarcomatoid carcinoma. Typically such tumors are polypoid and exophytic. Microscopically the tumor consists of well-differentiated squamous cell carcinoma merging with a spindle cell component forming fascicles. Such tumors are also called carcinosarcomas, spindle cell carcinomas or pseudosarcomas. Immunohistochemically, the spindle cells stain with the antibodies to keratins, but some also have features of myofibroblasts and react with antibodies to vimentin, smooth muscle cell actin and desmin. **(p. 629–630)**

A60. D

Type A or immune chronic gastritis is an autoimmune disease caused by antibodies to proton pump on chief cells of the gastric mucosa. It typically affects the fundus but spares the antrum. Atrophy of the gastric glands causes hypochlorhydria or achlorhydria and a reactive elevation of gastrin in blood. **(p. 651)**

A61. C

Gastric carcinoma of the diffuse type (signet ring carcinoma) occurs as a familial tumor. Germline truncating mutations of the E-cadherin gene have been found in these families. Because of the high penetrance of this mutated gene some authors have proposed prophylactic gastrectomy in these individuals. The same mutation is found in 30% of sporadic diffuse-type carcinomas, but not in intestinal-type gastric adenocarcinomas. **(p. 665)**

A62. A

Epstein–Barr virus gene transcripts are found in almost all cases of gastric lymphoepithelioma-like carcinoma, similar to those developing in the nasopharynx. It is worth noting that EBV can also be detected in 6–16% of gastric adenocarcinomas of the conventional type. **(p. 667)**

A63. B

Enterochromaffin-like (ECL) cells account for most of the gastric WDENT. They are usually multiple, often polypoid, and distributed throughout the fundus. They are not immunoreactive for any of the standard gastrointestinal pancreatic hormones and are usually accompanied by hyperplasia of argyrophilic cells in the adjacent mucosa. **(p. 673)**

A64. E

Gastrointestinal stromal tumor (GIST) is accompanied by a somatic mutation of c-*kit*, a tyrosine kinase receptor. GISTs react with the antibodies to CD117, which is also expressed on the interstitial cells of Cajal. **(p. 678)**

A65. C

AP12–MLT fusion, the result of t(11,18) translocation, is found in approximately 50% of all gastric low-grade MALT lymphomas, but not in other forms of lymphoma or chronic inflammation. Other microscopic features supporting the diagnosis of MALT lymphoma are the finding of cytologic atypia, occasional Dutcher bodies and lymphoepithelial lesions. **(p. 681)**

A66. D

Enteropathy-associated T-cell lymphoma is in most instances a complication of celiac disease. Tumor cells have phenotypic features of cytotoxic T cells. **(p. 717)**

A67. A

Crohn's disease is a transmural inflammation that often leads to the formation of intestinal adhesions and enteroenteric fistulas. **(p. 721)**

A68. D

Gangliocytic paraganglioma occurs almost exclusively in the second portion of the duodenum, usually in proximity to the ampulla of Vater. Occasionally this tumor may be found distally in the small intestine and even in the appendix. **(p. 733–734)**

A69. A

Most pleomorphic adenomas occur in the parotid gland. The submaxillary gland is involved ten times less often and the sublingual gland and the intraoral glands are involved even less often. **(p. 879)**

A70. C

Mucoepidermoid carcinoma is the most common malignant salivary gland tumor in children, in whom it may represent a second malignancy. **(p. 890)**

A71. D

Cat-scratch disease is characterized by a primary cutaneous lesion and enlargement of regional lymph nodes, usually axillary or cervical. Early lesions of lymph nodes have histiocytic proliferation and follicular hyperplasia, intermediate lesions have granulomatous changes, and late lesions have abscesses of various sizes. These abscesses are very suggestive of the diagnosis because of their pattern of central, sometimes stellate, necrosis with neutrophils, surrounded by a palisading of histiocytes. However, similar abscesses can be seen in lymphogranuloma venereum. **(p. 1900)**

A72. E

The lymph node abnormalities in AIDS patients include mycobacterial and other opportunistic infections, Kaposi's sarcoma, malignant lymphomas of Hodgkin's or non-Hodgkin's type, and florid reactive hyperplasia. The latter change is the most common. It may be accompanied by collections of monocytoid B-cells in the sinuses, neutrophils, and features of dermatopathic lymphadenopathy. **(p. 1901)**

A73. D

In nodular lymphocyte-predominant Hodgkin's lymphoma the predominant cell is a small B lymphocyte, with or without an accompanying population of benign-appearing histiocytes. The lymph node architecture is partially or totally effaced, and the infiltrate has a variously well-developed nodular pattern of growth. Classic Reed–Sternberg cells are absent. One sees instead a variable but usually large number of a type of Reed–Sternberg cell, the L&H cell or 'popcorn' cell, characterized by a folded, multilobed nucleus with smaller nucleoli. L&H cells express the pan-B-cell markers but are consistently negative for T-cell markers. They may express CD30 or EMA, and they generally lack CD15 expression. **(p. 1922)**

A74. C

Depending on the relative proportion of small and large cells, follicular lymphomas are subdivided into three categories. Patients in the first category are often asymptomatic, usually have generalized disease, and have a good prognosis. Tumors in the third category are more commonly localized at the time of presentation but run a more aggressive clinical course and are more likely to lose their nodular pattern of growth and become diffuse. The prognosis of tumors in the second category is intermediate between these two, but closer to the first. **(p. 1940)**

A75. A

The metastatic carcinomas that most closely simulate a malignant lymphoid process are nasopharyngeal lymphoepithelioma and lobular carcinoma of the breast. The first may masquerade clinically and pathologically as Hodgkin's lymphoma because of its common presentation in a young adult, with painless unilateral cervical lymphadenopathy and the presence of a polymorphic population (including eosinophils) on microscopic examination. The second may be confused with malignant lymphomas of one type or another. This is particularly true of the type composed of small uniform cells with only occasional signet ring formations, which can look remarkably lymphocyte-like. **(p. 1976)**

A76. D

The diseases most commonly associated with spontaneous rupture of the spleen are infectious mononucleosis, malaria, typhoid fever, subacute bacterial endocarditis, peliosis lienis, malignant lymphomas, leukemias, and primary non-lymphoid splenic neoplasms. Blunt trauma to the abdomen and surgical intervention within the abdominal cavity are the two most common factors responsible for rupture of the normal spleen. **(p. 2020)**

A77. E

Malignant lymphoma is by far the most common malignant tumor involving the spleen. Although usually affected as part of a generalized process, in some cases the spleen represents the only detectable site of disease. **(p. 2027)**

A78. D

Hepatosplenic γ/δ T-cell lymphoma typically presents with hepatosplenomegaly, fever and weight loss in young males, and carries a poor prognosis. Grossly, the spleen is usually very large, with a uniform cut surface in which the malpighian follicles cannot be identified. Microscopically, the neoplastic infiltration involves the cords and sinuses and is composed of medium-sized lymphoid cells with oval or folded nuclei, moderately condensed chromatin and pale cytoplasm. At the molecular level there is usually clonal rearrangement of the γ or δ chain of the T-cell receptor gene. **(p. 2030)**

A79. A

The spleen is the most common site of extranodal organ involvement by Hodgkin's lymphoma, but primary Hodgkin's lymphoma of the spleen is extremely rare. By far the most common type is nodular sclerosis, but others may be seen as well. **(p. 2030)**

A80. B

The distinctive enzyme histochemical feature of hairy cell leukemia is the presence of tartrate-resistant acid phosphatase; this enzyme can now be demonstrated immunohistochemically. **(p. 2032)**

A81. D

In the most severe form of aplastic anemia the intertrabecular marrow space is occupied predominantly by adipose tissue with scattered lymphocytes, plasma cells, tissue mast cells and hemosiderin-laden macrophages. In less severe processes there is an increased amount of fat tissue and scattered small collections of erythroblasts, granulocytes and megakaryocytes. The blood findings in aplastic anemia are characterized by varying degrees of pancytopenia. **(p. 2053)**

A82. B

A finding referred to as abnormal localization of immature precursors (ALIP), characterized by aggregates (three to five cells) and clusters (more than five cells) of myeloblasts and promyelocytes in central areas of the marrow tissue away from the endosteal surface of the bone trabeculae and vascular structures, has been described in the myelodysplastic syndromes. **(p. 2067)**

A83. C

Chronic myeloid leukemia is generally characterized by an elevated leukocyte count with basophilia, decreased neutrophil alkaline phosphatase, and the presence of the Philadelphia chromosome and/or molecular evidence of the *bcr-abl* hybrid gene in the hematopoietic cells. **(p. 2068)**

A84. A

Richter's syndrome is the occurrence of a pleomorphic lymphoma in a patient with a prior history of B-CLL or another low-grade B-cell lymphoproliferative disorder, such as plasmacytoid lymphoma. **(p. 2075)**

A85. B

A highly specific antibody to human mast cell tryptase that may be used on decalcified and B5-fixed paraffin-embedded specimens is very useful for identification of mast cell lesions. Other antibodies that react with mast cells include antibodies to α-antitrypsin, α-antichymotrypsin, CD68 and CD117 (c-*kit*). **(p. 2110)**

A86. A

Bacterial osteomyelitis may be caused by a large variety of microorganisms. About 70–90 of cases are due to coagulase-positive staphylococci. Other organisms involved are *Klebsiella, Aerobacter, Proteus, Pseudomonas*, streptococcus, pneumococcus, gonococcus, meningococcus, *Brucella* and *Salmonella*. **(p. 2140)**

A87. A

Most osteosarcomas arising de novo are located in the metaphyseal area of the long bones, particularly the lower end of the femur, the upper end of the tibia and the upper end of the humerus. **(p. 2150)**

A88. D

Multiple enchondromas having a predominantly unilateral distribution are referred to as Ollier's disease. The association of multiple enchondromas with soft tissue hemangiomas is known as Maffucci's syndrome. **(p. 2158)**

A89. B

Chordoma is usually seen in patients in the fifth and sixth decades, but occurs in all ages and in both sexes. The sacrococcygeal tumors are more common in the fifth and sixth decade of life, whereas many of the spheno-occipital neoplasms occur in children and adolescents. **(p. 2183)**

A90. A

In Langerhans' cell hisitocytosis a specific intracytoplasmic organelle, known as Langerhans' or Birbeck's granule, which is present in this figure, is regularly present on electron microscopic examination. **(p. 2197)**

A91. B

Morton's neuroma can be regarded as a subtype of traumatic neuroma cause by repeated mild trauma to the region. Its typical location is the interdigital plantar nerve between the third and fourth toes. **(p. 2263)**

A92. E

Myxoid liposarcoma is the most common type of liposarcoma. It shows a marked predilection of the lower extremities, particularly the thigh. Microscopically, it has few or no mitotic figures and is characterized by proliferating lipoblasts in different stages of differentiation, a prominent anastomosing capillary network, and a mucoid matrix rich in hyaluronidase-sensitive acid mucopolysaccharides. **(p. 2280)**

A93. B

The classic location of glomus tumor is the subungual region, but it can occur elsewhere in the skin, soft tissues (particularly the flexor surface of the arms and about the knee), nerves, stomach, nasal cavity and trachea. **(p. 2288)**

A94. B

Sarcoma botryoides is currently regarded as a variation in the pattern of growth of embryonal rhabdomyosarcoma. Microscopically, the tumor cells are small and spindle shaped. A feature of diagnostic value is the presence of highly cellular areas usually surrounding blood vessels alternating with parvicellular regions that have abundant mucoid intercellular material. A highly characteristic feature of the polypoid ('botryoid') tumors is the presence of a dense zone of undifferentiated tumor cells immediately beneath the epithelium, a formation known as Nicholson's cambium layer. **(p. 2304)**

A95. B

Epithelioid sarcomas are most commonly located on the extremities, particularly the hands and fingers. A high proportion of myxomas arise within skeletal muscle, especially in the thigh region. Alveolar soft part sarcoma involves most often the deep soft tissues of the thigh and leg. The classic location of granular cell tumor is the tongue. Liposarcomas occur most frequently in the lower extremities. **(p. 2321)**

A96. A

The immunohistochemical profile of intra-abdominal desmoplastic small cell tumor is distinctive in the sense that it displays simultaneous expression of epithelial (keratin, EMA), muscular (desmin) and neural (neuron-specific enolase) markers. **(p. 2383)**

A97. D

The appendix is the primary site of origin of pseudomyxoma in the vast majority of cases in both men and women. The associated mucinous ovarian tumors, when present, are most likely additional implants from the appendiceal lesions rather than independent synchronous neoplasms. **(p. 2387)**

A98. C

Adipose tissue tumors are the most frequent primary retroperitoneal soft tissue neoplasms. They are particularly prone to arise and grow in the perirenal region. **(p. 2396)**

A99. A

Tailgut cyst (retrorectal cystic hamartoma) presents in the presacrococcygeal area, usually in adult patients as a multiloculated cyst lined by squamous, transitional or glandular epithelium. **(p. 2401)**

A100. B

Pilonidal sinuses appear as small openings in the intergluteal fold about 3.5–5 cm posterior to the anal orifice. Hairs are sometimes seen protruding from them. The opening is continued by a sinus tract, which is directed upward in the vast majority of cases. **(p. 2402)**

A101. A

Metastases to the vulva most often stem from primary carcinomas of the cervix (almost 50%). Other common primary sites are the endometrium, kidneys, or the lower gastrointestinal tract. The labium majus is the most common location of such metastases. **(p. 1497)**

A102. E

Adenoid cystic carcinoma is a specific variant of cervical adenocarcinoma that tends to occur in elderly multigravid black women and is associated with a particularly poor prognosis. It may be cribriform (the most common pattern) or grow in a predominantly solid fashion. **(p. 1543)**

A103. D

Among the various morphologic variants, the papillary serous and clear cell types are the most aggressive, the former having a definite tendency for upper abdominal spread. Adenosquamous carcinomas are also highly malignant, but this is probably only a reflection of the fact that they are poorly differentiated tumors. Conversely, the excellent prognosis associated with grade I endometrioid adenocarcinoma, adenoacanthoma and secretory carcinoma probably relates to their well-differentiated nature. **(p. 1594)**

A104. C

Yolk sac tumor (endodermal sinus tumor) is generally a neoplasm of children and young adults, although it has also been described in the elderly. The serum α-fetoprotein level is invariably elevated, whereas the chorionic gonadotropin levels are normal. **(p. 1683)**

A105. E

Amnion nodosum is the result of fetal renal agenesis and is associated with oligohydramnios. It presents as small plaques on the amniotic surface, formed by squamous cells and fibrin. **(p. 1749)**

A106. A

Microscopically, the most important diagnostic feature of sclerosing adenosis is its architecture as seen at very low magnification. The nodule retains a round or oval lobular configuration and is more cellular centrally than peripherally. **(p. 1776)**

A107. B

According to the three-grade system based on cytologic criteria, classic comedocarcinoma becomes grade 3 ductal carcinoma in situ (DCIS), classic solid/cribriform/ micropapillary lesions become grade 1 DCIS, and those showing intermediate cytologic features are reported as grade 2 DCIS. **(p. 1789)**

A108. C

Tubular carcinoma simulates a benign condition because of the well-differentiated nature of the glands, the absence of necrosis or mitoses, and scanty pleomorphism. The clues to the diagnosis are the haphazard arrangement of the glands in the stroma with the absence of any organoid configuration; frequent invasion of fat at the periphery of the lesion; the cellular nature of the stroma; irregular and often angulated contours of the glands; open lumina with basophilic secretion; apocrine-type 'snouts' in the apical cytoplasm; formation of trabecular bars; lack of a myoepithelial cell component; lack of basement membrane; and occurrence in two-thirds or more of cases of typical intraductal carcinoma in ducts within or outside the lesion. **(p. 1805)**

A109. D

Overexpression of HER2/*neu* is an excellent predictor of response to Herceptin but a weak predictor of response to chemotherapy. **(p. 1826)**

A110. B

Angiosarcoma (malignant hemangioendothelioma) of the breast characteristically occurs in young women. **(p. 1831)**

A111. C

The morphologic characteristics of psoriasis are those of incomplete keratinization manifested as parakeratosis. Acanthosis, in which there is a regular elongation of the rete ridges, seen as pegs in two dimensions, is prominent. Above the tips of the dermal papillae the layer of epidermal cells is distinctly attenuated, a feature known as 'suprapapillary thinning.' Within the dermal papillae the capillaries are prominent. There is also a polymorphic infiltrate composed of lymphocytes, macrophages and neutrophils. Transmigration of polymorphonuclear leukocytes through the reactive epidermis into the parakeratotic scale results in the formation of Munro microabscesses. **(p. 104)**

A112. E

At sites of trauma, chronic irritation and ulcers, the reparative hyperplasia of the epidermis may produce seemingly invasive tongues of epithelial cells. This abnormality, known as pseudoepitheliomatous (pseudocarcinomatous) hyperplasia, can also be caused by mycotic infections, bromoderma, pyoderma vegetans, tuberculosis, syphilis, granular cell tumor and melanocytic lesions. **(p. 136)**

A113. A

Pilomatrixoma is a nodular, subepidermal benign tumor arising from a hair matrix. Microscopically, it is composed of solid nests of small basaloid cells that may lead to a mistaken diagnosis of basal cell carcinoma, particularly on cytologic examination. The key feature is the fact that these basaloid cells undergo abrupt keratinization, leading to the formation of 'ghost' and 'shadow' cells. **(p. 153)**

A114. B

Blue nevus of the ordinary type is characterized by an ill-defined deep dermal proliferation of elongated and/or dendritic dermal melanocytes, sometimes extending into the subcutis. Melanin pigment is usually abundant. **(p. 156)**

A115. C

Desmoplastic melanoma is a subtype of spindle cell melanoma, characterized by positivity of tumor cells for S-100 protein but negativity for HMB-45, Melan-A, or any of the other more specific melanoma markers. **(p. 166)**

A116. A

Glottic tumors tend to remain localized for long periods because of the surrounding cartilaginous wall and the paucity of lymphatic vessels. **(p. 342)**

A117. B

Bronchiectasis refers to the permanent dilatation of bronchial lumina, usually associated with destruction of some elements of the bronchial wall and inflammatory changes in the surrounding lung parenchyma. **(p. 370)**

A118. D

Pneumocystis carinii pneumonia is a fungal opportunistic infection. Most cases are seen in individuals who are chronically debilitated and immunosuppressed, such as those receiving therapy for neoplastic disease or affected with AIDS. **(p. 381)**

A119. D

The non-mucinous type of bronchoalveolar carcinoma present grossly as gray-white foci of parenchymal consolidation. **(p. 395)**

A120. C

Clear cell tumor ('sugar tumor') is made up of large cells with clear to eosinophilic granular cytoplasm crowded with glycogen granules. Immunohistochemically, there is diffuse positivity for HMB-45, HMB-50 and cathepsin B; focal reactivity for S-100 protein; and inconstant positivity for neuron-specific enolase (NSE) and synaptophysin. **(p. 419)**

A121. A

In patients with myasthenia gravis the thymus shows follicular hyperplasia as the only abnormality in about 65% of cases, a thymoma in 10%, and no gross or overt microscopic abnormalities in 25% of cases. **(p. 466)**

A122. A

Type A thymoma (spindle cell, medullary) is a tumor composed of a population of neoplastic thymic epithelial cells having a spindle/oval shape, lacking nuclear atypia, and accompanied by few or no non-neoplastic lymphocytes. **(p. 469)**

A123. D

Microscopically, thymic carcinoid tumor exhibits ribbon and festoon formation, rosette-like glands with central lumina, 'balls' of cells with central necrosis and calcification, marked vascularization, and frequent lymphatic and blood vessel invasion. **(p. 483)**

A124. C

Malignant lymphoma can present as an anterior, superior or middle mediastinal mass, in this order of frequency. It represents the most common primary neoplasm of the middle portion of the mediastinum. **(p. 489)**

A125. B

Mediastinal large cell lymphoma can present as a mass in the thymus with or without lymph node involvement. Most patients are young women. The tumor frequently presents with signs and symptoms of superior vena cava syndrome. **(p. 491)**